PROGRESS IN BRAIN RESEARCH

VOLUME 104

NEUROPEPTIDES IN THE SPINAL CORD

Other Volumes in PROGRESS IN BRAIN RESEARCH

PROGRESS IN BRAIN RESEARCH

VOLUME 104

NEUROPEPTIDES IN THE SPINAL CORD

EDITED BY

F. NYBERG

Department of Pharmaceutical Biosciences, Upsala University, Uppsala, Sweden

H.S. SHARMA

Department of Neuropathology, University Hospital, Uppsala, Sweden

Z. WIESENFELD-HALLIN

Division of Clinical Neurophysiology, Karolinska Institute, Huddinge University Hospital, Huddinge, Sweden

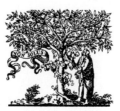

ELSEVIER
AMSTERDAM – LAUSANNE – NEW YORK – OXFORD – SHANNON – TOKYO
1995

ISBN 0-444-81719-0 (volume)
ISBN 0-444-80104-9 (series)

Published by:
Elsevier Science B.V.
P.O. Box 211
1000 AE Amsterdam
The Netherlands

Library of Congress Catalogue-in-Publication Data

Neuropeptides in the spinal cord / edited by F. Nyberg, H.S. Sharma, Z. Wiesenfeld-Hallin.
    p. cm. -- (Progress in brain research ; v. 104)
Includes bibliographical references and index.
ISBN 0-444-80104-9 (series : alk. paper). -- ISBN 0-044-81719-0
(alk. paper)
    1. Neuropeptides--Physiological effect. 2. Neuropeptides-
-Pathophysiology. 3. Spinal cord--Physiology. 4. Spinal cord-
-Pathophysiology. I. Nyberg, F. II. Sharma, H.S. (Hari Shanker)
III. Wiesenfeld-Hallin, Z. IV. Series.
    [DNLM: 1. Neuropeptides--physiology. 2. Receptors, Neuropeptide-
physiology. 3. Spinal Cord--physiology. W1 PR667J v. 104 1995 (P)
/ WL 104 N494293 1995]
QP376.P7 vol. 104
[QP552.N39]
612.8'2 s--dc20[612.8'3]
DNLM/DLC
for Library of Congress   95-602
                                                                     CIP

Printed in The Netherlands on acid-free paper

List of Contributors

U. Arvidsson, Department of Neuroscience, Doktorsringen 17, Karolinska Institutet, 171 77 Stockholm, Sweden

D. Besse, Neurobiology and Anesthesiology Branch, National Institute of Dental Research, National Institutes of Health, Bethesda, MD 20892, USA and Unité de Recherches de Physiopharmacologie du Système Nerveux de l'INSERM (U 161) and Laboratoire de Physiopharmacologie de la Douleur de l'EPHE, 2, rue d'Alésia, 75014 Paris, France

J.M. Besson, Unit de Recherches de Physiopharmacologie du Système Nerveux de l'INSERM (U 161) and Laboratoire de Physiopharmacologie de la Douleur de l'EPHE, 2, rue d'Alésia, 75014 Paris, France

L. Brodin, The Nobel Institute for Neurophysiology, Department of Neuroscience, Karolinska Institutet, S-171 77 Stockholm, Sweden

R. Cerne, Department of Veterinary Physiology and Pharmacology, Iowa State University, Ames, IA 50011, USA

G. Cheng, Department of Veterinary Physiology and Pharmacology, Iowa State University, Ames, IA 50011, USA

E. Csuhai, Department of Biochemistry, University of Kentucky, Chandler Medical Center, 800 Rose Street, Lexington, KY 40536-0084, USA

S. Cullheim, Department of Neuroscience, Doktorsringen 17, Karolinska Institutet, 171 77 Stockholm, Sweden

A.C. Cuello, Department of Pharmacology and Therapeutics, McGill University, 3655 Drummond Street, Montréal, Québec, Canada H3G 1Y6

A. Dray, Department of Pharmacology, Sandoz Institute for Medical Research, 5 Gower Place, London, WC1E 6BN, England, UK

A.W. Duggan, Department of Preclinical Veterinary Sciences, University of Edinburgh, Royal (Dick) School of Veterinary Studies, Summerhall, Edinburgh, EH9 1QH, Scotland, UK

U. Eriksson, Department of Pharmaceutical Biosciences, Biomedical Center, Uppsala University, Uppsala, Sweden.

A.J. Fox, Department of Thoracic Medicine, National Heart and Lung Institute, Dovehouse Street, London, England, UK

C.A. Haas, Institute of Anatomy I, University of Freiburg, Freiburg, Germany

U. Hanesch, Physiologisches Institut, Universität Würzburg, Röntgenring 9, D-97070 Würzburg, Germany

C.J. Helke, Department of Pharmacology, Uniformed Services University of the Health Sciences, 4301 Jones Bridge Road, Bethesda, MD 20814-4799, USA

J.L. Henry, Departments of Physiology and Psychiatry, McGill University, Montréal, Québec, Canada

T. Herdegen, University of Heidelberg, II. Institute of Physiology, Im Neuenheimer Feld 326, 69120 Heidelberg, Germany

L.B. Hersh, Department of Biochemistry, University of Kentucky, Chandler Medical Center, 800 Rose Street, Lexington, KY 40536-0084, USA

S.P. Hunt, Division of Neurobiology, Laboratory of Molecular Biology, MRC Centre, Hills Road, Cambridge, England, CB2 2QH, UK

S. Jeftinija, Department of Anatomy, Iowa State University, Ames, IA 50010, USA

P. Kogner, Paediatric Oncology Unit, Department of Paediatrics, and Peptide Research Laboratory, Department of Clinical Chemistry, Karolinska Hospital, S-171 76 Stockholm, Sweden

Lj. Kojić, Department of Veterinary Physiology and Pharmacology, Iowa State University, Ames, IA 50011, USA

M. Kolaj, Department of Veterinary Physiology and Pharmacology, Iowa State University, Ames, IA 50011, USA

G.W. Kreutzberg, Department of Neuromorphology, Max-Planck-Institute for Psychiatry, 82152 Martinsried, Germany

D. Larhammar, Department of Medical Genetics, Uppsala University, Box 589, S-751 23 Uppsala, Sweden

S.N. Lawson, Department of Physiology, School of Medical Sciences, University Walk, Bristol, BS8 1TD, England, UK

P. Le Grevés, Department of Pharmaceutical Biosciences, Biomedical Center, Uppsala University, Uppsala, Sweden.

A. Lecci, Pharmacology Department, A. Menarini Pharmaceuticals, Via Sette Santi 3, 50131 Florence, Italy

S.S. Little, Department of Biochemistry, University of Kentucky, Chandler Medical Center, 800 Rose Street, Lexington, KY 40536-0084, USA

M.C. Lombard, Unité de Recherches de Physiopharmacologie du Système Nerveux de l'IN-SERM (U 161) and Laboratoire de Physiopharmacologie de la Douleur de l'EPHE, 2, rue d'Alésia, 75014 Paris, France

C.A. Maggi, Pharmacology Department, A. Menarini Pharmaceuticals, Via Sette Santi 3, 50131 Florence, Italy

R. Munglani, Department of Anaesthesia, University of Cambridge Clinical School, Addenbrookes Hospital, Hills Road, Cambridge, England CB2 2QQ, UK

F. Nyberg, Department of Pharmaceutical Biosciences, Biomedical Center, Uppsala University, Uppsala, Sweden

Y. Olsson, Laboratory of Neuropathology, University Hospital, Uppsala University, Uppsala, Sweden

S. Persson, Department of Pharmaceutical Biosciences, Biomedical Center, Uppsala University, Uppsala, Sweden. Department of Medical Inflammation Research, Lund University, Lund, Sweden

V. Pieribone, Laboratory of Molecular and Cellular Neuroscience, The Rockefeller University, New York, NY 10021, USA

V. Radhakrishnan, Departments of Physiology & Psychiatry, McGill University, Montréal, Québec, Canada

G. Raivich, Department of Neuromorphology, Max-Planck-Institute for Psychiatry, 82152 Martinsried, Germany

M. Randić, Department of Veterinary Physiology and Pharmacology, Iowa State University, Ames, IA 50011, USA

M. Reddington, Department of Neuromorphology, Max-Planck-Institute for Psychiatry, 82152 Martinsried, Germany

K. Ren, Neurobiology and Anesthesiology Branch, National Institute of Dental Research, National Institutes of Health, Bethesda, MD 20892, USA

A. Ribeiro-da-Silva, Department of Pharmacology & Therapeutics, McGill University, 3655 Drummond Street, Montréal, Québec, Canada H3G 1Y6

V.H. Routh, Department of Pharmacology, Uniformed Services University of the Health Sciences, 4301 Jones Bridge Road, Bethesda, MD 20814-4799, USA

M.A. Ruda, Neurobiology and Anesthesiology Branch, National Institute of Dental Research, National Institutes of Health, Bethesda, MD 20892, USA

H.-G. Schaible, Physiologisches Institut, Universität Würzburg, Röntgenring 9, D-97070 Würzburg, Germany

H.S. Sharma, Laboratory of Neuropathology, University Hospital and Department of Pharmaceutical Biosciences, Biomedical Center, Uppsala University, Uppsala, Sweden

J. Silberring, Department of Clinical Neurosciences, Karolinska Institute, Stockholm, Sweden.

C. Söderberg, Department of Medical Genetics, Uppsala University, Box 589, S-751 23 Uppsala, Sweden

S.W.N. Thompson, Department of Pharmacology, Sandoz Institute for Medical Research, 5 Gower Place, London, WC1E 6BN, UK

M. Thörnwall, Department of Pharmaceutical Biosciences, Biomedical Center, Uppsala University, Uppsala, Sweden

L. Urban, Department of Pharmacology, Sandoz Institute for Medical Research, 5 Gower Place, London, WC1E 6BN, England, UK

M.R. Vasko, Departments of Pharmacology and Toxicology, Anesthesia and Medicine, Indiana University School of Medicine, Indianapolis, IN 46202-5120, USA

R.A. Wang, Department of Veterinary Physiology and Pharmacology, Iowa State University, Ames, IA 50011, USA

J. Westman, Department of Human Anatomy, Biomedical Centre, Uppsala University, Uppsala, Sweden

Z. Wiesenfeld-Hallin, Karolinska Institute, Department of Medical Laboratory Sciences and Technology, Division of Clinical Neurophysiology, Huddinge University Hospital, Huddinge, Sweden

M. Zimmermann, University of Heidelberg, II. Institute of Physiology, Im Neuenheimer Feld 326, 69120 Heidelberg, Germany

Preface

Neuropeptides in the spinal cord: past, present and future

This is, to our knowledge, the first book devoted exclusively to examining the role of neuropeptides in the spinal cord. Great progress has been made recently in our understanding of the role of neuropeptides in neurotransmission. Receptors for a variety of neuropeptides have been cloned and the pharmacological and physiological function of these neuroactive substances are under vigorous investigation. Particular interest has been shown in the development of highly selective receptor agonists and antagonists by a large number of research laboratories, as well as the pharmaceutical industry, which will give us tools to study the function of endogenous neuropeptides in health and disease. Because the general organization of the spinal cord is well conserved among species and neuropeptides appear to have a major role in spinal neurotransmission, we consider it timely to present a compendium of recent research in this field.

Neuropeptides, like the classical neurotransmitters, are well preserved from the evolutionary point of view. The spinal cord of primitive vertebrates, which have evolved separately from mammals for hundreds of millions of years, have neuropeptides with highly similar amino acid sequences when compared with mammals, including primates (Brodin et al., Chapter 4). The anatomical distribution of neuropeptides in lamprey and mammalian spinal cord has also many similarities. Such observations suggest that there may be a general similarity of function across many species, although major species differences between the distribution of neuropeptides and their receptors, as well as the affinity of agonists and antagonists to receptors, have also been described. Thus, it is important to establish interspecies similarities and differences.

The anatomical and immunohistological localization of neuropeptides in primary afferents and the spinal cord has revealed a complex pattern of coexistence between neuropeptides and classical neurotransmitters under normal and pathological conditions. The plasticity of this organization under pathological conditions can be related to functional plasticity (Hökfelt et al., 1994). The organization of peptidergic interneurons and terminals of descending tracks in the dorsal horn of the spinal cord studied at the electronmicroscopic level has greatly increased our understanding of the processing of somatosensory input, especially that evoked by nociceptive stimuli (Ribeiro-da-Silva and Cuello, Chapter 3). Similarly, peptide expression under normal and pathological conditions in motoneurons has been studied in great detail and can be related to functional plasticity (Cullheim and Arvidsson, Chapter 2; Raivich et al., Chapter 1).

The first tachykinin discovered, substance P, was isolated by von Euler and Gaddum in 1931 and was suggested to have a role in sensory transmission by Lembeck in 1953. Three tachykinin peptides have been identified and their receptors have been isolated (Nakanishi, 1991). Through receptor binding studies a great deal is now known about the distribution and function of these peptides in the spinal cord (Routh and Helke, Chapter 6). Similarly, at least three subtypes of opioid receptors have been identified, μ, δ and κ and their respective receptors have also recently been cloned. Binding of selective agonists to opioid receptors has yielded much information on their role in the processing of sensory information under normal and pathological circumstances (Lombard et al., Chapter 5).

Neuropeptides are converted and degraded by a number of enzymes and peptidases. There is a great need for the isolation and characterization of neuropeptide processing and degrading enzymes (Persson et al., Chapter 7; Csuhai et al., Chapter 8). Inhibitors of neuropeptide degrading enzymes may be useful drugs. For example, inhibitors of the degradation of endogenous opioid peptides could be useful analgesics in the future.

A wide variety of approaches have been used to study the sensory and motor function of neuropeptides in the spinal cord. A large section in this volume is devoted to describing results obtained with a great number of techniques. Combined electrophysiological and morphological techniques are used to try to elucidate the relationship between peptide content and physiological properties of primary afferents (Lawson, Chapter 10), as well as the role of prostaglandins in the release of neuropeptides (Vasko, Chapter 21). *Ex vivo* methods have been used to characterize the role of peptides released from primary afferents in the development of the sensitization of the dorsal horn of the spinal cord (Urban et al., Chapter 14), as well as the interaction of neuropeptides and excitatory amino acids (Randic et al., Chapter 14). Electrophysiological studies on the role of sensory neuropeptides in spinal cord have also been carried out *in vivo* under normal and pathological conditions (Radhakrishnan and Henry, Chapter 11; Wiesenfeld-Hallin, Chapter 15; Olsson et al., Chapter 22; Sharma et al., Chapter 23). An elegant technique has been developed to measure the release of neuropeptides into the spinal cord *in vivo* (Duggan, Chapter 12). On the motor side the role of tachykinins in the micturition reflex has also been elucidated (Lecci and Maggi, Chapter 9).

The induction of the expression of proto-oncogenes as a sign of neuronal activity, primarily involving nociception, has been studied *in vitro* as well as *in vivo* in the spinal cord (Murglani and Hunt, Chapter 16; Herdegen and Zimmermann, Chapter 17). The regulation of the expression of proto-oncogenes and neuropeptides that may be related to their expression during inflammation is described by Ruda et al. (Chapter 20). Neuropeptide levels in primary afferents are also altered during inflammation (Hanesch and Schaible, Chapter 19). The expression of neuropeptides in neuroblastomas and ganglioneuromas is another example of the presence of such molecules in pathology (Kogner, Chapter 18).

We hope that this volume will help to stimulate further research in the field of neuropeptides which will lead to better understanding of this role in health and disease.

F. Nyberg
H.S. Sharma
Z. Wiesenfeld-Hallin

References

Hökfelt, T., Zhang, X. and Wiesenfeld-Hallin, Z. (1994) Messenger plasticity in primary sensory neurons following axotomy and its functional implications. *Trends Neurosci.*, 17: 22–30.

Lembeck, F. (1953) Zur Frage der zentralen Übertragung afferenter Impulse. III. Mitteilung. Das Vorkommen und die Bedeutung der Substanz P in den dorsalen Wurzeln des Rückenmarks. *Naunyn-Schmiedebergs Arch. Pharmakol.*, 219: 197–213.

Nakanishi, S. (1991) Mammalian tachykinin receptors. *Annu. Rev. Neurosci.*, 14: 123–136.

Von Euler, U.S. and Gaddum, J.H. (1931) An unidentified depressor substance in certain tissue extracts. *J. Physiol. (London), 72:74–87.*

Contents

SECTION I

Neuropeptides: Distribution and Plasticity

F. Nyberg, H.S. Sharma and Z. Wiesenfeld-Hallin (Eds.)
Progress in Brain Research, Vol 104
© 1995 Elsevier Science BV. All rights reserved.

CHAPTER 1

Peptides in motoneurons

G. Raivich[1], M. Reddington[1], C.A. Haas[2] and G.W. Kreutzberg[1]

[1]*Department of Neuromorphology, Max-Planck-Institute for Psychiatry, 82152 Martinsried, Germany and*
[2]*Institute of Anatomy I, University of Freiburg, Freiburg, Germany*

Introduction

Although motoneurons are primarily known for cholinergic neurotransmission there is increasing interest in the role of neuropeptides. In the anterior spinal cord, motoneurons receive a variety of peptidergic inputs coming from sensory, spinal and supraspinal sources. Alpha- and γ-motoneurons also express a steadily increasing list of different neuropeptides such as calcitonin gene-related peptide (CGRP), galanin, cholecystokinin, substance P and proopiomelanocortin- or POMC-derived peptides. As a group, the motoneuronal neuropeptides are developmentally regulated in a strikingly similar fashion: they reach a peak during the onset or the main phase of synaptogenesis and decline to much lower levels in the adult. They also become re-expressed after axotomy and during regeneration. This ontogenetic and post-traumatic regulation profile, as well as functional evidence, have emphasized the role of motoneuron neuropeptides as differentiation factors which are important in the formation or re-establishment of neuromuscular interaction. However, some neuropeptides may also play a role in the physiological control of muscle function in the normal, adult organism.

The aim of this review is to summarize the data on the localization, function and regulation of neuropeptides in motoneurons during development, in the adult and in pathology. Since many experiments on neuropeptide regulation were first performed or have only been performed on cranial motoneurons, data on neuropeptides in brainstem motor nuclei are included. We also include information on other functionally important molecules like agrin, acetylcholine receptor-inducing activity (ARIA) and other growth factors, which are synthesized by motoneurons and may influence the cholinergic and peptidergic signal transmission between motoneurons and their target, the skeletal muscle.

Motoneuron neuropeptides

Calcitonin gene-related peptide (CGRP)

At present, the calcitonin gene-related peptides (CGRPs) are the most extensively analysed neuropeptides in the developing, adult and regenerating motoneurons in a variety of species including frog, chick, rat, guinea pig, cat, monkey and human. Calcitonin gene-related peptides are two closely homologous 37-amino acid neuromodulator proteins (α and β) which differ only in one amino acid in the rat and three in the human (Rosenfeld et al., 1983; Morris et al., 1984; Amara et al., 1985; Steenbergh et al., 1985). α-Calcitonin gene-related peptide (α-CGRP) was initially discovered as an alternative splicing product of the already identified calcitonin gene and provided the first demonstration of regulated alternative mRNA processing in the mammalian neuroendocrine system (Rosenfeld et al., 1981). Although α-CGRP and calcitonin are structurally related, there is only an approximately 20% homology in the amino acid sequence and little cross-reactivity towards specific CGRP and calcitonin receptors (Wimalawansa, 1992). Molecular cloning has also identified a second, calcitonin/CGRP-related gene, now referred to as the β-CGRP gene (Amara et al., 1985). This second CGRP gene does not exhibit the phenomenon of alternative processing and gives rise to the β-CGRP peptide (Emeson et al., 1992). In addition to very similar action profiles of α- and β-CGRP, the close homology should also be noted for methodological reasons, since most antibodies used in immunohistochemical studies may not differentiate between the two peptides (Wimalawansa, 1992).

Expression, distribution and colocalization of CGRP in motoneurons

Both α- and β-CGRP mRNA types are normally expressed in low to moderate levels on a fraction of adult cranial and spinal motoneurons, with α-CGRP being more abundant (Gibson et al., 1988a; Saika et al., 1991; Rosenfeld et al., 1992). Overall, there is considerable variation in the intensity of expression and percentage of CGRP-positive motoneurons in different motoneuron pools (Amara et al., 1985, Popper and Mycevych, 1989a; Kresse et al., 1992; Rosenfeld et al., 1992). Similar differences have also been observed with CGRP immunocytochemistry (Skofitsch and Jacobowitz, 1985; Takami et al., 1985; Batten et al., 1989; Popper and Micevych, 1990; Arvidsson et al., 1991; Csillik et al., 1993; Forger et al., 1993). Interestingly, the expression of CGRP on visceral motoneurons also varies with respect to location. CGRP is absent on purely visceromotor cranial nuclei like dorsal motor vagal nucleus and Edinger-Westphal nucleus (Skofitsch et al., 1985; Takami et al., 1985); in the functionally mixed nucleus ambiguus, CGRP is only present on motoneurons which innervate skeletal muscle but not on the preganglionic autonomic neurons (McWilliam et al., 1989; Lee et al., 1992). In contrast, high levels of CGRP immunoreactivity are detected on the spinal neurons innervating sympathetic and parasympathetic ganglia (Senba and Tohyama, 1988; Yamamoto et al., 1989). This variability in CGRP expression is apparently mediated by the target tissue. Although the dorsal medial vagal nucleus is normally CGRP-negative, a strong expression of CGRP is observed on these visceral motoneurons after an anatomically incorrect reconnection to the skeletal muscle normally innervated by the hypoglossal nerve (Batten et al., 1992).

CGRP-positive neurons in the ventral spinal cord and brainstem motor nuclei also express choline acetyltransferase (ChAT) and acetylcholinesterase (AChE), the classical motoneuron marker enzymes (Takami et al., 1985; Batten et al., 1988, 1989; Cortés et al., 1990; Hietanen et al., 1990), indicating the expression of CGRP on motoneurons. Colocalization with CGRP was also demonstrated for cholecystokinin (CCK) on the comparatively small subpopulation of adult CCK-positive motoneurons (Cortés et al., 1990), and for somatostatin and vasoactive intestinal peptide (VIP) during embryonic development (Villar et al., 1988). CGRP and galanin immunoreactivities are apparently mutually exclusive in cranial motoneurons (Moore, 1989). In spinal motoneurons, a subpopulation of CGRP-positive neurons also contains galanin (Johnson et et al., 1992). Interestingly, the CGRP-positive and negative somatic motoneurons appear to differ with respect to their synaptic input. According to Hietanen et al. (1990), only the CGRP-negative motoneurons receive enkephalin-immunoreactive synaptic terminals. No correlation was observed, however, in the fraction of CGRP-positive neurons in identified motor nuclei with respect to the overall fiber type composition of the target muscle (Arvidsson et al., 1993). It remains to be seen if this lack of correlation is also present at the level of individual myotubes and the neuromuscular junction.

Physiological function of motoneuron CGRP

CGRP plays an important role in the regulation of motor function at the developing or regenerating neuromuscular junction. During development, CGRP promotes myotube differentiation and the upregulation of nicotinic acetylcholine receptors, particularly at the level of the α-subunit (New and Mudge, 1986; Fontaine et al., 1986; Moss et al., 1991; Changeux et al., 1992). CGRP also enhances the burst duration of stimulated acetylcholine receptors (Owens and Kullberg, 1993; Lu et al., 1993). In vitro, these actions of CGRP in cultured muscle cells are mediated by a rapid increase in cAMP levels via activation of adenylate cyclase (Jennings and Mudge, 1989; Kirilovsky et al., 1989) and the ensuing phosphorylation of acetylcholine receptors on the α- and δ-subunits (Miles et al., 1989; Changeux et al., 1992; Lu et al., 1993). CGRP prevents motoneurite sprouting in the inactivated developing (Kubke and Landmesser, 1991) and adult skeletal muscle (Tsujimoto and Kuno, 1988). In the normal adult skeletal muscle, CGRP also enhances the force of twitch muscle contraction by approximately 30–50% (Ohhashi and Jacobowitz, 1988; Uchida et al., 1990).

The issue as to whether motoneuron CGRP is also normally active at the adult neuromuscular junction is still largely unsettled. Most normal junctions in the adult muscle are CGRP-negative or contain CGRP in very low amounts (Mora et al., 1989; Matteoli et al., 1990; Li and Dahlström, 1992; Csillik et al., 1993). Junctional CGRP immunoreactivity is present on specialized subpopulations of skeletal muscle which border visceral tissue (tongue, upper esophagus, m. bulbocavernosus, m. sphincter ani externus) and on the inner paw muscles like m. flexor digiti brevis (Moore, 1989; Csillik et al., 1993). Moderate levels of CGRP are also present on neuromuscular junctions in intrafusal fibers (Matteoli et al., 1990; Forsgren et al., 1992), suggesting ongoing involvement in γ-motoneuron function. Local blockade of neurotrasmission with bupivacaine causes a slow accumulation of CGRP in the normally negative neuromuscular junctions (Csillik et al., 1993). This could imply steady release of minute amounts of CGRP from the normal motoneuron terminals, but upregulation of CGRP synthesis in response

to a signal from inactivated muscle is also possible (Popper et al., 1992).

In agreement with its putative function at the neuromuscular junction, CGRP synthesized in the motoneuron cell body is transported anterogradely to the target muscles (Bööj et al., 1989; Kashihara et al., 1989; Li et al., 1992; Raivich et al., 1992), with CGRP receptors concentrated at the muscle endplate (Popper and Micevych, 1989b). Only a small fraction of anterogradely transported CGRP is also transported retrogradely, implying effective peripheral release (Bööj et al., 1989; Kashihara et al., 1989; Raivich et al., 1992). Despite coexistence with acetylcholine (ACh) in motoneurite terminals, CGRP is released much less readily than acetylcholine (Matteoli et al., 1988; Uchida et al., 1990; Csillik et al., 1993). This may be due to differential storage: acetylcholine is concentrated in small synaptic vesicles, CGRP in large dense-core vesicles (Matteoli et al., 1988). As shown by Csillik et al. (1993) the release of CGRP from this location depends on a very prolonged, supramaximal stimulation of the motor axons. This mode of release argues against a role for CGRP in every neuromuscular excitation, although it could implicate this neuropeptide in promoting training effects on strongly exercised muscle.

CGRP regulation in developing, adult and regenerating motoneurons

The onset of CGRP expression in embryonic motoneurons coincides with their initial innervation of specific target muscles (New and Mudge, 1986; Villar et al., 1988). There is a rapid build-up in CGRP levels both in the motoneurons and neurite terminals during the following period of natural motoneuron cell death and the differentiation of the neuromuscular junction, reaching maximal levels at embryonic days 12–16 (E12–E16) in chick (Esquerada et al., 1989; Mason and Mudge, 1992) and during the first postnatal week in rat (Matteoli et al., 1990; Forger et al., 1993). This developmental maximum of CGRP expression is followed by a gradual decline during further maturation, leading to an almost complete disappearance from most neuromuscular junctions and motoneurons in the adult animal (Bööj et al., 1989; Matteoli et al., 1990; Csillik et al., 1993).

A summary of experimental data reported in the literature suggests that skeletal muscle, the peripheral target of motoneurons, is the primary source of developmentally regulated factors that enhance, and later inhibit CGRP synthesis. In vitro, culture in presence of embryonic muscle extract, will maintain high levels of motoneuron CGRP (Juurlink et al., 1990) and in vivo, muscle innervation or reinnervation coincides with CGRP upregulation (New and Mudge, 1986; Villar et al., 1988; Dumoulin et al., 1991). Programmed neuron cell death also coincides with the developmental CGRP increase, but its role appears to be indirect. Prevention of motoneuronal death with tubocurarine, an ACh receptor blocker that inhibits neuromuscular excitation (Pittman and Oppenheim, 1978), does not interfere with the early

phase of CGRP expression at E10 (Mason and Mudge, 1992). However, it completely abolishes CGRP at later stages at E14–E16 (Esquerada et al., 1989). It is possible that muscle innervation by surviving supernumerary motoneurons enhances the developmentally regulated synthesis of putative muscle-derived factors, which inhibit motoneuron CGRP synthesis.

Peripheral axotomy causes a rapid and massive re-expression or re-upregulation of α-CGRP mRNA and CGRP immunoreactivity on adult cranial and spinal motoneurons (Moore, 1989; Streit et al., 1989; Arvidsson et al., 1990; Haas et al., 1990; Dumoulin et al., 1991; Saika et al., 1991; Caldero et al., 1992; Grothe, 1993; Borke et al., 1993; Herdegen et al., 1993; Wang et al., 1993) (Fig. 1). The expression of β-CGRP, already expressed at lower levels (Gibson et al., 1988a; Rosenfeld et al., 1992), is further reduced (Noguchi et al., 1990; Saika et al., 1991). This differential regulation of α- and β-CGRP sug-

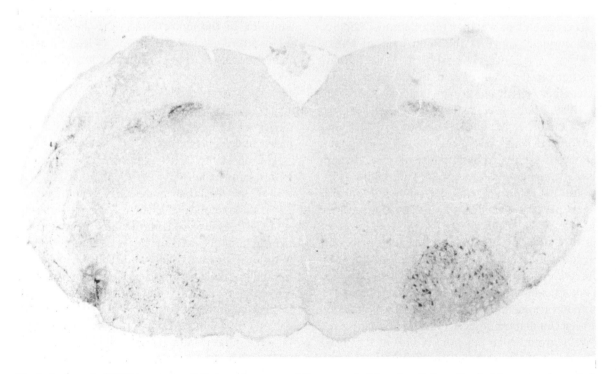

Fig. 1. Increase in CGRP immunoreactivity in motoneurons of the mouse facial nucleus 3 days after facial nerve axotomy. Left: control site; right: operated side.

gests that the post-axotomy increase in CGRP immunoreactivity is due to enhanced α-CGRP synthesis (Saika et al., 1991). Upregulation of α-CGRP also occurs if axonal flow is transiently interrupted by transport blockers like colchicine or vinblastine, suggesting that these substances interfere with the retrograde transport of inhibitory factors from the periphery (Moore, 1989; Rethelyi et al., 1991; Katoh et al., 1992). Later changes in CGRP expression depend on the type of injury. High levels of α-CGRP mRNA and immunoreactivity are maintained after peripheral nerve crush and ensuing regeneration, disappearing during successful reinnervation of peripheral muscles (Saika et al., 1991; Caldero et al., 1992; Borke et al., 1993). After transection, the expression of CGRP is clearly biphasic, returning to normally low levels during the first week after trauma (Arvidsson et al., 1990; Haas et al., 1990; Saika et al., 1991; Borke et al., 1993; Grothe, 1993) and increasing again at the onset of muscle reinnervation (Dumoulin et al., 1991; Borke et al., 1993; Grothe et al., 1993). Transection, and even more the resection of peripheral nerves clearly delay the process of neurite regeneration compared to nerve crush (see, e.g., Borke et al., 1993) and the absence of the biphasic CGRP expression after crush may therefore simply reflect a merging of the post-axotomy and reinnervation phases of CGRP upregulation. In both cases, after crush or transection, successful neurite regeneration elicits a massive, but transient induction of CGRP immunoreactivity on motoneurites reinnervating muscle endplates (Csillik et al., 1993), underlining the apparent importance of CGRP in the reestablishment as well as in the development of neuromuscular interactions (Matteoli et al., 1990).

CGRP expression in spinal motoneurons is also regulated by integrating supraspinal, sensory and hormone input. Removal of supraspinal, descending afferents by spinal cord transection decreases CGRP levels in the cell body (Arvidsson et al., 1989; Marlier et al., 1990) and in the anterograde transport to the periphery (Li et al., 1992). Unilateral removal of sensory afferents by rhizotomy

will counteract this effect (Hökfelt et al., 1992). Interestingly, CGRP immunoreactivity also disappears on surviving motoneurons in spinal cord autopsies from cases of amyotrophic lateral sclerosis, with associated degeneration of supraspinal input (Gibson et al., 1988b). The chemical nature of the supraspinal afferents that maintain CGRP synthesis in motoneurons is still unclear. Although serotoninergic fibers comprise a large fraction of descending supraspinal input, a selective destruction of serotoninergic afferents with 5,7-dihydroxytryptamine will in fact enhance CGRP synthesis (Hökfelt et al., 1992).

Finally, the expression of CGRP in sexually-dimorphic motor nuclei, like the spinal nucleus of the bulbocavernosus (SNB), is also regulated by androgens (Popper et al., 1992; Forger et al., 1993). The onset of CGRP immunoreactivity in rat SNB is clearly delayed, apparently reflecting low levels of circulating androgens in postnatal animals (Forger et al., 1993). In the adult rat, however, a reduction in androgens by castration will cause a strong upregulation in α-CGRP mRNA and peptide immunoreactivity (Popper and Micevych, 1989; Popper et al., 1992). Although these actions may seem contradictory, it is possible that androgens have a pleiotrophic influence: first enhancing the synthesis of developmentally-regulated factors that promote CGRP induction and later, in more mature muscle, factors that repress the synthesis of this motoneuron neuropeptide.

Non-muscle CGRP targets and mechanisms of action

In addition to skeletal muscle, CGRP has been shown to interact with many different cells including endothelial cells, macrophages and lymphocytes, neurons and glial cells. The most prevalent response is a stimulation of adenylate cyclase (Poyner, 1992). In relation to the actions of CGRP synthesized by motoneurons, the skeletal muscle appears to be the primary target; during regeneration further potential targets are Schwann cells in the injured peripheral nerve, and astrocytes and microglia at central sites. The functional roles of CGRP on muscle cell function have been referred to already.

The Schwann cells are a likely target for CGRP derived from regenerating motoneurites. CGRP immunoreactivity is concentrated on the tips of the outgrowing neurites which interact with adjacent bands of Schwann cells during nerve regeneration. Only a small proportion of anterogradely transported CGRP is returned to neuronal cell bodies, implying efficient release by regenerating neurites into the extracellular space in the injured peripheral nerve (Raivich et al., 1992). Sciatic nerve axotomy also lead to an increased number of CGRP binding sites in the distal, denervated part of the nerve, again suggesting local action of endoneural CGRP on the activated Schwann cells (Raivich et al., 1992). Cultured Schwann cells have receptors for CGRP and their activation leads to an elevation of cyclic AMP levels in these cells (Mudge et al., 1991). Although CGRP alone is not mitogenic for Schwann cells, elevation of cAMP does enhance the mitogenic action of established Schwann cell mitogens like fibroblast growth factors/FGF or platelet-derived growth factor/PDGF (Davis and Stroobant, 1990). Interestingly, motoneurons also synthesize FGF and PDGF (see below). Reinnervation of the distal, denervated peripheral nerve leads to a brisk phase of Schwann cell activation and proliferation (Pellegrino and Spencer, 1985; Raivich et al., 1992) and coexpression of FGF and PDGF with CGRP may enhance the mitogenic potential of these Schwann cell growth factors.

In addition to the cellular changes observed in the periphery, motoneuron axotomy also leads to an activation of adjacent astrocytes and proliferation of activated microglia in the central nervous system (Graeber and Kreutzberg, 1986; Graeber et al., 1988). A putative role for glial cells as targets of CGRP action after neuronal injury was first suggested by studies showing that specific, high-affinity CGRP binding was not decreased in the rat facial nucleus after the selective destruction of facial motoneurons with the toxic lectin, ricin (Dumoulin, 1991). The presence of glial CGRP receptors was confirmed by studies on the effects of CGRP on cultured astrocytes, where this neuropeptide lead to rapid morphological changes known as stellation, accompanied by a 30-fold increase in cyclic AMP (Lazar et al., 1991). The stimulation by CGRP of astrocyte adenylate cyclase is followed by an induction of the immediate early genes, c-*fos* and *jun*B, but not of c-*jun* (Haas et al., 1991a,b). A similar induction of *fos* and *jun*B has also been observed on cultured microglia (Priller, Haas, Reddington, unpublished observations). Overall, these data present an outline of the CGRP signal transduction cascade, beginning with receptor activation, followed by that of adenylate cyclase and the induction of some immediate early-gene products like *fos* and *jun*B, which would, in turn, stimulate the transcription of as yet unidentified target genes.

The possible roles for CGRP in normal and injured motoneurons are illustrated in Fig. 2.

Galanin

Galanin is a 29-amino acid peptide that was first isolated from porcine intestine by Tatemoto et al. (1983). It has been shown to be widely distributed in the mammalian nervous system (Ch'ng et al., 1985; Melander et al., 1986). However, little or no galanin or galanin mRNA is expressed in normal adult motoneurons (Moore, 1989; Saika et al., 1991; Kordower et al., 1992; Zhang et al., 1993a,b).

In contrast to the adult, high levels of peptide immunoreactivity and message are observed during development and following motoneuron injury. During development, peptide immunoreactivity was first observed in presumptive motoneuron pools at E15 in the rat, with a steady increase in the number of galanin-positive motoneurons up to the first postnatal days (Marti et al., 1987). Similar upregulation was also observed in the human fetus, between the 6th and 14th embryonic weeks (Marti et al., 1987). As in the case of CGRP, the number of positive motoneurons then rapidly declined to the very low adult levels.

Axotomy has been shown to induce a re-expression of galanin in facial (Moore, 1989), vagal (Rutherford, 1992) and spinal motoneurons

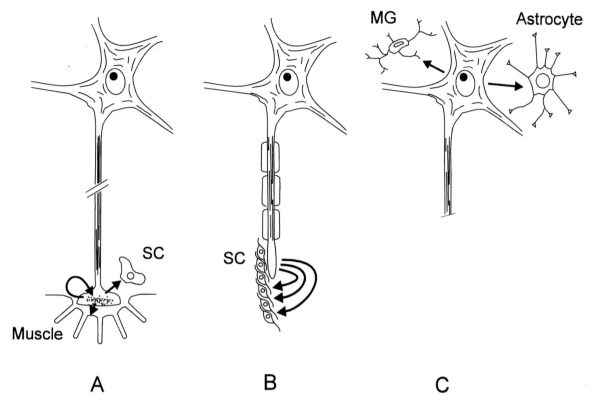

Fig. 2. Possible functions of CGRP in motoneurons. A. Under normal conditions, CGRP is released from motor nerve terminals, where it could act on muscle, on the adjacent perijunctional Schwann cells and, as a feedback regulator, on the release of neurotransmitter from the nerve endings. B. Following axotomy, CGRP released from neurites can act on Schwann cells in the injured peripheral nerve. C. In the central nervous system, CGRP might act on perineuronal astrocytes and microglia and play a role in their activation following motoneuron injury. SC, Schwann cells; MG, microglia. Arrows indicate possible sites of release and action.

(Zhang et al., 1993a,b). A similar induction was also observed for galanin mRNA (Saika et al., 1991; Zhang et al., 1993a,b). Interestingly, interruption of axonal flow with colchicine also leads to the re-expression of galanin (Moore, 1989). This similarity to the regulation of CGRP, could again point to the presence of inhibitory factors, which are normally transported from muscle to the motoneuron cell body and suppress the normal expression of motoneuron neuropeptides.

Immunocytochemical studies after axotomy showed galanin immunoreactivity both in the large α- and in the small, γ-motoneurons (Zhang et al., 1993a). Its colocalization with other neuropeptides appears to be differ in various regions. In the brainstem motor nuclei, Moore (1989) reported that motoneurons expressed either galanin or CGRP but not both. In the spinal cord, however, some motoneurons clearly express both CGRP and galanin (Johnson et al., 1992; Zhang et al., 1993a), whereas others only express one of the peptides. This presumably reflects different roles for these neuropeptides, although the function of galanin in motoneurons is currently unknown.

Cholecystokinin (CCK)

The discovery of gastrin-like peptides in the brain by Vanderhaegen et al. (1975) led to studies on the distribution and function of these peptides in the central nervous system. The major form of these peptides in the nervous system is the C-terminal octapeptide of cholecystokinin (CCK-8). Initial studies on the immunohistochemical distribution of CCK-like immunoreactivity (CCK-LI) revealed a widespread distribution, including motoneurons (Schroder, 1983). However, positive results using immunohistochemical approaches to CCK localization must be approached critically due to the possibility of cross-reaction with other peptides, including CGRP (Ju et al., 1986). Other investigators have been unable to demonstrate CCK-LI in motoneuron perikarya, even after colchicine treatment or nerve resection (Kubota et al., 1983; Fuji et al., 1985; Saika et al., 1991).

More recently, in situ hybridization techniques have been used to approach the distribution of CCK in the nervous system. Several studies have reported the presence of CCK mRNA in motoneurons of the spinal cord and various cranial nerve nuclei, including the motor trigeminal, facial and hypoglossal nuclei (Ingram et al., 1989; Sutin and Jacobowitz, 1990; Cortés et al., 1990; Abelson and Micevych, 1991; Schiffmann et al., 1991). Some species differences have been observed. For instance, numerous spinal cord motoneurons express CCK mRNA in the rat and monkey, whereas few positive motoneurons were observed in guinea pig spinal cord (Cortés et al., 1990; Verge et al., 1993; Zhang et al., 1993b). Using antisera specific for CCK, an accumulation of this peptide has been reported proximal to a ligation of the rat sciatic nerve, supporting the view that CCK mRNA is translated into peptide and that this is transported into the motoneuron axon (Cortés et al., 1991).

The effects of axotomy on CCK mRNA expression differ in different regions and species. Crushing the rat facial nerve results in an increase in the proportion of motoneurons positive for CCK mRNA from 7% in controls to about 30% in the facial nucleus ipsilateral to the crush (Saika et al., 1991). This reaction is transient, the highest number of positive neurons being observed 7–14 days after lesion. Resection of the facial nerve leads to an even larger response, with 60% of motoneurons CCK mRNA-positive after 7 days, and it persists as long as 8 weeks after resection. In contrast to the axotomy of the facial nerve, transection of rat sciatic nerve or ventral root leads to a *decrease* in CCK mRNA in spinal motoneurons (Piehl et al., 1993). In the monkey, transection of the sciatic nerve had no effect on the number of CCK mRNA-positive motoneurons in the spinal cord (Zhang et al., 1993b). Finally, Taquet et al. (1992) reported that lesion of primary afferent fibres by dorsal rhizotomy in adult rats led to an increase in CCK-LI in the ipsilateral ventral horn, suggesting that expression of CCK in motoneurons is under the control of primary afferent input.

The above observations suggest that CCK might have different functions in different motoneuron systems. CCK is a modulator of acetylcholine release at frog neuromuscular junctions (Akasu et al., 1986) and has a trophic effect on cultured rat ventral spinal cord (Iwasaki et al., 1989). It is therefore possible that it plays roles both in neurotransmission and in motoneuron regeneration.

Other neuropeptides

In addition to CGRP, galanin and CCK, several other neuropeptides have been reported to occur in motoneurons, although these have not been extensively studied to date. Substance P-like immunoreactivity (SP-LI) has been observed in large dense-core vesicles in frog motoneurons and their terminals (Matteoli et al., 1990), but studies in the rat and monkey failed to detect SP-LI (Zhang et al., 1993a,b). However, in both mammalian species, substance P mRNA has been detected in spinal motoneurons after axotomy (Zhang et al., 1993a,b). SP-LI is transiently expressed in motoneurons of the rat and human spinal cord during ontogenesis (Marti et al., 1987).

Vasoactive intestinal polypeptide (VIP) has been demonstrated using immunocytochemistry in motoneuron perikarya in the rat and chick spinal cords (Villar et al., 1988; Li et al., 1992; Zhang et al., 1993a). VIP mRNA has also been found to increase in rat spinal motoneurons following sciatic nerve lesion (Zhang et al., 1993a).

Increases in the mRNAs for somatostatin and neuropeptide Y have also been reported in motoneurons of the spinal cord after axotomy in the rat (Zhang et al., 1993) but not in the monkey (Zhang et al., 1993b). As described for other neuropeptides, the developmental profile of motoneuronal somatostatin and neuropeptide Y is transient (Marti et al., 1987). Since somatostatin has been shown to prevent natural cell death occurring during development of chick spinal cord motoneurons (Weill, 1991), this peptide might enhance neuronal survival during ontogenesis and during regeneration.

The peptides, α-melanotropin (α-MSH) and β-endorphin, both of which are derived from pro-opiomelanocortin (POMC), have been detected in motoneurons. Although POMC-derived peptides are expressed in motoneurons of immature mice, little or no expression is observed in normal adults (Haynes and Smith, 1985; Hughes and Smith, 1988). However, motoneuronal POMC-peptides are increased in adult dystrophic mice (Haynes and Smith, 1985). After sciatic nerve lesion in the rat, an increased number of POMC-immunoreactive motoneuron profiles is observed on the denervated muscle (Hughes and Smith, 1989). POMC-LI is also observed in rat motoneurons during chemically induced neurotoxicity (Hughes et al., 1992). The POMC-derived peptides might therefore play a general role in the response of motoneurons to injury caused by different factors.

The neuropeptides discussed so far all increase their expression following injury. In contrast, it was found in a recent study that enkephalin mRNA *decreases* in spinal motoneurons following axotomy of the sciatic nerve in both rat and monkey (Zhang et al., 1993a,b).

Motoneuron proteins with possible involvement in neurotransmitter and neuropeptide function

In addition to the neuropeptides reviewed above, motoneurons also contain a number of functional proteins which may be involved in the development and ongoing function of the neuromuscular junction, modulating the muscle response to acetylcholine and to the various motoneuron neuropeptides. There is a steadily growing list of these regulatory substances which include agrin, acetylcholine receptor-inducing activity or ARIA/neuregulin and a number of growth factors like transferrin, insulin-like growth factor I (IGF1), platelet-derived growth factors (PDGFs) and fibroblast growth factors (FGFs).

Agrin, a 200-kDa glycoprotein, is the most prominent member of this list (for recent reviews see Nastuk and Fallon, 1993; McMahan et al., 1992). It is a soluble protein that is synthesised and secreted by motoneurons and that induces the aggregation of ACh receptors at the site of the initial neurite-muscle contacts. Agrin is deposited at the basement membrane of developing neuromuscular junctions, where it binds very firmly (Magill-Solc and McMahan, 1988). Its action is mediated by specific muscle agrin receptors on the postsynaptic muscle membrane (Nastuk et al., 1991) and involves the induction of tyrosine kinase activity (Wallace et al., 1991). Agrin is a relatively complex molecule. Binding to the muscle receptor and the aggregating activity apparently reside on the C-terminal part of the molecule which contains a number of EGF- and laminin-like repeats (Ruegg et al., 1992). The N-terminal part contains 9 cystein-rich related modules with significant sequence homology to a group of extracellular, growth factor-scavenging glycoproteins including follistatin, osteonectin/SPARC and SC1 (Patthy and Nikolics, 1993). This N-terminal part may be involved in regulating growth factor-mediated junctional differentiation of the presynaptic motoneurite and the muscle endplate (see below).

The receptor-aggregating action of agrin is physiologically important as it concentrates acetylcholine neurotransmission just at the narrow patch of neuromuscular junction, ensuring rapid response and high sensitivity due to very limited diffusion distance. In vitro, it also mediates the rapid aggregation of agrin receptors, acetylcholinesterase and butyrylcholinesterase and, with some delay, a relatively large list of cytoskeletal proteins and extracellular matrix components (for a review see Nastuk and Fallon, 1993). In view of these data, agrin or a similar substance, may also mediate the aggregation of CGRP receptors at the adult neuromuscular junction (Popper and Micevych, 1989b). As shown by Kuno and his colleagues, sensory neurites are responsible for most of muscle CGRP, while only 5–30% of total CGRP is of motoneuronal origin (Kashihara et al., 1989; Sakaguchi et al., 1991, 1992). Concentration of CGRP receptors at the neuromuscular junction would thus not only enhance the sensitivity to CGRP released from the presynaptic neurite terminal but also dampen the effects of sensory CGRP. A similar effect may also be involved in mediating the activity of other motoneurite neuropeptides.

Acetylcholine receptor-inducing activity or ARIA is a 42-kDa glycoprotein which is a member of the neuroregulins. This family of growth factors is derived by alternative splicing from a single neuregulin gene (Falls et al., 1993; Marchionni et al., 1993) and apparently acts on the same receptor tyrosine kinase, also known as c-*neu* or c-*erb*B2 protooncogene (Prigent and Lemoine, 1992; Corfas et al., 1993; Raivich and Kreutzberg, 1994). The onset of ARIA synthesis in motoneurons is very early, starting before the onset of neuromuscular interaction and continuing through adulthood (Falls et al., 1993). In vitro, ARIA enhances acetylcholine receptor synthesis (Usdin and Fischbach, 1986), similar to that of CGRP (New and Mudge, 1986; Fontaine et al., 1986). However, the effects of ARIA and CGRP differ in their transduction mechanism and action profile: CGRP enhances almost selectively the expression of the α-subunit (Moss et al., 1991; Changeux et al., 1992), ARIA exerts a broader action, leading to a moderate, 2-fold upregulation of α-, χ- and δ-subunits, and a massive, up to 10-fold, increase in the ϵ-subunit (Martinou et al., 1991). Postnatal muscle development leads to a dramatic change in kinetic properties of acetylcholine receptor channels (Schuetze and Role,

1987; Brehm, 1989) that are accompanied by a change in their receptor subunit composition from $\alpha_2\beta\delta\chi$ to $\alpha_2\beta\delta\epsilon$ (Mishina et al., 1986; Gu and Hall, 1988). The strongly stimulatory effects of ARIA on ϵ-subunit synthesis have highlighted the possible role of ARIA on the developmental transition of acetylcholine receptors from embryonic to adult type (Martinou et al., 1991). However, there is a temporal mismatch: ARIA is produced throughout motoneuron development (Falls et al., 1993), while acetylcholine receptor transition is a late postnatal event (Gu and Hall, 1988). Since CGRP selectively enhances the synthesis of α- but not of ϵ-receptor subunits, it is possible that high postnatal levels of CGRP interfere with receptor transition, so that it takes place as the motoneurite levels of CGRP begin to decline (Matteoli et al., 1990).

Finally, adult motoneurons also express and/or contain a large number of different growth factors like transferrin (Oh et al., 1986; Mescher, 1992), insulin-like growth factor 1 (IGF1) (Andersson et al., 1986; Hansson et al., 1987), α-platelet-derived growth factor (α-PDGF) (Yeh et al., 1991) and acidic and basic fibroblast growth factors also known as FGF1 and FGF2 (Elde et al., 1991; Otsuka et al., 1993). Anterograde transport to motoneurite terminals has also been shown for IGF1 (Hansson et al., 1987), transferrin (Kiffmeyer et al., 1991; Mescher, 1992) and FGF2 (Otsuka et al., 1993). In all three cases, only a fraction of anterogradely transported material is returned, suggesting effective release at neuromuscular junctions. During development, these growth factors have a very broad action profile, supporting growth and differentiation of muscle cells, motoneurons and Schwann cells as well as many other cell types (Aizenmann et al., 1986; Walicke and Baird, 1988; Davis and Stroobant, 1990; Stewart et al., 1991; Ang et al., 1992; Caroni and Becker, 1992). The possible physiological function of these motoneuron-derived growth factors in the adult is still unclear, although they may be involved in maintaining the high level of differentiation on the axonal, Schwann cell and muscle components of the neuromuscular junction. The presence of growth factor-binding domains in the motoneuron-secreted agrin molecule, also hints at a potentially important role for the regulation of growth factor levels at the functionally dense interphase between motoneurite and skeletal muscle (Patthy and Nikolics, 1993).

Peptidergic input onto motoneurons

In addition to their expression by motoneurons described above, neuropeptides also modulate motoneuron activity via peptidergic input from a variety of sources. Terminal varicosities containing substance P, for instance, are found making contact with motoneurons in the ventral spinal cord and in brain stem motor nuclei (Hökfelt et al., 1975a,b, 1976; Ljungdahl et al., 1978; Johansson et al., 1981; Gibson et al., 1984; Atsumi et al., 1985; Connaughton et al., 1986; Hietanen et al., 1990; Tallaksen et al., 1993). Spinal cord motoneurons receive substance P input from both spinal projections of medullary neurons (Nicholas et al., 1992) and from the dorsal horn (Gibson et al., 1984) and specific binding sites for substance P have been located on the target motoneurons (Helke et al., 1986). Colocalisation of substance P in these pathways has been reported with serotonin and the acidic amino acids (Hökfelt et al., 1978; Björklund et al., 1979; Chan-Palay, 1979; Singer et al., 1979; Nicholas et al., 1992; Tallaksen et al., 1993). Functionally, substance P depolarizes motoneurons and modulates synaptic activity by setting the level of excitability of motoneurons and thus altering the efficacy of transmission (Krivoy et al., 1980; Nicoll et al., 1980; White, 1985).

Some motoneurons receiving input from substance P-positive pathways are also innervated by enkephalinergic neurons (Tashiro et al., 1989). As in the case of substance P, colocalisation of enkephalin with serotonin has been reported (Arvidsson et al., 1992). However, whereas substance P-positive terminals are found on both CGRP-positive and -negative motoneurons in the rat spinal cord, enkephalinergic input is mainly found surrounding CGRP-negative cells

(Hietanen et al., 1990). Further, in the rat hypoglossal nucleus, substance P immunoreactive fibres make multiple axosomatic contacts while enkephalin immunoreactive terminals make contact mainly with large and small dendrites (Connaughton et al., 1986) indicating different functional roles for these neuropeptides.

The thyrotropin-releasing hormone (TRH) is a hypothalamic peptide that is also present in networks of terminals arising from supraspinal sites (e.g., the bulbospinal tract) and terminating on motoneurons of the spinal cord (Hökfelt et al., 1975c; Johansson et al., 1980, 1981). All motor nuclear groups appear to be innervated by TRH, frequently in association with α-motoneurons (Lechan et al., 1984). Like substance P, TRH depolarizes spinal and brain stem motoneurons in several species (Nicoll, 1978; Suzue et al., 1981; Takahashi, 1985) and also facilitates glutamate- or NMDA-induced excitability (White, 1985; Lacey et al., 1989), possibly by interacting with NMDA receptors (Rekling, 1992). The excitatory actions of TRH are probably mediated postsynaptically via block of a novel K^+ conductance (Nistri et al., 1990; Rekling, 1990; Bayliss et al., 1992) similar to that affected by substance P (Fisher and Nistri, 1993), although a presynaptic site of action has also been suggested (Lacey et al., 1989; Behbehani et al., 1990). TRH is colocalized with both substance P and serotonin (Johansson et al., 1981) and it interacts synergistically with serotonin to excite spinal motoneurons (Clarke et al., 1985). The excitability of motoneurons is thus probably controlled by an interaction between serotonin, TRH and substance P. In addition, TRH has trophic effects on motoneurons of the ventral spinal cord in vitro (Schmidt-Achert et al., 1984).

Finally, several other neuropeptides have been implicated in the regulation of motoneuron function on the basis of either pharmacological or immunocytochemical studies, including vasopressin (Suzue et al., 1981; Raggenbass et al., 1991; Widmer et al., 1992), β-MSH (Krivoy and Zimmermann, 1977; Krivoy et al., 1985), dynorphin (Klein et al., 1991) and neuropeptide Y (Kawano et al., 1993).

References

Abelson, L. and Micevych, P.E. (1991) Distribution of prepro-cholecystokinin mRNA in motoneurons of the rat brainstem and spinal cord. *Mol. Brain Res.*, 10: 327–335.

Aizenmann, Y., Wiechsel, M. and DeVellis, J. (1986) Changes in insulin and transferrin requirements of pure brain neuronal cultures during embryonic development. *Proc. Natl. Acad. Sci. USA*, 83: 2263–2266.

Akasu, T., Tsurusaki, M. and Ariyoshi, M. (1986) Presynaptic effects of cholecystokinin octapeptide on neuromuscular transmission in the frog. *Neurosci. Lett.*, 67: 329–333.

Amara, S.G., Arriza, J.L., Leff, S.E., Swanson, L.W., Evans, R.M. and Rosenfeld, M.G. (1985) Expression in brain of a messenger RNA encoding a novel neuropeptide homologous to calcitonin gene-related peptide. *Science*, 229: 1094–1097.

Andersson, I., Billig, H., Fryklund, L., Hansson, H., Isaksson, O., Isgaard, J., Nilsson, A., Rozell, B., Skotter, A. and Stemme, S. (1986) Localization of IGF-1 in adult rats: immunohistochemical studies. *Acta Phys. Scand.*, 126: 311–312.

Ang, L.C., Bhaumick, B., Munoz, D.G., Sass, J. and Juurlink, B.H. (1992) Effects of astrocytes, insulin and insulin-like growth factor I on the survival of motoneurons in vitro. *J. Neurol. Sci.*, 109: 168–172.

Arvidsson, U., Cullheim, S., Ulfhake, B., Hökfelt, T. and Terenius, L. (1989) Altered levels of calcitonin gene-related peptide (CGRP)-like immunoreactivity of cat lumbar motoneurons after chronic spinal cord transection. *Brain Res.*, 489: 387–391.

Arvidsson, U., Johnson, H., Piehl, F., Cullheim, S., Hökfelt, T. and Risling, M. (1990) Peripheral nerve section induces increased levels of calcitonin gene-related peptide (CGRP)-like immunoreactivity in axotomized motoneurons. *Exp. Brain Res.*, 79: 212–216.

Arvidsson, U., Ulfhake, B., Cullheim, S., Terenius, L. and Hökfelt, T. (1991) Calcitonin gene-related peptide in monkey spinal cord and medulla oblongata. *Brain Res.*, 558: 330–334.

Arvidsson, U., Cullheim, S., Ulfhake, B., Ramirez, V., Dagerlind, A. and Luppi, P.H. (1992) Distribution of enkephalin and its relation to serotonin in cat and monkey spinal cord and brain stem. *Synapse*, 11: 85–104.

Arvidsson, U., Piehl, F., Johnson, H., Ulfhake, B., Cullheim, S. and Hökfelt, T. (1993) The peptidergic motoneurone. *Neuroreport*, 4: 849–856.

Atsumi, S., Sakamoto, H., Yokota, S. and Fujiwara, T. (1985) Substance p and 5-hydroxytryptamine immunoreactive presynaptic boutons in presumed alpha-motoneurons in the chicken ventral horn. *Arch. Histol. Jpn.*, 48: 159–172.

Batten, T.F., Appenteng, K. and Saha, S. (1988) Visualisation of CGRP and ChAT-like immunoreactivity in identified trigeminal neurones by combined peroxidase and alkaline phosphatase enzymatic reactions. *Brain Res.*, 447: 314–324.

Batten, T.F., Lo, V.K., Maqbool, A. and McWilliam, P.N. (1989) Distribution of calcitonin gene-related peptide-like immunoreactivity in the medulla oblongata of the cat, in relation to choline acetyltransferase-immunoreactive motoneurones and substance P-immunoreactive fibres. *J. Chem. Neuroanat.*, 2: 163–176.

Batten, T.F., Maqbool, A. and McWilliam, P.N. (1992) CGRP in brain stem motoneurons. Dependent on target innervated? *Ann. NY Acad. Sci.*, 60: 458–460.

Bayliss, D.A., Viana, F. and Berger, A.J. (1992) Mechanisms underlying excitatory effects of thyrotropin-releasing hormone on rat hypoglossal motoneurons in vitro. *J. Neurophys.*, 68: 1733–1745.

Behbehani, M.M., Pun, R.Y., Means, E.D. and Anderson, D.K. (1990) Thyrotropin-releasing hormone has profound presynaptic action on cultured spinal cord neurons. *Synapse*, 6: 169–174.

Björklund, A., Emson, P., Gilbert, R. and Skagerberg, G. (1979) Further evidence for the possible coexistence of 5-hydroxytryptamine and substance P in medullary raphe neurones of rat brain. *Br. J. Pharmacol.*, 66: 112–113.

Borke, R.C., Curtis, M. and Ginsberg, C. (1993) Choline acetyltransferase and calcitonin gene-related peptide immunoreactivity in motoneurons after different types of nerve injury. *J. Neurocytol.*, 22: 141–153.

Bööj, S., Goldstein, M., Fischer, C.R. and Dahlstroem, A. (1989) Calcitonin gene-related peptide and chromogranin A: presence and intra-axonal transport in lumbar motor neurons in the rat, a comparison with synaptic vesicle antigens in immunohistochemical studies. *Neuroscience*, 30: 479–501.

Brehm, P. (1989) Resolving the structural basis for developmental changes in muscle ACh receptor function: it takes nerve. *Trends Neurosci.*, 12: 174–177.

Caldero, J., Casanovas, A., Sorribas, A. and Esquerda, J.E. (1992) Calcitonin gene-related peptide in rat spinal cord motoneurons: subcellular distribution and changes induced by axotomy. *Neuroscience*, 48: 449–461.

Caroni, P. and Becker, M. (1992) The downregulation of growth-associated proteins in motoneurons at the onset of synapse elimination is controlled by muscle activity and IGF1. *J. Neurosci.*, 12: 3849–3861.

Ch'ng, J., Christofides, N., Anand, P., Gibson, S., Allen, Y., Su, H., Tatemoto, K., Morrison, J., Polak, J. and Bloom, S. (1985) Distribution of galanin immunoreactivity in the central nervous system and responses of galanin-containing pathways to injury. *Neuroscience*, 16: 343–354.

Chan-Palay, V. (1979) Combined immunocytochemistry and autoradiography after in vivo injections of monoclonal antibody to substance P and ^{3}H-serotonin: coexistence of two putative transmitters in single raphe cells and fiber plexuses. *Anat. Embryol.*, 156: 241–254.

Changeux, J.P., Duclert, A. and Sekine, S. (1992) Calcitonin gene-related peptides and neuromuscular interactions. *Ann. NY Acad. Sci.*, 78: 361–378.

Clarke, K.A., Parker, A.J. and Stirk, G.C. (1985) Potentiation of motoneurone excitability by combined administration of 5-HT agonist and TRH analogue. *Neuropeptides*, 6: 269–282.

Connaughton, M., Priestley, J.V., Sofroniew, M.V., Eckenstein, F. and Cuello, A.C. (1986) Inputs to motoneurones in the hypoglossal nucleus of the rat: light and electron microscopic immunocytochemistry for choline acetyltransferase, substance P and enkephalins using monoclonal antibodies. *Neuroscience*, 17: 205–224.

Corfas, G., Falls, D.L. and Fischbach, G.D. (1993) ARIA, a protein that stimulates acetylcholine receptor synthesis, also induces tyrosine phosphorylation of a 185-kDa muscle transmembrane protein. *Proc. Natl. Acad. Sci. USA*, 90: 1624–1628.

Cortés, R., Arvidsson, U., Schalling, M., Ceccatelli, S. and Hökfelt, T. (1990) In situ hybridization studies on mRNAs for cholecystokinin, calcitonin gene-related peptide and choline acetyltransferase in the lower brain stem, spinal cord and dorsal root ganglia of rat and guinea pig with special reference to motoneurons. *J. Chem. Neuroanat.*, 3: 467–485.

Cortés, R., Aman, K., Arvidsson, U., Terenius, L., Frey, P., Rehfeld, J.F., Walsh, J.H. and Hökfelt, T. (1991) Immunohistochemical study of cholecystokinin peptide in rat spinal motoneurons. *Synapse*, 9: 103–110.

Csillik, B., Tajti, L., Kovacs, T., Kukla, E., Rakic, P. and Knyiharcsillik, E. (1993) Distribution of calcitonin gene-related peptide in vertebrate neuromuscular junctions: relationship to the acetylcholine receptor. *J. Histochem. Cytochem.*, 41: 1547–1555.

Davis, J. and Stroobant, P. (1990) Platelet-derived growth factors and fibroblaast growth factors are mitogens for rat Schwann cells. *J. Cell Biol.*, 110: 1353–1360.

Dumoulin, F.L. (1991) Calcitonin Gene-Related Peptide (CGRP) in der Regeneration motorischer und sensorischer Neurone der Ratte. *M.D. Thesis, Technical University of Munich.*

Dumoulin, F.L., Raivich, G., Streit, W.J. and Kreutzberg, G.W. (1991) Differential regulation of calcitonin gene-related peptide (CGRP) in regenerating rat facial nucleus and dorsal root ganglion. *Eur. J. Neurosci.*, 3: 338–342.

Elde, R., Cao, Y., Cintra, A., Brelie, T., Pelto-Huikko, M., Junttila, T., Fuxe, K., Pettersson, R. and Hökfelt, T. (1991) Prominent expression of acidic fibroblast growth factor in motor and sensory neurons. *Neuron*, 7: 349–364.

Emeson, R., Yeakley, J., Hedjran, F., Merillat, N., Lenz, J. and Rosenfeld, M. (1992) Posttranscriptional regulation of calcitonin/CGRP gene expression. *Ann. NY Acad. Sci.*, 657: 18–35.

Esquerda, J.E., Ciutat, D. and Comella, J.X. (1989) Absence of histochemical immunoreactivity to calcitonin gene-related peptide (CGRP) in spinal cord motoneurons from (+)-tubocurarine-treated chick embryos. *Neurosci. Lett.*, 105: 1–6.

Falls, D.L., Rosen, K.M., Corfas, G., Lane, W.S. and Fischbach, G.D. (1993) ARIA, a protein that stimulates acetylcholine receptor synthesis, is a member of the neu ligand family. *Cell*, 72: 801–815.

Fisher, N.D. and Nistri, A. (1993) Substance P and TRH share a common effector pathway in rat spinal motoneurones: an in vitro electrophysiological investigation. *Neurosci. Lett.*, 153: 115–119.

Fontaine, B., Klarsfeld, A., Hökfelt, T. and Changeux, J.P. (1986) Calcitonin gene-related peptide, a peptide present in spinal cord motoneurons, increases the number of acetylcholine receptors in primary cultures of chick embryo myotubes. *Neurosci. Lett.*, 71: 59–65.

Forger, N.G., Hodges, L.L. and Breedlove, S.M. (1993) Ontogeny of calcitonin gene-related peptide immunoreactivity in rat lumbar motoneurons: delayed appearance and sexual dimorphism in the spinal nucleus of the bulbocavernosus. *J. Comp. Neurol.*, 330: 514–520.

Forsgren, S., Bergh, A., Carlsson, E. and Thornell, L.E. (1992) Studies on the distribution of calcitonin gene-related peptide-like and substance-P-like immunoreactivities in rat hind limb muscles. *Histochem. J.*, 24: 345–353.

Fuji, K., Snba, E., Fujii, S., Nomura, I., Wu, J., Ueda, Y. and Tohyama, M. (1985) Distribution, ontogeny and projections of cholecytokinin-8, vasoactive intestinal polypeptide and γ-aminobutyrate-containing neuron systems in the rat spinal cord: an immunohistochemical analysis. *Neuroscience*, 14: 881–894.

Gibson, S.J., Bloom, S.R. and Polak, J.M. (1984) A novel substance P pathway linking the dorsal and ventral horn in the upper lumbar segments of the rat spinal cord. *Brain Res.*, 301: 243–251.

Gibson, S.J., Polak, J.M., Giaid, A., Hamid, Q.A., Kar, S., Jones, P.M. and Denny, P. (1988a) Calcitonin gene-related peptide messenger RNA is expressed in sensory neurones of the dorsal root ganglia and also in spinal motoneurones in man and rat. *Neurosci. Lett.*, 91: 283–288.

Gibson, S.J., Polak, J.M., Katagiri, T., Su, H., Weller, R.O. and Brownell, D.B. (1988b) A comparison of the distributions of eight peptides in spinal cord from normal controls and cases of motor neurone disease with special reference to Onuf's nucleus. *Brain Res.*, 474: 255–278.

Graeber, M. and Kreutzberg, G. (1986) Astrocytes increase in glial fibrillary acidic protein during retrograde changes of facial motor neurons. *J. Neurocytol.*, 15: 363–373.

Graeber, M. and Tetzlaff, W. and Kreutzberg, G.W. (1988)

Microglial cells but not astrocytes undergo mitosis following rat facial nerve axotomy. *Neurosci. Lett.*, 85: 317–321.

Grothe, C. (1993) Biphasic increase of calcitonin gene-related peptide-like immunoreactivity in rat hypoglossal motoneurons after nerve transection. *Acta Histochem.*, 94: 20–24.

Gu, Y. and Hall, Z.W. (1988) Immunological evidence for a change in subunits of the acetylcholine receptor in developing and denervated rat muscle. *Neuron*, 1: 117–125.

Haas, C.A., Streit, W.J. and Kreutzberg, G.W. (1990) Rat facial motoneurons express increased levels of calcitonin gene-related peptide messenger RNA in response to axotomy. *J. Neurosci. Res.*, 27: 270–275.

Haas, C.A., Reddington, M. and Kreutzberg, G.W. (1991a) Calcitonin gene-related peptide stimulates the induction of c-*fos* gene expression in rat astrocyte cultures. *Eur. J. Neurosci.*, 3: 708–712.

Haas, C., Reddington, M. and Kreutzberg, G. (1991b) Calcitonin gene-related peptide elicits differential expression of early response genes in cultured astrocytes. *Eur. J. Neurosci.*, Suppl. 4: 1040.

Hansson, H., Rozell, B. and Skottner, A. (1987) Rapid axoplasmic transport of insulin-like growth factor 1 in the sciatic nerve of adult rats. *Cell Tissue Res.*, 247: 241–247.

Haynes, L.W. (1990) Immunocytochemical detection of beta-endorphin in mouse spinal motoneurons cocultured with astrocytes from spinal cord and forebrain. *Mol. Chem. Neuropathol.*, 12: 27–35.

Haynes, L.W. and Smith, M.E. (1985) Presence of immunoreactive alpha-melanotropin and beta-endorphin in spinal motoneurones of the dystrophic mouse. *Neurosci. Lett.*, 58: 13–18.

Helke, C.J., Charlton, C.G. and Wiley, R.G. (1986) Studies on the cellular localization of spinal cord substance P receptors. *Neuroscience*, 19: 523–533.

Herdegen, T., Fiallos, E.C., Bravo, R. and Zimmermann, M. (1993) Colocalisation and covariation of c-JUN transcription factor with galanin in primary afferent neurons and with CGRP in spinal motoneurons following transection of rat sciatic nerve. *Mol. Brain Res.*, 17: 147–154.

Hietanen, M., Pelto, H.M. and Rechardt, L. (1990) Immunocytochemical study of the relations of acetylcholinesterase, enkephalin-, substance P-, choline acetyltransferase- and calcitonin gene-related peptide-immunoreactive structures in the ventral horn of rat spinal cord. *Histochemistry*, 93: 473–477.

Hökfelt, T., Kellereth, J.O., Nilsson, G. and Pernow, B. (1975a) Substance P: localization in the central nervous system and in some primary sensory neurons. *Science*, 190: 889–890.

Hökfelt, T., Kellerth, J.O., Nilsson, G. and Pernow, B. (1975b) Experimental immunohistochemical studies on the localization and distribution of sunstance p in cat primary sensory neurons. *Brain Res.*, 100: 235–252.

Hökfelt, T., Johansson, O., Kellereth, J.O., Ljungdahl, A., Nilsson, G., Nygards, A. and Pernow, B. (1975c) Thy-rotropin releasing hormone (TRH)-containing nerve terminals in certain brain stem nuclei and in the spinal cord. *Neurosci. Lett.*, 1: 133–139.

Hökfelt, T., Elde, R., Johansson, O., Luft, R., Nilsson, G. and Arimura, A. (1976) Immunohistochemical evidence for separate populations of somatostatin-containing and substance P-containing primary afferent neurons in the rat. *Neuroscience*, 1: 131–136.

Hökfelt, T., Ljungdahl, A., Steinbusch, H., Verhofstad, A., Nilsson, G., Brodin, E., Pernow, B. and Goldstein, M. (1978) Immunohistochemical evidence of substance P-like immunoreactivity in some 5-hydroxytryptamine-containing neurons in the rat central nervous system. *Neuroscience*, 3: 517–538.

Hökfelt, T., Arvidsson, U., Ceccatelli, S., Cortés, R. and Cullheim, S. (1992) Calcitonin gene-related peptide in the brain, spinal cord, and some peripheral systems. *Ann. NY Acad. Sci.*, 657: 119–134.

Hughes, S. and Smith, M.E. (1988) Effect of nerve section on beta-endorphin and alpha-melanotropin immunoreactivity in motor nerves of normal and dystrophic mice. *Neurosci. Lett.*, 92: 1–7.

Hughes, S. and Smith, M.E. (1989) Pro-opiomelanocortin-derived peptides in transected and contralateral motor nerves of the rat. *J. Chem. Neuroanat.*, 2: 227–237.

Hughes, S., Smith, M.E., Simpson, M.G. and Allen, S.L. (1992) Effect of IDPN on the expression of POMC-derived peptides in rat motoneurones. *Peptides*, 13: 1021–1023.

Ingram, S., Krause, R., Baldino, J., Jr., Skeen, L. and Lewis, M. (1989) Neuronal localization of cholecystokinin mRNA in the rat brain by using in situ hybridization histochemistry. *J. Comp. Neurol.*, 287: 260–272.

Iwasaki, Y., Kinosita, M. and Ikeda, K. (1989) Neurotrophic effect of cholecystokinin on ventral spinal cord in culture. *Neurol. Res.*, 11: 231–232.

Jennings, C.G.B. and Mudge, A.W. (1989) Chick myotubes in culture express high-affinity receptors for calcitonin gene-related peptide. *Brain Res.*, 504: 199–205.

Johansson, O., Hökfelt, T., Jeffcoate, S., White, N. and Sternberger, L. (1980) Ultrastructural localization of TRH-like immunoreactivity. *Exp. Brain Res.*, 38: 1–10.

Johansson, O., Hökfelt, T., Pernow, B., Jeffcoate, S., White, N., Steinbusch, H., Verhofstad, A., Emson, P. and Spindel, E. (1981) Immunohistochemical support for three putative transmitters in one neuron: coexistence of 5-hydroxytryptamine, substance P- and thyrotropin releasing hormone-like immunoreactivity in medullary neurons projecting to the spinal cord. *Neuroscience*, 6: 1857–1881.

Johnson, H., Hökfelt, T. and Ulfhake, B. (1992) Galanin-like and CGRP-like immunoreactivity coexist in rat spinal motoneurons. *Neuroreport*, 3: 303–306.

Ju, G., Hökfelt, T., Fischer, J., Frey, P., Rehfeld, J. and Dockray, G. (1986) Does cholecystokinin-like immunoreactivity in the rat primary sensory neurons represent calcitonin gene-related peptide? *Neurosci. Lett.*, 68: 305–310.

Juurlink, B. and Devon, R.M. (1990) Calcitonin gene-related peptide identifies spinal motoneurons in vitro. *J. Neurosci. Res.*, 26: 238–241.

Kashihara, Y., Sakaguchi, M. and Kuno, M. (1989) Axonal transport and distribution of endogenous calcitonin gene-related peptide in rat peripheral nerve. *J. Neurosci.*, 9: 3796–3802.

Katoh, K., Tohyama, M., Noguchi, K. and Senba, E. (1992) Axonal flow blockade induces alpha-CGRP mRNA expression in rat motoneurons. *Brain Res.*, 599: 153–157.

Kawano, M., Sugita, O., Inagaki, S., Furuyama, T. and Takagi, H. (1993) Neuropeptide Y innervation in the spinal nucleus of bulbocavernosus of the rat. *Neurosci. Lett.*, 152: 158–160.

Kiffmeyer, W.R., Tomusk, E.V. and Mescher, A.L. (1991) Axonal transport and release of transferrin in nerves of regenerating amphibian limbs. *Dev. Biol.*, 147: 392–402.

Kirilovsky, J., Duclert, A., Fontaine, B., Devillers-Thiery, A., Osterlund, M. and Changeux, J.P. (1989) Acetylcholine receptor expression in primary cultures of embryonic chick myotubes. 2. Comparison between the effects of spinal cord cells and calcitonin gene-related peptide. *Neuroscience*, 32: 289–296.

Klein, C.M., Sorkin, L.S., Chung, K. and Coggeshall, R.E. (1991) Unmyelinated primary afferent fiber stimulation depletes dynorphin A (1–8) immunoreactivity in rat ventral horn. *Brain Res.*, 566: 70–76.

Kordower, J., Le, H. and Mufson, E. (1992) Galanin immunoreactivity in the primate central nervous system. *J. Comp. Neurol.*, 319: 479–500.

Kresse, A., Jacobowitz, D. and Skofitsch, G. (1992) Distribution of calcitonin gene-related peptide in the central nervous system of the rat by immunocytochemistry and in situ hybridisation histochemistry. *Ann. NY Acad. Sci.*, 657: 455–457.

Krivoy, W.A. and Zimmermann, E. (1977) An effect of beta-melanocyte stimulating hormone (beta-MSH) on alpha-motoneurones of cat spinal cord. *Eur. J. Pharmacol.*, 46: 315–322.

Krivoy, W.A., Couch, J.R., Stewart, J.M. and Zimmermann, E. (1980) Modulation of cat monosynaptic reflexes by substance P. *Brain Res.*, 202: 365–372.

Krivoy, W.A., Couch, J.R. and Stewart, J.M. (1985) Modulation of spinal synaptic transmission by beta-melanocyte stimulating hormone (beta-MSH). *Psychoneuroendocrinology*, 10: 103–108.

Kubke, M. and Landmesser, L. (1991) Exogenous CGRP partially prevents the dTC induced increase in intramuscular nerve branching in embryonic chicken. *Soc. Neurosci. Abstr.*, 17: 735.

Kubota, Y., Inagaki, S., Shiosaka, S., Cho, H., Tateishi, K., Hashimura, E., Hamaoka, T. and Tohyama, M. (1983) The distribution of cholecystokinin octapeptide-like structures

in the lower brain stem of the rat: an immunohistochemical analysis. *Neuroscience*, 9: 587–604.

Lacey, G., Nistri, A. and Rhys, M.E. (1989) Large enhancement of excitatory postsynaptic potentials and currents by thyrotropin-releasing hormone (TRH) in frog spinal motoneurones. *Brain Res.*, 488: 80–88.

Lazar, P., Reddington, M., Streit, W., Raivich, G. and Kreutzberg, G.W. (1991) The action of calcitonin gene-related peptide on astrocyte morphology and cyclic AMP accumulation in astrocyte cultures from neonatal rat brain. *Neurosci. Lett.*, 130: 99–102.

Lechan, R.M., Snapper, S.B., Jacobson, S. and Jackson, I.M. (1984) The distribution of thyrotropin-releasing hormone (TRH) in the rhesus monkey spinal cord. *Peptides*, 5, Suppl. 1, 185–194.

Lee, B.H., Lynn, R.B., Lee, H.S., Miselis, R.R. and Altschuler, S.M. (1992) Calcitonin gene-related peptide in nucleus ambiguus motoneurons in rat: viscerotopic organization. *J. Comp. Neurol.*, 320: 531–543.

Lhungdahl, A., Hökfelt, T. and Nilsson, G. (1978) Distribution of substance p-like immunoreactivity in the central nervous system of the rat. I. Cell bodies and nerve terminals. *Neuroscience*, 3: 861–943.

Li, J.Y. and Dahlstroem, A.B. (1992) Development of calcitonin-gene-related peptide, chromogranin A, and synaptic vesicle markers in rat motor endplates, studied using immunofluorescence and confocal laser scanning. *Muscle Nerve*, 15: 984–992.

Li, J.Y., Kling, P.A. and Dahlstroem, A. (1992) Influence of spinal cord transection on the presence and axonal transport of CGRP-, chromogranin A-, VIP-, synapsin I-, and synaptophysin-like immunoreactivities in rat motor nerve. *J. Neurobiol.*, 23: 1094–1100.

Lu, B., Fu, W.M., Greengard, P. and Poo, M.M. (1993) Calcitonin gene-related peptide potentiates synaptic responses at developing neuromuscular junction. *Nature*, 363: 76–79.

Magill-Solc, C. and McMahan, U. (1988) Motor neurons conatin agrin-like molecules. *J. Cell Biol.*, 107: 1825–1833.

Marchionni, M.A., Goodearl, A.D., Chen, M.S., Bermingham, M.O., Kirk, C., Hendricks, M., Danehy, F., Misumi, D., Sudhalter, J. and Kobayashi, K., et al. (1993) Glial growth factors are alternatively spliced erbB2 ligands expressed in the nervous system. *Nature*, 362: 312–318.

Marlier, L., Rajaofetra, N., Peretti, R.R., Kachidian, P. and Poulat, P. (1990) Calcitonin gene-related peptide staining intensity is reduced in rat lumbar motoneurons after spinal cord transection: a quantitative immunocytochemical study. *Exp. Brain Res.*, 82: 40–47.

Marti, E., Gibson, S., Polak, J., Facer, P., Springall, D., Van Aswegen, G., Aitchison, M. and Koltzenburg, M. (1987) Ontogeny of peptide- and amine-containing neurones in motor, sensory and autonomic regions of rat and human spinal cord, dorsal root ganglia and rat skin. *J. Comp. Neurol.*, 266: 332–359.

Martinou, J.C., Falls, D.L., Fischbach, G.D. and Merlie, J.P. (1991) Acetylcholine receptor-inducing activity stimulates expression of the epsilon-subunit gene of the muscle acetylcholine receptor. *Proc. Natl. Acad. Sci. USA*, 88: 7669–7673.

Mason, I.J. and Mudge, A.W. (1992) Onset of CGRP expression and its restriction to a subset of spinal motor neuron pools in the chick embryo is not affected by treatment with curare. *Neurosci. Lett.*, 138: 128–132.

Matteoli, M., Haimann, C. and De, C.P. (1990) Substance P-like immunoreactivity at the frog neuromuscular junction. *Neuroscience*, 37: 271–275.

McMahan, U.J., Horton, S.E., Werle, M.J., Honig, L.S., Kroeger, S. and Ruegg, M.A. (1992) Agrin isoforms and their role in synaptogenesis. *Curr. Opin. Cell Biol.*, 4: 869–874.

McWilliam, P.N., Maqbool, A. and Batten, T.F. (1989) Distribution of calcitonin gene-related peptide-like immunoreactivity in the nucleus ambiguus of the cat. *J. Comp. Neurol.*, 282: 206–214.

Melander, T., Hökfelt, T. and Rökaeus, A. (1986) Distribution of galanin-like immunoreactivity in the rat central nervous system. *J. Comp. Neurol.*, 248: 475–517.

Mescher, A. (1992) Trophic activity of regenerating peripheral nerves. *Comments Dev. Neurobiol.*, 1: 373–390.

Miles, K., Greengard, P. and Huganir, R.L. (1989) Calcitonin gene-related peptide regulates phosphorylation of the nicotinic acetylcholine receptor in rat myotubes. *Neuron*, 2: 1517–1524.

Mishina, M., Takai, T., Imoto, K., Noda, M., Takahashi, T., Numa, S., Methfessel, C. and Sakmann, B. (1986) Molecular distinction between fetal and adult forms of muscle acetylcholine receptor. *Nature*, 321: 406–411.

Moore, R. (1989) Cranial motor neurons contain either galanin- or calcitonin gene-related peptide-like immunoreactivity. *J. Comp. Neurol.*, 282: 512–522.

Mora, M., Marchi, M., Polak, J.M., Gibson, S.J. and Cornelio, F. (1989) Calcitonin gene-related peptide immunoreactivity at the human neuromuscular junction. *Brain Res.*, 492: 404–407.

Morris, H., Panico, M., Etienne, T., Tippins, J., Girgis, S. and MacIntyre, J. (1984) Isolation and characterization of human calcitonin gene-related peptide. *Nature*, 308: 746–748.

Moss, S.J., Harkness, P.C., Mason, I.J., Barnard, E.A. and Mudge, A.W. (1991) Evidence that CGRP and cAMP increase transcription of AChR alpha-subunit gene, but not of other subunit genes. *J. Mol. Neurosci.*, 3: 101–108.

Mudge, A. (1991) CGRP in development and regeneration. *Eur. J. Neurosci.*, Suppl. 4: 4013.

Nastuk, M. and Fallon, J. (1993) Agrins and the molecular choreography of synapse formation. *Trends Neurosci.*, 16: 72–76.

Nastuk, M.A., Lieth, E., Ma, J.Y., Cardasis, C.A., Moynihan, E.B., McKechnie, B.A. and Fallon, J.R. (1991) The putative agrin receptor binds ligand in a calcium-dependent manner

and aggregates during agrin-induced acetylcholine receptor clustering. *Neuron*, 7: 807–818.

New, H.V. and Mudge, A.W. (1986) Calcitonin gene-related peptide regulates muscle acetylcholine receptor synthesis. *Nature*, 323: 809–811.

Nicholas, A.P., Pieribone, V.A., Arvidsson, U. and Hökfelt, T. (1992) Serotonin-, substance P- and glutamate/aspartate-like immunoreactivities in medullo-spinal pathways of rat and primate. *Neuroscience*, 48: 545–559.

Nicoll, R.A. (1978) The action of thyrotropin-releasing hormone, substance P and related peptides on frog spinal motoneurons. *J. Pharmacol. Exp. Ther.*, 207: 817–824.

Nicoll, R.A., Alger, B.E. and Jahr, C.E. (1980) Peptides as putative excitatory neurotransmitters: carnosine, enkephalin, substance P and TRH. *Proc. Roy. Soc. London Ser. B.*, 210: 133–149.

Nistri, A., Fisher, N.D. and Gurnell, M. (1990) Block by the neuropeptide TRH of an apparently novel K^+ conductance of rat motoneurones. *Neurosci. Lett.*, 120: 25–30.

Noguchi, K., Senba, E., Morita, Y., Sato, M. and Tohyama, M. (1990) α-CGRP and β-CGRP mRNAs are differentially regulated in the rat spinal cord and dorsal root ganglion. *Mol. Brain Res.*, 7: 299–304.

Oh, T., Markelonis, G., Royal, G. and Bregman, B. (1986) Immunocytochemical distribution of transferrin and its receptor in the developing chicken nervous system. *Dev. Brain Res.*, 30: 207–220.

Ohhashi, T. and Jacobowitz, D. (1988) Effects of calcitonin gene-related peptide on neuromuscular transmission in the isolated rat diaphragm. *Peptides*, 9: 613.

Otsuka, H., Matsuda, S., Fujita, H., Matsuda, Y., Shibata, T. and Uryu, K. (1993) Localization of basic fibroblast growth factor (bFGF)-like immunoreactivity in neural circuits innervating the gastrocnemius muscle, with reference to the direction of bFGF transport. *Arch. Histol. Cytol.*, 56: 207–215.

Owens, J.L. and Kullberg, R.W. (1993) Calcitonin-gene-related peptide lengthens acetylcholine-receptor channel open time in developing muscle. *Receptors Channels*, 1: 165–171.

Patthy, L. and Nikolics, K. (1993) Functions of agrin and agrin-related proteins. *Trends Neurosci.*, 16: 76–81.

Pellegrino, R. and Spencer, P. (1985) Schwann cell mitosis in response to regenerating peripheral axons in vivo. *Brain Res.*, 341: 16–25.

Piehl, F., Arvidsson, U., Johnson, H., Cullheim, S., Dagerlind, A., Ulfhake, B., Cao, Y., Elde, R., Pettersson, R.F., Terenius, L. and Hökfelt, T. (1993) GAP-43, aFGF, CCK and alpha-CGRP and beta-CGRP in rat spinal motoneurons subjected to axotomy and/or dorsal root severance. *Eur. J. Neurosci.*, 5: 1321–1333.

Pittman, R. and Oppenheim, R. (1978) Neuromuscular blockade increases motoneurone survival during normal cell death in the chick embryo. *Nature*, 271: 364–366.

Popper, P. and Micevych, P.E. (1989a) The effect of castration on calcitonin gene-related peptide in spinal motor neurons. *Neuroendocrinology*, 50: 338–343.

Popper, P. and Micevych, P.E. (1989b) Localization of calcitonin gene-related peptide and its receptors in a striated muscle. *Brain Res.*, 496: 180–186.

Popper, P. and Micevych, P.E. (1990) Steroid Regulation of calcitonin gene-related peptide messenger RNA expression in motoneurons of the spinal nucleus of the bulbocavernosus. *Mol. Brain Res.*, 8: 159–166.

Popper, P., Ulibarri, C. and Micevych, P.E. (1992) The role of target muscles in the expression of calcitonin gene-related peptide mRNA in the spinal nucleus of the bulbocavernosus. *Mol. Brain Res.*, 13: 43–51.

Poyner, D.R. (1992) Calcitonin gene-related peptide: multiple actions, multiple receptors. *Pharmacol. Ther.*, 56: 23–51.

Prigent, S.A. and Lemoine, N.R. (1992) The type 1 (EGFR-related) family of growth factor receptors and their ligands. *Prog. Growth Factor Res.*, 4: 1–24.

Raggenbass, M., Goumaz, M., Sermasi, E., Tribollet, E. and Dreifuss, J.J. (1991) Vasopressin generates a persistent voltage-dependent sodium current in a mammalian motoneuron. *J. Neurosci.*, 11: 1609–1616.

Raivich, G. and Kreutzberg, G. (1994) Pathophysiology of glial growth factor receptors. *Glia*, 11: 129–146.

Raivich, G., Dumoulin, F., Streit, W. and Kreutzberg, G. (1992) Calcitonin gene-related peptide (CGRP) in the regenerating sciatic nerve. *Restorat. Neurol. Neurosci*, 4: 107–115.

Rekling, J.C. (1990) Excitatory effects of thyrotropin-releasing hormone (TRH) in hypoglossal motoneurons. *Brain Res.*, 510: 175–179.

Rekling, J.C. (1992) Interaction between thyrotropin-releasing hormone (TRH) and NMDA-receptor-mediated responses in hypoglossal motoneurones. *Brain Res.*, 578: 289–296.

Rethelyi, M., Mohapatra, N.K., Metz, C.B., Petrusz, P. and Lund, P.K. (1991) Colchicine enhances mRNAs encoding the precursor of calcitonin gene-related peptide in brainstem motoneurons. *Neuroscience*, 42: 531–539.

Rosenfeld, M.G., Amara, S.G., Roos, B.A., Ong, E.S. and Evans, R.M. (1981) Altered expression of the calcitonin gene associated with RNA polymorphism. *Nature*, 290: 63–65.

Rosenfeld, M., Mermod, J., Amara, S., Swanson, L., Sawachenko, P., Rivier, H., Vale, W. and Evans, R. (1983) Production of novel neuropeptide encoded by the calcitonin gene via tissue specific RNA processing. *Nature*, 308: 746–748.

Rosenfeld, M., Emeson, R., Yeakley, J., Merillat, N., Hedjran, F., Lenz, J. and Delsert, C. (1992) Calcitonin gene-related peptide: a neuropeptide generated as a consequence of tissue-specific, developmentally regulated alternative RNA processing events. *Ann. NY Acad. Sci.*, 657: 1–17.

Ruegg, M.A., Tsim, K.W., Horton, S.E., Kroeger, S., Escher,

G., Gensch, E.M. and McMahan, U.J. (1992) The agrin gene codes for a family of basal lamina proteins that differ in function and distribution. *Neuron*, 8: 691–699.

Rutherfurd, S.D., Widdop, R.E., Louis, W.J. and Gundlach, A.L. (1992) Preprogalanin mRNA is increased in vagal motor neurons following axotomy. *Mol. Brain Res.*, 14: 261–266.

Saika, T., Senba, E., Noguchi, K., Sato, M., Kubo, T., Matsunaga, T. and Tohyama, M. (1991) Changes in expression of peptides in rat facial motoneurons after facial nerve crushing and resection. *Mol. Brain Res.*, 11: 187–196.

Sakaguchi, M., Inaishi, Y., Kashihara, Y. and Kuno, M. (1991) Release of calcitonin gene-related peptide from nerve terminals in rat skeletal muscle. *J. Physiol.*, 434: 257–270.

Sakaguchi, M., Inaishi, Y., Kashihara, Y. and Kuno, M. (1992) Degeneration of motor nerve fibers enhances the expression of calcitonin gene-related peptide in rat sensory neurons. *Neurosci. Lett.*, 137: 61–64.

Schiffmann, S.N., Teugels, E., Halleux, P., Menu, R. and Vanderhaeghen, J.J. (1991) Cholecystokinin mRNA detection in rat spinal cord motoneurons but not in dorsal root ganglia neurons. *Neurosci. Lett.*, 123: 123–126.

Schmidt-Achert, K., Askanas, V. and Engel, W. (1984) Thyrotropin-releasing hormone enhances choline acetyltransferase and creatine kinase in cultured spinal ventral horn neurons. *J. Neurochem.*, 43: 586–589.

Schroder, H. (1983) Localization of cholecytokinin-like immunoreactivity in the rat spinal cord, with particular reference to the autonomic innervation of the pelvic organs. *J. Comp. Neurol.*, 217: 176–186.

Senba, E. and Tohyama, M. (1988) Calcitonin gene-related peptide containing autonomic efferent pathways to the pelvic ganglia of the rat. *Brain Res.*, 449: 386–390.

Singer, E., Sperk, G., Placheta, P. and Leeman, S. (1979) Reduction of substance P levels in the ventral cervical spinal cord of the rat after intracisternal 5,7-dihydroxytryptamine injection. *Brain Res.*, 174: 362–365.

Skofitsch, G. and Jacobowitz, D. (1985) Calcitonin gene-related peptide: detailed immunohistochemical distribution in the central nervous system. *Peptides*, 6: 721–745.

Steenbergh, P., Höppener, J., Zandberg, J., Lips, C. and Jansz, H. (1985) A second human calcitonin/CGRP gene. *FEBS Lett.*, 183: 403–407.

Stewart, H., Eccleston, P.A., Jessen, K.R. and Mirsky, R. (1991) Interaction between camp elevation, identified growth-factors, and serum components in regulating schwann-cell growth. *J. Neurosci. Res.*, 30:

Strand, F.L., Saintcome, C., Lee, T.S., Lee, S.J., Kume, J. and Zuccarelli, L.A. (1993) ACTH/MSH(4–10) analog BIM-22015 aids regeneration via neurotrophic and myotrophic attributes. *Peptides*, 14: 287–296.

Streit, W., Dumoulin, F., Raivich, G. and Kreutzberg, G. (1989) Calcitonin gene-related peptide increases in rat facial motoneurons after peripheral nerve transection. *Neurosci. Lett.*, 101: 143–148.

Sutin, E. and Jacobowitz, D. (1990) Detection of CCk mRNA in the motor nucleus of the rat trigeminal nerve with in situ hybridisation histochemistry. *Mol. Brain Res.*, 8: 63–68.

Suzue, T., Yanaihara, N. and Otsuka, M. (1981) Actions of vasopressin, gastrin releasing peptide and other peptides on neurons on newborn rat spinal cord in vitro. *Neurosci. Lett.*, 26: 137–142.

Takahashi, T. (1985) Thyrotropin-releasing hormone mimics descending slow synaptic potentials in rat spinal motoneurons. *Proc. Roy. Soc. London Ser. B.*, 225: 391–398.

Takami, K., Kawai, Y., Uchida, S., Tohyama, M., Shiotani, Y., Yoshida, H., Emson, P.C., Girgis, S., Hillyard, C.J. and MacIntyre, I. (1985) Effect of calcitonin gene-related peptide on contraction of striated muscle in the mouse. *Neurosci. Lett.*, 60: 227–230.

Tallaksen, G.S., Elde, R. and Wessendorf, M.W. (1993) Regional distribution of serotonin and substance P co-existing in nerve fibers and terminals in the brainstem of the rat. *Neuroscience*, 53: 1127–1142.

Taquet, H., Plachot, J.J., Pohl, M., Collin, E., Benoliel, J.J. and Bourgoin, S. (1992) Increased calcitonin gene-related peptide- and cholecystokinin-like immunoreactivities in spinal motoneurones after dorsal rhizotomy. *J. Neural Trans.*, 88: 127–141.

Tashiro, T., Satoda, T., Matsushima, R. and Mizuno, N. (1989) Convergence of serotonin-, enkephalin- and substance P-like immunoreactive afferent fibers on single pudendal motoneurons in Onuf's nucleus of the cat: a light microscope study combining the triple immunocytochemical staining technique with the retrograde HRP-tracing method. *Brain Res.*, 481: 392–398.

Tatemoto, K., Roekaeus, A., Joernvall, H., McDonald, T.J. and Mutt, V. (1983) Galanin: a novel biologically active peptide from porcine intestine. *FEBS Lett.*, 164: 124–128.

Tsujimoto, T. and Kuno, M. (1988) Calcitonin gene-related peptide prevents disuse-induced sprouting of rat motor nerve terminals. *J. Neurosci.*, 8: 3951–3957.

Uchida, S., Yamomoto, H., Iio, S., Matsumoto, N., Wang, X., Yonehara, N., Imai, Y., Inoki, R. and Yoshida, H. (1990) Release of calcitonin gene-related peptide-like immunoreactive substance from neuromuscular junction by nerve excitation and its action on striated muscle. *J. Neurochem.*, 54: 1000.

Usdin, T.B. and Fischbach, G.D. (1986) Purification and characterization of a polypeptide from chick brain that promotes the accumulation of acetylcholine receptors in chick myotubes. *J. Cell Biol.*, 103: 493–507.

Vanderhaegen, J.-J., Signeau, J. and Gepts, W. (1975) New peptide in vertebrate CNS reacting with anti-gastrin antibodies. *Nature*, 257: 604–605.

Verge, V.M., Wiesenfeld, H.Z. and Hökfelt, T. (1993) Cholecystokinin in mammalian primary sensory neurons and spinal cord in-situ hybridization studies in rat and monkey. *Eur. J. Neurosci.*, 5: 240–250.

Villar, M.J., Huchet, M., Hökfelt, T., Changeux, J.P., Fahrenkrug, J. and Brown, J.C. (1988) Existence and coexistence of calcitonin gene-related peptide, vasoactive intestinal polypeptide- and somatostatin-like immunoreactivities in spinal cord motoneurons of developing embryos and post-hatch chicks. *Neurosci. Lett.*, 86: 114–118.

Villar, M.J., Roa, M., Huchet, M., Changeux, J.P., Valentino, K.L. and Hökfelt, T. (1991) Occurrence of neuropeptide K-like immunoreactivity in ventral horn cells of the chicken spinal cord during development. *Brain Res.*, 541: 149–153.

Walicke, P. and Baird, A. (1988) Trophic effects of fibroblast growth factor on neural tissue. *Progr. Brain Res.*, 78: 333–338.

Wallace, B.G., Qu, Z. and Huganir, R.L. (1991) Agrin induces phosphorylation of the nicotinic acetylcholine receptor. *Neuron*, 6: 869–78.

Wang, X.H., Iannuzzelli, P.G. and Murphy, E.H. (1993) Calcitonin gene-related peptide increases following axotomy of trochlear motoneurons. *Exp. Neurol.*, 123: 157–66.

Weill, C.L. (1991) Somatostatin (SRIF) prevents natural motoneuron cell death in embryonic chick spinal cord. *Dev. Neurosci.*, 13: 377–381.

White, S.R. (1985) A comparison of the effects of serotonin, substance P and thyrotropin-releasing hormone on excitability of rat spinal motoneurons in vivo. *Brain Res.*, 335: 63–70.

Widmer, H., Dreifuss, J.J. and Raggenbass, M. (1992) N-Methyl-D-aspartate and vasopressin activate distinct voltage-dependent inward currents in facial motoneurones. *Brain Res.*, 593: 215–220.

Wimalawamsa, S. (1992) Isolation, purification and biochemical characterization of calcitonin gene-related peptide receptors. *Ann. NY Acad. Sci.*, 657: 70–87.

Yamamoto, M. and Kondo, H. (1989) Calcitonin gene-related peptide (Cgrp)-immunoreactive nerve varicosities in synaptic contact with sensory neurons in the trigeminal ganglion of rats. *Neurosci. Lett.*, 104: 253–257.

Yamamoto, K., Senba, E., Matsunaga, T. and Tohyama, M. (1989) Calcitonin gene-related peptide containing sympathetic preganglionic and sensory neurons projecting to the superior cervical ganglion of the rat. *Brain Res.*, 487: 158–164.

Yeh, H., Ruit, K., Wang, Y., Parks, W., Snider, W. and Deuel, T. (1991) PDGF A-chain is expressed by mammalian neurons during development. *Cell*, 64: 209–216.

Zhang, X., Verge, V.M., Wiesenfeld, H.Z., Piehl, F. and Hökfelt, T. (1993a) Expression of neuropeptides and neuropeptide mRNAs in spinal cord after axotomy in the rat, with special reference to motoneurons and galanin. *Exp. Brain Res.*, 93: 450–461.

Zhang, X., Ju, G., Elde, R. and Hökfelt, T. (1993b) Effect of peripheral nerve cut on neuropeptides in dorsal root ganglia and the spinal cord of monkey with special reference to galanin. *J. Neurocytol.*, 22: 342–381.

F. Nyberg, H.S. Sharma and Z. Wiesenfeld-Hallin (Eds.)
Progress in Brain Research, Vol 104
© 1995 Elsevier Science BV. All rights reserved.

CHAPTER 2

The peptidergic innervation of spinal motoneurons via the bulbospinal 5-hydroxytryptamine pathway

S. Cullheim and U. Arvidsson

Department of Neuroscience, Doktorsringen 17, Karolinska Institutet, 171 77 Stockholm, Sweden

Introduction

The spinal motoneuron constitutes the final link between the nervous system and the skeletal muscles of the trunk and limb, and it has thus been referred to as the 'final common path' for the nervous regulation of motor activity. Large motoneurons of α type, innervating the extrafusal muscle fibers and smaller γ-motoneurons, innervating intrafusal muscle fibers of muscle spindles are intermingled in nuclei in the ventral grey matter of the spinal cord referred to as lamina IX by Rexed (1954). Morphological study of spinal α-motoneurons after intracellular staining with horseradish peroxidase (HRP) (Cullheim and Kellerth, 1976) has revealed a very extensive dendritic arbour of these neurons (Ulfhake and Kellerth, 1981; Cullheim et al., 1987), producing a total receptive area of about 0.5 mm²/cell and thus making room for 50–100 000 nerve terminals to contact a single motoneuron (Ulfhake and Cullheim, 1988). The knowledge about origin and transmitter content of the synaptic inputs to the motoneurons has remained rather limited for quite some time. In recent years, however, a considerable amount of information on transmitter-identified inputs to spinal motoneurons has been gained by use of various immunohistochemical, in situ hybridization and electrophysiological techniques. In these studies, it has become evident, that 5-hydroxytryptamine (5-HT)-containing nerve fibers constitute a major input to lamina IX of the spinal cord. Since it is now also clear, that the peptidergic innervation of the ventral horn is achieved mainly via these fibers, we will in this review concentrate on a description of the 5-HT system and coexisting peptides in the ventral spinal cord.

After the original description of the 5-hydroxytryptamine (5-HT) innervation of the rat spinal cord by Fuxe (1965), several studies have dealt with the distribution of 5-HT fibers in the cord and their origin. The general view, based on chemical and surgical manipulations, has been that 5-HT-containing fibers in all parts of the spinal cord originate from supraspinal levels, in particular the raphe nuclei in the brain stem (Fig. 1A; Carlsson et al., 1964; Dahlström and Fuxe, 1964; Clineschmidt et al., 1971; Magnusson, 1973; Stanton et al., 1975; Oliveras et al., 1977; Steinbusch, 1981; Skagerberg and Björklund, 1985; Arvidsson et al., 1990a) (see, however, below in the following section). Subsequently, a concept has emerged, which states that the bulbospinal 5-HT neurons can be subdivided into two major systems, one containing several neuropeptides with ventral projections, involved in motor control and a second, dorsally projecting one with so far no coexisting peptides described, and related to processing of sensory information (Wessendorf and Elde, 1987; Arvidsson et al., 1990a). Here we will deal with the coexistence situation in the ventral 5-HT system in some detail and will also

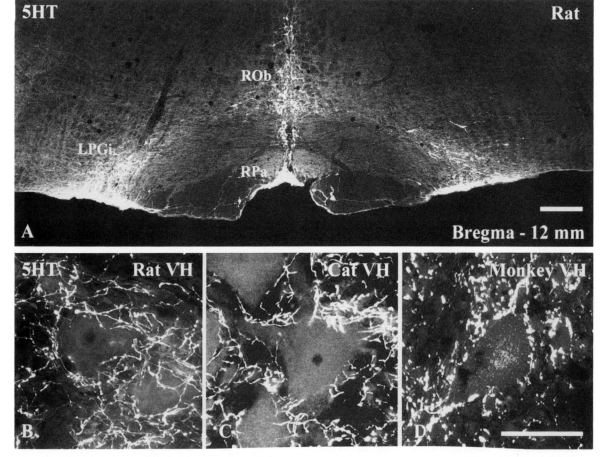

Fig. 1. Confocal microscopy images of sections from the rat brain stem (A; Bregma - 12 mm according to Paxinos and Watson, 1986) and spinal cord ventral horn (VH) from rat (B), cat (C) and monkey (D) single-stained for goat anti-serotonin (5-HT) followed by cyanine 3.18-conjugated donkey anti-goat IgG. (A) In order to visualize 5-HT neurons the animal received an injection of a MAO inhibitor and L-tryptophan. Note distribution of 5-HT-positive cell bodies in the midline raphe nuclei, nucleus raphe pallidus (RPa) and nucleus raphe obscurus (ROb), as well as in groups adjacent to the midline, e.g., lateral paragigantocellular nucleus (LPGi). The 5-HT neurons in these anatomical areas project to the motor nuclei in the spinal cord ventral horn. B–D. 5-HT immunoreactive varicosities and fibers in the motor nuclei in the spinal cord ventral horn. Note dense innervation of 5-HT around large cell bodies, presumably motoneurons, in all three species. In the monkey (D), a denser innervation is seen around the soma in comparison to both rat (B) and cat (C). Scale bars = 500 μm in A and 50 μm in D.

include some recent data on the presence of growth-related proteins in this system (coexisting substances are listed in Table 1). Possible functional consequences of this multitude of neuronal messengers in the 5-HT system will also be considered.

Distribution of 5-HT and coexisting compounds in the ventral horn of the spinal cord

5-HT

In 1965 Fuxe had already noted that the 5-HT

TABLE I

Coexistence of 5-HT and peptides, substances related to growth and trophism, peptide receptors and amino acids in the brain stem raphe nuclei and spinal cord ventral horn

Colocalization	Species	References	
		Brain stem raphe nuclei	Spinal cord ventral horn
Coexistence with peptides			
5HT/SP	Rat	Chan-Palay et al., 1978; Hökfelt et al., 1978; Johansson et al., 1981; Priestly and Cuello, 1982; Bowker et al., 1983; Sasek et al., 1990; Ozaki et al., 1992	Pelletier et al., 1981; Gilbert et al., 1982; Wessendorf and Elde, 1985, 1987; Okado et al., 1991; Sakamoto and Atsumi, 1991; Ozaki et al., 1992; Johnson et al., 1993; Wu et al., 1993
	Cat	Lovick and Hunt, 1983; Marson and Loewy, 1985; Ciriello et al., 1988; Marson, 1989; Dean et al., 1993; Arvidsson et al., 1994a	Tashiro and Ruda, 1988; Arvidsson et al., 1990a; Okado et al., 1991; Ramírez-León et al., 1994
	Monkey	—	Bowker et al., 1986b; Okada et al., 1991; Sakamoto and Atsumi, 1991; Arvidsson et al., 1992c
5HT/TRH	Rat	Johansson et al., 1991; Helke et al., 1986; Sasek et al., 1990; Kachidian et al., 1991; Johnson et al., 1993	Gilberth et al., 1982; Johnson et al., 1993; Wu et al., 1993
	Cat	Dean et al., 1993; Arvidsson et al., 1994a	Arvidsson et al., 1990a; Ramírez-León et al., 1994
	Monkey	—	Arvidsson et al., 1992c
5HT/SP/TRH	Rat	Johansson et al., 1991; Staines et al., 1988; Sasek et al., 1990; Wessendorf et al., 1990	Staines et al., 1988; Wessendorf et al., 1990; Wessendorf and Brelje 1993
	Cat	Dean et al., 1993; Arvidsson et al., 1994a	—
5HT/ENK	Rat	Millhorn et al., 1989; Sasek and Helke, 1989; Wessendorf et al., 1990; Kachidian et al., 1991; Tanaka et al., 1993	—
	Cat	Glazer et al., 1981; Hund and Lovick, 1982; Charnay et al., 1984; Lèger et al., 1986; Arvidsson et al., 1992a	Tashiro et al., 1988; Arvidsson et al., 1992a
	Monkey	—	Tashiro et al., 1990; Arvidsson et al., 1992a
5HT/GAL	Rat	Melander et al., 1986	Johnson et al., 1993
	Cat	—	Arvidsson et al., 1991a
5HT/CGRP	Monkey	Arvidsson et al., 1990c; 1991b	Arvidsson et al., 1990c
5HT/CCK	Rat	Kubota et al., 1983	—
5HT/SOM	Rat	Finley et al., 1981	—

TABLE I (*continued*)

Colocalization	Species	References	
		Brain stem raphe nuclei	Spinal cord ventral horn
Coexistence with substances related to growth and trophism			
5HT/GAP43	Rat	Kruger et al., 1993; Yao et al., 1993	Ch'ng et al., 1994
	Monkey	Arvidsson et al., 1992b	Arvidsson et al., 1992b
5HT/trkC	Monkey	—	Arvidsson et al., 1994b
5HT/bFGF	Rat	Chadi et al., 1993	—
Coexistence with peptide receptors			
5HT/δ-opioid receptor	Rat	—	Arvidsson et al., 1995
Coexistence with amino acids			
5HT/GABA	Rat	Belin et al., 1983; Millhorn et al., 1987; Kachidian et al., 1991	—
5HT?GLU	Rat	Nicholas et al., 1992	Nicholas et al., 1992
	Monkey	—	Nicholas et al., 1992

Abbreviations: 5HT, 5-hydroxytryptamine (serotonin); bFGF, basic fibroblast growth factor; CCK, cholecystokinin; CGRP, calcitonin gene-related peptide; ENK, enkephalin; GAL, galanin; GABA, γ-aminobutyric acid; GAP43, growth-associated protein-43; GLU, glutamate; SOM, somatostatin, SP, substance P; TRH, thyrotropin-releasing hormone; trkC, tyrosine kinase C.

innervation of the ventral horn is quite substantial. In fact, a quantitative analysis of this innervation in the cat has revealed that the number of 5-HT-immunoreactive (IR) varicosities, most likely representing nerve terminals, in the unilateral motor nuclei of one single spinal cord segment (L7) is $55-110 \times 10^6$ (Arvidsson et al., 1990a). The innervation density differs somewhat between different parts of the motor nuclei, however, in that the most ventral part contains 50% more 5-HT-IR varicosities than the dorsal part. This is in agreement with what has been reported qualitatively for the rat (Fuxe, 1965), chicken (Okado et al., 1988) and various other mammals (Kojima and Sano, 1983). Since motoneurons innervating proximal hind limb muscles are the most ventrally located ones in the L7 segment, it may be concluded that such motoneurons receive a denser innervation of 5-HT fibers than distal hind limb motoneurons. With respect to the distribution of 5-HT-IR nerve terminals on the receptive domains of the motoneurons, there is a distinct difference between species (see Fig. 1B–D). Thus, in the cat, 5-HT-LI is mainly observed in fibers and varicosities distributed in the neuropil, while only few IR varicosities are found in close contact with the soma and juxtasomatic domain of large cells (Arvidsson et al., 1990a). In the monkey, however, the 5-HT-IR fibers appear to almost encapsulate the large cell bodies and their proximal dendrites (Kojima and Sano, 1983; Kojima et al., 1983; Arvidsson et al., 1990c).

Substance P and thyrotropin-releasing hormone

It has been known for quite some time that the bulbospinal 5-HT system contains a number of peptides. Thus, colocalization of 5-HT and substance P (SP) was early demonstrated in the raphe nuclei of the rat (Chan-Palay et al., 1978; Hökfelt et al., 1978) and, somewhat later, the distribution patterns were found to be very similar for 5-HT, SP- and thyrotropin-releasing hormone (TRH)-IR fibers in the rat ventral horn, suggesting a possible colocalization of these compounds in the cord (Johansson et al., 1981). Further evidence for this coexistence in the rat was provided by the fact that treatment with 5,7-dihydrotryptamine leads to an almost complete disappearance of 5-HT-, SP- and TRH-LI in the ventral horn (Hökfelt et al., 1978; Johansson et al., 1981; Gilbert et al., 1982). In both cat (Arvidsson et al., 1990a) and monkey (Arvidsson et al., 1990c, 1992c), a distribution similar to that of 5-HT is encountered for both SP (Fig. 3C,D) and TRH. In the cat, the estimated number of SP-IR varicosities in the unilateral L7 motor nucleus is $55-110 \times 10^6$, i.e., the same number as found for 5-HT-IR varicosities, while the corresponding figure for TRH-IR

varicosities is $45-90 \times 10^6$ (Arvidsson et al., 1990a). In the ventral quadrants of the cat spinal cord, the amount of SP and TRH has been estimated with biochemical methods to be about 3–5 and 0.2–0.4 ng/mg protein, respectively (Arvidsson et al., 1990a). Combining these data gives a concentration of SP and TRH in IR varicosities of about 0.3–0.6 and 0.1–0.2 mM, respectively.

From the high degree of coexistence noted in the cat motor nuclei for 5-HT, SP and TRH, it can be calculated that at least 70% of the 5-HT-IR varicosities should also contain both SP-and TRH-LI. A difference between SP and TRH in relation to 5-HT seems to be at hand in the cat, however, in that all TRH-IR fibers in the motor nuclei seem to be part of the 5-HT system, while a distinct population (about 10% of total) of SP-IR fibers is not immunoreactive to 5-HT (Arvidsson et al., 1990a). In this context, it should be mentioned that, with triple-labelling proce-

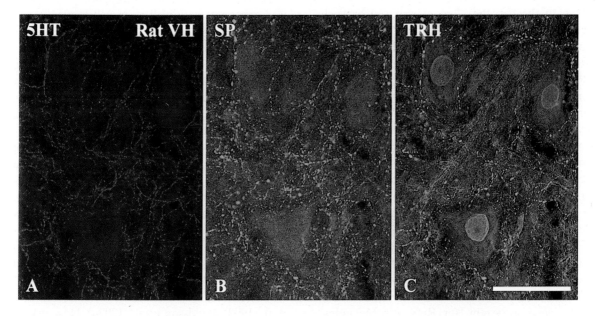

Fig. 2. Confocal microscopy images of sections from the rat lumbar spinal cord ventral horn (rat VH) triple stained for goat anti-serotonin (5-HT) (A), rat anti-substance P (B) and rabbit anti-preprothyrotropin-releasing hormone[160–169] (a marker for thyrotropin-releasing hormone (TRH)) (C) followed by lissamine rhodamine-conjugated donkey anti-goat IgG, fluorescein-conjugated donkey anti-rabbit IgG and cyanine 5.18-conjugated donkey anti-rat IgG (pseudocolored blue from deep red). All three compounds can be seen in varicosities in the neuropil of the ventral horn. Note varicosities and fibers that contain immunoreactivity for all three substances. Arrows in A–C are pointing to a triple-labelled fiber close to a large cell body. Scale bar = 50 μm.

dures, it has been shown that 5-HT-, SP- and TRH-LI coexist to a high degree in one and the same nerve fiber in the ventral horn (Staines et al., 1988; Wessendorf et al., 1990) (see also Fig. 2A–C).

The high degree of coexistence of 5-HT-, SP- and TRH-LI in the ventral horn should mean that the ultrastructural features of IR nerve terminals are very much alike, and fine structure analysis in the cat has confirmed this (Ulfhake et al., 1987). Thus, 5-HT-, SP- and TRH-IR terminals all contain small, pleomorphic agranular vesicles, as well as large vesicles with a dense core. Two subtypes of IR terminals can be distinguished, however, one with a large number of dense core vesicles, and another with only few such vesicles. According to analysis of vesicle contents in various preparations, the studied terminals should harbour 5-HT in both types of vesicle, while the peptides are confined to the large, dense core type (Hökfelt, 1968; Lundberg et al., 1981; Pelletier et al.,, 1981; Fried et al., 1985). In the cat, the element apposed by such terminals is almost always a dendrite. In the monkey ventral horn, ultrastructural analysis of SP-IR (de Lanerolle and Lamotte, 1982) and TRH-IR material (Arvidsson et al., 1992c) has demonstrated immunoreactive nerve terminals in contact with both dendrites of variable size and cell bodies. Also, in the monkey, contacts lacking synaptic specializations are encountered. In common for both cat and monkey is the peripheral localization of large dense core vesicles in labelled terminals.

Galanin

Galanin (GAL), a 29-amino acid peptide originally isolated from porcine intestine (Tatemoto et al., 1983), has been found with a wide distribution in the nervous system (for Refs. see Melander, 1986a), including the spinal cord (Rökaeus et al., 1984; Ch'ng et al., 1985; Skofitsch and Jacobowitz, 1985b; Melander et al., 1986a; Ju et al., 1987a,b; Tuchscherer and Seybold, 1989). In these reports, which are primarily based on findings in the rat,

no or only a few GAL-IR fibers are found in the spinal motor nuclei. However, in the aged rat a dense innervation of GAL-IR fibers is seen in the neuropil around the motoneuron (Johnson et al., 1993). In the cat, there seems to be a relatively dense network of GAL-IR fibers and varicosities in the spinal motor nuclei (Fig. 3A,B; Arvidsson et al., 1991a). Morerover, such fibers in both the aged rat and cat are to a large extent found to co-contain 5-HT-LI. In the cat, 90–95% of the GAL-IR fibers in this area are immunoreactive also to 5-HT, while 60–80% of the 5-HT-IR fibers contain GAL-LI. At the ultrastructural level, GAL-IR boutons containing small spherical vesicles and large dense core vesicles make synaptic or non-synaptic contacts with dendrites in the cat motor nuclei (Arvidsson et al., 1991a).

Enkephalin

The pentapeptide enkephalin (ENK) has been described in nerve fibers throughout the spinal cord grey matter as well as in cell bodies in the dorsal horn and around the central canal (for Refs. see Björklund and Hökfelt, 1988). The density of ENK-IR fibers has been reported to be rather low in somatic spinal motor nuclei, while a much denser innervation has been found in Onuf's nucleus (Finley et al., 1981; Cruz and Basbaum, 1985; Ramírez-León et al., 1994). The same relation between motor nuclei has been found in both cat and monkey, but in the cat there seems to be a somewhat denser general innervation of ENK-IR fibers (Arvidsson et al., 1992a). Sections from the cat processed for both ENK and 5-HT has revealed scattered fibers harboring both compounds (roughly 5% of the 5-HT containing fibers) in the motor nuclei (Tashiro et al., 1988; Arvidsson et al., 1992a). A similar low degree of coexistence has been encountered also in the monkey (Tashiro et al., 1990; Arvidsson et al., 1992a). However, in the monkey, some medium-sized cell bodies in the periphery of the motor nucleus are almost encapsulated by ENK-IR fibers, which invariably contain 5-HT-LI (Arvidsson et al., 1992a). So far, there is no evidence available for a coexistence of

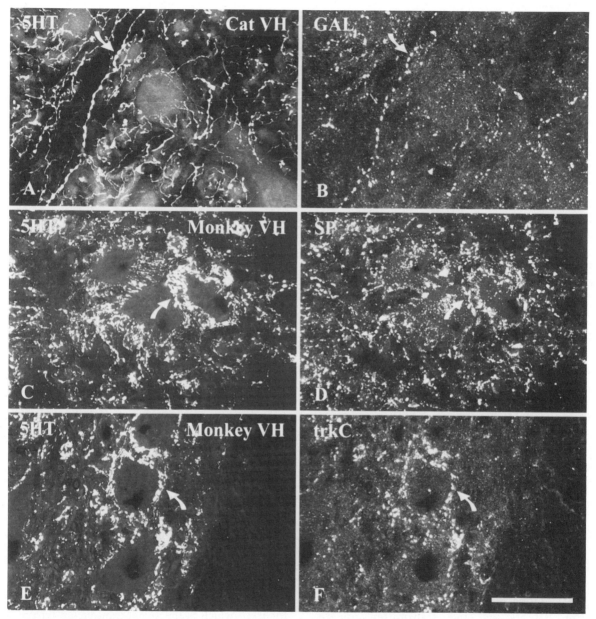

Fig. 3. Examples of compounds coexisting with 5-HT immunopositive terminals in cat and monkey spinal cord ventral horn (VH). Confocal microscopy images of sections from the cat (A,B) and monkey (C–F) double-stained for goat anti-serotonin (5-HT; A,C,E) and rabbit anti-galanin (B) or rat anti-substance P (D) or rabbit anti-trkC (F) followed by lissamine rhodamine-conjugated donkey anti-goat IgG and fluorescein-conjugated donkey anti-rat IgG or lissamine rhodamine-conjugated donkey anti-goat IgG and fluorescein-conjugated donkey anti-rabbit IgG. A,B. Note presence of galanin-like immunoreactivity in 5-HT-positive fibers in the cat spinal cord motor nucleus (arrow). C–F. In the monkey, substance P is present in some 5-HT terminals (arrow). However, there is also a subset of substance P fibers lacking 5-HT and 5-HT fibers lacking substance P. E,F. The coexistence with the neurotrophin receptor trkC is demonstrated (see arrow; trkC is the receptor for neurotrophin-3). Scale bar = 50 μm.

5-HT and ENK in the rat spinal cord ventral horn.

Calcitonin gene-related peptide

Calcitonin gene-related peptide (CGRP) (Amara et al., 1982; Rosenfeld et al., 1983), a 37-amino acid peptide synthesized from the calcitonin gene by alternative processing of the primary transcript, is yet another neuropeptide, which is widely distributed in the CNS and PNS (Rosenfeld et al., 1983; Gibson et al., 1984; Skofitch and Jacobowitz, 1985a,c; Kruger et al., 1988). In the spinal cord ventral horn, this peptide has primarily been associated with motoneurons, which normally harbor CGRP (Rosenfeld et al., 1983). It has been shown, that the CGRP levels in motoneurons are sensitive to experimental perturbations, such as axotomy and deafferentation (Arvidsson et al., 1989, 1990b; Moore, 1989; Streit et al., 1989; Piehl et al., 1991; for further Refs. see Arvidsson et al., 1993). In the monkey, but not in other species studied so far, there is in addition a dense CGRP-IR innervation of the motor nuclei (Arvidsson et al., 1990c, 1991b). Thus, CGRP-IR fibers and varicosities are seen in close apposition to the large cell bodies in a pattern similar to what has been described for 5-HT, SP and TRH. Double-labelling experiments have indeed revealed a high degree of coexistence of 5-HT- and CGRP-LI (Arvidsson et al., 1990c)

Growth-associated protein-43

The growth-associated protein (GAP)-43 is a phosphoprotein proposed to be involved in axonal growth during development, regeneration, long-term potentiation and transmitter release (Lovinger et al., 1986; Benowitz et al., 1988; Dekker et al., 1989; Skene, 1989). A role for GAP-43 in the monoaminergic system has been suggested from the findings of Bendotti et al. (1991), who demonstrated mRNA coding for GAP-43 in the dorsal raphe nucleus, which harbors 5-HT-containing neurons. In the spinal cord of both monkey and cat, fibers containing GAP-

43-LI are seen in close apposition to cell bodies of motoneurons (Arvidsson et al., 1992b). In the monkey motor nuclei, a high degree of coexistence of GAP-43- and 5-HT-LI can be seen, while no such coexistence is found in the cat ventral horn, nor in other parts of the cord in either cat or monkey (Arvidsson et al., 1992b). In the rat, GAP-43 has recently been reported to be present in descending 5-HT fibers not only in the ventral horn, but also in the intermediolateral nucleus as well as in the dorsal horn (Ching et al., 1994). In situ hybridization has revealed mRNA coding for GAP-43 in neurons in the midline raphe nuclei and nucleus reticularis lateralis, which are known to harbor 5-HT-containing cells (Arvidsson et al., 1992b; Kruger et al., 1993; Yao et al., 1993). In near adjacent sections through the midline raphe nuclei, an overlap between neurons coding for GAP-43 and 5-HT has been demonstrated, as shown by use of a probe against aromatic L-amino acid decarboxylase (Arvidsson et al., 1992). These results support a role for GAP-43 in the bulbospinal pathway, at least in monkey and rat.

trkC

The neurotrophins represent a family of structurally related molecules implicated in processes involving cell differentiation, migration, survival and synapse formation in the nervous system (for Refs. see Thoenen, 1991; Korsching, 1993). The signal-transducing tyrosine kinase receptors for the neurotrophins are encoded by members of the trk family of proto-oncogenes, and three loci have hitherto been identified: trkA, trkB and trkC. In the monkey spinal cord, immunolabelling for trkC, which is the signal-transducing tyrosine kinase receptor for neurotrophin-3 (NT-3), is present in dense, intensely immunolabelled nerve fiber networks in the autonomic intermediolateral and Onuf's nuclei, while less intensely labelled fibres surround somatic motoneurons at all spinal cord levels (Arvidsson et al., 1994b). The majority of these fibers are also immunoreactive to 5-HT (see Fig. 3E,F).

Amino acid transmitter subsances

The primary scope of the present review is to deal with neuropeptides in the descending 5-HT pathway. It should be mentioned, however, that 5-HT-IR raphe neurons have been reported to be immunoreactive also for glutamate (Nicholas et al., 1992) and γ-aminobutyric acid (GABA) (Belin et al., 1983; Millhorn et al., 1987). The possibility that glutamate is a co-transmitter in the 5-HT system has gained further support in a recent in vitro study, in which postnatal rat serotonergic neurons in microculture were demonstrated to be able to evoke excitatory glutamatergic potentials in themselves or in target neurons (Johnson, 1994). Thus, the functional transmitter repertoire of the descending 5-HT pathway with projections to the ventral horn may well also include amino acid transmitter substances. The implications of this chemical complexity for motor function remain to be elucidated.

Origin of 5-HT nerve terminals in the spinal cord

As mentioned in the Introduction, the general concept regarding the origin of 5-HT fibers in the spinal cord is that it has a supraspinal location. However, there are some reports on the presence of a small number of segmental 5-HT cell bodies around the central canal and in the superficial dorsal horn in monkey (La Motte et al., 1982; Bowker, 1986a) and rat (Björklund et al., 1970; Newton and Hamill, 1988; Newton et al., 1986). A minor contribution of 5-HT nerve endings in the ventral horn from these local neurons can at present not be excluded in these species, but it is clear that the vast majority of the 5-HT nerve terminals in the cord has indeed a supraspinal origin in the raphe nuclei. With regard to the origin of the two major subdivisions of the 5-HT system, based on their contents of peptides and growth-related proteins, as well as their different projections in the cord, it has been shown that neurons in the raphe magnus nucleus project preferentially to the dorsal horn, whereas the ventral horn receives its 5-HT input from the

raphe obscurus and raphe pallidus nuclei (e.g., Skagerberg and Björklund, 1985; Holstege and Kuypers, 1987). This is then also mirrored in the distribution of peptides in 5-HT neurons, in that a large proportion of such neurons in the caudally located raphe obscurus and raphe pallidus nuclei, as shown in the cat, contain SP (Lovick and Hunt, 1983; Marson and Loewy, 1985; Ciriello et al., 1988; Marson, 1989; Dean et al., 1993; Arvidsson et al., 1994a) and TRH (Dean et al., 1993; Arvidsson et al., 1994a), while no such cells have been verified in the raphe magnus nucleus (Marson, 1989).

Lesion experiments

The different origins of peptidergic nerve terminals in the ventral versus the dorsal horn are illustrated by experiments in the cat, in which a transection of the cord was performed at the thoracic level. Thus, in the motor nuclei below the lesion, all TRH-LI disappeared, indicating a suprasegmental location of TRH-IR cell bodies (Arvidsson et al., 1990a). This is quite consistent with the total TRH/5-HT coexistence in this region. In the dorsal horn, however, the TRH-IR fiber plexus evidently originates from local neurons (cat: Ulfhake et al., 1987b; rat: Harkness and Brownfield, 1986), with no effects detectable after spinal cord transection.

In contrast to what is found for 5-HT- and TRH-LI, a substantial number of SP-IR varicosities remains in the ventral horn after a spinal cord transection (Arvidsson et al., 1990a). This is the case also after a combination of spinal cord transection and dorsal rhizotomy. These findings indicate that SP-IR fibers seen in the motor nuclei derive from sources in the spinal cord in addition to the descending 5-HT pathway. However, the remaining number of SP-IR varicosities is much higher than expected from the double-labelling experiments in unoperated animals, indicating that part of the SP-IR innervation seen after the lesion derives from sprouting local neurons. This hypothesis is supported by the demonstration of an increased number of SP-IR cell bodies in several laminae in the cord after lesion (Arvidsson et al., 1990a). In the dorsal horn, the SP-IR fiber plexus remains intact after spinal cord transection. After combining the transection with a dorsal rhizotomy the immunoreactivity decreases, but never disappears, supporting the idea that the SP fiber plexus in the dorsal horn derives from both primary afferent neurons and intrinsic neurons in the cord (Ljungdahl et al., 1978; Tessler et al., 1980, 1981, 1984; Ruda et al., 1986; see further chapters in this volume).

With regard to the neuropeptide in the ventral 5-HT system that seems to be particularly abundant in the cat (i.e., GAL), a spinal cord transection in this species totally abolishes the GAL-IR staining in the ventral horn, in parallel with what is found for 5-HT and TRH (Arvidsson et al., 1991a). In the dorsal horn no alteration of the staining pattern for GAL is detected, indicating that there are no GAL projections from supraspinal levels in this region of the cord.

Also, the ENK-LI in the cat motor nuclei is affected by a spinal cord transection, in that there is a definite decrease in staining for ENK-LI, indicating that also part of this innervation derives from supraspinal levels (Arvidsson et al., 1992a). However, as mentioned above, ENK does not seem to be as closely related to 5-HT as SP, TRH and GAL in the ventral horn and possible supraspinal sources for ENK other than the 5-HT system should be considered. In fact, an alternative explanation for the described effects of the transection could be a down-regulation in a local ENK spinal system as a result of deafferentation. In the dorsal horn, no effects on the ENK-LI are induced by this lesion.

Brain stem studies

The strong link between the presence of neuropeptides and 5-HT in the ventral horn of the spinal cord suggested by the studies of coexistence patterns in the cord and the lesion experiments mentioned above, is further strengthened in brain stem studies. Thus, early immunohistochemical studies have revealed that 5-HT neurons may also contain SP (Chan-Palay et al., 1978; Hökfelt et al., 1978), TRH (Johansson et al., 1981), ENK (Glazer et el., 1981) and GAL (Melander et al., 1986). In addition, somatostatin-IR (Finley et al., 1981) and cholecystokinin (CCK)-IR (Kubota et al., 1983) cell bodies have been demonstrated in the medullary raphe nuclei, but in these cases no coexistence has been established. Later, it has been demonstrated that one and the same neuronal cell body in midline raphe nuclei could stain for 5-HT as well as the two peptides SP and TRH (Johansson et al., 1981; Staines et al., 1988; Sasek et al., 1990; Wessendorf et al., 1990; Dean et al., 1993; Arvidsson et al., 1994a). When comparing different nuclei harbouring 5-HT cell bodies, studies in colchicine-treated rats (Johansson et al., 1981) have shown that, in nucleus raphe magnus (NRM) and nucleus raphe obscurus (NRO), the number of neurons containing 5-HT is twice as many as those containing SP or TRH, whereas in nucleus raphe pallidus (NRP), there is a more even distribution of the three neuroactive compounds. In the colchicine-treated cat, a large part (45–90%) of the 5-HT-IR cells in the caudal raphe nuclei and the lateral reticular nucleus is also immunoreactive to SP and/or TRH (Arvidsson et al., 1994a), with a tendency for a lower degree of coexistence in the more rostral raphe nuclei.

Also, after colchicine treatment in cats, numerous ENK-IR neurons are detectable in the raphe nuclei and NRL, with the highest density of positive cells found in NRP and NRO (Glazer et al., 1981; Hunt and Lovick, 1982; Charney et al., 1984; Lèger et al., 1986; Millhorn et al., 1989; Arvidsson et al., 1992a). Furthermore, cell bodies in the raphe nuclei or NRL may stain for both ENK and 5-HT, and quantitative studies on this co-localization (Hunt and Lovick, 1982) have shown that 38–63% of the neurons in NRM and NRP harbour immunoreactivity for both compounds. These results are somewhat surprising, in light of the relatively low degree (5%) of coexistence between 5-HT- and ENK-LI found in nerve fibers in the spinal cord (Arvidsson et al., 1992a). There are several possible reasons for this apparent discrepancy between cell bodies and nerve terminals. One is that ENK is transported anterogradely only to a limited extent in 5-HT neurons, or that the transported amounts are in general too low for detection in the fibers. An alternative, but less plausible explanation would be that the studied cells in the brain stem do not project to the cord. Lastly, and more speculatively, 5-HT and ENK may be routed differentially into subsets of axonal arborizations in the cord.

Yet another possible explanation for the different co-localization patterns of 5-HT and ENK in the brain stem and the spinal cord is linked with the colchicine pretreatment of the studied animals. Thus, in non-colchicine-treated animals, few or no ENK-IR cell bodies are encountered in the brain stem (Arvidsson et al., 1992a). The ENK-LI seen in raphe neurons after colchicine treatment can then be a result of a colchicine-induced increase of ENK mRNA synthesis, with a subsequent accumulation of ENK peptide, thus representing a peptide that is normally not found in these cells or is only encountered in low amounts. In this context, one should also consider the possibility that ENK levels are particularly sensitive to experimental perturbations of the motor system. This is suggested by the finding that, after a ventral funiculus lesion in the cord, accomplishing a central axotomy of motoneurons, ENK-LI is increased in the lesioned motor nuclei, in contrast to all other neuroactive substances examined (Lindå et al., 1990). In this context it is also of interest that δ-opioid receptor-LI is present on 5-HT terminals apposing motoneurons, implicating that ENK, which is the endogenous ligand for the δ-opioid receptor may modulate the release of 5-HT and coexisting peptides from these fibers (Arvidsson et al., 1995).

The problem with the use of colchicine treatment for detection of neuroactive peptides is further exemplified with the search for GAL in 5-HT cell bodies. Thus, it has been shown that midline raphe neurons in the rat normally express low or undetectable levels of GAL mRNA (Cortés et al., 1990). After colchicine treatment, GAL mRNA expression increases in these neurons, indicating

an influence on GAL synthesis in raphe neurons by colchicine. In the cat, GAL-LI has been demonstrated without colchicine treatment (Arvidsson et al., 1991a), and should therefore not be artifactually induced. With the technique used (peroxidase-antiperoxidase; PAP) in the latter study, direct coexistence between GAL and 5-HT in raphe neurons could not be verified, even if the very high degree of coexistence between these compounds in nerve fibers in the motor nuclei supports this indirectly. In the monkey, there is also evidence for a colocalization between 5-HT and GAL in the bulbospinal system (Arvidsson et al., unpublished data).

Using PAP and in situ hybridization techniques, neurons containing CGRP peptide and mRNA encoding CGRP can be demonstrated in NRP, NRO, NRM and NRL of the monkey (Arvidsson et al., 1990c, 1991b). The highest density of CGRP-IR cell bodies is found in NRP and NRO. From adjacent sections it is possible to demonstrate the presence of both preprotachykinin (PPT) mRNA and CGRP mRNA in one and the same midline raphe neuron suggesting coexistence of SP and CGRP (Arvidsson et al., 1990c), thereby in turn also indicating coexistence of 5-HT and CGRP.

With regard to the presence of substances related to axon growth and plasticity (GAP-43 and trkC) in the 5-HT system, suggested from studies of the spinal cord (Arvidsson et al., 1992b, 1994b; Kruger et al., 1993; Yao et al., 1993), brain stem studies have provided further support for this possibility. Thus, cell bodies expressing mRNA encoding for GAP-43 (Arvidsson et al., 1992b; Kruger et al., 1993; Yao et al., 1993) and trkC (Tessarollo et al., 1993; Arvidsson et al., unpublished data) have been demonstrated in the medullary midline raphe nuclei.

Functional aspects on the innervation of motoneurons by 5-HT and coexisting compounds

It is obvious from the foregoing presentation, that those nerve terminals of the descending 5-HT system, which impinge on the motoneuron also contain several peptides and substances related to plasticity. Moreover, it is also clear that the vast majority of peptide-containing nerve terminals in the motor nuclei originate from the 5-HT system. A discussion of possible peptidergic effects on spinal motoneurons must then necessarily also consider any effects of 5-HT.

5-HT

5-HT has been reported to have excitatory effects on motoneuron activity (Barasi and Robert, 1974; Myslinsky and Anderson, 1978; Roberts and Wright, 1978; McCall and Aghajanian, 1979; Parry and Roberts, 1980; White and Neuman, 1980, 1983; Bell and Matsumiya, 1981; VanderMaelen and Aghajanian, 1982; Clarke et al., 1985; White, 1985; Holtman et al., 1986; Van Dongen et al., 1986). Since iontophoresis of 5-HT does not by itself excite motoneurons, but dramatically potentiates the action of excitatory amino acids (McCall and Aghajanian, 1979; VanderMaelen and Aghajanian, 1982; White and Neuman, 1980, 1983), a 'gain-setting' role has been proposed for the descending 5-HT innervation of motoneurons. 5-HT would then regulate the amplification of synaptic excitation (McCall and Aghajanian, 1979; Kuypers and Huisman, 1982; VanderMaelen and Aghajanian, 1982). The recent findings that 5-HT-IR neurons may also be immunoreactive for glutamate (Nicholas et al., 1992), and that glutamate may be co-released with 5-HT in such neurons (Johnson, 1994) raise the possibility that the 5-HT system exerts powerful excitatory effects on the motoneurons by its own repertoire of transmitters.

Studies in the unanesthetized decerebrate cat (Crone et al., 1988; Hounsgaard et al., 1988) have provided further insight into possible mechanisms for such actions of 5-HT in mammalian spinal motoneurons. Thus, by use of intracellular microelectrodes, it has been shown that short-lasting depolarizing current pulses can induce plateau potentials in the motoneurons, which trigger a self-sustained firing of these cells. This firing can then be terminated by hyperpolarizing current

pulses. The two levels of excitability have been referred to as 'bistable' behaviour of the motoneurons. It has been suggested that the plateau potential is due to a voltage-dependent non-inactivating Ca^{2+}-conductance, induced by activity in the descending 5-HT pathway (Hounsgaard et al., 1988). Such a mechanism may be of value in the control of posture by maintaining tonic activity with a minimum of ongoing synaptic excitation (Conway et al., 1988). The 'gain-setting' by the 5-HT system may also provide a motivational drive in the excitation of movements (Kuypers and Huisman, 1982). One may further speculate that the 'bistable' behaviour may be of relevance for alternating motoneuron activity during locomotion. Membrane potential oscillations in motoneurons would then, in an alternating manner, trigger 'on' and 'off' responses with regard to the plateau potential, thereby increasing the firing frequency during the active phase.

With the approach of studying the electrophysiological activity of 5-HT neurons in cats exposed to a variety of behavioural, environmental and physiological conditions, a more general hypothesis regarding 5-HT and motor control has been developed (Jacobs and Fornal, 1993). Thus, since there is an increased activity of 5-HT neurons in the brain in association with motor outputs, such as increased muscle tone and responses mediated by central pattern generators, the primary functions of the 5-HT system may be to facilitate motor output and simultaneously suppress sensory processing that might disrupt this output.

It has also been proposed that the descending 5-HT system imposes developmental changes on the spinal network that controls locomotion (Sillar, 1994). For example, pharmacological deletion of serotonergic fibres near the time of hatching causes a significant reduction in non-serotonergic axo-somatic synapses on spinal motoneurons (Okado et al., 1992). A similar finding was obtained in adults, suggesting that 5-HT may sustain synaptic connectivity in mature animals, in addition to controlling the development of spinal synaptic connections. Moreover, physiological data suggest that the transition from a simple embryonic motor pattern to a more flexible adult-like form is linked to the ingrowth of descending 5-HT fibers in the spinal cord (Sillar, 1994).

Peptides and growth-related substances

With this background information regarding the effects of the 5-HT system on motoneurons, what is the role for accompanying neuropeptides and growth-related substances? It has been questioned, whether these peptides are of functional significance, or represent a class of molecules which have served as transmitter substances during early evolution, but later have been replaced by other transmitters, leaving the peptides as remnants from the past (see, e.g., Hökfelt et al., 1987; Hökfelt, 1991). However, in light of the precise colocalization patterns in the 5-HT system and also the distinct differences in peptide contents between species, it is difficult to see that these patterns represent non-significant remnants of evolutionary processes. Moreover, it seems unlikely that 5-HT neurons would pay the high metabolic price of producing substances in the cell body and transport them to the nerve terminals with no evidence for a reuptake after release, if these substances were of no functional significance.

As mentioned above, 5-HT by itself seems to have an excitatory action on motoneurons. This effect may be enhanced by synergistic actions of TRH and SP. Thus, evidence has been provided that SP may block the inhibitory 5-HT autoreceptor, and thereby increase the transmission at 5-HT/SP synapses (Mitchell and Fleetwood-Walker, 1981). Also, it has been suggested that the release of transmitter substances is dependent on the frequency and/or firing pattern of nerve impulse activity (Lundberg and Hökfelt, 1983; Hökfelt et al., 1987; Iverfeldt et al., 1989). It may then be possible that, at a low firing frequency, only 5-HT is released from small, agranular synaptic vesicles while, at high frequencies, in addition to 5-HT, peptides are also released from the large dense-cored vesicles. It should be noted,

however, that the peptide content of 5-HT terminals on cat motoneurons does not necessarily exert an excitatory action. Thus, in several systems, GAL has been found to have an action of inhibitory nature, for example in antagonizing the facilitory effect of SP on the nociceptive flexor reflex in the rat (Xu et al., 1990). Any corresponding effects on the motoneuron obviously make the peptidergic actions in the 5-HT system even more complex. With regard to the CGRP content of 5-HT terminals in the monkey, any effects of this peptide on motoneuron excitability remain to be elucidated.

Another putative function for neuropeptides is linked with the ability of neurons to alter their functional properties in response to intracellular biochemical changes, which in turn are induced by synaptic or hormonal actions on the neurons. Such neuromodulatory effects may allow the neurons to adapt to a changing environment on a long-term basis. In this context, it is of interest that the response of the 5-HT system with its battery of peptides differs significantly from that of amino acid-containing nerve terminals in the motor nuclei, following a cut lesion in the ventral funiculus, which accomplishes a central axotomy of motoneurons (Risling et al., 1983). In this situation, the innervation of 5-HT and accompanying peptides seems virtually unchanged with even an increase of ENK-LI (Lindå et al., 1990), while nerve terminals containing amino acid immunoreactivity are clearly diminished in number (Lindå et al., in preparation). Furthermore, in the monkey not only peptides, but also GAP-43 and trkC, seem to be present in 5-HT nerve terminals on spinal motoneurons. The presence of GAP-43 in neurons has been related to plastic events, such as development and regeneration (e.g., Skene, 1989), as well as long-term potentiation amd memory function (Nelson and Routtenberg, 1985; Lovinger et al., 1986), and trkC is the signal-transducing tyrosine kinase receptor for at least one member of the neurotrophin family, i.e., neurotrophin-3. It may, therefore, be speculated that the 5-HT system in the monkey in some way takes part in a 'motor memory' involving plastic changes of the motoneurons. That such changes may indeed occur is supported by recent findings in studies of the monosynaptic stretch reflex in the monkey spinal cord. Even this simple reflex can be operantly conditioned, and the 'memory traces' responsible for the change in behaviour seem to be located at the level of the Ia afferent terminal and/or the motoneuron itself (Wolpaw and Carp, 1990). Whether the 5-HT system with its transmitter complexity in the ventral horn takes part in this type of long-term changes of motoneuron properties remains to be elucidated.

Concluding remarks

The organisation of the peptidergic innervation of the spinal cord differs significantly between the ventral and dorsal horns, in that the ventral horn, in particular the motor nuclei, receives its major peptidergic input via the bulbospinal 5-HT pathway, while the dorsal horn, in particular the superficial part, is innervated by peptidergic nerve terminals preferentially via primary afferent fibers and local dorsal horn neurons. 5-HT fibers with a dorsal projection do not seem to harbour any known neuropeptide. The demonstrated multitude of coexisting neuropeptides and growth-related substances in 5-HT terminals in the motor nuclei suggests an action of this system, which is more complex than that which can be inferred from 5-HT effects only. One may speculate, that such an action is related to motor plasticity at the spinal cord level, involving also the spinal motoneuron. The demonstrated species differences in contents of neuropeptides and growth-related substances in the 5-HT system may then reflect different potentials for this system to exert an influence related to plasticity. It will be necessary to make use of a variety of in vivo and in vitro techniques to explore these possibilities.

References

Amara, S.G., Jonas, V., Rosenfeld, M.G., Ong, E.S. and Evans, R.M. (1982) Alternative RNA processing in calcitonin gene expression generates mRNAs encoding different polypeptide products. *Nature*, 298: 240–244.

Arvidsson, U., Cullheim, S., Ulfhake, B., Hökfelt, T. and Terenius, L. (1989) Altered levels of calcitonin gene-related peptide (CGRP)-like immunoreactivity of cat lumbar motoneurons after chronic spinal cord transection. *Brain Res.*, 489: 387–391.

Arvidsson, U., Cullheim, S., Ulfhake, B., Bennett, G.W., Fone, K.C.F., Cuello, A.C., Verhofstad, A.A.J., Visser, T.J. and Hökfelt, T. (1990a) 5-Hydroxytryptamine, substance P and thyrotropin-releasing hormone in the adult cat spinal cord segment L7: immunohistochemical and chemical studies. *Synapse*, 6: 237–270.

Arvidsson, U., Johnson, H., Piehl, F., Cullheim, S., Hökfelt, T., Risling, M., Terenius, L. and Ulfhake, B. (1990b) Peripheral nerve section induces increased levels of calcitonin gene-related peptide (CGRP)-like immunoreactivity in axotomized motoneurons. *Exp. Brain Res.*, 79: 212–216.

Arvidsson, U., Schalling, M., Cullheim, S., Ulfhake, B., Terenius, L., Verhofstad, A. and Hökfelt, T. (1990c) Evidence for coexistence between calcitonin gene-related peptide and serotonin in the bulbospinal pathway in the monkey. *Brain Res.*, 532: 47–57.

Arvidsson, U., Ulfhake, B., Cullheim, S., Hökfelt, T. and Theodorsson, E. (1991a) Distribution of ^{125}I-galanin binding sites, immunoreactive galanin and its coexistence with 5-hydroxytryptamine in the cat spinal cord: biochemical, histochemical and experimental studies at the light and electron microscopic level. *J. Comp. Neurol.*, 308: 115–138.

Arvidsson, U., Ulfhake, B., Cullheim, S., Terenius, L. and Hökfelt, T. (1991b) Calcitonin gene-related peptide in monkey spinal cord and medulla oblongata. *Brain Res.*, 558: 330–334.

Arvidsson, U., Cullheim, S., Ulfhake, B., Ramirez, V., Dagerlind, A., Luppi, P.H., Kitahama, K., Jouvet, M., Terenius, L., Åman, K. and Hökfelt, T. (1992a) Distribution of enkephalin and its relation to serotonin in cat and monkey spinal cord and brain stem. *Synapse*, 11: 85–104.

Arvidsson, U., Risling, M., Cullheim, S., Dagerlind, Å., Lindå, H., Shupliakov, O., Ulfhake, B. and Hökfelt, T. (1992b) On the distribution of GAP-43 and its relation to serotonin in adult monkey and cat spinal cord and lower brainstem. *Eur. J. Neurosci.*, 4: 777–784.

Arvidsson, U., Ulfhake, B., Cullheim, S., Shupliakov, O., Brodin, E., Franck, J., Bennett, G.W., Fone, K.C., Visser, T.J. and Hökfelt, T. (1992c) Thyrotropin-releasing hormone (TRH)-like immunoreactivity in the grey monkey (*Macaca fascicularis*) spinal cord and medulla oblongata with special emphasis on the bulbospinal tract. *J. Comp. Neurol.*, 322: 293–310.

Arvidsson, U., Piehl, F., Johnson, H., Ulfhake, B., Cullheim, S. and Hökfelt, T. (1993) The peptidergic motoneurone. *NeuroReport*, 4: 849–856.

Arvidsson, U., Cullheim, S., Ulfhake, B., Luppi, P.-H., Kitahama, K., Jouvet, M. and Hökfelt, T. (1994a) Quantitative and qualitative aspects on the distribution of 5-HT and its coexistence with substance P and TRH in cat ventral medullary neurons. *J. Chem. Neuroanat.*, 7: 3–12.

Arvidsson, U., Dado, R.J., Law, P.Y., Loh, H.H., Elde, R. and Wessendorf, M.W. (1995) Immunohistochemical localization of delta-opioid receptor: relationship to biogenic amines and enkephalin in brain stem and spinal cord. *J Neurosci.*, in press.

Arvidsson, U., Risling, M., Frisén, J., Piehl, F., Fried, K., Hökfelt, T. and Cullheim, S. (1994b) trkC-like immunoreactivity in the primate descending serotoninergic system. *Eur. J. Neurosci.*, 6: 230–236.

Barasi, S. and Robert, M.H.T. (1974) The modification of lumbar motoneurone excitability by stimulation of a putative 5HT pathway. *Br. J. Pharmacol..*, 52: 339–348.

Belin, M.F., Nanopoulos, D., Didier, M., Aguera, M., Steinbusch, H., Verhofstad, A., Maitre, M. and Pujol, J.-F. (1983) Immunohistochemical evidence for the presence of gamma-aminobutyric acid and serotonin in one nerve cell. A study on the raphe nuclei of the rat using antibodies to glutamate decarboxylase and serotonin. *Brain Res.*, 275: 329–339.

Bell, J.A. and Matsumiya, T. (1981) Inhibitory effects of dorsal horn and excitant effects of ventral horn intraspinal microinjections of norepinephrine and serotonin in the cat. *Life Sci.*, 29: 1507–1514.

Bendotti, C., Servadio, A. and Samanin, R. (1991) Distribution of GAP-43 mRNA in the brain stem of adult rats as evidenced by in situ hybridization: localization within monoaminergic neurons. *J. Neurosci.*, 11: 600–607.

Benowitz, L.I., Apostolides, P.J., Perrone-Bizzozero, N.I., Finklestein, S.P. and Zwiers, H. (1988) Anatomical distribution of the growth-associated proteins GAP-43/B-50 in the adult rat brain. *J. Neurosci.*, 8: 339–352.

Björklund, A. and Hökfelt, T. (1988) Handbook of chemical neuroanatomy. In: A. Björklund, T. Hökfelt and C. Owman (Eds.), *The Peripheral Nervous System*, Elsevier, Amsterdam, New York.

Björklund, A., Falck, B. and Stenevi, V. (1970) On the possible existence of a new intraneuronal monoamine in the spinal cord of the rat. *J. Pharmacol. Exp. Ther.*, 175: 525–532.

Bowker, R.M. (1986a) Intrinsic 5HT-immunoreactive neurons in the spinal cord of the fetal non-human primate. *Dev. Brain Res.*, 28: 137–143.

Bowker, R.M. (1986b) Serotonergic and peptidergic inputs to the primate ventral spinal cord as visualized with multiple chromagens on the same tissue section. *Brain Res.*, 375: 345–350.

Bowker, R.M., Westlund, K.N., Sullivan, M.C., Wilber, J.F. and Coulter, J.D. (1983) Descending serotonergic, peptidergic and cholinergic pathways from the raphe nuclei: a multiple transmitter complex. *Brain Res.*, 288: 33–48.

Carlsson, A., Falck, B., Fuxe, K. and Hillarp, N. Å. (1964) Cellular localization of monoamines in the spinal cord. *Acta Physiol. Scand.*, 60: 112–119.

Ch'ng, J.L.C., Christofides, N.D., Anand, P., Gibson, S.J., Allen, Y.S., Su, H.C., Tatemoto, K., Morrison, J.F.B., Polak, J.M. and Bloom, S.R. (1985) Distribution of galanin immunoreactivity in the central nervous system and responses of galanin-containing neuronal pathways to injury. *Neuroscience*, 16: 343–354.

Chadi, G., Tinner, B., Agnati, L.F. and Fuxe, K. (1993) Basic fibroblast growth factor (bFGF, FGF-2) immunoreactivity exists in the noradrenaline, adrenaline and 5-HT nerve cells of the rat brain. *Neurosci. Lett.*, 160: 171–176.

Chan-Palay, V., Jonsson, G. and Palay, S.L. (1978) Serotonin and substance P coexist in neurons of the rat's central nervous system. *Proc. Natl. Acad. Sci. USA*, 75: 1582–1586.

Charnay, Y., Paulin, C., Dray, F. and Dubois, P.M. (1984) Distribution of enkephalin in human fetus and infant spinal cord: an immunofluorescence study. *J. Comp. Neurol.*, 223: 415–423.

Ching, Y.P., Averill, S., Wilkin, G.P., Wotherspoon, G. and Priestly, J.V. (1994) Serotoninergic terminals express a growth associated (GAP-43) in the adult rat spinal cord. *Neurosci. Lett.*, 167: 67–72.

Ciriello, J., Caverson, M.M., Calaresu, F.R. and Krukoff, T.L. (1988) Neuropeptide and serotonin immunoreactive neurons in the cat ventrolateral medulla. *Brain Res.*, 440: 53–66.

Clarke, K.A., Parker, A.J. and Stirk, G.C. (1985) Potentiation of motoneurone excitability by combined administration of 5-HT agonist and TRH analogue. *Neuropeptides*, 6: 269–282.

Clineschmidt, B.V., Pierce, J.E. and Lovenberg, W. (1971) Tryptophan hydroxylase and serotonin in spinal cord and brain after chronic transection. *J. Neurochem.*, 18: 1593–1596.

Conway, B.A., Hultborn, H., Kiehn, O. and Minty, I. (1988) Plateau potentials in alpha-motoneurones induced by intravenous injection of L-DOPA and clonidine in the spinal cat. *J. Physiol.*, 405: 369–384.

Cortés, R., Ceccatelli, S., Schalling, M. and Hökfelt, T. (1990) Differential effects of intraventricular colchicine administration on the expression of mRNAs for neuropeptides and neurotransmitter enzymes, with special emphasis on galanin: an in situ hybridization study. *Synapse*, 6: 369–391.

Crone, C., Hultborn, H., Kiehn, O., Mazieres, L. and Wigström, H. (1988) Maintained changes in motoneuronal excitability by short-lasting inputs in the decerebrate cat. *J. Physiol.*, 405: 321–343.

Cruz, L. and Basbaum, A.I. (1985) Multiple opioid peptides and the modulation of pain: Immunohistochemical analysis of dynorphin and enkephalin in the trigeminal nucleus caudalis and spinal cord of the cat. *J. Comp. Neurol.*, 240: 331–348.

Cullheim, S. and Kellerth, J.-O. (1976) Combined light and electron microscopic tracing of neurons, including axons

36

and synaptic terminals, after intracellular injection of horseradish peroxidase. *Neurosci. Lett.*, 2: 307–313.

Cullheim, S. Fleshman, J.W., Glenn, L.L. and Burke, R. (1987) Membrane area and dendritic structure in type-identified triceps surae alpha-motoneurons. *J. Comp. Neurol.*, 255: 68–81.

Dahlström, A. and Fuxe, K. (1964) Evidence for the existence of monoamine neurons in the central nervous system. I. Demonstration of monoamines in cell bodies of brain stem neurons. *Acta Physiol. Scand.*, 62: 1–55.

Dean, C., Marson, L. and Kampine, J.P. (1993) Distribution and co-localization of 5-hydroxytryptamine, thyrotropin-releasing hormone and substance P in the cat medulla. *Neuroscience*, 57: 811–822.

De Lanerolle, N.C. and LaMotte, C.C. (1982) The morphological relationships between substance P immunoreactive processes and ventral horn neurons in the human and monkey spinal cord. *J. Comp. Neurol.*, 207: 305–313.

Dekker, L.V., De Graan, P.N.E., Oestreicher, A.B., Versteeg, D.H.G. and Gispen, W.H. (1989) Inhibition of noradrenaline release by antibodies to B-50 (GAP-43). *Nature*, 342: 74–76.

Finley, J.C., Maderdrut, J.L., Roger, L.J. and Petrusz, P. (1981) The immunocytochemical localization of somatostatin-containing neurons in the rat central nervous system. *Neuroscience*, 6: 2173–2192.

Fried, G., Terenius, L., Hökfelt, T. and Goldstein, M. (1985) Evidence for differential localization of noradrenaline and neuropeptide Y in neuronal storage vesicles isolated from rat vas deferens. *J. Neurosci.*, 5: 450–458.

Fuxe, K. (1965) Evidence for the existence of monoamine neurons in the central nervous system-IV. The distribution of monoamine terminals in the central nervous system. *Acta Physiol. Scand.*, 64: 37–85.

Gibson, S.J., Polak, J.M., Bloom, S.R., Sabate, I.M., Mulderry, P.M., Ghatei., M.A., McGregor, G.P., Morrison, J.F.B., Kelly, J.S., Evans, R.M. and Rosenfeld, M.G. (1984) Calcitonin gene-related peptide immunoreactivity in the spinal cord of man and of eight other species. *J. Neurosci.*, 4: 3101–3111.

Gilbert, R.F.T., Emson, P.C., Hunt, S.P., Bennett, G.W., Marsden, C.A., Sandberg, B.E.B., Steinbusch, H.W.M. and Verhofstad, A.A.J. (1982) The effects of momoamine neurotoxins on peptides in the rat spinal cord. *Neuroscience*, 7: 69–87.

Glazer, E.J., Steinbusch, H., Verhofstad, A. and Basbaum, A.I. (1981) Serotonin neurons in nucleus raphe dorsalis and paragigantocellularis of the cat contain enkephalin. *J. Physiol.*, 77: 241–245.

Harkness, D.H. and Brownfield, M.S. (1986) A thyrotropin-releasing hormone containing system in the rat dorsal horn separate from serotonin. *Brain Res.*, 384: 323–333.

Helke, C.J., Sayson, S.C., Keeler, J.R. and Charlton, C.G. (1986) Thyrotropin-releasing hormone-immunoreactive

neurons project from the ventral medulla to the intermediolateral cell column: partial coexistence with serotonin. *Brain Res.*, 381: 1–7.

Hökfelt, T. (1968) In vitro studies on central and peripheral monoamine neurons at the ultrastructural level. *Z. Zellforsch. Mikrosk. Anat.*, 91: 1–74.

Hökfelt, T. (1991) Neuropeptides in perspective: the last ten years. *Neuron*, 7: 867–879.

Hökfelt, T., Ljungdahl, Å., Steinbusch, H., Verhofstad, A., Nilsson, G., Brodin, E., Pernow, B. and Goldstein, M. (1978) Immunohistochemical evidence of substance P-like immunoreactivity in some 5-hydroxytryptamine-containing neurons in the rat central nervous system. *Neuroscience*, 3: 517–538.

Hökfelt, T., Millhorn, D., Seroogy, K., Tsuruo, Y., Ceccatelli, S., Lindh, B., Meister, B., Melander, T., Schalling, M., Bartfai, T. and Terenius, L. (1987) Coexistence of peptides with classical neurotransmitters. *Experientia*, 43: 768–780.

Holstege, J.C. and Kuypers, H.G.J.M. (1987) Brainstem projections to spinal motoneurons: an update. *Neuroscience*, 23: 809–821.

Holtman, J.R., Jr., Dick, T.E. and Berger, A.J. (1986) Involvement of serotonin in the excitation of phrenic motoneurons evoked by stimulation of the raphe obscurus. *J. Neurosci.*, 6: 1185–1193.

Hounsgaard, J., Hultborn, H., Jespersen, B. and Kiehn, O. (1988) Bistability of alpha-motoneurones in the decerebrate cat and in the acute spinal cat after intravenous 5-hydroxytryptophan. *J. Physiol.*, 345–367.

Hunt, S.P. and Lovick, T.A. (1982) The distribution of serotonin, met-enkephalin and beta-lipotropin-like immunoreactivity in neuronal perikarya of the cat brainstem. *Neurosci. Lett.*, 30: 139–145.

Iverfeldt, K., Serfszs, P., Diaz Arnesto, L. and Bartfai, T. (1989) Differential release of coexisting neurotransmitters: frequency dependence of the efflux of substance P, thyrotropin releasing hormone and [^{3}H]serotonin from tissue slices of rat ventral spinal cord. *Acta Physiol. Scand.*, 137: 63–71.

Jacobs, B.L. and Fornal, C.A. (1993) 5-HT and motor control: a hypothesis. *Trends Neurosci.*, 16: 346–352.

Johansson, O., Hökfelt, T., Pernow, B., Jeffcoate, S.L., White, N., Steinbusch, H.M.W., Verhofstad, A.A.J., Emson, P.C. and Spindel, E. (1981) Immunohistochemical support for three putative transmitters in one neuron: coexistence of 5-hydroxytryptamine-, substance P- and thyrotropin releasing hormone-like immuno-reactivity in medullary neurons projecting to the spinal cord. *Neuroscience*, 6: 1857–1881.

Johnson, H., Ulfhake, B., Dagerlind, Å., Bennett, G.W., Fone, K.C.F. and Hökfelt, T. (1993) The serotoninergic bulbospinal system and brainstem-spinal cord content of serotonin-, TRH-, and substance P-like immunoreactivity in the aged rat with special reference to the spinal cord motor nucleus. *Synapse*, 15: 63–89.

Johnson, M.D. (1994) Synaptic glutamate release by postnatal rat serotonergic neurons in microculture. *Neuron*, 12: 433–442.

Ju, G., Hökfelt, T., Brodin, E., Fahrenkrug, J., Fischer, J.A., Frey, P., Elde, R.P. and Brown, J.C. (1987a) Primary sensory neurons of the rat showing calcitonin gene-related peptide immunoreactivity and their relation to substance P-, somatostatin-, galanin-, vasoactive intestinal polypeptide- and cholecystokinin-immunoreactive ganglion cells. *Cell Tissue Res.*, 247: 417–431.

Ju, G., Melander, T., Ceccatelli, S., Hökfelt, T. and Frey, P. (1987b) Immunohistochemical evidence for a spinothalamic pathway co-containing cholecystokinin- and galanin-like immunoreactivities in the rat. *Neuroscience*, 20: 439–456.

Kachidian, P., Poulat, P., Marlier, L. and Privat, A. (1991) Immunohistochemical evidence for the coexistence of substance P, thyrotropin-releasing hormone, GABA, methionine-enkephalin, and leucin-enkephalin in the serotonergic neurons of the caudal raphe nuclei: a dual labeling in the rat. *J. Neurosci. Res.*, 30: 521–530.

Kojima, M. and Sano, Y. (1983) The organization of serotonin fibers in the anterior column of the mammalian spinal cord. *Anat. Embryol.*, 167: 1–11.

Kojima, M., Takeuchi, Y., Goto, M. and Sano, Y. (1983) Immunohistochemical study on the localization of serotonin fibers and terminals in the spinal cord of the monkey (*Macaca fuscata*). Cell Tissue Res., 229: 23–36.

Korsching, S. (1993) The neurotrophic factor concept: a reexamination. *J. Neurosci.*, 13: 2739–2748.

Kruger, L., Mantyh, P.W., Sternini, C., Brecha, N.C. and Mantyh, C.R. (1988) Calcitonin gene-related peptide (CGRP) in the rat central nervous system: patterns of immunoreactivity and receptor binding sites. *Brain Res.*, 463: 223–244.

Kruger, L., Bendotti, C., Rivolta, R. and Samanin, R. (1993) Distribution of GAP-43 mRNA in the adult rat brain. *J. Comp. Neurol.*, 333: 417–434.

Kubota, Y., Inagaki, S., Shiosaka, S., Cho, S.J., Tateishi, K., Hashimura, E., Hamaoka, T. and Tohyama, M. (1983) The distribution of cholecystokinin octapeptide-like structures in the lower brain stem of the rat: an immunohistochemical analysis. *Neuroscience*, 9: 587–604.

Kuypers, H.J.G.M. and Huisman, A.M. (1982) The new anatomy of the descending brain pathways. In: B. Sjölund, B. and A. Björklund (Eds.), *Brain Stem Control of Spinal Mechanisms*, Elsevier Biomedical Press, Amsterdam, pp. 29–54.

LaMotte, C.C., Johns, D.R. and De Lanerolle, N.C. (1982) Immunohistochemical evidence of indolamine neurons in monkey spinal cord. *J. Comp. Neurol.*, 206: 359–370.

Lèger, L., Charnay, Y., Dubois, P.M. and Jouvet, M. (1986) Distribution of enkephalin-immunoreactive cell bodies in relation to serotonin-containing neurons in the raphe nu-

clei of the cat: immunohistochemical evidence for the coexistence of enkephalins and serotonin in certain cells. *Brain Res.*, 362: 63–73.

Lindå, H., Cullheim, S., Risling, M., Arvidsson, U., Mossberg, K., Ulfhake, B., Terenius, L. and Hökfelt, T. (1990) Enkephalin-like immunoreactivity levels increase in the motor nucleus after an intramedullar axotomy of motoneurons in the adult cat spinal cord. *Brain. Res.*, 534: 352–356.

Ljungdahl, Å., Hökfelt, T. and Nilsson, G. (1978) Distribution of substance P-like immunoreactivity in the central nervous system of the rat. I. Cell bodies and nerve terminals. *Neuroscience*, 3: 861–943.

Lovick, T.A. and Hunt, S.P. (1983) Substance P-immunoreactive and serotonin-containing neurones in the ventral brainstem of the cat. *Neurosci. Lett.*, 36: 223–228.

Lovinger, D.M., Colley, P.A., Akers, R., Nelson, F. and Routtenberg, A. (1986) Direct relation of long-term synaptic potentiation to phosphorylation of membrane protein F1, a substrate for membrane protein kinase C. *Brain Res.*, 399: 205–211.

Lundberg, J.M., Fried, G., Fahrenkrug, J., Holmstedt, B., Hökfelt, T., Lagercrantz, H., Lundgren, G. and Änggård, A. (1981) Subcellular fractionation of cat submandibular gland: comparative studies on the distribution of acetylcholine and vasoactive intestinal polypeptide (VIP). *Neuroscience*, 6: 1001–1010.

Lundberg, J.M. and Hökfelt, T. (1983) Coexistence of peptides and classical neurotransmitters. *TINS*, 6: 325–333.

Magnusson, T. (1973) Effect of chronic transection on dopamine, noradrenaline and 5-hydroxytryptamine in the rat spinal cord. *Naunyn-Schmiedebergs Arch. Pharmacol.*, 278: 13–22.

Marson, L. (1989) Evidence for colocalization of substance P and 5-hydroxytryptamine in spinally projecting neurons from the cat medulla oblongata. *Neurosci. Lett.*, 96: 54–59.

Marson, L. and Loewy, A.D. (1985) Topographic organization of substance P and monoamine cells in the ventral medulla of the cat. *J. Autonom. Nerv. Syst.*, 14: 271–285.

McCall, R.B. and Aghajanian, G.K. (1979) Serotonergic facilitation of facial motoneuron excitation. *Brain Res.*, 169: 11–27.

Melander, T., Hökfelt, T. and Rökaeus, Å. (1986) Distribution of galaninlike immunoreactivity in the rat central nervous system. *J. Comp. Neurol.*, 248: 475–517.

Millhorn, D.E., Hökfelt, T., Seroogy, K., Oertel, W., Verhofstad, A.A.J. and Wu, J.-Y. (1987) Immunohistochemical evidence for colocalization of gamma-aminobutyric acid and serotonin in neurons of the ventral medulla oblongata projecting to the spinal cord. *Brain Res.*, 410: 179–185.

Millhorn, D.E., Hökfelt, T., Verhofstad, A.A.J. and Terenius, L. (1989) Individual cells in the raphe nuclei of the medulla oblongata in the rat that contain immunoreactivities for both serotonin and enkephalin project to the spinal cord. *Exp. Brain Res.*, 75: 536–542.

38

Mitchell, R. and Fleetwood-Walker, S. (1981) Substance P, but not TRH, modulates the 5-HT autoreceptor in ventral lumbar spinal cord. *Eur. J. Pharmacol.*, 76: 119–120.

Moore, R.Y. (1989) Cranial motor neurons contain either galanin- or calcitonin gene-related peptide like immunore-activty. *J. Comp. Neurol.*, 282: 512–522.

Myslinsky, N.R. and Anderson, E.G. (1978) The effect of serotonin precursors on alpha- and gamma-motoneuron activity. *J. Pharmac. Exp. Ther.*, 204: 19–26.

Nelson, R.B. and Routtenberg, A. (1985) Characterization of protein F1 (47kDa, 4.5pl): A kinase C substrate directly related to neuronal plasticity. *Exp. Neurol.*, 89: 213–224.

Newton, B.W. and Hamill, R.W. (1988) The morphology and distribution of rat serotoninergic intraspinal neurons: an immunohistochemical study. *Brain Res. Bull.*, 20: 349–360.

Newton, B.W., Maley, B.E. and Hamill, R.W. (1986) Immunohistochemical demonstration of serotonin neurons in autonomic regions of the rat spinal cord. *Brain Res.*, 376: 155–163.

Nicholas, A.P., Pieribone, V.A., Arvidsson, U. and Hökfelt, T. (1992) Serotonin-, substance P- and glutamate/aspartate-like immunoreactivities in medullo-spinal pathways of rat and primate. *Neuroscience*, 48: 545–559.

Okado, N., Homma, S., Ishihara, R., Sako, H. and Kohno, K. (1988) Differential innervation of specific motor neuron pools by serotonergic fibers in the chick spinal cord. *Neurosci. Lett.*, 94: 29–32.

Okado, N., Matsukawa, M., Noritake, S., Ozaki, S., Hamada, S., Arita, M. and Kudo, N. (1991) Species differences in the distribution and coexistence ratio of serotonin and substance P in the monkey, cat, rat and chick spinal cord. *Neurosci Lett.*, 132: 155–8.

Okado, M., Cheng, L., Tanatsuga, Y., Hamada, S. and Hamaguchi, K. (1992) Synaptic loss following removal of serotoninergic fibers in newly hatched and adult chickens. *J. Neurobiol.*, 24: 687–698.

Oliveras, J.L., Bourgoin, S., Hery, F., Besson, J.M. and Hamon, M. (1977) The topographical distribution of serotoninergic terminals in the spinal cord of the cat: biochemical mapping by the combined use of microdissection and microassay procedures. *Brain Res.*, 138: 393–406.

Ozaki, S., Kudo, N. and Okado, N. (1992) Immunohistochemical study on development of serotonin-, substance P-, and enkephalin-positive fibers in the rat spinal motor nucleus. *J. Comp. Neurol.*, 325: 462–470.

Parry, O. and Roberts, M.H.T. (1980) The responses of motoneurons to 5-hydroxytryptamine. *Neuropharmacology*, 19: 515–518.

Paxinos, G. and Watson, C. (1986) *The Rat Brain in Stereotaxic Coordinates*, Second Edition, Academic Press, New York.

Pelletier, G., Steinbusch, H.W.M. and Verhofstad, A.A.J. (1981) Immunoreactive substance P and serotonin present in the same dense-core vesicles. *Nature*, 293: 71–72.

Piehl, F., Arvidsson, U., Johnson, H., Cullheim, S., Villar, M., Dagerlind, Å., Terenius, L., Hökfelt, T. and Ulfhake, B. (1991) Calcitonin gene-related peptide (CGRP)-like immunoreactivity and CGRP mRNA in rat spinal cord motoneurons after different types of lesions. *Eur. J. Neurosci.*, 3: 737–757.

Priestley, J.V. and Cuello, A.C. (1982) Coexistence of neuroactive substances as revealed by immunohistochemistry with monoclonal antibodies. In: A.C. Cuello, (Ed.), *Cotransmission*, Macmillan Press, London, pp. 165–188.

Ramírez-León, V., Ulfhake, B., Arvidsson, U., Verhofstad, A.A.J. and Hökfelt, T. (1994) Serotoninergic, peptidergic and GABAergic innervation of the ventrolateral and dorsolateral motor nuclei in the cat S1/S2 segments: an immunofluorescence study. *J. Chem. Neuroanat.*, 7: 87–103.

Rexed, B. (1954) The cytoarchitectonic organization of the spinal cord in the cat. *J. Comp. Neurol.*, 96: 415–496.

Risling, M., Cullheim, S. and Hildebrand, C. (1983) Reinnervation of the ventral root L7 from ventral horn neurons following intramedullary axotomy in adult cats. *Brain Res.*, 280: 15–23.

Roberts, M.H.T. and Wright, D.M. (1978) Effect of a substance P analogue and 5-hydroxytryptamine on motoneurone excitability following dorsal root section in the rat. *J. Physiol.*, 285: 21–22P.

Rökaeus, Å., Melander, T., Hökfelt, T., Lundberg, J.M., Tatemoto, K., Carlquist, M. and Mutt, V. (1984) A galanin-like peptide in the central nervous system and intestine of the rat. *Neurosci. Lett.*, 47: 161–166.

Rosenfeld, M.G., Mermod, J.-J., Amara, S.G., Swanson, L.W., Sawchenko, P.E., Rivier, J., Vale, W.W. and Evans, R.M. (1983) Production of a novel neuropeptide encoded by the calcitonin gene via tissue-specific RNA processing. *Nature*, 304: 129–135.

Ruda, M.A., Bennett, G.J. and Dubner, R. (1986) Neurochemistry and neural circuitry in the dorsal horn. In: P.C. Emson, M.N. Rossor, and M. Tohyama, (Eds.), *Progress in Brain Research*, Elsevier, Amsterdam, pp. 219–268.

Sakamoto, H. and Atsumi, S. (1991) Species differences in the coexistence of 5-hydroxytryptamine and substance P in presynaptic boutons in the cervical ventral horn. *Cell Tissue Res.*, 264: 221–230.

Sasek, C.A. and Helke, C.J. (1989) Enkephalin-immunoreactive neuronal projections from the medulla oblongata to the intermediolateral cell column: relationship to substance P-immunoreactive neurons. *J. Comp. Neurol.*, 287: 484–94.

Sasek, C.A., Wessendorf, M.W. and Helke, C.J. (1990) Evidence for co-existence of thyrotropin-releasing hormone, substance P and serotonin in ventral medullary neurons that project to the intermediolateral cell column in the rat. *Neuroscience*, 35: 105–119.

Sillar, K.T. (1994) Synaptic specificity: development of locomotor rhythmicity. *Curr. Opin. Neurobiol.*, 4: 101–107.

Skagerberg, G. and Björklund, A. (1985) Topographic principles in the spinal projections of serotonergic and non-serotonergic brainstem neurons in the rat. *Neuroscience*, 15: 445–480.

Skene, J.H.P. (1989) Axonal growth-associated protein. *Annu. Rev. Neurosci.*, 12: 127–156.

Skofitsch, G. and Jacobowitz, D.M. (1985a) Calcitonin gene-related peptide: detailed immunohistochemical distribution in the central nervous system. *Peptides*, 6: 721–745.

Skofitsch, G. and Jacobowitz, D.M. (1985b) Galanin-like immunoreactivity in capsaicin sensory neurons and ganglia. *Brain Res. Bull.*, 15: 191–195.

Skofitsch, G. and Jacobowitz, D.M. (1985c) Quantitative distribution of calcitonin gene-related peptide in the rat central nervous system. *Peptides*, 6: 721–745.

Staines, W.A., Meister, B., Melander, T., Nagy, J.I. and Hökfelt, T. (1988) Three-color immunofluorescence histochemistry allowing triple labeling within a single section. *J. Histochem. Cytochem.*, 36: 145–151.

Stanton, E.S., Smolen, P.M., Nashold, B.S., Dreyer, D.A. and Davis, J.N. (1975) Segmental analysis of spinal cord after thoracic transection in dog. *Brain Res.*, 89: 93–98.

Steinbusch, H.W.M. (1981) Distribution of serotonin-immunoreactivity in the central nervous system of the rat-Cell bodies and terminals. *Neuroscience*, 6: 557–618.

Streit, W.J., Dumoulin, F.L., Raivich, G. and Kreutzberg, G.W. (1989) Calcitonin gene-related peptide increases in rat facial motoneurons after peripheral nerve transection. *Neurosci. Lett.*, 101: 143–148.

Tanaka, M., Okamura, H., Yanaihara, N., Tanaka, Y. and Ibata, Y. (1993) Differential expression of serotonin and :Met:enkephalin-Arg6-Gly7-Leu8 in neurons of the rat brain stem. *Brain Res. Bull.*, 30: 561–570.

Tashiro, T. and Ruda, M.A. (1988) Immunocytochemical identification of axons containing coexistent serotonin and substance P in the cat lumbar spinal cord. *Peptides*, 9: 383–391.

Tashiro, T., Satoda, T., Takahashi, O., Matsushima, R. and Mizuno, N. (1988) Distribution of axons exhibiting both enkephalin- and serotonin-like immunoreactivities in the lumbar cord segments: an immunohistochemical study in the cat. *Brain Res.*, 440: 357–362.

Tashiro, T., Satoda, T., Matsushima, R. and Mizuno, N. (1990) Distribution of axons showing both enkephalin- and serotonin-like immunoreactivities in the lumbar cord segments of the Japanese monkey (*Macaca fuscata*). *Brain Res.*, 512: 143–146.

Tatemoto, K., Rökaeus, Å., Jörnvall, H., McDonald, T.J. and Mutt, V. (1983) Galanin: a novel biologically active peptide from porcine intestine. *FEBS Lett.*, 164: 124–128.

Tessarollo, L., Tsoulfas, P., Martin-Zanca, D., Gilbert, D.J., Jenkins, N.A., Copeland, N.G. and Parada, L.F. (1993) trkC, a receptor for neurotrophin-3, is widely expressed in the developing nervous system and in non-neuronal tissues. *Development*, 118: 463–475.

Tessler, A., Glazer, E., Artymyshyn, R., Murray, M. and Goldberger, M.E. (1980) Recovery of substance P in the cat spinal cord after unilateral lumbosacral deafferentation. *Brain Res.*, 191: 459–470.

Tessler, A., Himes, B.T., Artymyshyn, R., Murray, M. and Goldberger, M.E. (1981) Spinal neurons mediate return of substance P following deafferentation of cat spinal cord. *Brain Res.*, 230: 263–281.

Tessler, A., Himes, B.T., Soper, K., Murray, M., Goldberger, M.E. and Reichlin, S. (1984) Recovery of substance P but no somatostatin in the cat spinal cord after unilateral lumbosacral dorsal rhizotomy: a quantitative study. *Brain Res.*, 305: 95–102.

Thoenen, H. (1991) The changing scene of neurotrophic factors. *TINS*, 14: 165–170.

Tuchscherer, M.M. and Seybold, V.S. (1989) A quantitative study of the coexistence of peptide in varicosities within the superficial laminae of the dorsal horn of the rat spinal cord. *J. Neurosci.*, 9: 195–205.

Ulfhake, B. and Cullheim, S. (1988) Postnatal development of cat hind limb motoneurons. III. Changes in size of motoneurons supplying the triceps surae muscle. *J. Comp. Neurol.*, 278: 103–120.

Ulfhake, B. and Kellerth, J.-O. (1981) A quantitative light microscopic study of the dendrites of cat spinal alpha motoneurons after intracellular staining with horseradish peroxidase. *J. Comp. Neurol.*, 202: 571–583.

Ulfhake, B., Arvidsson, U., Cullheim, S., Hökfelt, T., Brodin, E., Verhofstad, A. and Visser, T. (1987a) An ultrastructural study of 5-hydroxytryptamine-, thyrotropin-releasing hormone- and substance P-immunoreactive axonal boutons in the motor nucleus of spinal cord segments L7-S1 in the adult cat. *Neuroscience*, 23: 917–929.

Ulfhake, B., Arvidsson, U., Cullheim, S., Hökfelt, T. and Visser, T.J. (1987b) Thyrotropin-releasing hormone (TRH)-immunoreactive boutons and nerve cell bodies in the dorsal horn of the cat L7 spinal cord. *Neurosci. Lett.*, 73: 3–8.

VanderMaelen, C.P. and Aghajanian, G.K. (1982) Intracellular studies on the effects of systemic administration of serotonin agonists on rat facial motoneurons. *Eur. J. Pharmacol.*, 78: 233–236.

Van Dongen, P.A.M., Grillner, S. and Hökfelt, T. (1986) 5-Hydroxytryptamine (serotonin) causes a reduction in the afterhyperpolarization following the action potential in lamprey motoneurons and premotor interneurons. *Brain Res.*, 366: 320–325.

Wessendorf, M.W. and Brelje, T.C. (1993) Multicolor fluorescence microscopy using the laser-scanning confocal microscope. *Neuroprotocols*, 2: 121–140.

Wessendorf, M.W. and Elde, R.P. (1985) Characterization of an immunofluorescence technique for the demonstration of coexisting neurotransmitters within nerve fibers and terminals. *J. Histochem. Cytochem*, 33: 984–994.

Wessendorf, M.W. and Elde, R. (1987) The coexistence of serotonin- and substance P-like immunoreactivity in the spinal cord of the rat as shown by immunofluorescent double labeling. *J. Neurosci.*, 7: 2352–2363.

Wessendorf, M.W., Apple, N.M., Molitor, T.W. and Elde, R.P. (1990) A method for immunofluorescent demonstration of three coexisting neurotransmitters in rat brain and spinal cord, using the fluorophores fluorescein, lissamine rhodamine, and 7-amino-4-methylcoumarin-3-acetic acid. *J. Histochem. Cytochem.*, 38: 1859–1877.

White, S.R. (1985) Serotonin and co-localized peptides: effects on spinal motoneuron excitability. *Peptides*, 6: 123–127.

White, S.R. and Neuman, R.S. (1980) Facilitation of spinal motoneurone excitability by 5-hydroxytryptamine and noradrenaline. *Brain Res.*, 188: 119–127.

White, S.R. and Neuman, S.R. (1983) Pharmacological antagonism of facilitatory but not inhibitory effects of sertonin and norepinephrine on excitability of spinal motoneurones. *Neuropharmacology*, 22: 489–494.

Wolpaw, J.R. and Carp, J.S. (1990) Memory traces in spinal cord. *TINS*, 13: 137–142.

Wu, W., Elde, R. and Wessendorf, M.W. (1993) Organization of the serotonergic innervation of spinal neurons in rats. III. Differential serotonergic innervation of somatic and parasympathetic preganglionic motoneurons as determined by patterns of co-existing peptides. *Neuroscience*, 55: 223–233.

Yao, G.L., Kiyama, H. and Tohyama, M. (1993) Distribution of GAP-43 (B50/F1) mRNA in the adult rat brain by in situ hybridization using an alkaline phosphatase labeled probe. *Brain Res. Mol. Brain Res.*, 18: 1–16.

Xu, X.-J., Wiesenfeld-Hallin, Z., Villar, M.J. and Hökfelt, T. (1990) Intrathecal galanin antagonizes the facilitatory effect of substance P on the nociceptive flexor reflex in the rat. *Acta Physiol. Scand.*, 137: 463–463.

F. Nyberg, H.S. Sharma and Z. Wiesenfeld-Hallin (Eds.)
Progress in Brain Research, Vol 104
© 1995 Elsevier Science BV. All rights reserved.

CHAPTER 3

Organization of peptidergic neurons in the dorsal horn of the spinal cord: anatomical and functional correlates

A. Ribeiro-da-Silva and A. Claudio Cuello

*Department of Pharmacology and Therapeutics, McGill University, 3655 Drummond Street, Montréal,
Québec, Canada H3G 1Y6*

Neuropeptides as spinal cord transmitter candidates

It is frequently stated that, in contrast to classical transmitters, neuropeptides usually have actions of slow onset and long duration, and they are not removed from their target sites by reuptake mechanisms. However, more recent ideas put greater emphasis on similarities rather than on differences because classical transmitters can share some of the characteristics attributed to neuropeptides, such as a rather prolonged effect (Otsuka and Yoshioka, 1993). Frequently, neuropeptides are co-localized with the more classical transmitters and/or with other neuropeptides. There is an extensive literature on neuropeptides in the dorsal horn of the spinal cord (for reviews see Yaksh and Aimone, 1989; Willis and Coggeshall, 1991). Major interest in this issue was triggered by the classical study of Jessel and Iversen (1977) demonstrating that opiates inhibit the release of substance P in the substantia gelatinosa of the trigeminal nucleus in vitro. The hypothesis was advanced that enkephalin (ENK) might inhibit the release of substance P from primary sensory fibres in the substantia gelatinosa through axo-axonic synapses. Unfortunately, such a synaptic arrangement was never confirmed in subsequent studies applying either double-labelling high resolution immunocytochemistry or the combination of that technique with intracellular filling of dorsal horn nociceptive neurons after physiological characterization.

Neuropeptide-containing nerve cell bodies and fibres in the dorsal horn of the spinal cord

Immunoreactivities for a considerable number of peptides have been described in the dorsal horn of the spinal cord. A detailed review of the chemical neuroanatomy of the dorsal horn is beyond the scope of this chapter. For reviews, the reader is referred to Willis and Coggeshall (1991) and Todd and Spike (1993). Here, we will focus mainly on three peptides, substance P, ENK and calcitonin gene-related peptide (CGRP), although we will briefly mention some of the others. Figure 1 represents a diagrammatic resumé of our views on the participation of peptidergic neurons in the circuits of the rat dorsal horn.

Substance P

There is now considerable evidence of the involvement of substance P in the processing of sensory information in the region of the first sensory synapse (for reviews see Henry, 1982; Cuello, 1987; Otsuka and Yanagisawa, 1990). Im-

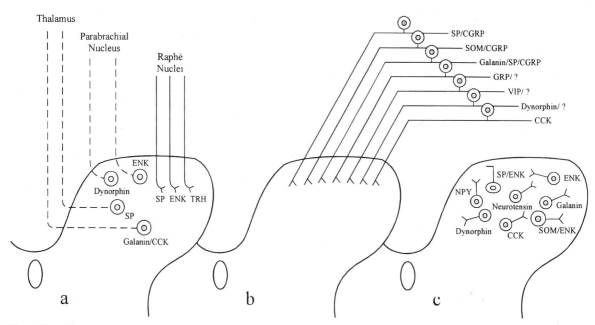

Fig. 1. Simplified schematic representation of the origin of peptide immunoreactivity in the dorsal horn of rat spinal cord. For the sake of clarity, there was no concern for accuracy in the laminar localization of the structures. (a) Projecting neurons and descending fibres; (b) primary sensory fibres; (c) local circuit neurons. SP, substance P; ENK, enkephalin; TRH, thyrotropin-releasing hormone; CCK, cholecystokinin; SOM, somatostatin; NPY, neuropeptide tyrosine; VIP, vasoactive intestinal polypeptide.

munocytochemically, it has been shown to occur in either unmyelinated or thinly myelinated sensory fibres that terminate mainly in Laminae I and outer II (Hökfelt et al., 1975; Cuello et al., 1978). It is important to note that there is also a significant substance P primary sensory input to Lamina V, where clusters of immunoreactive fibres are separated by areas almost entirely devoid of substance P immunoreactivity (Ruda et al., 1986).

With regard to interpreting substance P immunoreactivity in the dorsal horn, two problems are involved. One concerns whether or not the substance being recognized is really substance P, as some antibodies cross-react with the other mammalian neurokinins (neurokinins A and B). Therefore, in most studies, when discussing substance P immunoreactivity, the authors are actually referring to neurokinin immunoreactivity. The other concern is that, even assuming that the detected substance P immunoreactivity corre-

sponds to real substance P, there is ample evidence that it is not entirely of sensory origin (for review see Ruda et al., 1986), as substance P is found in some dorsal horn neurons (Ljungdahl et al., 1978; Hunt et al., 1981) and in descending pathways from the brain stem (Hökfelt et al., 1978; Gilbert et al., 1982; Tashiro and Ruda, 1988). Perhaps as much as 50% of the immunoreactivity in the superficial laminae might originate from neurons intrinsic to the CNS, mostly located in the spinal cord.

There is restricted information in relation to substance P-immunoreactive (IR) neurons in the spinal cord. They are known to occur in most laminae (Ljungdahl et al., 1978; Todd and Spike, 1993). In Lamina I, they represent flattened neurons, a category of cell that frequently projects to the thalamus (Lima et al., 1993). The projection of substance P-IR neurons to the thalamus has been demonstrated in the rat by combining tract-tracing techniques with immunocytochemistry

(Battaglia and Rustioni, 1992). One characteristic of substance P-IR neurons in Lamina II is that virtually all of them display a co-localization with ENK immunoreactivity (Senba et al., 1988; Ribeiro-da-Silva et al., 1991c). It is very likely that many of these cells co-localizing both peptides may represent stalked cells (Ribeiro-da-Silva et al., 1991c). Substance P immunoreactivity occurs in neurons of the raphe nuclei projecting to the spinal cord (Menétrey and Basbaum, 1987). However, the contribution of such fibres to the immunoreactivity in the dorsal horn is probably quite small because, after the application of monoamine neurotoxins, the loss of substance P immunoreactivity is restricted to the ventral horn (Gilbert et al., 1982). Moreover, double-labelling immunocytochemical studies reveal that, in both cat and rat, the number of axons co-localizing substance P and serotonin immunoreactivities is quite low in the superficial dorsal horn (Pearson and Jennes, 1988; Tashiro and Ruda, 1988; Arvidsson et al., 1990). In relation to the other two neurokinins, neurokinin A originates from the same gene and is co-localized with substance P in sensory neurons and probably also in dorsal horn cells (for review see Helke et al., 1990). In contrast, neurokinin B is encoded by a different gene. In situ hybridization histochemistry showed that neurokinin B mRNA occurs mostly in Lamina III, in contrast to cells expressing substance P mRNA, which prevail in Laminae I–II (Warden and Young, 1988; for review see Helke et al., 1990).

Enkephalin (ENK)

Since their discovery, the endogenous opioid peptides have been considered as important candidates for presynaptic interactions in the dorsal horn of the spinal cord. The opioid peptides Met- and Leu-ENK occur in high concentrations in Laminae I and II of the spinal cord (see, e.g., Hökfelt et al., 1977; Hunt et al., 1981), and have been demonstrated in nerve cell bodies in Laminae I–III (Del Fiacco and Cuello, 1980; Hunt et al., 1981; Bennett et al., 1982; Glazer and Bas-

baum, 1984; Miller and Seybold, 1987). It seems likely that virtually all ENK immunoreactivity comes from neurons intrinsic to the dorsal horn. ENK has been localized in serotonergic neurons of the raphe nuclei that project to the spinal cord, but most of such fibres terminate in the ventral horn (Tashiro et al., 1988; Menétrey and Basbaum, 1987; Arvidsson et al., 1992). Also, some ENK immunoreactivity has been suggested to originate from primary sensory fibres. However, ENK has never been detected in a significant number of neurons in the dorsal root ganglia (Garry et al., 1989). Relative to dorsal horn cell populations possessing ENK immunoreactivity, in Lamina II immunoreactivity occurs in both stalked and islet cells, in cat and rat (Bennett et al., 1982; Todd and Spike, 1993). In Lamina I, most ENK-IR cells correspond to pyramidal neurons (Lima et al., 1993). It should be noted that approximately half of the neurons from Lamina I that project to the parabrachial nucleus in the rat are ENK-IR (Standaert et al., 1986). An important characteristic of ENK immunoreactivity in the dorsal horn is its co-localization with other neurochemicals, including substance P (see above), somatostatin (Todd and Spike, 1992) and GABA (Todd et al., 1992b).

CGRP

Immunoreactivity for CGRP has been shown to occur in dorsal root ganglia and in primary sensory fibres which project mainly to the superficial laminae of the spinal cord (Kaway et al., 1985; Lee et al., 1985; Traub et al., 1990). One of the interesting features of CGRP immunoreactivity in sensory systems is its co-localization with substance P. In reality, substance P immunoreactivity is almost invariably co-localized with CGRP immunoreactivity in dorsal root ganglion cells, although CGRP immunoreactivity occurs in a considerably higher percentage of these cells than does substance P (Ju et al., 1987a). Another interesting feature of CGRP immunoreactivity in the dorsal horn is its virtual disappearance after dorsal rhizotomy (Chung et al., 1988; Traub et al.,

1989). This finding suggests that all CGRP immunoreactivity in the dorsal horn originates from primary sensory fibres, a finding that is confirmed by in situ hybridization studies which do not reveal any dorsal horn neurons synthesizing the peptide (Réthelyi et al., 1989). Therefore, it seems legitimate to use the co-localization of CGRP and substance P in the same terminal as a marker of primary sensory origin. It should be pointed out, however, that CGRP immunoreactivity occurs in bulbospinal neurons, although they do not seem to project to the dorsal horn (Orazzo et al., 1993).

Dynorphin

The opioid peptides, dynorphin A and B, occur in the dorsal horn. Immunoreactivity for these peptides has been described in Laminae I and II in rat, cat and monkey (for review see Todd and Spike, 1993). The origin seems to be mainly neurons intrinsic to the dorsal horn, which occur in Laminae I and outer Lamina II. Some Lamina I neurons project to the parabrachial nucleus (Standaert et al., 1986) or the solitary tract nucleus (Leah et al., 1988). These neurons are apparently distinct from ENK-IR neurons (Standaert et al., 1986). However, in contrast to ENK, dynorphin also originates from primary sensory fibres, particularly at sacral levels (Basbaum et al., 1986; Ruda et al., 1988). A minor component of dynorphin immunoreactivity may originate from bulbospinal fibres (Ménétrey and Basbaum, 1987).

Somatostatin (SOM)

Immunoreactivity for SOM originates mostly from neurons intrinsic to the dorsal horn, although an important component is of sensory origin. SOM-IR fibres occur in Laminae I and II, and nerve cells bodies can be found mostly in Lamina II (Alvarez and Priestley, 1990a; Ribeiro-da-Silva and Cuello, 1990). These neurons have the morphology of islet cells and some co-localize ENK immunoreactivity (Todd and Spike, 1992).

Neurotensin

Immunoreactivity for neurotension has been de-

scribed in fibres in Laminae I–II and perikarya mainly of ventral Lamina II (Seybold and Elde, 1982; Todd et al., 1992a). The morphology is of islet cells (Seybold and Elde, 1982), although such cells do not co-localize ENK or GABA immunoreactivities (Proudlock et al., 1993).

Galanin

This neuropeptide occurs both in the spinal ganglion, where it is co-localized with substance P and CGRP immunoreactivities (Ju et al., 1987a), and in Laminae I–II of the spinal cord (Zhang et al., 1993a). In Laminae I–II, there are many galanin-IR perikarya (Melander et al., 1986).

Vasoactive intestinal polypeptide (VIP)

This peptide occurs mostly at the level of lumbar and sacral spinal cord (Laminae I–II) and is associated with visceral primary sensory fibres (Gibson et al., 1981; Honda et al., 1983). Most immunoreactivity originates from sensory fibres, although there are a few immunopositive cells in Laminae I–II (Hökfelt et al., 1987).

Neuropeptide tyrosine (NPY)

There is a rather dense network of NPY-IR fibres in Laminae I–III (for review see Todd and Spike, 1993). Probably most of this immunoreactivity originates from sources intrinsic to the spinal cord. There are NPY-IR perikarya in Laminae I–III, but mostly in Lamina II (for review see Todd and Spike, 1993). It should be noted, however, that NPY immunoreactivity in sensory fibres is greatly increased after peripheral nerve lesions (Wakisaka et al., 1991; Zhang et al., 1994).

Cholecystokinin (CCK)

Immunoreactivity for this peptide in the dorsal horn was originally thought to originate from primary sensory fibres. However, most of the immunoreactivity detected in the original studies probably resulted from a cross-reactivity with CGRP (see Ju et al., 1986). However, real CCK is expressed by sensory fibres after peripheral axotomy (Verge et al., 1993) as detected by in situ hybridization studies. In the normal spinal cord, CCK immunoreactivity occurs mainly in neurons of Lamina II. In rat, some spinothalamic tract neurons contain a co-localization of galanin and CCK immunoreactivities (Ju et al., 1987b; Verge et al., 1993).

Others

Immunoreactivities for other neuropeptides, such as gastrin-releasing peptide (GRP), neuropeptide FF, thyrotropin-releasing hormone (TRH) and neuromedin B, have been described in the dorsal horn. However, discussing them here is beyond the scope of this review. Interested readers should consult, e.g., Tood and Spike (1993).

Peptide-containing synaptic arrangements in the dorsal horn of the spinal cord

Our knowledge of the dorsal horn synaptic circuits in which neuropeptides are actually involved is still rather incomplete. The synaptic circuitry can only be established with certainty using ultrastructural techniques. In this regard, some recent studies applying high resolution methods have provided important new clues on peptidergic synapses. Studies combining the intracellular filling of physiologically characterized neurons with ultrastructural immunocytochemistry have been particularly important in the integration of high resolution chemical neuroanatomy with function. Those studies are described in the section entitled *Physiological implications of peptidergic synapses*. This section is a short description of some recent findings relative to dorsal horn circuitry involving neuropeptides, with emphasis on substance P, CGRP, SOM and ENK.

Substance P

At the ultrastructural level, it is well known that substance P immunoreactivity occurs as the central bouton in a certain number of synaptic glomeruli in Lamina II in cat and monkey (DiF-

iglia et al., 1982; de Lanerolle and LaMotte, 1983; Ruda, 1986). Contrary to early assumptions, we were able to demonstrate that, in rat, about 10% of substance P immunoreactivity in ventral Lamina II occurs in the central boutons of synaptic glomeruli (Ribeiro-da-Silva et al., 1989). Although this number is not high, the information is meaningful because such profiles are of known sensory origin (Coimbra et al., 1984; Murray and Goldberger, 1986). This origin has been confirmed using a combination of post-embedding immunogold immunostaining and HRP-tracing of the sensory fibres (De Biasi and Rustioni, 1988; Merighi et al., 1992). Most of the substance P-IR boutons in the superficial dorsal horn are clearly non-glomerular. Some of these non-glomerular profiles have been shown to be presynaptic to Lamina I spinothalamic neurons after retrograde labelling (Priestley and Cuello, 1989) (Figs. 2 and 3). These synapses might be particularly important in nociceptive pathways. However, the actual physiological significance of these synaptic arrangements can only be established by the direct correlation of ultrastructure with physiological data. In this regard, there has been some recent progress (see below).

CGRP

At the ultrastructural level, this peptide occurs mostly in non-glomerular varicosities in the dorsal horn of the spinal cord of rat and monkey, although a few varicosities are of the glomerular type (Carlton et al., 1988; Ribeiro-da-Silva and Cuello, 1991). We have recently studied the co-localization of CGRP and substance P in the rat. In glomeruli, approximately 20% of the central varicosities of type I glomeruli possessed CGRP immunoreactivity, where it is co-localized with either substance P (14% of the type I population) or SOM (approximately 6%) (for review see Ribeiro-da-Silva, 1995). It is interesting to note that substance P and SOM immunoreactivities were only occasionally co-localized and that the finding of substance P or SOM immunoreactivity in the central varicosities of glomeruli in the absence of CGRP immunoreactivity almost never

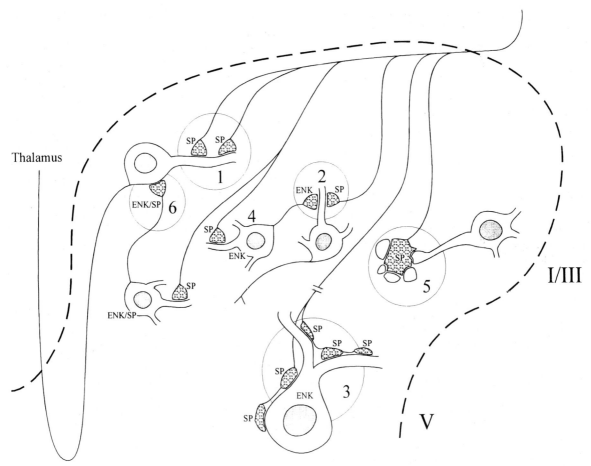

Fig. 2. Diagrammatic representation of the main types of dorsal horn circuits involving neuropeptides. Each type of circuit is ascribed a number and, when circled, are illustrated in one of the figures that follow. (1) Lamina I spinothalamic neuron postsynaptic to substance P-IR fibres (see Figure 3). (2) dendrite from dorsal horn neuron contacted both by a substance P sensory fibre and by an enkephalinergic profile (see Figure 4). (3) Repetitive synapses of substance P-IR fibres on the same wide dynamic range neuron from Lamina V (see Fig. 5). (4) Enkephalinergic neuron postsynaptic to SP-IR boutons (not illustrated for Lamina II neurons; for a similar arrangement in Lamina V see Fig. 6). (5) Substance P-IR central varicosity in a glomerulus presynaptic to a dendrite of a dorsal horn neuron (see Fig. 7). (6) Profile double-labelled for substance P and ENK immunoreactivities presynaptic to dorsal horn neuron (see Figs. 4 and 7). SP, substance P; ENK, enkephalin.

occurred. The co-localization of CGRP with these and other neuropeptides has been studied in detail recently using a post-embedding immunogold protocol (Zhang et al., 1993b).

Somatostatin

SOM immunoreactivity was detected in about 6% of the central varicosities of type I synaptic glomeruli (Ribeiro-da-Silva and Cuello, 1990). Those boutons virtually never co-localized substance P immunoreactivity, but always possessed CGRP immunoreactivity (manuscript in preparation). As seen for CGRP and substance P, most of the SOM-IR boutons are non-glomerular. SOM immunoreactivity also occurred in surrounding dendritic profiles of glomeruli, either with or without synaptic vesicles (Alvarez and Priestley,

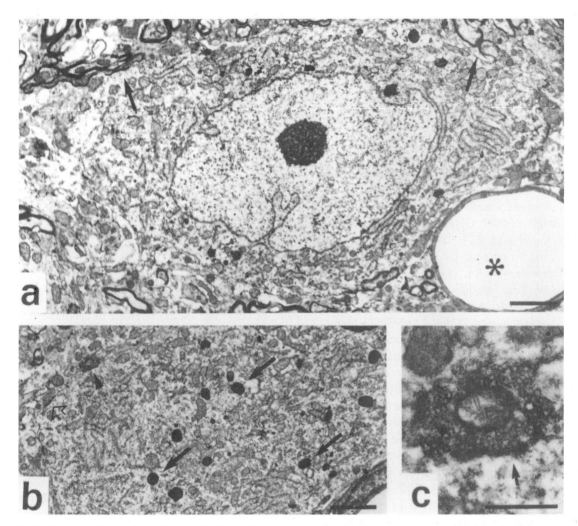

Fig. 3. Electron micrographs of Lamina I of the trigeminal subnucleus caudalis (homologous of Lamina I of the spinal cord) double-labelled for substance P immunoreactivity and for HRP retrogradely transported after injection in thalamus. (a,b) Low magnification micrographs showing the appearance of a retrogradely labelled cell at two levels cut through the Vibratome section. In (a), the asterisk indicates a blood vessel and arrows point to the edge of white matter (spinal tract of the trigeminal nerve). Arrows in (b) indicate the dense HRP bodies. (c) Enlargement of the substance P-immunostained bouton that is indicated with an arrowhead in (b) and which is presynaptic to the cell. Scale bars = 2 μm (a,b), 0.5 μm (c). (Reproduced with permission from Priestley and Cuello, 1989.)

1990b; Ribeiro-da-Silva and Cuello, 1990). It is very likely that SOM and ENK immunoreactivities co-localize in some of those profiles, as such co-localization has been detected in perikarya at the light microscopic level by Todd and Spike (1992).

The above observations on three sensory neu-ropeptides reinforce the notion that the modality of termination of peptidergic fibres in the dorsal horn is mostly non-glomerular. The physiological role of those that are glomerular is not clear, although such an arrangement provides a tool to activate several dorsal horn neurons by means of a single sensory bouton. It should also be stressed that a feature of glomeruli with neuropeptides in their central varicosity is their relatively simple synaptic architecture. In fact, the central (peptidergic) varicosity is virtually never postsynaptic to other profiles.

Enkephalin (ENK)

Immunoreactivity for ENK has been demonstrated in glomerular peripheral profiles in the substantia gelatinosa of the cat, monkey and rat, including some which contain synaptic vesicles (Bennett et al., 1982; Glazer and Basbaum, 1983; Ribeiro-da-Silva et al., 1991c), but, again, no real evidence of presynaptic interactions on the central glomerular bouton could be demonstrated. Double-labelling studies combining radio-immunocytochemistry and diaminobenzidine-based immunocytochemistry (Cuello, 1983a; Ribeiro-da-Silva et al., 1991c) have demonstrated that sometimes ENK- and substance P-IR varicosities establish separate synapses on a common dendrite (Figs. 2 and 4). Furthermore, substance P-IR central glomerular boutons are presynaptic to ENK-IR dendrites in the rat (Ribeiro-da-Silva et al., 1991c). These results, obtained in the rat, were confirmed in the cat (Ribeiro-da-Silva et al., 1991a,b) and demonstrate, together with data indicated below, that substance P-IR central boutons in glomeruli excite dendrites of enkephalinergic interneurons in the substantia gelatinosa, and that the axons of such neurons inhibit the dendrites of neurons that had been excited by substance P (see Fig. 2). These high resolution chemical neuroanatomy studies would, therefore, indicate that the enkephalinergic 'gating' of substance P-mediated sensory information occurs at a postsynaptic site. Cho and Basbaum (1989) also failed to detect a significant number of dynorphin B-immunostained structures presynaptic to sensory fibres (identified by degeneration after dorsal rhizotomy). In contrast, there is evidence that retrogradely labelled spinothalamic neurons receive direct synapses from ENK-IR boutons (Ruda, 1982; Ruda et al., 1984; Priestley and Cuello, 1989). Therefore, based on anatomical criteria, it seems likely that opioid peptides interact with peptidergic sensory fibres postsynaptically. However, the possibility of a presynaptic mechanism cannot be ruled out as ENK may act on peptidergic sensory fibres at a non-synaptic site (Cuello, 1983b), since these fibres are known to possess opiate receptor sites (e.g., see Gouardères et al., 1991). A particularly significant finding was the co-localization of substance P and ENK immunoreactivities in a considerable number of cells and axonal boutons of Laminae I–II in both rat (Ribeiro-da-Silva et al., 1991c) and cat (Ribeiro-da-Silva et al., 1991b) (see Figs. 2, 4 and 7). Probably, some of the cells co-localizing both peptides represent stalked cells (Ribeiro-da-Silva et al., 1991c). Concerning the localization of ENK immunoreactivity in glomeruli, it never occurred in profiles presynaptic to peptidergic central varicosities, but was detected in both surrounding axonal and dendritic profiles of glomeruli that did not have peptide immunoreactivity in the central bouton. In many of these profiles, GABA immunoreactivity was detected as co-localizing with ENK immunoreactivity (Ribeiro-da-Silva et al., 1993).

Physiological implications of peptidergic synapses

There are a few studies in which high resolution immunocytochemistry has been combined with

---

Fig. 4 Ultrastructural features of substance P/ENK double-labelling in Lamina I. (a) A large dendrite (D) is postsynaptic to profiles which contain only substance P immunoreactivity (open arrow) or ENK immunoreactivity (arrow). (b) A profile co-localizing substance P/ENK immunoreactivities (double arrow) is apposed to a medium-sized dendrite (D) establishing an asymmetric contact with it (small arrow). Note also a profile immunolabelled only for substance P (open arrow). (c) A double-labelled dome-shaped profile (double arrow) establishes an asymmetric contact (arrows) with a small dendritic spine. Scale bar in all micrographs = 0.5 μm. (Reproduced with permission from Ribeiro-da-Silva et al., 1991c.)

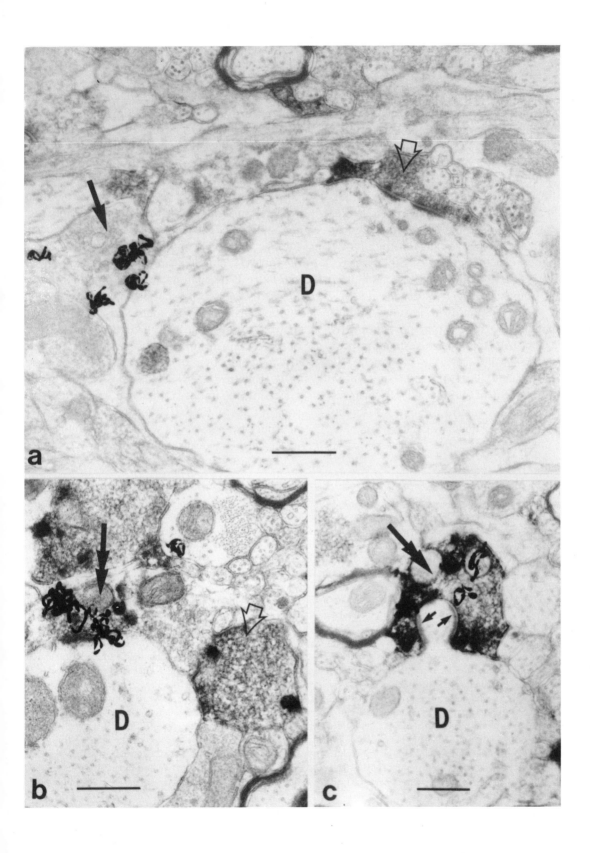

the intracellular characterization and filling of either primary sensory fibres or dorsal horn neurons. This basic approach has been used by a number of investigators in the spinal cord of cats and monkeys (Maxwell and Noble, 1987; Ulfhake et al., 1987; Maxwell et al., 1990, 1991; Westlund et al., 1990; Todd et al., 1991; Carlton et al., 1992; Alvarez et al., 1992, 1993). This is an area in which we have made some advances in the cat, in collaboration with J.L. Henry and colleagues (De Koninck et al., 1992; Ribeiro-da-Silva et al., 1992a; Cuello et al., 1993). The most significant finding from our studies has been the demonstration of a correlation between the type of physiological response of dorsal horn neurons and the amount of innervation from substance P-IR profiles. In fact, cells with strong responses to noxious stimuli receive abundant synapses from substance P-IR varicosities, but cells that do not respond to noxious stimulation hardly receive any substance P-IR input (De Koninck et al., 1992). Interestingly, the number and pattern of substance P-IR synapses appear to be proportional to the intensity of the nociceptive response. Wide dynamic range neurons with moderate nociceptive responses receive fewer substance P-IR synapses than wide dynamic range cells with strong nociceptive responses (De Koninck et al., 1992; Cuello et al., 1993, and manuscript in preparation). These findings are illustrated in Figs. 2 and 5 and in Table I.

Interestingly, most of the nociceptive neurons which were strongly innervated by substance P-IR boutons possessed ENK immunoreactivity (Ribeiro-da-Silva et al., 1992a; Cuello et al., 1993). The peptidergic synaptic input to these neurons was investigated and a considerable number of the substance P-IR boutons were shown to co-localize with ENK immunoreactivity (Figs. 2 and 6; Table I), although approximately half of the substance P-IR boutons were not immunoreactive for ENK (Table I). In contrast, approximately half of the substance P-IR boutons apposed to such neurons co-localized with CGRP and, therefore, probably represent the substance P-IR primary sensory component of the synaptic input to these cells (Ribeiro-da-Silva et al., 1992b, and manuscript in preparation). It can be speculated that some of these ENK-IR dorsal horn nociceptive neurons also possess substance P immunoreactivity, as such co-localization has been detected in

Fig. 5 Dorsal horn neuron responding with a slow, prolonged EPSP after noxious cutaneous stimulation. (A, right) Camera lucida reconstruction of the cell body, located in Lamina V, that was associated with a discrete area of substance P-IR fibres (see C). (Left) Response of the neuron to low-threshold mechanical stimulation (hair, H). The period of application of each of two stimuli is represented by the horizontal bars below the trace. (Inset) Enlargement, on a faster time scale, of a typical burst of action potentials riding on EPSPs during the stimulus. (Centre) The cutaneous receptive field of the neuron is represented on the schematic diagram: darkened area represents the low-threshold touch receptive field and larger hatched area represents the high-threshold pinch receptive field. (B) Response of the neuron to high-threshold mechanical stimulation (pinch; P). The period of the stimulus is represented by the horizontal bar below the trace. Note the marked depolarization during the noxious stimulus associated with action potential inactivation. Note also the prolonged depolarization after the end of the stimulus associated with increased firing frequency. (C) Light microscopic photograph of a parasagittal, 4-μm thick, Epon-flat-embedded section showing part of the neuronal cell body. Note the numerous substance P-IR profiles apposed to the cell body (arrows). The cell body was located within a region of intense immunoreactivity corresponding to one of the clusters of substance P-IR fibres commonly found in Lamina V. Scale bar = 20 μm. (D) Electron microscopic photographs of an ultrathin section taken from the 4-μm thick section shown in C. Note the two substance P-containing varicosities (arrows) apposed to the cell body. Synapses between these varicosities and the cell body could be demonstrated in adjacent sections (data not shown). Asterisks indicate non-immunoreactive axonal varicosities. Scale bar = 1 μm. (E) Electron micrographs of an ultrathin section taken from the 4-μm thick section in E'. The portion of the dendrite shown in E corresponds to the curved portion of the dendrite shown in E' (the two arrows on the left of E' indicate the two boutons pointed to by two of the arrows in E). The immunoreactive profiles (arrows) belong to an axon that appears to wrap in a spiral-like fashion around the dendrite (arrows in E') of the cell and make several contacts with the dendrite. Asterisks indicate non-immunoreactive varicosities apposed to the dendrite. Scale bar = 1 μm. E''. Details of the synapse (open arrow) established by the profile on the right in E (right arrow in E), obtained from an adjacent ultrathin section. Scale bars in E' = 20 μm; in E'' = 0.5 μm. (Reproduced from De Koninck et al., 1992.)

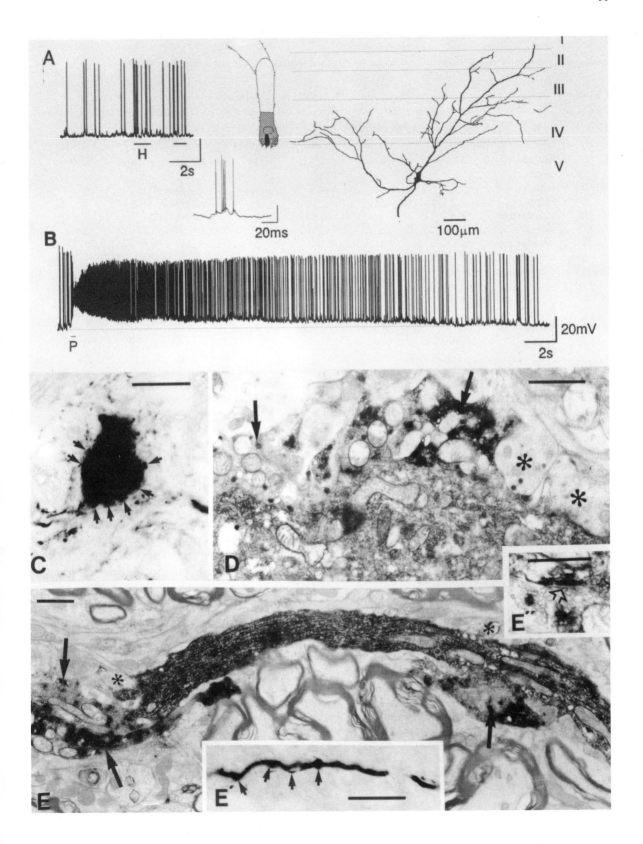

TABLE I

Summary of substance P and ENK inputs to functionally classified neurons labelled intracellularly with HRP

Lamina	Cell type	Number of cells	Nociceptive after-depolarization	ENK-only input (%)	Substance P and ENK input (%)	Total substance P input (%)	ENK immunoreactivity of cell
I	nociceptive specific	3	+ + +	19	14	31	+
IIi–III	wide dynamic range	2	+ + +	n/c	n/c	20 (Li-IIo) 6 (LIIi–III)	+
III–III	wide dynamic range	1	+ +	n/c	n/c	18 (Li-IIo) 5 (LIIi–III)	–
III–IV	non-nociceptive	2	–	18	2	4	–
III–IV	non-nociceptive	1	–	n/c	n/c	3	–
IV–V	wide dynamic range	1	+	n/c	n/c	2 (LIII) 10 (LV)	–
IV–V	wide dynamic ramge	1	+	n/c	n/c	12	–
V	wide dynamic range	2	+ + + + +	27	9	25	+

Results represent average percentages of immunoreactive varicosities in the total number of boutons apposed to the cell body and dendrites per cell type. Synaptic contacts were present in approximately 30% of the immunoreactive boutons apposed to the cells, independent of their neurochemical characteristics. Number of varicosities counted per cell = approx. 300. n/c = not counted. (Reproduced from Cuello et al., 1993.)

the cat dorsal horn (see above). Because knowledge of the physiological characteristics of dorsal horn neurons co-localizing both peptides is particularly important, we trust that this information will soon be available from our own and other laboratories.

Conclusions

Our understanding of the synaptology of the dorsal horn of the spinal cord is still rather incomplete. However, based on direct analysis of transmitter-specific circuits at the ultrastructural level, we would like to advance the following tentative conclusions.

(1) From the available morphological evidence, the postulated enkephalinergic 'gating' of peptidergic nociceptive primary sensory information should occur at postsynaptic sites. However, the possibility of a presynaptic mechanism cannot be ruled out; such gating may occur non-synaptically.

Fig. 6 Demonstration of ENK immunoreactivity in the neuron shown in Figure 5. (a) Light micrograph of 4-μm thick section. Curved arrow points to proximal dendrite shown in (b), arrowhead to elongated dendrite shown in (c) and small arrow to small dendrite shown in (d). Scale bar = 20 μm. (b) Dendritic trunk close to the cell body shows immunoreactivity for ENK (silver grains). A varicosity with substance P immunoreactivity (B) is presynaptic to the double-labelled dendrite. Scale bar = 1 μm. (c) Elongated dendritic profile of the cell shows immunoreactivity for ENK (silver grains). An axonal varicosity immunoreactive exclusively for substance P (B) is presynaptic to the dendrite. Scale bar = 1 μm. (d). Small dendritic process of the cell (arrow) shows immunoreactivity for ENK (silver grains) and is contacted by a substance P-IR bouton (B). A dendritic spine from the same cell is also overlaid by silver grains (small arrow). Radioautograms were exposed for 3 months and developed with D19b. Scale bar = 1 μm. (Reproduced with permission from Ribeiro-da-Silva et al., 1992a.)

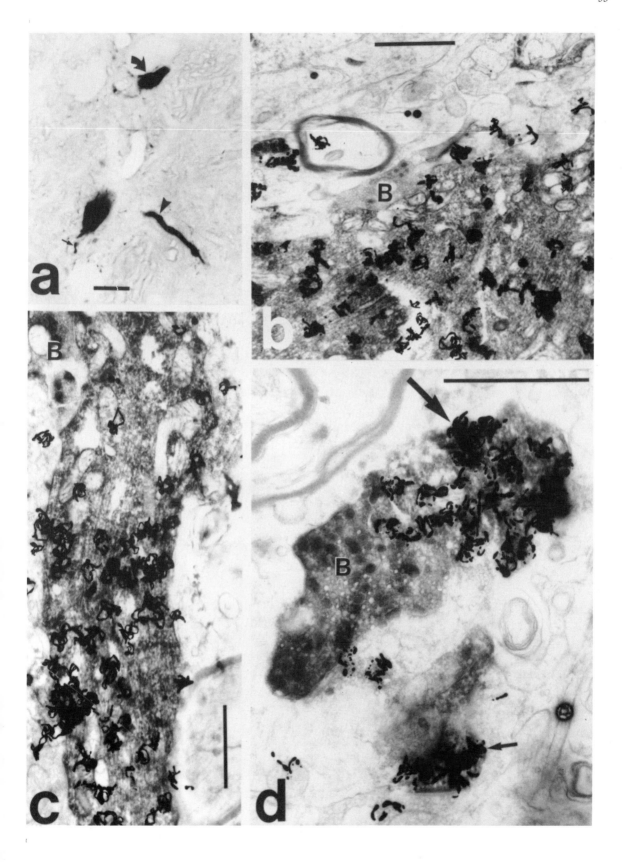

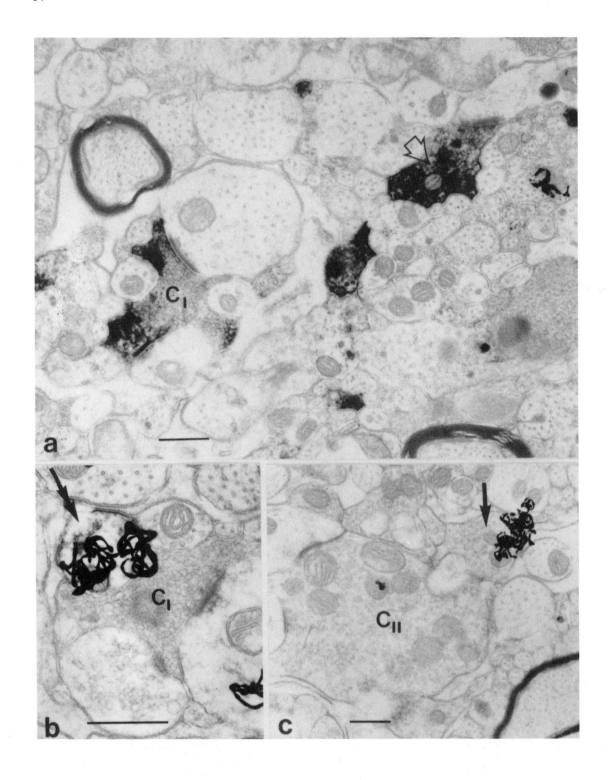

(2) In contrast, enkephalinergic neurons intrinsic to the dorsal horn are sometimes pre-synaptic to the central element of synaptic glomeruli which do not display peptide immunoreactivity in the central bouton. This would indicate that ENK acts both pre- and postsynaptically in the modulation of non-peptidergic primary sensory information.

(3) The responsiveness of dorsal horn neurons to noxious stimulation is directly related to the number of primary sensory peptidergic (particularly substance P) varicosities that are presynaptic to them.

(4) In neurons with strong nociceptive responses, the number of substance P-IR terminals establishing synapses on them is very high (up to 40 % of the total number of synapses). Frequently, the same fibre contacts the cell through several varicosities, in a repetitive manner (see Figs. 2 and 5).

(5) The termination of peptidergic primary sensory fibres in the spinal cord occurs mostly outside of synaptic glomeruli.

(6) When peptidergic primary sensory boutons participate in glomeruli, these display a simplified architecture. In them, the central (peptidergic) bouton is virtually never postsynaptic to other profiles. This would indicate that axo-axonic or dendro-axonic interactions are unlikely to take place in the modulation of information conveyed by peptidergic sensory fibres.

Acknowledgements

Research was support by grants from NIH (A.C. Cuello) and Canadian MRC (A. Ribeiro-da-Silva). The research involving the combination of intracellular recording from dorsal horn neurons with ultrastructural immunocytochemistry was carried out in collaboration with Drs. J.L. Henry and Y. de Koninck. We are grateful to Mrs. Marie Ballak and to Mr. Sylvain L. Côté for excellent technical support, and to Mr. Alan Forster for photographic expertise. We also acknowledge the editorial assistance of Ms. Susan Grant and Mrs. Oralia Mackprang-Arauz.

References

Alvarez, F.J. and Priestley, J.V. (1990a) Anatomy of somatostatin-immunoreactive fibres and cell bodies in the rat trigeminal subnucleus caudalis. *Neuroscience*, 38: 343–357.

Alvarez, F.J. and Priestley, J.V. (1990b) Ultrastructure of somatostatin-immunoreactive nerve terminals in laminae I and II of the rat trigeminal subnucleus caudalis. *Neuroscience*, 38: 359–371.

Alvarez, F.J., Kavookjian, A.M. and Light, A.R. (1992) Synaptic interactions between GABA-immunoreactive profiles and the terminals of functionally defined myelinated nociceptors in the monkey and cat spinal cord. *J. Neurosci.*, 12: 2901–2917.

Alvarez, F.J., Kavookjian, A.M. and Light, A.R. (1993) Ultrastructural morphology, synaptic relationships and CGRP immunoreactivity of physiologically identified C-fiber terminals in the monkey spinal cord. *J. Comp. Neurol.*, 329: 472–490.

Arvidsson, U., Cullheim, S., Ulfhake, B., Bennett, G.W., Fone, K.C., Cuello, A.C., Verhofstad, A.A., Visser, T.J. and Hökfelt, T. (1990) 5-Hydroxytryptamine, substance P and thyrotropin-releasing hormone in the adult cat spinal cord segment L7: immunohistochemical and chemical studies. *Synapse*, 6: 237–270.

Arvidsson, U., Cullheim, S., Ulfhake, B., Ramírez, V., Dagerlind, Å., Luppi, P.-H., Kitahama, K., Jouvet, M., Terenius, L., Åman, K. and Hökfelt, T. (1992) Distribution of enkephalin and its relation to serotonin in cat and monkey spinal cord and brain stem. *Synapse*, 11: 85–104.

Fig. 7 Ultrastructural features of immunolabelled profiles in synaptic glomeruli of Lamina IIB. The sections were incubated for the demonstration of both substance P- and ENK-IR sites. (a) A central varicosity of a type I synaptic glomerulus (C_I) and a non-glomerular scalloped terminal (open arrow) are both immunoreactive for only substance P; terminals with these morphological characteristics are consistent with a primary sensory origin (see text). (b) A double-labelled (double arrow) dendrite in a type I synaptic glomerulus. C_I, central varicosity of a type I synaptic glomerulus. (c) A peripheral axonal varicosity (arrow) of a type II glomerulus is only immunoreactive for ENK. C_{II}, central varicosity of a type II glomerulus. Scale bars = 0.5 μm. (Reproduced with permission from Ribeiro-da-Silva et al., 1991c.)

56

Basbaum, A.I., Cruz, L. and Weber, E. (1986) Immunoreactive dynorphin B in sacral primary afferent fibers of the cat. *J. Neurosci.*, 6: 127–133.

Battaglia, G. and Rustioni, A. (1992) Substance P innervation of the rat and cat thalamus. II. Cells of origin in the spinal cord. *J. Comp. Neurol.*, 315: 473–486.

Bennett, G.J., Ruda, M.A., Gobel, S. and Dubner, R. (1982) Enkephalin immunoreactive stalked cells and lamina IIb islet cells in cat substantia gelatinosa. *Brain Res.*, 240: 162–166.

Carlton, S.M., Mcneill, D.L., Chung, K. and Coggeshall, R.E. (1988) Organization of calcitonin gene-related peptide-immunoreactive terminals in the primate dorsal horn. *J. Comp. Neurol.*, 276: 527–536.

Carlton, S.M., Westlund, K.N., Zhang, D. and Willis, W.D. (1992) GABA-immunoreactive terminals synapse on primate spinothalamic tract cells. *J. Comp. Neurol.*, 322: 528–537.

Cho, H.J. and Basbaum, A.I. (1989) Ultrastructural analysis of dynorphin B-immunoreactive cells and terminals in the superficial dorsal horn of the deafferented spinal cord of the rat. *J. Comp. Neurol.*, 281: 193–205.

Chung, K., Lee, W.T. and Carlton, S.M. (1988) The effects of dorsal rhizotomy and spinal cord isolation on calcitonin gene-related peptide-labeled terminals in the rat lumbar dorsal horn. *Neurosci. Lett.*, 90: 27–32.

Coimbra, A., Ribeiro-da-Silva, A. and Pignatelli, D. (1984) Effects of dorsal rhizotomy on the several types of primary afferent terminals in laminae I–III of the rat spinal cord. An electron microscope study. *Anat. Embryol (Berlin)* 170:279–287.

Cuello, A.C. (1983a) Central distribution of opioid peptides. *Br. Med. Bull.*, 39: 11–16.

Cuello, A.C. (1983b) Nonclassical neuronal communications. *Fed. Proc.*, 42: 2912–2922.

Cuello, A.C. (1987) Peptides as neuromodulators in primary sensory neurons. *Neuropharmacology*, 26: 971–979.

Cuello, A.C., Del Fiacco, M. and Paxinos, G. (1978) The central and peripheral ends of the substance P-containing sensory neurones in the rat trigeminal system. *Brain Res.*, 152: 499–509.

Cuello, A.C., Ribeiro-da-Silva, A., Ma, W., De Koninck, Y. and Henry, J.L. (1993) Organization of substance P primary sensory neurons: ultrastructural and physiological correlates. *Regul. Peptides*, 46: 155–164.

De Biasi, S. and Rustioni, A. (1988) Glutamate and substance P coexist in primary afferent terminals in the superficial laminae of spinal cord. *Proc. Natl. Acad. Sci. USA*, 85: 7820–7824.

De Koninck, Y., Ribeiro-da-Silva, A., Henry, J.L. and Cuello, A.C. (1992) Spinal neurons exhibiting a specific nociceptive response receive abundant substance P-containing synaptic contacts. *Proc. Natl. Acad. Sci. USA*, 89: 5073–5077.

de Lanerolle, N.C. and LaMotte, C.C. (1983) Ultrastructure of

chemically defined neuron systems in the dorsal horn of the monkey. I. Substance P immunoreactivity. *Brain Res.*, 274: 31–49.

Del Fiacco, M. and Cuello, A.C. (1980) Substance P-and enkephalin-containing neurones in the rat trigeminal system. *Neuroscience*, 5: 803–815.

DiFiglia, M., Aronin, N. and Leeman, S.E. (1982) Light microscopic and ultrastructural localization of immunoreactive substance P in the dorsal horn of the monkey spinal cord. *Neuroscience*, 7: 1127–1139.

Garry, M.G., Miller, K.E. and Seybold, V.S. (1989) Lumbar dorsal root ganglia of the cat: a quantitative study of peptide immunoreactivity and cell size. *J. Comp. Neurol.*, 284: 36–47.

Gibson, S.J., Polak, J.M., Bloom, S.R. and Wall, P.D. (1981) The distribution of nine peptides in rat spinal cord with special emphasis on the substantia gelatinosa and the area around the central canal (lamina X). J. Comp. Neurol., 201: 65–79.

Gilbert, R.F., Emson, P.C., Hunt, S.P., Bennett, G.W., Marsden, C.A., Sandberg, B.E., Steinbusch, H.W. and Verhofstad, A.A. (1982) The effects of monoamine neurotoxins on peptides in the rat spinal cord. *Neuroscience*, 7: 69–87.

Glazer, E.J. and Basbaum, A.I. (1983) Opioid neurons and pain modulation: an ultrastructural analysis of enkephalin in cat superficial dorsal horn. *Neuroscience*, 10: 357–376.

Glazer, E.J. and Basbaum, A.I. (1984) Axons which take up [^{3}H]serotonin are presynaptic to enkephalin immunoreactive neurons in cat dorsal horn. *Brain Res.*, 298: 386–391.

Gouardères, C., Beaudet, A., Zajac, J.-M., Cros, J. and Quirion, R. (1991) High resolution radioautographic localization of [^{125}I]FK-33.824-labelled mu opioid receptors in the spinal cord of normal and deafferented rats. *Neuroscience*, 43: 197–209.

Helke, C.J., Krause, J.E., Mantyh, P.W., Couture, R. and Bannon, M.J. (1990) Diversity of mammalian tachykinin peptidergic neurons: multiple peptides, receptors and regulatory mechanisms. FASEB J., 4: 1606–1615.

Henry, J.L. (1982) Relation of substance P to pain transmission: neurophysiological evidence. In: *Substance P in the Nervous System* (Ciba Foundation Symposium No. 91). Pitman, London, pp. 206–224.

Honda, C.N., Réthelyi, M. and Petrusz, P. (1983) Preferential immunohistochemical localization of vasoactive intestinal polypeptide (VIP) in the sacral spinal cord of the cat: light and electron microscopic observations. *J. Neurosci.*, 3: 2183–2196.

Hökfelt, T., Kellerth, J.O., Nilsson, G. and Pernow, B. (1975) Substance P: localization in the central nervous system and in some primary sensory neurons. *Science*, 190: 889–890.

Hökfelt, T., Ljungdahl, A., Terenius, L., Elde, R. and Nilsson, G. (1977) Immunohistochemical analysis of peptide pathways possibly related to pain and analgesia: enkephalin and substance P. *Proc. Natl. Acad. Sci. USA*, 74: 3081–3085.

Hökfelt, T., Ljungdahl, A., Steinbusch, H.W., Verhofstad, A.N., Nilsson, G., Brodin, E., Pernow, B. and Goldstein, M. (1978) Immunohistochemical evidence of substance P-like immunoreactivity in some 5-hydroxytryptamine-containing neurons in the rat central nervous system. *Neuroscience*, 3: 517–538.

Hökfelt, T., Fahrenkrug, J., Ju, G., Ceccatelli, S., Tsuruo, Y., Meister, B., Mutt, V., Rundgren, M., Brodin, E., Terenius, L., Hulting, A.-L., Werner, S., Björklund, H. and Vale, W. (1987) Analysis of peptide histidine-isoleucine/vasoactive intestinal polypeptide-immunoreactive neurons in the central nervous system with special reference to their relation to corticotropin releasing factor- and enkephalin-like immunoreactivities in the paraventricular hypothalamic nucleus. *Neuroscience*, 23: 827–857.

Hunt, S.P., Kelly, J.S., Emson, P.C., Kimmol, J.R., Miller, R.J. and Wu, J.-Y. (1981) An immunohistochemical study of neuronal populations containing neuropeptides or gamma-aminobutyrate within the superficial layers of the rat dorsal horn. *Neuroscience*, 6: 1883–1898.

Jessell, T.M. and Iversen, L.L. (1977) Opiate analgesics inhibit substance P release from rat trigeminal nucleus. *Nature*, 268: 549–551.

Ju, G., Hökfelt, T., Fischer, J.A., Frey, P., Rehfeld, J.F. and Dockray, G.J. (1986) Does cholecystokinin-like immunoreactivity in rat primary sensory neurons represent calcitonin gene-related peptide. *Neurosci. Lett.*, 68: 305–310.

Ju, G., Hökfelt, T., Brodin, E., Fahrenkrug, J., Fischer, J.A., Frey, P., Elde, R.P. and Brown, J.C. (1987a) Primary sensory neurons of the rat showing calcitonin gene-related peptide immunoreactivity and their relation to substance P-, somatostatin-, galanin-, vasoactive intestinal polypeptide- and cholecystokinin-immunoreactive ganglion cells. *Cell Tissue Res.*, 247: 417–431.

Ju, G., Melander, T., Ceccatelli, S., Hökfelt, T. and Prey, P. (1987b) Immunohistochemical evidence for a spinothalamic pathway co-containing cholecistokinin- and galanin-like immunoreactivities in the rat. *Neuroscience*, 20: 439–456.

Kaway, Y., Takami, K., Shiosaka, S., Emson, P.C., Hillyard, C.J., Girgis, S., MacIntyre, I. and Tohyama, M. (1985) Topographic localization of calcitonin gene-related peptide in the rat brain: an immunohistochemical analysis. *Neuroscience*, 15: 747–763.

Leah, J., Menétrey, D. and De Pommery, J. (1988) Neuropeptides in long ascending spinal tract cells in the rat: evidence for parallel processing of ascending information. *Neuroscience*, 24: 195–207.

Lee, Y., Kaway, Y., Shiosaka, S., Takami, K., Kiyama, H., Hillyard, C.J., Girgis, S., MacIntyre, I., Emson, P.C. and Tohyama, M. (1985) Coexistence of calcitonin gene-related peptide and substance P-like peptide in single cells of the trigeminal ganglion of the rat: immunohistochemical analysis. *Brain Res.*, 330: 194–196.

Lima, D., Avelino, A. and Coimbra, A. (1993) Morphological characterization of marginal (lamina I) neurons immunoreactive for substance P, enkephalin, dynorphin and gamma-aminobutyric acid in the rat spinal cord. *J. Chem. Neuroanat.*, 6: 43–52.

Ljungdahl, A., Hökfelt, T. and Nilsson, G. (1978) Distribution of substance P-like immunoreactivity in the central nervous system of the rat. I. Cell bodies and nerve terminals. *Neuroscience*, 3: 861–943.

Maxwell, D.J. and Noble, R. (1987) Relationship between hair-follicle afferent terminations and glutamic acid decarboxylase-containing boutons in cat's spinal cord. *Brain Res.*, 408: 308–312.

Maxwell, D.J., Christie, W.M., Short, A.D. and Brown, A.G. (1990) Direct observations of synapses between GABA-immunoreactive boutons and muscle afferent terminals in lamina VI of the cat's spinal cord. *Brain Res.*, 530: 215–222.

Maxwell, D.J., Christie, W.M., Short, A.D. and Brown, A.G. (1991) Direct observation of synapses between GABA-immunoreactive boutons and identified spinocervical tract neurons in the cat's spinal cord. *J. Comp. Neurol.*, 307: 375–392.

Melander, T., Hökfelt, T. and Rökaeus, A. (1986) Distribution of galanin-like immunoreactivity in the rat central nervous system. *J. Comp. Neurol.*, 248: 475–517.

Menétrey, D. and Basbaum, A.I. (1987) The distribution of substance P-, enkephalin- and dynorphin-immunoreactive neurons in the medulla of the rat and their contribution to bulbospinal pathways. *Neuroscience*, 23: 173–187.

Merighi, A., Cruz, F. and Coimbra, A. (1992) Immunocytochemical staining of neuropeptides in terminal arborization of primary afferent fibers anterogradely labeled and identified at light and electron microscopic levels. *J. Neurosci. Methods*, 42: 105–113.

Miller, K.E. and Seybold, V.S. (1987) Comparison of met-enkephalin-, dynorphin A- and neurotensin immunoreactive neurons in the cat and rat spinal cords: I. Lumbar cord. *J. Comp. Neurol.*, 255: 293–304.

Murray, M. and Goldberger, M.E. (1986) Replacement of synaptic terminals in lamina II and Clarke's nucleus after unilateral lumbosacral dorsal rhizotomy in adult cats. *J. Neurosci.*, 6: 3205–3217.

Orazzo, C., Pieribone, V.A., Ceccatelli, S., Terenius, L. and Hökfelt, T. (1993) CGRP-like immunoreactivity in A11 dopamine neurons projecting to the spinal cord and a note on CGRP-CCK cross-reactivity. *Brain Res.*, 600: 39–48.

Otsuka, M. and Yanagisawa, M. (1990) Pain and neurotransmitters. *Cell. Mol. Neurobiol.*, 10: 293–302.

Otsuka, M. and Yoshioka, K. (1993) Neurotransmitter functions of mammalian tachykinins. *Physiol. Rev.*, 73: 229–308.

Pearson, J.C. and Jennes, L. (1988) Localization of serotonin- and substance P-like immunofluorescence in the caudal spinal trigeminal nucleus of the rat. *Neurosci. Lett.*, 88: 151–156.

58

Priestley, J.V. and Cuello, A.C. (1989) Ultrastructural and neurochemical analysis of synaptic input to trigemino-thalamic projection neurones in lamina I of the rat: a combined immunocytochemical and retrograde labelling study. *J. Comp. Neurol.*, 285: 467–486.

Proudlock, F., Spike, R.C. and Todd, A.J. (1993) Immunocytochemical study of somatostatin, neurotensin, GABA and glycine in rat spinal dorsal horn. *J. Comp. Neurol.*, 327: 289–297.

Réthelyi, M., Metz, C.B. and Lund, P.K. (1989) Distribution of neurons expressing calcitonin gene-related peptide mR-NAS in the brain stem, spinal cord and dorsal root ganglia of rat and guinea-pig. *Neuroscience*, 29: 225–239.

Ribeiro-da-Silva, A. (1995) Substantia gelatinosa of spinal cord. In: G. Paxinos (Ed.) *The Rat Nervous System*, Academic Press, Sydney, pp 47–59.

Ribeiro-da-Silva, A. and Cuello, A.C. (1990) Ultrastructural evidence for the occurrence of two distinct somatostatin-containing systems in the substantia gelatinosa of rat spinal cord. *J. Chem. Neuroanat.*, 3: 141–153.

Ribeiro-da-Silva, A. and Cuello, A.C. (1991) Co-localization of substance P and calcitonin gene-related peptide immunore-activities in the rat dorsal horn. An ultrastructural double-labelling study. *Abstr. IBRO Third World Congr. Neurosci.*, 195.

Ribeiro-da-Silva, A., Tagari, P. and Cuello, A.C. (1989) Morphological characterization of substance P-like immunore-active glomeruli in the superficial dorsal horn of the rat spinal cord and trigeminal subnucleus caudalis: a quantitative study. *J. Comp. Neurol.*, 281: 497–415.

Ribeiro-da-Silva, A., De Koninck, Y., Henry, J.L. and Cuello, A.C. (1991a) Co-localization of substance P and enkephalin immunoreactivities in synaptic boutons apposed onto physiologically identified dorsal horn neurones: an ultrastructural multiple-labelling study. *Soc. Neurosci. Abstr.*, 17: 1007

Ribeiro-da-Silva, A., De Koninck, Y., Henry, J.L. and Cuello, A.C. (1991b) Co-localization of substance P and enkephalin immunoreactivities in synaptic boutons of the cat superficial dorsal horn. An ultrastructural double-labelling study. *Abstr. IBRO Third World Congr. Neurosci.*, 195.

Ribeiro-da-Silva, A., Pioro, E.P. and Cuello, A.C. (1991c) Substance P- and enkephalin-like immunoreactivities are colocalized in certain neurons of the substantia gelatinosa of the rat spinal cord. An ultrastructural double-labeling study. *J. Neurosci.*, 11: 1068–1080.

Ribeiro-da-Silva, A., De Koninck, Y., Cuello, A.C. and Henry, J.L. (1992a) Enkephalin-immunoreactive nociceptive neurons in the cat spinal cord. *NeuroReport*, 3: 25–28.

Ribeiro-da-Silva, A., Ma, W., De Koninck, Y., Cuello, A.C. and Henry, J.L. (1992b) Nociceptive spinal dorsal horn neurons receive abundant synaptic contacts from sensory fibres co-localizing substace P and CGRP immunoreactivi-

ties. An ultrastructural triple-labelling study in the cat. *Soc. Neurosci. Abstr.*, 18: 291

Ribeiro-da-Silva, A., Ballak, M. and Cuello, A.C. (1993) GABA immunoreactivity is co-localized with enkephalin or CHAT immunoreactivities in the dorsal horn of the rat spinal cord. An ultrastructural double-labeling study. *Soc. Neurosci. Abstr.*, 19: 1196

Ruda, M.A. (1982) Opiates and pain pathways: demonstration of enkephalin synapses on dorsal horn projection neurons. *Science*, 215: 1523–1525.

Ruda, M.A. (1986) The pattern and place of nociceptive modulation in the dorsal horn. A discussion of the anatomically characterized neural circuitry of enkephalin, serotonin and substance P. In: T.L. Yaksh (Ed.) *Spinal Afferent Processing*, Plenum Press, New York, pp. 141–164.

Ruda, M.A., Coffield, J. and Dubner, R. (1984) Demonstration of postsynaptic opioid modulation of thalamic projection neurons by the combined techniques of retrograde horseradish peroxidase and enkephalin immunocytochemistry. *J. Neurosci.*, 4: 2117–2132.

Ruda, M.A., Bennett, G.J. and Dubner, R. (1986) Neurochemistry and neural circuitry in the dorsal horn. *Prog. Brain Res.*, 66: 219–268.

Ruda, M.A., Iadarola, M.J., Cohen, L.V. and Young, W.S. (1988) In situ hybridization histochemistry and immunocytochemistry reveal an increase in spinal dynorphin biosynthesis in a rat model of peripheral inflammation and hyperalgesia. *Proc. Natl. Acad. Sci. USA*, 85: 622–626.

Senba, E., Yanaihara, C., Yanaihara, N. and Tohyama, M. (1988) Co-localization of substance P and Met-enkephalin-Arg[6]-Gly[7]-Leu[8] in the intraspinal neurons of the rat, with special reference to the neurons in the substantia gelatinosa. *Brain Res.*, 453: 110–116.

Seybold, V.S. and Elde, R.P. (1982) Neurotensin immunoreactivity in the superficial laminae of the dorsal horn of the rat. I. Light microscopic studies of cell bodies and proximal dendrites. *J. Comp. Neurol.*, 205: 89–100.

Standaert, D.G., Watson, S.J., Houghten, R.A. and Saper, C.B. (1986) Opoioid peptide immunoreactivity in spinal and trigeminal dorsal horn neurons projecting to the parabrachial nucleus in the rat. *J. Neurosci.*, 6: 1220–1226.

Tashiro, T. and Ruda, M.A. (1988) Immunocytochemical identification of axons containing coexistent serotonin and substance P in the cat lumbar spinal cord. *Peptides*, 9: 383–391.

Tashiro, T., Satoda, T., Takahashi, O., Matsushima, R. and Mizuno, N. (1988) Distribution of axons exhibiting both enkephalin- and serotonin-like immunoreactivities in the lumbar cord segments: an immunohistochemical study in the cat. *Brain Res.*, 440: 357–362.

Todd, A.J. and Spike, R.C. (1992) Co-localization of Met-enkephalin and somatostatin in the spinal cord of the rat. *Neurosci. Lett.*, 145: 71–74.

Todd, A.J. and Spike, R.C. (1993) The localization of classical transmitters and neuropeptides within neurons in laminae I–III of the mammalian spinal dorsal horn. *Prog. Neurobiol.*, 41: 609–638.

Todd, A.J., Maxwell, D.J. and Brown, A.G. (1991) Relationships between hair-follicle afferent axons and glycine-immunoreactive profiles in cat spinal dorsal horn. *Brain Res.*, 564: 132–137.

Todd, A.J., Russell, G. and Spike, R.C. (1992a) Immunocytochemical evidence that GABA and neurotensin exist in different neurons in laminae II and III of rat spinal dorsal horn. *Neuroscience*, 47: 685–691.

Todd, A.J., Spike, R.C., Russell, G. and Johnston, H.M. (1992b) Immunohistochemical evidence that Met-enkephalin and GABA coexist in some neurones in rat dorsal horn. *Brain Res.*, 584: 149–156.

Traub, R.J., Iadarola, M.J. and Ruda, M.A. (1989) Effect of multiple dorsal rhizotomies on calcitonin gene-related peptide-like immunoreactivity in the lumbosacral dorsal spinal cord of the cat: a radioimmunoassay analysis. *Peptides*, 10: 979–983.

Traub, R.J., Allen, B., Humphrey, E. and Ruda, M.A. (1990) Analysis of calcitonin gene-related peptide-like immunoreactivity in the cat dorsal spinal cord and dorsal root ganglia provide evidence for a multisegmental projection of nociceptive C-fiber primary afferents. *J. Comp. Neurol.*, 302: 562–574.

Ulfhake, B., Cullheim, S., Hökfelt, T. and Visser, T.J. (1987) The combined use of immunohistochemistry and intracellular staining with horseradish peroxidase for light and electron microscopic studies of transmitter-identified inputs to functionally characterized neurons. *Brain Res.*, 419: 387–391.

Verge, V.M.K., Wiesenfeld-Hallin, Z. and Hökfelt, T. (1993) Cholecystokinin in mammalian primary sensory neurons and spinal cord: in situ hybridization studies in rat and monkey. *Eur. J. Neurosci.*, 5: 240–250.

Wakisaka, S., Kajander, K.C. and Bennett, G.J. (1991) Increased neuropeptide Y (NPY)-like immunoreactivity in rat sensory neurons following peripheral axotomy. *Neurosci. Lett.*, 124: 200–203.

Warden, M.K. and Young, W.S. (1988) Distribution of cells containing mRNAs encoding substance P and neurokinin B in the rat central nervous system. *J. Comp. Neurol.*, 272: 90–113.

Westlund, K.N., Carlton, S.M., Zhang, D. and Willis, W.D. (1990) Direct catecholaminergic innervation of primate spinothalamic tract neurons. *J. Comp. Neurol.*, 299: 178–186.

Willis, W.D. and Coggeshall, R.E. (1991) *Sensory Mechanisms of the Spinal Cord*, Plenum Press, New York.

Yaksh, T.L. and Aimone, L.D. (1989) The central pharmacology of pain transmission. In P.D. Wall and R. Melzack (Eds.) *Textbook of Pain*, Churchill Livingstone, Edinburgh, London, Melbourne and New York, pp. 181–205.

Zhang, X., Ju, G., Elde, R. and Hökfelt, T. (1993a) Effect of peripheral nerve cut on neuropeptides in dorsal root ganglia and the spinal cord of monkey with special reference to galanin. *J. Neurocytol.*, 22: 342–381.

Zhang, X., Nicholas, A.P. and Hökfelt, T. (1993b) Ultrastructural studies on peptides in the dorsal horn of the spinal cord. I. Co-existence of galanin with other peptides in primary afferents in normal rats. *Neuroscience*, 57: 365–384.

Zhang, X., Wiesenfeld-Hallin, Z. and Hökfelt, T. (1994) Effect of peripheral axotomy on expression of neuropeptide Y receptor mRNA in rat lumbar dorsal root ganglia. *Eur. J. Neurosci.*, 6: 43–57.

F. Nyberg, H.S. Sharma and Z. Wiesenfeld-Hallin (Eds.)
Progress in Brain Research, Vol 104

CHAPTER 4

Peptidergic neurons in the vertebrate spinal cord: evolutionary trends

L. Brodin[1], C. Söderberg[2], V. Pieribone[3] and D. Larhammar[2]

[1]*The Nobel Institute for Neurophysiology, Department of Neuroscience, Karolinska Institutet, S-171 77 Stockholm, Sweden,*
[2]*Department of Medical Pharmacology, Uppsala University, Box 594, S-751 24 Uppsala, Sweden and*
[3]*Laboratory of Molecular and Cellular Neuroscience, The Rockefeller University, New York, NY 10021, USA*

Introduction

How did the peptidergic neuron systems in the mammalian CNS evolve? Were they present in the earliest vertebrates, like many of the non-peptide transmitter systems, or did they appear at later stages? Are the peptidergic systems similarly organized in all species, or do they differ? The answers to these questions would not only shed light on the evolution of the vertebrate CNS, but they would most certainly also improve our understanding of the functional role of peptidergic neurons. In some instances, comparisons of peptide sequences between species have made it possible to deduce the mutational events during the evolution of a neuropeptide. However, in order to understand how a specific system of peptidergic neurons has evolved, it is necessary to jointly compare its molecular features, anatomical organization, co-transmitters, target cells, etc. Due to the anatomical differences between mammals and non-mammals, such comprehensive comparative analyses may be difficult to apply to certain CNS regions, like the forebrain. In contrast, the spinal cord is well suited for this type of study, as its general outline can be recognized in all vertebrate classes, ranging from cyclostomes to primates (Petras, 1976; Fritsch and Northcutt, 1993). Moreover, the organization, connectivity and pharmacology of many spinal neuron systems have been thoroughly analysed in several different vertebrates, thus providing a well-established framework for comparative studies (see, e.g., Simpson, 1976; Rovainen, 1979; Roberts et al., 1986; Brodin and Grillner, 1990; Daw et al., 1993).

In this review we will attempt to illustrate some trends in the evolution of spinal peptidergic neurons, by comparing the molecular and anatomical features of systems, which have been characterized in mammals as well as in non-mammals (for other reviews relating to this topic, see Lazarus et al., 1985; Fasolo et al., 1988; Andersen et al., 1992; Larhammar et al., 1993a,b).

Neuropeptide Y: highly conserved structure and expression pattern in sensory systems

Neuropeptide Y (NPY) is a 36-amino acid peptide (Tatemoto et al., 1982), which is abundant and widespread in the central and peripheral nervous system (McDonald, 1988). The NPY family of peptides includes also the gut endocrine peptide YY (PYY), and a pancreas hormone, which is termed pancreatic polypeptide (PP) in tetrapods, and peptide-tyrosine (PY) in teleost fishes (for review see, Larhammar et al., 1993b). The distinction between NPY and PYY in non-mammalian vertebrates for long remained unclear, mainly because of the similarities between their immunological and chemical properties. Extensive sequence analyses along with studies of the tissue distribution of NPY-related peptides have now resolved this issue, and shown that both peptides were already present in the earliest vertebrate ancestor (see below, Larhammar et al., 1993a; Söderberg et al., 1994).

Seventeen vertebrate NPY sequences are known, which display an impressive degree of sequence conservation (Fig. 1A). Most mammals have identical NPY sequences and the cartilaginous fish *Torpedo marmorata* sequence differs from the human sequence at only three positions. Since the *Torpedo* sequence has no unique positions as compared to bony fishes and tetrapods, it is likely to be identical to NPY of the common ancestor of fish and mammals (Blomqvist et al., 1992). The most distant NPY sequence as compared to mammalian NPY has been deduced from a cDNA clone of the river lamprey (*Lampetra fluviatilis*; Söderberg et al., 1994). Lampreys are our most distant relatives in the vertebrate tree and are considered to have retained many ancestral features since their divergence from the an-

cestor of the jawed vertebrates (gnathostomes) approximately 450 million years ago (Hotton, 1976; Nieuwenhuys, 1977). Lamprey NPY displays 83% identity to human NPY (30 out of 36 positions; Fig. 1A). While peptides containing NPY-like sequences have also been isolated from molluscs and worms (Larhammar et al., 1993a), these have not been conclusively shown to be evolutionarily related to NPY (cf. also NPY-like immunoreactivity in invertebrates, Larhammar et al., 1993b).

The spinal cord of all vertebrates, ranging from lampreys to mammals, appears to contain high levels of NPY (de Quidt et al., 1990; Rawitch et al., 1992; Andersen et al., 1993; Söderberg et al., 1994). Several anatomical classes of NPY-immunoreactive neurons have been identified, but some caution is required in the interpretation of immunohistochemical data, due to the potential cross-reactivity between the different members of the NPY family (see discussion in Pieribone et al., 1992). In mammals, most of the NPY-immunoreactivity belongs to a system of dorsal horn interneurons (Fig. 2). Their cell bodies are located in the substantia gelatinosa and provide a dense local innervation of this area, which is similar at all levels of the spinal cord (Gibson et al., 1984; Sasek and Elde, 1985). At the lumbar level, a moderate number of NPY cells have also been detected in the ventral horn (Sasek and Elde, 1985). The intermediolateral column of the thoracic cord is innervated by NPY fibers, which probably derive from noradrenergic neurons in the brainstem (Everitt et al., 1984; de Quidt et al., 1990). After peripheral nerve lesions, NPY has also been detected in dorsal root ganglion cells (Wakisaka et al., 1991; Hökfelt, this volume).

Comparative studies have suggested that the NPY neuron system in the dorsal horn has been evolutionarily conserved. In an amphibian (*Rana ridibunda*, Danger et al., 1985), and two species of lampreys (Fig. 2; *Lampetra fluviatilis* and *Ichthyomyzon unicuspis*; Brodin et al., 1989b), NPY-containing cell bodies in the dorsal horn supply a dense local innervation of NPY-immunoreactive

A. Alignment of Neuropeptide Y (NPY) Sequences

```
                    1         10        20        30    36
                    |         |         |         |     |
NPY rat             YPSKPDNPGEDAPAEDMARYYSALRHYINLITRQRY
NPY human           -----------------------------------
NPY chicken         ------S----------------------------
NPY Xenopus laevis  ------------------K----------------
NPY goldfish        --T-------G----EL-K----------------
NPY Torpedo marm.   ----------G-----L-K----------------
NPY river lamprey   F-N---S-----------L---L--U---------
```

B. Alignment of Peptide YY (PYY) Sequences

```
                    1         10        20        30    36
                    |         |         |         |     |
PYY rat             YPAKPEAPGEDASPEELSRYYASLRHYLNLUTRQRY
PYY human           --I--------------N-----------------
PYY chicken         A--P---S--DA-----IAQ-FSA----I------
PYY Rana ridibunda  --P---N---------MTK-LTA----I------
PYY salmon          --P---N-----P----AK--TA----I--I-----
PYY spiny dogfish   --P---N-----P----AK--SA----I--I-----
PYY river lamprey   F-P--DN--DN----QMA--K-AU---I--I-----
```

Fig. 1. Sequences of neuropeptide Y-related peptides in different vertebrates. A. Alignment of neuropeptide Y from different species. The amino acids which differ from the rat sequence have been indicated. B. Alignment of peptide YY from different species. Note the larger degree of variability as compared to the NPY sequences (see text for references).

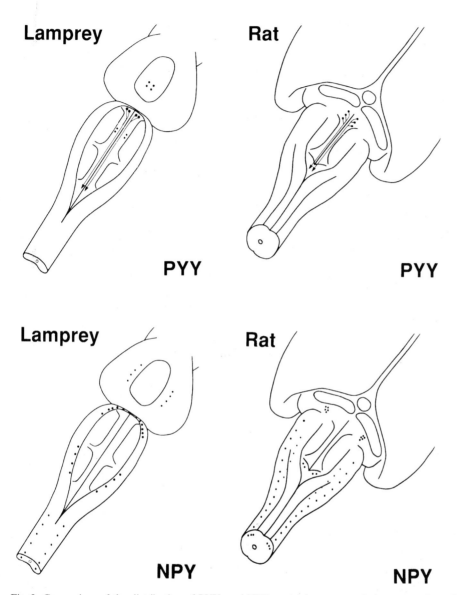

Fig. 2. Comparison of the distribution of PYY- and NPY-containing neurons in lamprey and rat. Schematic representation of the brainstem and spinal cord. In the diagrams of the rat brain, the cerebellum has been removed. In both rat and lamprey, a collection of large bulbospinal neurons, located in the medial part of the rostral medulla express PYY mRNA, along with immunoreactivity to PYY (Söderberg et al., 1989; Pieribone et al., 1992). The NPY neurons have a different distribution. In both rat and lamprey, cells containing NPY mRNA and NPY immunoreactivity occur in the dorsal horn and along the lateral edge of the lower brainstem. The NPY cells present in the dorsal medulla of rat (C3 adrenergic cell group), and the PYY mRNA expressing cells scattered in the lateral cell column of the lamprey spinal cord have been omitted from this diagram. (From Pieribone et al., 1992.)

fibers. In lamprey, the identity of the peptide has been verified with in situ hybridization (Söderberg et al., 1994). While this system is strategically located to influence sensory input to the spinal cord, termination areas of cranial nerve afferents also receive a dense NPY innervation, suggesting a similar role for NPY in the lower brainstem (Brodin et al., 1989; de Quidt et al., 1990; cf. also newt, Perroteau et al., 1988).

In primary cultures of rat dorsal root ganglion cells, NPY has been found to reduce voltage-gated calcium currents and to inhibit K^+-evoked release of substance P (Walker et al., 1988; Bleakman et al., 1991). This makes it likely that NPY can modulate transmitter release from sensory afferents in vivo, by influencing presynaptic calcium channels. It is as yet unclear if NPY exerts similar effects also in other vertebrates. Initial studies in lamprey have shown that NPY can depolarize mechanosensory neurons in situ (J. Tegnér, personal communication). As NPY can act via at least three distinct receptor types, which may be located either pre- or postsynaptically (Dumont et al., 1992; Grundemar et al., 1993), it would not seem unlikely that NPY has a complex action in the dorsal horn, of which the details perhaps differ between species. The anatomical conservation of the dorsal NPY system suggests, however, that NPY may have retained a basic role as a modulator of spinal sensory inflow throughout vertebrate evolution.

Peptide YY: conserved role as gut hormone and reticulospinal neuropeptide

Peptide YY (PYY) sequences are known for several vertebrates (Fig. 1B). For some of these, the identification as PYY has remained uncertain as they show higher identity to mammalian NPY than to mammalian PYY (cf. above). Comparison of a large set of vertebrate sequences showed that this is due to a more rapid divergence of mammalian PYY (Larhammar et al., 1993a). Overall, the PYY sequences display more variability than the NPY sequences, particularly in the mammalian lineage and in chicken. Nevertheless, frog and shark PYY are 83% identical and human and shark PYY are 75% identical. Even the latter percentage is in fact higher than for the endocrine peptides ACTH, insulin and calcitonin (see Larhammar et al., 1993b). The chicken sequence is the most divergent tetrapod sequence

and is the only peptide in the entire NPY family (some 60 sequences known) that is 37- instead of 36-amino acids long.

Peptide YY has been identified in two species of lampreys; one of these peptides was extracted from the intestine of the sea lamprey, *Petromyzon marinus* (Conlon et al., 1991), and the other was deduced from a cDNA clone from the river lamprey, *Lampetra fluviatilis* (Söderberg et al., 1994). Somewhat surprisingly, the PYY sequences are only 69% identical between these two lamprey species. The *Lampetra* peptide is about equally similar to mammalian NPY and PYY. By using oligonucleotide probes corresponding to the *Lampetra* cDNA clone, its identity as PYY could, however, be determined by analysis of its tissue distribution (Fig. 3; Söderberg, 1994; and below).

Peptide YY has primarily been considered as a gut hormone (de Quidt et al., 1990), but the demonstration of a PYY-immunoreactive reticulospinal system in rat (Fig. 2; Broomée et al., 1985; Ekman et al., 1986) and lamprey (Fig. 2; Brodin et al., 1989b), along with the demonstration of PYY-immunoreactivity in the frog and lizard CNS (Böttcher et al., 1985), suggested an additional role as a neuropeptide (cf. also Böttcher et al., 1993). In situ hybridization studies in both rat and lamprey (Fig. 3A,B) has confirmed that these neurons indeed contain PYY (Pieribone et al., 1992; Söderberg et al., 1994). The latter studies also showed that the expression of PYY mRNA in the CNS is far more abundant in lamprey than in rat. In both species the reticulospinal PYY cells are comparatively large, but fairly few in number. They are located in a restricted area near the midline in the most rostral part of the medulla oblongata (Figs. 2,3). The spinal projection of these neurons has been verified by retrograde tracing combined with immunohistochemistry (Fig. 4). As the rostral midline area of the lamprey medulla is known to contain glutamatergic neurons (Brodin et al., 1989a), it remains a possibility that the reticulospinal PYY neurons use glutamate as their fast transmitter. In the lamprey spinal cord, PYY mRNA also occurs in cell bodies scattered in the

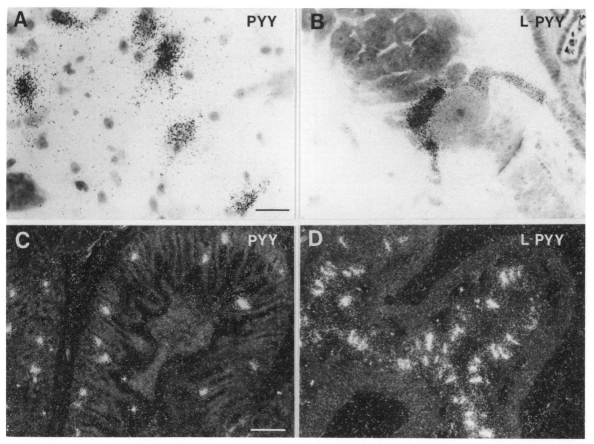

Fig. 3. Localization of PYY mRNA in rat and lamprey. Sections of the rostral medulla from rat (A) and lamprey (B) were hybridized with probes designed after cDNA sequences encoding PYY in each of the species. Hybridization occurs in large reticulospinal neurons in rat (A; Pieribone et al., 1992) and lamprey (B; Söderberg et al., 1994). The same probes also hybridize with numerous luminal cells in the gut of rat (C) as well as of lamprey (D). Scale bars 50 μm.

lateral cell column, while in the adult rat, no PYY mRNA has been detected outside the reticulospinal system (Pieribone et al., 1994). In the rat embryo, however, PYY mRNA has been detected in dorsal root ganglion cells (Jazin et al., 1993).

Taken together, these data indicate that PYY has served both as a gastrointestinal hormone and a neuropeptide from an early stage in vertebrate evolution. At present it is not possible to determine which of these functions that were first to emerge. In comparison to NPY, the structure of PYY shows a higher degree of variability between species, but the remarkable anatomical similarity of the reticulospinal PYY system between rat and lamprey, suggests the possibility that the functional role of PYY in this pathway has been conserved.

Cholecystokinin in motor and sensory systems: conserved and divergent patterns

The cholecystokinin (CCK)/gastrin family of peptides is characterized by a common C-terminal sequence, Trp-Met-Asp-Phe-NH$_2$ (Mutt and Jorpes, 1966; Vanderhaegen and Crawley, 1985), which is also present in the amphibian skin peptide caerulein (Wakabayashi et al., 1985). In mammals, CCK is abundantly expressed in the

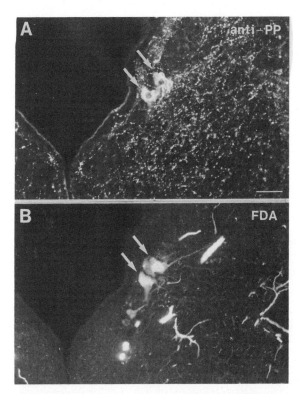

Fig. 4. Identification of peptide YY-containing reticulospinal neurons in lamprey by immunohistochemistry combined with retrograde tracing. A section from the rostral mesencephalon (anterior rhombencephalic reticular nucleus) taken from an animal which had received an injection of FITC-coupled dextranamine in the rostral spinal cord, was incubated with an antiserum directed against bovine pancreatic polypeptide. This antiserum cross-reacts with PYY in lamprey (Brodin et al., 1989). (A) shows the TRITC fluorescence, corresponding to PP immunoreactivity, and (B) shows the FITC fluorescence of the tracer. The identity of the peptide was further established with in situ hybridization (see Fig. 2). Scale bar = 50 μm. (From Brodin et al., 1989b.)

gut and CNS, while gastrin is expressed in the antrum (Dockray, 1979). Comparative studies indicate that CCK is phylogenetically old, while gastrin probably emerged at a more recent stage in vertebrate evolution. Thus, in amphibians (Johnsen and Rehfeld, 1992), bony fish (Sankaran et al., 1987) and cyclostomes (Holmquist et al., 1974), only one neural/gastrointestinal CCK/gastrin-related peptide has been identified. In amphibians this peptide has been termed 'gastrin',

as it was first isolated from the bullfrog antrum (*Rana catesbiana*; Johnsen and Rehfeld, 1992). However, nine out of its ten C-terminal residues are identical to human CCK, while only the C-terminal pentapeptide is shared with gastrin. According to immunochemical data this one and the same peptide occurs in high levels both in gut, brain and antrum, although the processing of the precursor appears to differ between tissues (Johnsen and Rehfeld, 1992). In chicken, and possibly in turtle, distinct CCKs and gastrins occur in the brain/gut and antrum, respectively (Fan et al., 1987; Dimaline and Lee, 1990; Johnsen and Rehfeld, 1992). Binding studies indicate that the receptors for CCK have evolved in parallel with the peptides. Thus, distinct brain and pancreas receptors for CCK appears to be present in birds and mammals, but not in amphibians (Vigna et al., 1986).

With the recent characterization of a peptide from a protochordate, the evolutionary history of the CCK/gastrin family can be traced to an even earlier stage. A peptide isolated from *Ciona intestinalis*, termed cionin, was found to be identical with CCK in eight out of its ten C-terminal residues (Johnsen et al., 1990; Monstein et al., 1993). The precursor sequence also shows considerable homology with CCK, while the degree of similarity with gastrin is relatively low. Moreover, cionin is expressed both in the gut and neural ganglion of Ciona (Monstein et al., 1993), which further links it to vertebrate CCK.

The presence of CCK in the spinal cord has been documented in several mammalian species (Larsson and Rehfeld, 1979; Vanderhaegen and Crawley, 1985), as well as in goldfish (Sankaran et al., 1985) and lamprey (Brodin et al., 1988). Immunohistochemical studies have been performed in many species, but it should be noted that some studies have proved to be erroneous, as CCK antisera tend to cross-react with unrelated peptides (for discussion see, Ju et al., 1986; Brodin et al., 1988; Hökfelt et al., 1988). In mammals, 'genuine' CCK immunoreactivity and/or CCK mRNA have been found to occur in no less than four classes of neuron, including reticulospinal neurons (Mantyh and Hunt, 1984), dorsal horn interneurons (Vanderhaegen et al., 1982; Fuji et al., 1985), dorsal root ganglion cells (Lind et al., 1988) and motoneurons (see below; Cortés et al., 1990, 1991). In comparative studies, both differences and similarities between species have been noted. For instance, a prominent CCK immunoreactivity (Lind et al., 1988), and expression of CCK mRNA (Seroogy et al., 1990) occur in dorsal root ganglion cells of guinea pig. In rat, however, no corresponding immunoreactivity or mRNA has been detected (Hökfelt et al., 1988; Seroogy et al., 1990), although both species show a similar expression of CCK mRNA in other CNS regions (Seroogy et al., 1990).

In contrast, studies of reticulospinal neurons have shown yet an example of a striking similarity between distantly related vertebrates (cf. above). Thus, in lampreys (*Lampetra fluviatilis* and *Ichthyomyzon unicuspis*; Brodin et al., 1988), like in rat (Mantyh and Hunt, 1984; Hökfelt et al., 1988), the medial portion of the caudal medulla oblongata contain a group of CCK-immunoreactive neurons (Fig. 5). These neurons have a spinal projection traversing in the ventral and lateral funiculi (Brodin et al., 1988; cf. rat, Fuji et al., 1985). The peptide present in these cells reacts with antibodies directed to the C-terminal (Fig. 5A), as well as to the N-terminal part of mammalian CCK-8 (Fig. 5B), while their descending fibers also react with an antiserum directed to the mid-portion of CCK-33 (Brodin et al., 1988). Immunohistochemical analyses of the *Xenopus* spinal cord have suggested that a similar CCK system is present also in amphibians (Pieribone et al., 1994), although the cells of origin of this projection have not been directly identified. In rat, a proportion of the descending CCK neurons also contain 5-HT (Mantyh and Hunt, 1984), while no such co-existence has been observed in other species (Brodin et al., 1988; Pieribone et al., 1994). With regard to CCK-containing interneurons, it is unclear to what an extent these are present in non-mammals. In lamprey, the entire CCK innervation appears to originate from the brainstem

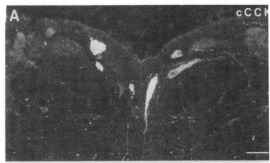
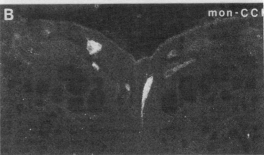

Fig. 5. Reticulospinal neurons in lamprey containing a CCl like peptide. A section from the lower medulla oblonga (posterior rhombencephalic reticular nucleus) was doubl stained with an antiserum directed to the C-terminal of CCK (cCCK) and a monoclonal antibody directed to the N-terminal of CCK-8 (mon-CCK). A shows the FITC-fluorescence indicating the C-terminal antiserum, and B shows the TRITC fluorescence corresponding to the N-terminal directed antibodies. Note the close overlap between the two types of immunoreactivity. (From Brodin et al., 1988b.)

(Brodin et al., 1988), while in stingray (*Daysatis sabina*) CCK-immunoreactive interneurons are present (Ritchie and Leonard, 1983). The identity of the peptide present in the latter neurons has, however, not yet been confirmed with sequence-specific antisera.

It is clear that CCK can exert potent effects in the spinal cord, but as yet, the information about its target neurons and cellular effects is limited. Locally or systemically applied CCK is known to have an antianalgesic effect in the rat spinal cord, which appears to be due to an antagonism of endogenous opioid mechanisms (for review, see Wiesenfeld-Hallin, this volume). Moreover, CCK can cause a depolarization of motoneurons (Long,

1993), but this effect can be blocked by NMDA receptor blockers, suggesting that it is indirect and mediated through the release of glutamate.

It can be concluded that CCK is a phylogenetically old peptide, which appears to have served dual roles as a neuropeptide and a gastrointestinal hormone even before the emergence of vertebrates (cf. PYY above). Its functional role in the spinal cord may possibly have been conserved in a reticulospinal projection, while certain species differences have also been documented.

Motoneuron peptides: ancient role of CGRP in neuromuscular transmission

In the above sections we have examined certain spinal cord peptides with regard to their primary sequence and expression pattern in different species. It should also be of interest to focus on a defined population of neurons, in order to find out whether or not these express the same peptide in different species. Cholinergic motoneurons and serotonergic raphespinal neurons are both suited for this purpose, as they occur in all classes of vertebrates, and show anatomical (Soller and Erulkar, 1979; Parent et al., 1984; Brodin et al., 1986; Brodin and Grillner, 1990; Tan and Miletic, 1990), as well as pharmacological (Hounsgaard et al., 1988, 1989; Venter et al., 1988; Wallén et al., 1989) similarities between species.

Mammalian motoneurons can express several peptides (see Kreutzberg, this volume), including calcitonin gene-related peptide (CGRP; Gibson et al., 1984b), CCK (Cortés et al., 1990, 1991) and galanin (Johnson et al., 1992). The present discussion will focus on the former, which has been most extensively studied. The occurrence of CGRP in motoneurons has been documented in several mammalian species (Gibson et al., 1984; Kreutzberg, this volume). The peptide has a wide-spread distribution among spinal and brainstem motoneurons, although subpopulations of cranial nerve motoneurons, which express galanin, may express little or no CGRP (Moore, 1989; cf. Johnson et al., 1992). While the sequence of CGRP (Rosenfeld et al., 1983) has not yet been determined in any non-mammal, immunochemical studies indicate that amphibian CGRP reacts with antisera to mammalian CGRP (Andersen et al., 1993; cf. Brauth and Reiner, 1991). In agreement with this mammalian CGRP has potent effects in the amphibian neuromuscular junction (see below). Immunohistochemical studies performed with mammalian antisera indicate that the expression of CGRP-like peptides in motoneurons is a widely distributed feature among vertebrates. Thus, spinal motoneurons in chicken (Villar et al., 1989), and different amphibians (Petkó and Santá, 1992; Csillik et al., 1993; Pieribone et al., 1994) exhibit CGRP-like immunoreactivity, while in lampreys a prominent CGRP-labelling has been observed in trigeminal motoneurons (L. Brodin, unpublished observation).

The experimental accessibility of muscle cells has stimulated many investigators to study the role of CGRP in neuromuscular transmission, and detailed functional studies have been carried out in rat, chicken and toad. These studies show that CGRP is transported to motor nerve terminals (Csillik et al., 1993) and released in a stimulus-dependent manner (Uchida et al., 1990). It binds to specific receptors on the muscle surface (Roa and Changeux, 1991), and elevates cAMP levels in muscle cells (Laufer and Changeux, 1987). Application of CGRP causes phosphorylation of ACh channels, which leads to an increased rate of ACh-induced desensitization, and thereby a down-regulation of the neuromuscular transmission (Mulle et al., 1988; Miles et al., 1989). In the developing neuromuscular junction, CGRP may instead up-regulate transmission, by causing a prolongation of the channel burst duration (*Xenopus laevis*; Lu et al., 1993). The basis for this difference is not fully understood, but it may be due to a difference in the subunit composition of the ACh channels between young and adult animals. In addition to these relatively rapid effects, CGRP may also have long-term effects, as an exposure of muscle cells to CGRP can increase the expression of ACh receptors (New and Mudge, 1986; Fontaine et al., 1986).

Taken together the experimental data thus implies that CGRP exerts a powerful regulatory influence in the developing and adult neuromuscular junction. As CGRP immunoreactivity has been detected in motoneurons of both cyclostomes, amphibians, birds and mammals, it seems likely that this role was established at an early stage in vertebrate evolution. With regard to other motoneuron peptides (Villar et al., 1989; Cortés et al., 1990, 1991; Johnson et al., 1992), much less comparative data is available. It is interesting to note, however, that CCK affects the neuromuscular transmission in amphibians, presumably via a presynaptic mechanism (Akasu et al., 1986).

Peptides in raphespinal 5-HT neurons: lack of evidence for evolutionary conservation

For a comparison, we will now consider the raphespinal 5-HT system. In mammals this system can be grossly divided into a ventral component, which innervates the ventral horn, and a dorsal component projecting to the dorsal horn. A range of neuropeptides have been detected in the ventrally projecting neurons, including substance P (SP), thyrotropin-releasing hormone (TRH), enkephalin, CCK, galanin and CGRP (for review, see Cullheim, this volume). Even among mammals, however, clear differences between species have been noted. For instance, quantitative analysis of the ventral horn have shown that more than 80% of the 5-HT-immunoreactive terminals in rat and cat exhibit SP-immunoreactivity, while in monkey only 20% of the terminals were found to be double-labelled (Wessendorf and Elde, 1987; Arvidsson et al., 1990a; Okado et al., 1991; cf. also Ni and Jonakait, 1989; Reddy et al., 1990). Moreover, in monkey a substantial proportion of the medullary 5-HT neurons express CGRP mRNA, and their terminals in the ventral horn exhibit the corresponding type of immunoreactivity (Arvidsson et al., 1990b). In rat and cat, however, similar immunohistochemical and in situ hybridization analyses have not provided evidence

for an expression of CGRP in raphespinal neurons (Cullheim, this volume).

In non-mammals, the analysis of the raphespinal 5-HT system has been hampered by the lack of sequence data for many of the relevant peptides, but immunohistochemical studies support the trend of marked species differences. For instance, fibers immunoreactive to SP and other tachykinins occur in the spinal cord of many species (see, e.g., Inagaki et al., 1981; Ritchie and Leonard, 1983; Wolters et al., 1986; cf. Lembeck et al., 1985), but double-labelling experiments performed in lampreys (Van Dongen et al., 1984; L. Brodin, unpublished observations), amphibians (Pieribone et al., 1994) and birds (Sakamoto and Atsumi, 1990; Okado et al., 1991), indicate that they are entirely distinct from the fibers containing 5-HT. Studies employing electronmicroscopic immunohistochemistry (Sakamoto and Atsumi, 1990) have reached the same conclusion. Moreover, spinal lesion experiments in toad, in which the build-up of immunoreactive material in descending fibers was analysed, further supports that the 5-HT and SP immunoreactivity occur in separate fiber populations (Pieribone et al., 1994). Other types of immunoreactivity, including that to galanin, CGRP, CCK, enkephalin and corticotropin-releasing factor was also localized to fibers lacking 5-HT (Pieribone et al., 1994), while the localization of TRH (see Zoller and Conway, 1989) yet remains to be studied. It should be noted, however, that co-expression of peptides and other transmitters is not an uncommon feature in non-mammals. For instance, the lamprey spinal cord has two additional classes of 5-HT neuron, midline interneurons and dorsal root ganglion cells, respectively. In contrast to the raphespinal neurons, both of these 5-HT systems co-contain immunoreactivity to peptides, including tachykinins and CGRP (Van Dongen et al., 1985, Brodin et al., 1988). Other examples of peptide co-storage in spinal neurons include that of GABA and somatostatin immunoreactivity (lamprey; Christenson et al., 1991), SP and galanin immunoreactivity (toad; Pieribone et al., 1994) and SP and CGRP immunoreactivity (frog; Venezio et al., 1987; cf. also Anderson and Reiner, 1990; Brodin et al., 1990).

Concluding remarks

As evident from this survey, our knowledge about the phylogenetic relationships of central peptidergic neuron systems is still fragmentary. This notwithstanding, a comparison of the most thoroughly examined systems can provide certain pieces of useful information. We have pointed out three systems, including NPY-containing dorsal horn neurons, CCK-containing reticulospinal neurons and CGRP-containing motoneurons, which may have been conserved from an early stage of vertebrate evolution. A fourth system, the PYY-containing reticulospinal projection, also appears to have been conserved anatomically, although the sequence of PYY shows a relatively large divergence between species. On the other hand, there are examples of systems in which the peptide content differs markedly between species, as for instance in the case of CCK-containing dorsal root ganglion cells and SP/CGRP-containing raphespinal neurons. As yet the comparative analyses of these systems have been confined to a limited number of species, and studies in other species will be required to determine the degree of conservation. If a given peptidergic system can be proven to have been strongly conserved during evolution it would seem reasonable to assume that it serves basic functions, which have been of vital importance during the course of evolution. Moreover, the function of such conserved systems can be explored in 'lower' vertebrates, some of which have a far less complex organization, and a better experimental amenability than the spinal cord of mammals.

Acknowledgements

The authors work was supported by the Swedish Medical Research Council (Project no. 10378) and the Swedish Natural Science Research Council (project B-BU 8524-317). We thank Dr. O. Shupliakov for valuable comments on the manuscript.

References

Akasu, T., Tsurusaki, M. and Ariyoshi, M. (1986) Presynaptic effects of cholecystokinin on neuromuscular transmission in the frog. *Neurosci. Lett.*, 464: 201–205.

Andersen, A., Tonon, M.C., Fasolo, A., Conlon, M., Pelletier, G. and Vaudry, H. (1993) Neuropeptides in the amphibian brain. *Int. Rev. Cytol.*, 138: 89–210.

Anderson, K.D. and Reiner, A.D. (1990) Extensive co-occurrence of substance P and dynorphin in striatal projection neurons: an evolutionary conserved feature of basal ganglia organization. *J. Comp. Neurol.*, 295: 339–369.

Arvidsson, U., Cullheim, S. Ulfhake, B., Bennett, G.W., Fone, K.C.F., Cuello, A.C., Verhofstad, A.A.J., Visser, T.J. and Hökfelt, T. (1990a) 5-Hydroxytryptamine, substance P, and thyrotropin-releasing hormone in the adult cat spinal cord segment L7: immunohistochemical and chemical studies. *Synapse*, 6: 237–270.

Arvidsson, U., Schalling, M., Cullheim, S., Ulfhake, B., Terenius, L., Verhofstad, A.A.J and Hökfelt, T. (1990b) Evidence for the coexistence between calcitonin gene-related peptide and serotonin in bulbospinal pathways in the monkey. *Brain Res.*, 532: 47–57.

Bleakman, D., Colmers, W.F., Fournier, A. and Miller, R.J. (1991) Neuropeptide Y inhibits Ca^{2+} influx into cultured dorsal root ganglion neurones of the rat via a Y2 receptor. *Br. J. Pharmacol.*, 103: 1781–1789.

Blomqvist, A.G., Söderberg, C., Lundell, I., Milner, R.J. and Larhammar D. (1992) Strong evolutionary conservation of neuropeptide Y: Sequences of chicken, goldfish, and *Torpedo marmorata* DNA clones. *Proc. Natl. Acad. Sci. USA*, 89: 2350–2354.

Böttcher, G., Ekblad, E., Ekman R., Håkanson, R. and Sundler, F. (1993) Peptide YY: a neuropeptide in the gut. Immunocytochemical and immunochemical evidence. *Neuroscience*, 55: 281–290.

Böttcher, G., Skagerberg, G., Ekman, R., Håkansson, R. and Sundler, F. (1985) PYY-like peptides in the central and peripheral nervous system of a frog and lizard. *Peptides*, 6(Suppl. 3): 215–221.

Brauth, S.E. and Reiner, A. (1991) Calcitonin gene-related peptide is an evolutionarily conserved marker within the amniote thalamo-telencephalic auditory pathway. *J. Comp. Neurol.*, 313: 227–239.

Brodin, L. and Grillner, S. (1990) The lamprey CNS: an experimentally amenable model for studies of synaptic interactions and integrative functions, In: H. Jansen (Ed.) *In Vitro Preparations from Vertebrate*, John Wiley and Sons, New York, pp. 103–153.

Brodin, L., Buchanan, J.T., Hökfelt, T. and Grillner, S. (1986) A spinal projection of 5-hydroxytryptamine neurons in the lamprey brainstem; evidence from combined retrograde tracing and immunohistochemistry. *Neurosci. Lett.*, 67: 53–57.

Brodin, L., Buchanan, J.T., Hökfelt, T., Grillner, S., Rehfeld, J.F., Frey, P., Verhofstad, A.A.J., Dockray, G.J. and Walsh, J.H. (1988) Immunohistochemical studies of cholecystokinin (CCK)-like peptides and their relation to 5-HT; CGRP and bombesin immunoreactivities in the brainstem and spinal cord of lampreys. *J. Comp. Neurol.*, 271: 1–18.

Brodin, L., Ohta, Y., Hökfelt, T. and Grillner, S. (1989a) Further evidence for excitatory amino acid transmission in lamprey reticulospinal neurons: retrograde labeling with [^{3}H]D-aspartate. *J. Comp. Neurol.*, 281: 225–233.

Brodin, L., Rawitch, A., Taylor, T.A., Ohta, Y., Ring, H., Hökfelt, T., Grillner, S. and Terenius, L. (1989b) Multiple forms of pancreatic polypeptide related compounds in the lamprey CNS: partial characterization and immunohistochemical localization in the brainstem and spinal cord. *J. Neurosci.*, 9: 3428–3442.

Brodin, L., Theodorson-Norheim, E., Christensson, J., Cullheim, S., Hökfelt, T., Brown, J., Buchan, A., Panula, P., Verhofstad, A.A.J. and Goldstein, M. (1990) Neurotensin-like peptides in the CNS of lampreys: chromatographic characterization and immunohistochemical localization with reference to the relation with monoaminergic markers. *Eur. J. Neurosci.*, 2: 1095–1109.

Broomée, M., Hökfelt, T. and Terenius, L. (1985) Peptide YY (PYY)-immunoreactive neurons in the lower brainstem and spinal cord of rat. *Acta Physiol. Scand.*, 125: 349–352.

Cameron, A.A., Plenderleith, M.B. and Snow, P.J. (1990) Organization of the spinal cord in four species of elasmobranch fish: cytoarchitecture and distribution of serotonin and selected neuropeptides. *J. Comp. Neurol.*, 297: 201–218.

Christenson, J., Alford, S., Hökfelt, T. and Grillner, S. (1991) Co-localized GABA and somatostatin use different ionic mechanisms to hyperpolarize target neurons in the lamprey spinal cord. *Neurosci. Lett.*, 134: 93–97.

Conlon, J.M., Björnholm, B., Jörgensen, F.S., Youson, J.H. and Schwartz, T.W. (1991) Primary structure and conformational analysis of peptide methionine-tyrosine, a peptide related to neuropeptide Y and peptide YY isolated from lamprey intestine. *Eur. J. Biochem.*, 199: 293–298.

Cortés, R., Arvidsson, U., Schalling, M., Ceccatelli, S. and Hökfelt, T. (1990) In situ hybridization studies on mRNA for cholecystokinin, calcitonin gene-related peptide and choline acetyltransferase in the lower brain stem, spinal cord and dorsal root ganglia of rat and guinea pig with special reference to motoneurons. *J. Chem. Neuroanat.*, 3: 467–485.

Cortés, R., Åman, K., Arvidsson, U., Terenius, L., Ceccatelli, S. and Hökfelt, T. (1991) Immunohistochemical study of cholecystokinin peptide in rat spinal motoneurons. *Synapse*, 9: 103–110.

Csillik, B., Tajti, L., Kovacs, T., Kukla, E., Rahic, P. and Knyihár-Csillik, E. (1993) Distribution of calcitonin gene-related peptide in vertebrate neuromuscular junctions: relationship to the acetylcholine receptor. *J. Histochem. Cytochem.*, 41: 1547–1555.

Danger, J.M., Guy, J., Benyamina, M., Leboulanger, F., Coté, J., Tonon, M.C., Pelletier, G. and Vaudry, H. (1985) Localization and identification of neuropeptide Y-like immunoreactivity in the frog brain. *Peptides* 6: 1225–1236.

Daw, N.W., Stein, P.S.G. and Fox, K. (1993) The role of NMDA receptors in information processing. *Annu. Rev. Neurosci.*, 16: 207–222.

Dimaline, R. and Lee, C.M. (1990) Chicken gastrin: a member of the gastrin/CCK family with novel structure-activity relationships. *Am. J. Physiol.*, 259: G882-G888.

Dockray, G.J. (1979) Comparative biochemistry and physiology of gut hormones. *Ann. Rev. Physiol.*, 41: 83–95.

Dumont Y., Martel J.-C., Fournier A., St-Pierre, S. and Quirion, R. (1992) Neuropeptide Y and neuropeptide Y receptor subtypes in brain and peripheral tissues. *Progr. Neurobiol.*, 38: 125–167.

Ekman, R., Wahlestedt, C., Böttcher, G., Sundler, F., Håkansson, R. and Panula, P. (1986) Peptide YY-like immunoreactivity in the central nervous system of the rat. *Regul. Peptides*, 16: 157–168.

Everitt, B.J., Hökfelt, T., Terenius, L., Tatemoto, K., Mutt, V. and Goldstein, M. (1984) Differential coexistence of neuropeptide Y (NPY)-like immunoreactivity with catecholamines in the central nervous system. *Neuroscience*, 11: 443–462.

Fan, Z.W., Eng, J., Moedel, M., Hulmes, J.D., Pan, Y.C.E. and Yalow, R.S. (1987) Cholecystokinin octapeptides purified from chinchilla and chicken brains. *Brain Res. Bull.*, 18: 757–760.

Fasolo, A., Panzica, G.C., Viglietti, C., Renda, T. and D'Este, L. (1988) Comparative chemical anatomy of the brain: concepts and methods. *Bas. Appl. Histochem.*, 32: 15–30.

Fontaine, B., Klarsfeld, A., Hökfelt, T. and Changeux, J.-P. (1986) Calcitonin gene-related peptide, a peptide present in spinal cord motoneurons, increases the number of acetylcholine receptors in primary cultures of chick embryo myotubes. *Neurosci. Lett.*, 71: 59–65.

Fritsch, B. and Northcutt, R.G., (1993) Cranial and spinal nerve organization in amphioxus and lampreys: evidence for an ancestral craniate pattern. *Acta Anat.*, 148:96–109.

Fuji, K.E., Senba, E., Fujii, S., Nomura, I., Wu, J.Y., Ueda Y. and Tohyama, M. (1985) Distribution and projections of cholecystokinin-8, vasoactive intestinal polypeptide and gamma amino butyrate-containing neuron systems in the rat spinal cord: an immunohistochemical study. *Neuroscience*, 14: 881–894.

Gibson, S.J., Polak, J.M., Allen, J.M., Adrian, T.E., Kelly, J.S. and Bloom, S.R. (1984a) The distribution of a novel brain peptide, neuropeptide Y, in the spinal cord of several mammals. *J. Comp. Neurol.*, 227: 78–91.

Gibson, S.J., Polak, J.M., Bloom, S.R., Sabate, I.M., Molderry, P.M., Ghatei, M.A., McGregor, G.P., Morrison, J.F., Kelly, S.J., Evans, R.M. and Rosenfeld, M. (1984b) Calcitonin gene-related peptide immunoreactivity in the spinal cord of man and of eight other species. *J. Neurosci.*, 4:3101–3111.

Grundemar L., Sheikh, S. and Wahlestedt, C. (1993) Characterization of receptor subtypes for neuropeptide Y and related peptides. In: C. Wahlestedt and W.F. Colmers (Eds.) *The Neurobiology of Neuropeptide Y and Related Peptides*, Humana Press, Clifton, NJ, pp. 197–239.

Hökfelt, T., Herrera-Marschitz, M., Seerogy, K., Ju, G., Holets, V., Schalling, M., Ungerstedt, U., Post, C., Rehfeld, J., Frey, P., Fischer, P., Dockray, G., Hamaoka, T., Walsh, J.H. and Goldstein, M. (1988) Immunohistochemical studies on cholecystokinin (CCK)-immunoreactive neurons in the rat using sequence-specific antisera and with special reference to the caudate nucleus and primary sensory neurons. *J. Chem. Neuroanat.*, 1: 11–52.

Hotton, N. (1976) Origin and radiation of poikilothermous vertebrates. In: R.B. Masterton, C.B.G. Campbell, M.E. Bitterman and N. Hotton (Eds.) *Evolution of Brain and Behavior in Vertebrates*, Erlbaum Publishers, New Jersey, pp 1–24.

Hounsgaard, J. and Kiehn, O. (1989) Serotonin-induced bistability of turtle motoneurones caused by a nifedipine-sensitive calcium plateau potential. *J. Physiol. (London)*, 414: 265–282.

Hounsgaard, J., Hultborn, H., Jespersen, B. and Kiehn, O. (1988) Bistability of alpha-motoneurones in the decerebrate rat and in the acute spinal cat after intravenous 5-hydroxytryptophan. *J. Physiol.*, 405: 345–367.

Inagaki, S., Senba, E., Shiosaka, S., Takagi, H., Kawai, Y., Takatsuki, K., Sakanaka, M., Matsuzaki T. and Tohyama M. (1981) Regional distribution of substance P-like immunoreactivity in the frog brain and spinal cord: immunohistochemical analysis. *J. Comp. Neurol.*, 201: 243–254.

Jazin, E.E., Zhang, X., Söderström, S., Williams, R., Hökfelt, T., Ebendal, T. and Larhammar, D. (1993) Expression of peptide YY and mRNA for the NPY/PYY receptor of the Y1 subtype in dorsal root ganglia during rat embryogenesis. *Dev. Brain Res.*, 76: 105–113.

Johnsen, A.H. and Rehfeld, J.F. (1990) Cionin: a disulfotyrosyl hybrid of cholecystokinin and gastrin from the neural ganglion of the protochordate Ciona intestinalis. *J. Biol. Chem.*, 265: 3054–3058.

Johnsen, A.H. and Rehfeld, J.F. (1992) Identification of cholecystokinin/gastrin peptides in frog and turtle. Evidence that cholecystokinin is phylogenetically older than gastrin. *Eur. J. Biochem.*, 207: 419–426.

Johnson, H., Hökfelt, T. and Ulfhake, B. (1992) Galanin- and CGRP-like immunoreactivity coexist in rat spinal motoneurons. *NeuroReport*, 3: 303–306.

Ju, G., Hökfelt, T., Fischer, J.A., Frey, P., Rehfeld J.F., and Dockray, G.J. (1986) Does cholecystokinin-like immunoreactivity in rat primary sensory neurons represent calcitonin gene-related peptide? *Neurosci. Lett.*, 68:305–310.

Larhammar, D., Blomqvist, A.G. and Söderberg, C. (1993a) Evolution of neuropeptide Y and its related peptides. *Comp. Biochem. Physiol.*, 106C: 743–752.

Larhammar, D., Söderberg, C. and Blomqvist, A.G. (1993b) Evolution of the neuropeptide Y family of peptides. In: C. Wahlestedt and W.F. Colmers (Eds.) *The Neurobiology of Neuropeptide Y and Related Peptides*, Humana Press, Clifton, NJ, pp. 1–41.

Larsson L.I. and Rehfeld, J. (1979) Localization and molecular heterogeneity of cholecystokinin in the central and peripheral nervous system. *Brain Res.*, 165: 201–218.

Laufer, R. and Changeux, J. (1987) Calcitonin gene-related peptide elevates cyclic AMP levels in chick skeletal muscle: possible neurotrophic role for a co-existing neuronal messenger. *EMBO J.*, 6: 901–906.

Lazarus, L.H., Wilson, W.E., Gaudino, G., Irons, B.J. and Guglietta, A. (1985) Evolutionary relationship between nonmammalian and mammalian peptides. *Peptides*, 6 (Suppl. 3): 295–307.

Lembeck, F., Bernatzky, G., Gamse, R. and Saria, A. (1985) Characterization of substance P-like immunoreactivity in submammalian species by high performance liquid chromatography. *Peptides*, 6: 231–236.

Lind, B., Hökfelt, T. and Elfvin, L.-G. (1988) Distribution and origin of peptide-containing nerve fibers in the celiac superior mesenteric ganglion of the guinea pig. *Neuroscience*, 26: 1037–1071.

Long, S.K. (1993) Cholecystokinin-induced ventral root depolarization of neonate rat hemicord in vitro. *Gen. Pharmacol.*, 24: 171–175.

Lu, B., Fu, W.-M., Greengard, P. and Poo, M.-M. (1993) Calcitonin gene-related peptide potentiates synaptic responses at developing neuromuscular junction. *Nature*, 363: 76–79.

McDonald, J.K. (1988) NPY and related substances. *CRC Crit. Rev. Neurobiol.*, 4: 97–135.

Mantyh, P.W. and Hunt, S.P. (1984) Evidence for cholecystokinin-like immunoreactive neurons in the rat medulla oblongata which project to the spinal cord. *Brain Res.*, 291: 49–54.

Miles, K., Greengard, P. and Huganir, R.L. (1989) Calcitonin gene-related peptide regulates phosphorylation of the nicotinic acetylcholine receptor in rat myotubes. *Neuron*, 2: 1517–1524.

Monstein, H.-J., Thorup, J.U., Folkesson, R., Johnsen, A. and Rehfeld, J. (1993) cDNA deduced procionin: structure and expression resemble that of procholecystokinin in mammals. *FEBS Lett.*, 311: 60–64.

Moore, R.Y. (1989) Cranial motor neurons contain either galanin- or calcitonin gene-related peptide-like immunoreactivity. *J. Comp. Neurol.*, 282: 512–522.

Mulle, C., Benoit, P., Pinset, C., Roa, M. and Changeux, J.P. (1988) Calcitonin gene-related peptide enhances the rate of desensitization of the nicotinic acetylcholine receptor in cultured mouse muscle cells. *Proc. Natl. Acad. Sci. USA*, 85: 774–776.

Mutt, V. and Jorpes, E. (1966) Isolation of aspartyl-phenylalanine amide from cholecystokinin-pancreozymin. *Biochem. Biophys. Res. Commun.*, 26: 392–397.

New, H.W. and Mudge, A.W. (1986) Calcitonin gene-related peptide regulates muscle acetylcholine receptor synthesis. *Nature*, 323: 809–811.

Ni, L. and Jonakait, G.M. (1989) Ontogeny of substance P-containing neurons in relation to serotonin-containing neurons in the central nervous system of the mouse. *Neuroscience*, 30: 257–269.

Nieuwenhuys, R. (1977) The brain of the lamprey in a comparative perspective. *Ann. NY Acad. Sci.*, 299: 97–145.

Okado, N., Matsukawa, M., Noritake, S., Ozaki, S., Hamada, S., Arita, M. and Kudo, N. (1991) Species differences in the distribution and coexistence ratio of serotonin and substance P in the monkey, cat, rat and chick spinal cord. *Neurosci. Lett.*, 132: 155–158.

Ozaki, S., Kudo, N. and Okado, N. (1991) Serotonin-positive fibers within the spinal motor nucleus of the newborn rat, with special reference to co-localization of substance P. *Neurosci. Lett.*, 16: 145–148.

Parent, A., Poitras, D. and Dubé, L. (1984) Comparative anatomy of central monoaminergic systems. In: A. Björklund and T. Hökfelt (Eds.) *Handbook of Chemical Neuroanatomy. Vol. 2: Classical Transmitters in the CNS, Part I.* Elsevier, Amsterdam, pp. 409–452.

Petkó, M. and Sánta, A. (1992) Distribution of calcitonin gene-related peptide immunoreactivity in the central nervous system of the frog, *Rana esculenta. Cell Tissue Res.*, 269: 525–534.

Petras, J.M. (1976) Comparative anatomy of the tetrapod spinal cord. In: R.B. Masterton, M.E. Bitterman, C.B.G. Campbell and N. Hotton (Eds.) *Evolution of Brain and Behavior in Vertebrates*, Erlbaum, New Jersey, pp. 345–382.

Pieribone, V.A., Brodin, L., Friberg, K., Dahlstrand, J., Söderberg, C., Larhammar, D. and Hökfelt, T. (1992) Differential expression of mRNAs for neuropeptide Y-related peptides in rat nervous tissues: possible evolutionary conservation. *J. Neurosci.*, 12: 3361–3371.

Pieribone, V., Brodin, L. and Hökfelt, T. (1994) Immunohistochemical analysis of the relation between 5-hydroxytryptamine- and neuropeptide-immunoreactive elements in the spinal cord of an amphibian (*Xenopus laevis*). *J. Comp. Neurol.*, 341: 492–506.

Rawitch, A.B., Pollock, H.G. and Brodin, L. (1992) A neuropeptide Y (NPY)-related peptide is present in the river lamprey CNS. *Neurosci. Lett.*, 140:165–168.

Reddy, V.K., Cassini, P., Ho, R.H. and Martin, G.F (1990) Origins and terminations of bulbospinal axons that contain serotonin and either enkephalin or substance-P in the North American opossum. *J. Comp. Neurol.*, 294: 96–108.

Ritchie, T.C. and Leonard, R.B. (1983) Immunohistochemical studies on the distribution and origin of candidate peptidergic primary afferent neurotransmitters in the spinal cord of an elasmobranch fish, the atlantic stingray (*Daysatis sabina*). *J. Comp. Neurol.*, 213: 414–425.

Rosenfeld, M.G., Mermod, J.-J., Amara, S.G. Swanson, L.W., Sawchenko, P.E., Rivier, J., Vale, W.W. and Evans, R.M. (1983) Production of a novel neuropeptide encoded by the calcitonin gene via tissue-specific RNA processing. *Nature*, 304:129–135.

Roa, M. and Changeux, J. (1991) Characterization and developmental regulation of a high-affinity binding site for calcitonin gene-related peptide on chick skeletal muscle membrane. *Neuroscience*, 41: 563–570.

Roberts, A., Soffe, S. and Dale, N. (1986) Spinal interneurones and swimming in frog embryos. In: S. Grillner, P.S.G. Stein, D.G. Stuart, H. Forssberg, R.M. Herman (Eds.) *Neurobiology of Vertebrate Locomotion*. MacMillan, London, pp. 279–306.

Rovainen, C.M. (1979) Neurobiology of lampreys. *Physiol. Rev.*, 59: 1007–1077.

Sakamoto, H. and Atsumi, S. (1991) Species differences in the coexistence of 5-hydroxytrypamine and substance P in presynaptic boutons in the cervical ventral horn. *Cell Tissue Res.*, 264: 221–230.

Sankaran, H., Wong, A., Khan, S.J., Peeke, H.V. and Raghypathy, E. (1987) Bioassayable cholecystokinin in the brain of the goldfish. *Neuropeptides*, 9: 103–111.

Sasek, C.A. and Elde, R.P. (1985) Distribution of neuropeptide Y-like immunoreactivity and its relationship to FMRF-amide-like immunoreactivity in the sixth lumbar and first sacral segments of the rat. *J. Neurosci.*, 5: 1729–1739.

Seerogy, K.B., Mohapatra, N.K., Lund, P.K., Réthelyi, M., McGehee, G.S. and Perl, E.R. (1990) Species-specific expression of cholecystokinin messenger RNA in rodent dorsal root ganglia. *Mol. Brain Res.*, 7: 171–176.

Simpson, J.I. (1976) Functional synaptology of the spinal cord. In: R. Llinas and W. Precht (Eds.) *Frog Neurobiology*, Springer, Berlin, pp. 728–749.

Söderberg, C., Pieribone V.A., Dahlstrand, J., Brodin, L. and Larhammar, D. (1994) Neuropeptide role of both peptide YY and neuropeptide Y in vertebrates suggested by abundant expression of both mRNAs in a cyclostome brain. *J. Neurosci. Res.*, 37: 633–640.

Soller, R.W. and Erulkar, S.D (1979) The bulbo-spinal indoleaminergic pathway in the frog. *Brain Res.*, 172: 259–276.

Tan, H. and Miletic, V. (1990) Bulbospinal serotoninergic pathways in the frog *Rana pipiens*. *J. Comp. Neurol.*, 292: 291–302.

Tatemoto, K. (1982) Neuropeptide Y: complete amino acid sequence of the brain peptide. *Proc. Natl. Acad. Sci. USA*, 79: 5485–5489.

Uchida, S., Yamanoto, H., Iio, S. and Matsumoto, N. (1990) Release of CGRP-like immunoreactive substance from neuromuscular junction by nerve excitation and its action on striated muscle. *J. Neurochem.*, 54: 1000–1003.

Van Dongen, P.A.M., Hökfelt, T., Grillner, S., Steinbusch, H.W.M., Verhofstad, A.A.J., Cuello, A.C. and Terenius, L. (1985) Immunohistochemical demonstration of some putative neurotransmitters in the lamprey spinal cord and spinal ganglia. 5-hydroxytryptamine-, tachykinin- and neuropeptide Y-like immunoreactive neurons and fibers. *J. Comp. Neurol.*, 234: 501–522.

Vanderhaegen, J.J. and Crawley, J. (1985) Neuronal cholecystokinin. *Ann. NY Acad. Sci.*, 448.

Vanderhaegen, J.J., Deschepper, C., Lotstra, F., Vierendels, G. and Schoenen, J. (1982) Immunohistochemical evidence for cholecystokinin-like peptides in neuronal cell bodies of the rat spinal cord. *Cell Tissue Res.*, 223: 463–467.

Venesio, T., Mulatero, B. and Fasolo, A. (1987) Co-existence of substance P and calcitonin gene-related peptide in the frog spinal cord. *Neurosci. Lett.*, 80: 246–250.

Venter, J.C., Di Porzio, U., Robinson, D.A., Shreeve, S.M., Lai, J., Kerlavage, A.R., Fracek, S.P., Lentes, K.U. and Fraser, C.M. (1988) Evolution of neurotransmitter receptor systems. *Progr. Neuorbiol.*, 30: 105–169.

Vigna, S.R. Thorndyke, M.C. and Williams, J.A. (1986) Evidence for a common evolutionary origin of brain and pancreas cholecystokinin receptors. *Proc. Natl. Acad. Sci. USA*, 83: 4355–4359.

Villar, M.J., Roa, M., Huchet, M., Hökfelt, T., Changeux, J.-P., Fahrenkrug, J., Brown, J.C., Epstein, M.C. and Hersh, L. (1989) Immunoreactive calcitonin gene-related peptide, vasoactive intestinal polypeptide and somatostatin in developing chicken spinal cord motoneurons. Distribution and role in regulation of cAMP in cultured muscle cells. *Eur. J. Neurosci.* 1: 269–287.

Wakabayashi, T., Kato, H. and Tachibana, S. (1985) Complete nucleotide sequence of mRNA for caerulein precursor for *Xenopus* skin: the mRNA contains an unusual repetitive structure. *Nucleic Acids Res.*, 25: 1817–1828.

Wakisaka, S., Kajander, K.C. and Bennett, G.J. (1991) Increased neuropeptide Y (NPY)-like immunoreactivity in rat sensory neurons following peripheral axotomy. *Neurosci. Lett.*, 124: 200–203.

Walker, M.W., Ewald, D.A., Perney, T.M. and Miller, R.J. (1988) Neuropeptide Y modulates neurotransmitter release and Ca^{2+} currents in rat sensory neurons. *J. Neurosci.*, 8: 2438–2446.

Wallén, P., Buchanan, J.T., Grillner, S., Christenson J., and Hökfelt, T. (1989) Effects of 5-hydroxytryptamine on the afterhyperpolarization, spike frequency regulation, and oscillatory membrane properties in lamprey spinal cord neurons. *J. Neurophysiol.*, 61: 759–768.

Wessendorf, M.W. and Elde, R.P. (1987) The co-existence of serotonin- and substance P-like immunoreactivity in the spinal cord of the rat as shown by immunofluorescence double labelling. *J. Neurosci.*, 7: 2352–2363.

Wolters, J.G., Ten Donkelaar, H.J. and Verhofstad A.A.J. (1986) Distribution of some peptides (substance P, Leu-enkephalin, Met-enkephalin), in the brainstem and spinal cord of a lizard, *Varanus exanthematicus. Neuroscience*, 18: 917–946.

Zoeller, R.T. and Conway, K.M. (1989) Neurons expressing Thyrotropin-releasing hormone-like messenger ribonucleic acid are widely distributed in *Xenopus laevis* brain. *Gen. Comp. Endocrinol.*, 76: 139–146.

SECTION II

Neuropeptide Receptors

F. Nyberg, H.S. Sharma and Z. Wiesenfeld-Hallin (Eds.)
Progress in Brain Research, Vol 104

CHAPTER 5

Opioid receptors in the superficial layers of the rat spinal cord: functional implications in pain processing

M.C. Lombard, D. Besse and J.M. Besson

Unité de Recherches de Physiopharmacologie du Système Nerveux de l'INSERM (U 161) and Laboratoire de Physiopharmacologie de la douleur de l'EPHE, 2, rue d'Alésia, 75014 Paris, France

Introduction

The role of opioids in nociceptive sensory processing in the spinal cord has been extensively reviewed (Duggan and North, 1984; Zieglgäns-berger, 1986; Besson and Chaouch, 1987; Dickenson, 1993; Duggan and Fleetwood-Walker, 1993). The superficial layers (I and II) of the dorsal horn which are the main termination sites of fine diameter primary afferent fibers are rich in endogenous opioid substances and are the main sites of action of morphine on the transmission of nociceptive messages at the spinal level. The aim of the present chapter is to focus essentially on opioid receptors in this region and on their functional implication in pain processing, reporting results of quantitative studies performed in the rat by our group.

In the first part of this study, we will try to answer the following questions. What are the respective proportions of the three main types of opioid receptors in the superficial layers of the dorsal horn? Are these proportions similar over the rostrocaudal axis of the spinal cord? What are their respective pre- and postsynaptic proportions? Can the rostrocaudal distribution of the thin primary afferent fibers arising from a single dorsal root be evaluated using opioid ligands as

markers? Is there a plasticity of opioid receptors in chronic deafferentation states?

In the second part, we will discuss the modifications of opioid binding sites density in relation to neuropathic pain.

Localization, distribution and plasticity of opioid receptors

General considerations

Numerous studies have demonstrated the presence of opioid receptors within the superficial dorsal horn of many species (see Refs. in Besse et al., 1990; Gouadères et al., 1991) including humans (Faull and Villiger, 1987). High proportions of these receptors are located on primary afferent fibers as demonstrated by the pioneering work of Lamotte et al. (1976), which showed a clear decrease in binding at this level after dorsal rhizotomy. Interestingly, following this report, several studies based on the administration of capsaicin in neonate rats (Gamse et al., 1979; Nagy et al., 1980) have shown that the opioid receptors are located on fine diameter primary afferent fibers. However, when we began our investigations, with a few exceptions, the majority of the previous studies did not provide data on the relative proportions of the three main types of opioid receptors μ, δ and κ, and no quantitative data were available concerning their pre- and postsynaptic locations. Moreover, difficulties arised when trying to compare the results of the different studies: a number of these investigations were binding studies, performed on membrane preparations where it is impossible to locate the site of binding, and most of the ligands used were not selective and did not allow a clear distinction between each type of receptor. Finally, in the studies considering deprivation of primary afferent fibers, the extent of the deafferentation lesions was, in many cases, rather restricted and the post-rhizotomy delay varied considerably between studies.

In an attempt to overcome the methodological differences mentioned above, we used highly selective ligands, [³H]DAMGO for μ receptors, [³H]DTLET for δ receptors, and [³H]ethylketocylazocine (EKC) in the presence of DAMGO and DTLET for κ receptors, with quantitative autoradiography and dorsal rhizotomies of various extents in the rat. The results consider: (1) the values of each ligand specific binding bilaterally in the dorsal horn superficial layers; and (2) the ratio of binding between the two sides. For further details concerning the methods, refer to the following papers: Zajac et al. (1989); Besse et al. (1990, 1991a,b, 1992, 1993a,b); Besson et al. (1990).

Relative proportions and distribution of opioid receptors over the rostrocaudal axis

In the dorsal horn superficial layers, the majority of opioid binding sites are μ sites, while δ sites are present in moderate density, with considerably fewer κ sites (Table I). This arrangement is found whatever the spinal cord level (i.e., cervical, thoracic, lumbar and sacral) (Fig. 1). Interestingly, the binding capacities for each of the three ligands are similar for each spinal cord level and consequently the specific opioid binding is homogeneous along the rostrocaudal axis (Table I). Consequently, the respective proportions of the three types of opioid receptors are remarkably homogeneous throughout the spinal cord (cervical, thoracic, lumbar and sacral levels) (Figs. 1 and 2). There is a high percentage of μ (70.4–74.3%), an intermediate percentage of δ (18.4–20%) and a low percentage of κ (7.3–9.5%) binding sites (Besse et al., 1991a). These results in the rat are in good agreement with the data presented by Stevens et al. (1991b) and Gouarderes et al. (1991). They are in contrast with former binding or autoradiographic studies reporting different proportions for the three types of opioid receptors and/or a rostrocaudal gradient of μ, δ and κ binding sites in the spinal cord of the same or other species (see Refs. in Besse et al., 1990; Gouadères et al., 1991) including hu-

TABLE I

Specific binding capacities of [³H]DAMGO, [³H]DTLET, [³H]EKC in the presence of 100 nM DAMGO and 100 nM DTLET at four rostrocaudal levels of the superficial dorsal horn, as determined by computerized densitometry

Spinal cord level	Specific binding capacity			Total opioid binding sites
	DAMGO	DTLET	EKC	
Cervical (C6–C8)	59.4 ± 2.9	14.8 ± 0.6	6.3 ± 0.7	80.5
Thoracic (T5–T7)	57.2 ± 4.9	16.2 ± 0.7	6.3 ± 0.6	79.6
Lumbar (L3–L5)	55.4 ± 5.7	15.8 ± 1.1	7.5 ± 0.2	78.6
Sacral (S2–S3)	59.9 ± 2.9	14.8 ± 0.4	5.8 ± 0.2	80.6

Values are expressed in fmol/mg of tissue equivalent and represent means ± S.E.M. ($n = 3$). The total opioid binding sites correspond to the sum of μ, δ and κ binding sites.

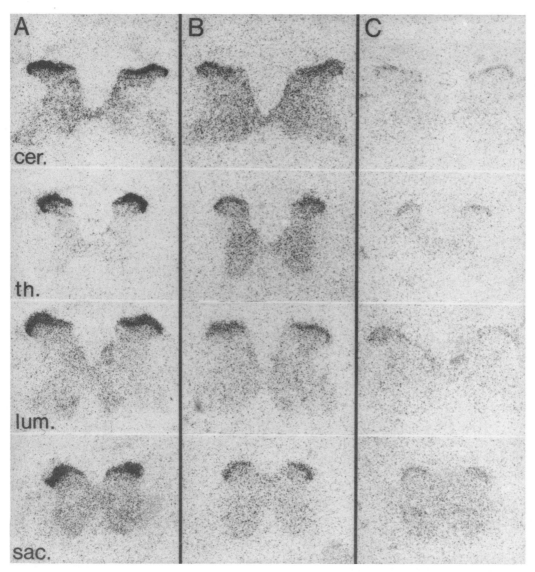

Fig. 1. Photographs of the autoradiographic distribution of the three ligands at different levels of the rat spinal cord: cervical (cer.), thoracic (th.), lumbar (lum.) and sacral (sac.). (A) Binding of [³H]DAMGO (μ sites). (B) Binding of [³H]DTLET (δ sites). (C) Binding of [³H]EKC in the presence of 100 nM DAMGO and 100 nM DTLET (κ sites).

mans (Czlonkowski et al., 1983; Gouardères et al., 1986). In human studies, Gouardères et al. (1986) reported very low levels, if any, of μ and δ opioid binding sites in lumbosacral spinal cord, the only specific sites being κ sites. In contrast, Czlonkowski et al. (1983) reported the existence of μ and δ opioid binding sites, in addition to κ

sites, at different segmental levels of the human spinal cord and a caudorostral gradient for the three types of site. There is no clear argument to explain these discrepancies. They may be due to the use of different ligands, tissue preparations, incubation conditions, postmortem delays. It is also possible that μ and δ sites are more labile

80

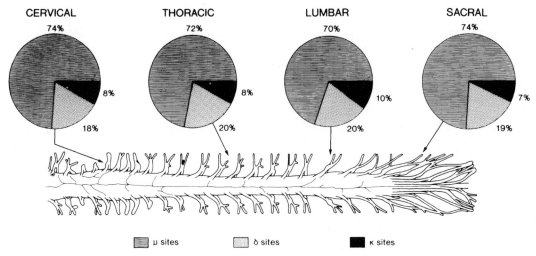

Fig. 2. Respective proportions of μ, δ and κ opioid binding sites in the superficial layers of the rat dorsal horn at cervical (C6–C8), thoracic (T5–T7), lumbar (L3–L5) and sacral (S2–S3) levels.

than κ sites. Further investigations using receptor autoradiography are still necessary to determine the exact comparative distribution of the various opioid receptors sub-types in human spinal cord. Nevertheless, and despite this controversy, hundreds of clinical reports claim that, in human, intrathecal administration of morphine (a preferentially μ binding sites agonist) is dramatically efficacious in relieving pain from different peripheral areas.

From the results we report above for the rat, several conclusions can be drawn:

● Since, in the superficial layers of the dorsal horn, opioid binding sites mainly reflect presynaptic sites (Lamotte et al., 1976; and see below) located on thin primary afferent fibers (Gamse et al., 1979; Nagy et al., 1980), our data suggest that there is an identical proportion of the three types of opioid receptor, whatever the peripheral location and/or origin of nociceptors.

● The high levels of μ, intermediate δ and low κ binding sites are in good agreement with several electrophysiological (Dickenson et al., 1987; Knox and Dickenson, 1987) and behavioral (see Yaksh et al., 1985; Leighton et al., 1988) studies

based on intrathecal administration of opioid substances showing that the antinociceptive effects of μ agonists were greater than those produced by κ agonists while, with δ ligands, intermediate effects were elicited.

● Although speculative, the similar densities of μ opioid receptors in the superficial layers of the dorsal horn along the length of the spinal cord support the idea that morphine could be equally effective in the relief of pain due to an excess of nociception arising from any part of the body. Despite the lack of systematic studies in animals trying to assess the efficacy of intrathecal administration of morphine at different levels of the neuraxis, clinical reports claim that a high percentage of cancer pain originating from various parts of the body can be adequately managed by intrathecal or epidural administration of morphine.

Pre- and postsynaptic proportion of opioid receptors

As mentioned above, a high proportion of opioid receptors are located on thin primary afferent fibers in the dorsal horn superficial layers. In order to define the optimal conditions to quantitatively evaluate pre- and postsynaptic opioid receptors, preliminary studies, based on dorsal rhizotomies, were carried out considering the influence of two parameters: the extent of the lesion and the post-lesion (PL) delay. These studies were done using unilateral dorsal rhizotomies of one, three, five, seven and nine roots at cervico-thoracic level. Quantitative measurements were performed in the C7 segment.

As shown in Fig. 3A, for μ binding sites, the decrease observed one week after the surgery in the side ipsilateral to the rhizotomy was clearly dependent on the extent of the lesion. All lesions induced a clear decrease of ipsilateral binding which was already significant after section of only one root (C7). This decrease in binding was also significant when comparing the effects of the section of one (C7) to three roots (C6–C8) and three to five roots (C5–T1). In contrast, no significant difference could be found when comparing the section of five to seven roots (C4–T2) and seven to nine roots (C3–T3). These results indicate that

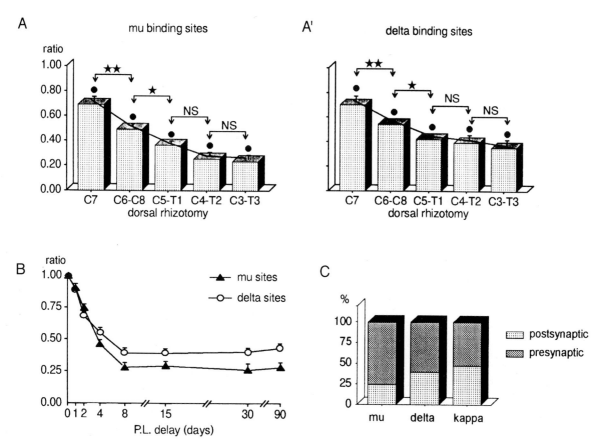

Fig. 3. (A and A') Rhizotomized/intact side ratio for μ (A) and δ (A') binding sites in Laminae I–II of the C7 segment, 1 week following unilateral dorsal rhizotomies of various extent (three rats per group). ● indicates significant difference in ratio ($P < 0.01$) as compared to intact animals; ★ $P < 0.05$ and ★★ $P < 0.01$ indicate significant differences between groups. (B) Curves showing the time-related decrease of the rhizotomized/intact side ratio for μ and δ sites in Laminae I–II of the C7 segment, following a unilateral dorsal rhizotomy of seven roots (C4–T2) (three rats per delay). Note that, for both types of binding sites, the maximal decrease is obtained at 8 days and that no further variation in ratio occurs for later delays. A significant difference between binding ratios of μ and δ sites is observed from 4 to 90 days post-lesion (PL). (C) Respective percentage of pre- and postsynaptic distribution of μ, δ and κ opioid binding sites in Laminae I–II of the spinal cord dorsal horn in the C7 segment.

after section of seven roots the C7 segment, which corresponds to the center of the deafferented zone, is totally deprived of primary afferent fibers. Similar data was obtained when considering δ binding sites (Fig. 3A′).

Taking into account the results obtained one week after the section of seven roots (C4–T2) we then considered the time-related modifications of μ and δ binding sites in this particular lesion following various survival times from 1 to 90 days. As illustrated in Fig. 3B, a decrease in binding was observed on the side ipsilateral to the lesion as early as the first day post-rhizotomy, the maximal loss being attained at 8 days PL. After 8 days PL, the residual binding remained stable over the period of analysis (90 days). The loss of μ receptors (71–74%) is significantly more pronounced than the loss of δ receptors (57–62%). This loss of binding is due to a decrease in the number of binding sites since the affinities of the remaining μ and δ sites are similar to those of the total receptor population in intact rats (Table II). We attribute the residual values to postsynaptic binding, whereas the decrease can be attributed to a loss of presynaptic sites.

Taken together, all these results indicate that a large unilateral lesion (seven roots) and a survival delay equal to or greater than 8 days are neces-sary, and sufficient conditions, for assessing with certainty, the relative proportions of pre- and postsynaptic opioid binding sites in the superficial dorsal horn. As illustrated in Fig. 3C, the presynaptic components of μ, δ and κ receptors are 76, 61 and 53%, respectively, the postsynaptic components being 24, 39 and 47%, respectively. It must be noted for the proportion of pre- and postsynaptic κ sites that the accuracy of the measurement is poor, since these sites are relatively weak ($< 10\%$) in the superficial dorsal horn.

The high proportion of μ and δ binding sites on primary afferent fibers favors a presynaptic action of opioids and, from a theoretical point of view, one can speculate that the depressive effects of morphine on the activity of dorsal horn nociceptive neurons would be considerably reduced after a large deafferentation lesion. This assertion is supported by the results of a comparative electrophysiological study we performed in order to evaluate the effects of morphine on the spontaneous hyperactivity of dorsal horn neurons in both intact and deafferented rats (Lombard and Besson, 1989). In this study, we reported that, in spinal decerebrate rats, 2 mg/kg i.v. of morphine was able to reduce by only 25% the spontaneous hyperactivity of dorsal horn neurons in-

TABLE II

Binding characteristics at equilibrium for [^{3}H] DAMGO and [^{3}H] DTLET in Laminae I–II of intact rats and rats with a unilateral (right) C4–T2 dorsal rhizotomy

	[^{3}H]DAMGO (0.5–24 nM)		[^{3}H]DTLET (0.5–24 nM)	
	K_d (nM)	B_{max} (fmol/mg)	K_d (nM)	B_{max} (fmol/mg)
Intact	1.3 ± 0.2	67.4 ± 4.1	2.3 ± 0.3	40.6 ± 3.5
Rhizotomized				
Left	1.4 ± 0.2	64.8 ± 2.0	2.0 ± 0.2	40.7 ± 1.0
Right	1.6 ± 0.2	24.5 ± 2.0^c	1.7 ± 0.4	$18.2 \pm 2.3^*$

Data were obtained by the linear regression of Scatchard and represent means $\pm$ S.E.M. ($n = 6$ for intact rats and 8 for rhizotomized rats). Degrees of correlation are comprised between $r = -0.948$ and $r = -0.999$.
$^*P < 0.001$ compared to values from intact rats.

duced by a large chronic dorsal rhizotomy (C5–T1), whereas the same dose was able to reduce by 50% the spontaneous activity of nociceptive neurons of polyarthritic rats. From this comparative electrophysiological study, it appeared that morphine was only half as effective in the deafferented rat compared with the normal arthritic rat. Thus the removal of presynaptic opioid receptors diminishes by about 50% the depressive effects of morphine on the spontaneous activity of nociceptive dorsal horn neurons.

Nevertheless, even after a large deafferentation lesion, it is clear that a reasonable amount of postsynaptic sites are still able to mediate some depressive effects of opioids. Thus it can be expected that increasing the dose of morphine will induce a more marked depressive effect on the activity of nociceptive dorsal horn neurons. In this respect, in the deafferented rats the effects of morphine on the spontaneous hyperactivity of dorsal neurons, although reduced, has been shown to be dependent on the dose, in a naloxone-reversible manner (Lombard and Besson, 1989). Several other lines of evidence are in favor of a postsynaptic action of morphine on dorsal horn neurons. As discussed by Wilcockson et al. (1986), electrophysiological studies have provided several possible postsynaptic actions of morphine: an inhibitory or blocking action on receptor-activated sodium channels (Barker et al., 1978, 1980; Zieglgänsberger and Bayer, 1976; Zieglgänsberger and Tulloch, 1979), an increased potassium conductance (Yoshimura and North, 1983) and an increased chloride conductance (Barker et al., 1980). Immunohistochemical studies have clearly established that some Laminae I and V dorsal horn neurons at the origin of the spinothalamic tract are directly contacted by enkephalin terminals (Ruda, 1982; Ruda et al., 1984). These connections are considerable in number since 67% of spinothalamic tract neurons in the monkey cervical cord have these terminals (Ruda et al., 1984). Finally, in freely moving mice, it has been shown that intrathecal morphine can suppress the behavioral syndrome (biting and scratching) elicited by intrathecal administration of substance

P (Hylden and Wilcox, 1983) or excitatory amino acids (Aanonsen and Wilcox, 1983). This latter result is in good agreement with the fact that iontophoretic morphine depresses the excitatory responses induced by glutamate on primate spinothalamic neurons (Wilcokson et al., 1986)

Opioid binding sites as markers for the distribution of thin primary afferent fibers in the superficial dorsal horn

Taking into account the fact that a high proportion of μ and δ opioid receptors are presynaptically located, we postulated that opioid binding sites could be possible markers for evaluating the anatomical distribution of the fine diameter afferent fibers in the superficial dorsal horn. In order to visualize and to quantify the distribution of these fibers arising from the C7 root, we used several experimental situations (Fig. 4B): control rats with the dorsal roots intact and lesioned rats with a unilateral dorsal rhizotomy of (a) the seven roots C4–T2, (b) the three roots above and below C7 (C7 spared) and (c) the C7 root alone. Binding measurements were made 8 days after the various lesions. The spinal cord distribution of μ and δ opioid binding sites belonging to the C7 dorsal root was then calculated according to the following methods: (a) subtraction of the data of the 'C7 cut' experimental situation from those in the 'intact' one and (b) subtraction of the data of the 'C4–T2 cut' experimental situation from those of the 'C7 spared' one. The combination of the results obtained with these two methods of calculation allowed assessment of the spinal distribution of μ and δ receptors belonging to the C7 dorsal root.

As shown in Fig. 4A, the distribution of μ sites belonging to the C7 root extends significantly in the segment of entry (C7), one segment caudal (C8) and two segments rostral (C6 and C5). More precisely, 40% of binding sites are found in the segment of entry, and the proportion reaches 80% if the two adjacent segments (C6–C8) are included. A similar distribution was observed for δ sites. This data is reminiscent of both anatomi-

84

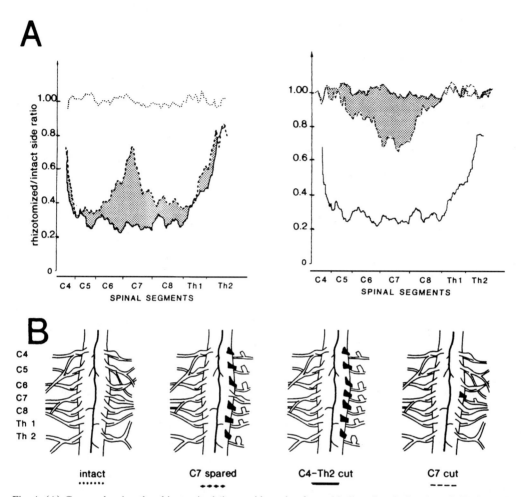

Fig. 4. (A) Curves showing the rhizotomized/intact side ratios for μ binding sites in Laminae I–II along the C4–Th2 cervical enlargement following unilateral dorsal rhizotomies of various extents illustrated by the diagrams in B (three rats per group). Measurements of binding were made every 120 mm. The curves on the left represent the ratios obtained in intact rats, rats with unilateral rhizotomy of C4–T2 and rats with rhizotomy of C4–T2 sparing C7. The curves on the right represent the ratios obtained in intact rats, rats with unilateral rhizotomy of C4–T2, and rats with unilateral rhizotomy of C7 alone. The shaded areas correspond to the component of μ binding sites belonging to the C7 dorsal root.

cal and electrophysiological investigations (Mc-Mahon and Wall, 1985; Sugiura et al., 1986; Traub et al., 1986; Traub and Mendell, 1988; Sugiura et al, 1989; Ardvidsson and Pfaller, 1990). In fact, the rostrocaudal projection of C-fibers is generally reported mainly over one to two segments rostral to the segment of entry, whereas the rostrocaudal projection of Aδ-fibers seems to be more widespread.

From these results it appears that for, a given spinal segment, there is a considerable overlap of the projections arising from two or three adjacent roots since, under our experimental conditions, 60% of the presynaptic receptors in the C7 segment did not belong to the C7 root. The functional relevance of this data can be assessed by clinical observations in humans. Indeed, it is well known that, according to neurosurgical reports, there is minimal hypoaesthesia after section of a single dorsal root of the brachial or lumbosacral plexus (White and Kjellberg, 1973). In contrast, at the time when dorsal rhizotomies were being proposed as a means to relieve pain originating from a localized peripheral area, it was reported that at least three consecutive dorsal roots must be sectioned in order to relieve pain (Ray, 1943). The clinical relevance of the preferential rostral projection of fine-diameter primary afferent fibers has not yet been established, but it may be an important consideration during neurosurgical procedures, namely selective posterior rhizotomy (Sindou et al., 1976) or the dorsal root entry zone lesion (Nashold and Ostdahl, 1979).

The results of this study, using opioid ligands as markers of fine diameter primary afferent fibers are in good agreement with those of another study by our group (Abbadie et al., 1992), which used *fos*-like immunoreactivity of dorsal horn neurons. Since the initial report from Hunt et al. (1987) demonstrating that various peripheral stimulation of primary sensory neurons, in the rat, causes the expression of c-*fos*-like protein immunoreactivity in nuclei of postsynaptic neurons of the spinal cord dorsal horn neurons, there is accumulating evidence that dorsal horn neurons receiving noxious inputs express c-*fos* when activated by noxious stimulation (see Refs. in Abbadie and Besson, 1993). In this respect, the C7-spared root preparation was used to evaluate, postsynaptically in the dorsal horn, the effects of a noxious stimulation, i.e., intraplantar injection of diluted formalin. Thus, in this experimental paradigm, it was possible to calculate the percentage of labelled neurons along the C4–T1 rostrocaudal spinal segment, activated via the fine diameter primary afferent fibers belonging only to the C7 dorsal root. As shown in Fig. 5A and B, there is a striking parallelism between the results of the two studies: in other words, the quantitative distribution of thin primary afferent fibers evaluated by opioid ligand binding is quite equivalent to the quantitative distribution of dorsal horn neurons expressing the protein c-*fos* in the superficial dorsal horn. The clinical relevance of these observations will be discussed later.

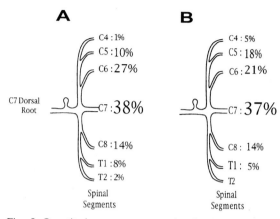

Fig. 5. Quantitative measurements in the C7-spared root preparation (section of C4–T2 sparing C7) of the rostrocaudal distribution of μ opioid binding sites associated with the fine diameter primary afferent fibers of the C7 dorsal root (A) and postsynaptic spinal neurons expressing c-*fos*-like protein following activation by formalin-evoked nociceptive inputs coming exclusively from the C7 dorsal root (B). Note the striking parallelism between the two distributions.

Plasticity of opioid receptors following dorsal rhizotomy

We have seen previously that, with a restricted lesion (i.e. after section of one dorsal root), the loss of opioid sites is relatively weak (60% of presynaptic sites remain, plus postsynaptic sites). Thus, in these conditions, one can speculate that morphine could still modulate the transmission of nociceptive messages at the spinal level. In addition the loss of opioid binding sites could be subject to compensatory regulation during chronic deafferentation states. To partly answer this latter question an experimental investigation was performed in order to gauge an eventual plasticity of opioid receptors, varying the extent of unilateral dorsal rhizotomies and the post-lesion delays (Besse et al., 1993)

In this study, several experimental groups were investigated: control animals with intact dorsal roots and lesioned animals with a unilateral dorsal rhizotomy of one to seven roots. Four different PL delays were studied: 1, 2, 4 and 12 weeks

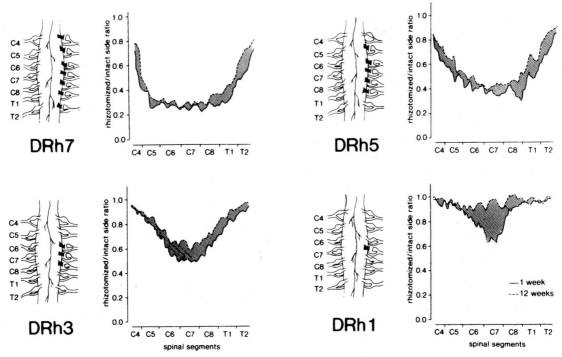

Fig. 6. Curves showing the rhizotomized/intact side ratios for μ binding sites in Laminae I–II along the C4–T2 cervical enlargement, 1 and 12 weeks after unilateral dorsal rhizotomies of seven to one roots (DRh7–DRh1, three rats per group). Measurements of binding were made every 120 mm. Hatched areas correspond to the recovery of binding at 12 weeks as compared to 1 week post-lesion.

for each lesion. The different lesions were performed so that all animals were the same age at the time of sacrifice. Figure 6 illustrates the changes in binding observed at 1 and 12 weeks PL. For the largest rhizotomies (seven or five roots), there is no significant difference in μ opioid binding after 1 and 12 weeks in the central C7 segment. For the more restricted rhizotomies (three or one root) there is a significant recovery of μ opioid binding toward values of the side contralateral to the lesion. For the latter two lesions, the percentages of recovery of binding at 12 weeks over the one-week level in the spinal segment central to the lesion (C7) were 18.1 ($P < 0.05$) and 85% ($P < 0.01$) for rhizotomy of three and one roots, respectively. In the case of the most restricted rhizotomy (one root), a significant recovery of binding was already present at 4 weeks (45%; $P < 0.05$). No difference in

binding could be measured between 1 and 2 weeks PL whatever the extent of the rhizotomy. Similar observations were made for δ sites.

Since no variation of binding was detected between 1 and 12 weeks PL in the central segment (C7) in the case of the large C4–T2 rhizotomy (seven roots), this data suggests that postsynaptic μ and δ sites are not significantly affected along the different PL delays. Consequently, the partial or almost total recovery of binding observed in this segment for the least extensive lesions (three and one roots) might be due to the presynaptic sites which are still present in a noticeable proportion at this level 1 week after these lesions. The recovery in binding could reflect either a simple receptor up-regulation producing an increase in receptor density in already existing terminals, or sprouting of terminals of fine primary afferent fibers arising from intact roots (see Refs. in Murray, 1992). The hypothesis of collateral sprouting, which is in good agreement with the anatomical study of McNeill et al. (1990) showing synaptogenesis in Laminae I and IIo of primary afferent CGRP immunoreactive terminals after chronic partial denervation, is very attractive. This assessment is supported by the fact that the magnitude of the recovery of binding is closely related to the degree of deafferentation: the less deprived of afferents a spinal segment is, the more pronounced the recovery in this segment. Primary afferent fibers projecting in Laminae I–II of the cervical dorsal horn have a rostrocaudal extent that does not exceed two segments above and below the segment of entry (see above and Refs. in Fitzgerald, 1989), and consequently the degree of deafferentation in a given spinal segment is dependent on the number of dorsal roots sectioned rostrally and caudally.

Our results are coherent with the concept that primary afferent fibers still present in partially deafferented regions, are capable, at least to a certain degree, of anatomical adjustments in response to injury. Moreover, the presence of an increased number of opioid binding sites in chronic lesions compared to acute ones suggests an increased capacity for opioid controls.

Changes in opioid binding sites in the dorsal horn and neuropathic pain

Many clinical anecdotal observations have reported an absence of efficacy of opioids in cases of neuropathic pain. Actually, few systematic investigations have been conducted; the conclusions were generally that neuropathic pain was insensitive to morphine. However, it has also been reported that patients with certain neuropathies may benefit from long-term opioid treatment. Thus, this subject is highly controversial (see Refs. in Arner and Meyerson, 1991; Foley and Portenoy, 1991). Clearly, it is of both theoretical and practical importance to determine if certain types of pain are indeed resistant to opiate treatment and, if so, why?

In order to explain the lack of, or the reduction in efficacy of morphine on neuropathic pain consecutive to peripheral lesions or plexus avulsion, three main hypotheses have been advanced (Devor et al., 1991).

The first hypothesis suggests that neuropathic pains are so severe that even morphine produces an insufficient analgesia. In other words, are opiates incapable of providing significant relief for pain above a certain intensity level? In this respect, there are suggestions in the literature that the pain response to transient noxious stimuli may be less sensitive to morphine than responses to sustained noxious stimuli. If this is true, lancinating pain and other paroxysmal transients which are common features of neuropathic sensation will respond poorly to morphine.

The second hypothesis is based on the observation of Campbell and co-workers (1988). These authors reported that sensory signals carried centrally along low threshold $A\beta$ fibers could be responsible for pain in some neuropathic conditions. Unlike small diameter nociceptive afferents, these fibers have few, if any, presynaptic opioid receptors and therefore the pain they evoke would be insensitive to morphine. This hypothesis is supported by an electrophysiological investigation we performed several years ago. In this experiment, the effects of morphine were evaluated on the responses of dorsal neurons to sural nerve stimulation: the responses to large myelinated $A\alpha\beta$ afferents were not influenced but there was a major reduction in responses due to the activation of both $A\delta$ and especially C-fibers (Le Bars et al., 1976). The specificity of such effects of intravenous opiates has been demonstrated in terms of isomerism, dose-dependency and reversal of the depression by naloxone.

The third hypothesis is relevant to the presence of a high proportion of opioid receptors on thin primary afferent fibers entering the spinal cord (see first part of this chapter). It is speculated that peripheral nerve lesions or posterior root avulsion induce a clear decrease in opioid binding sites. Thus fewer opiate receptors might yield a weaker opioid response. In this chapter, we want to discuss this third hypothesis.

Following dorsal rhizotomies of large extent (seven roots), the dramatic loss of opioid binding sites located on thin primary afferent fibers may explain why morphine is more effective in combating pain arising from nociceptors than pain due to large deafferentation lesions. This assertion is supported by the results of our a comparative electrophysiological study evaluating the effects of morphine on the spontaneous hyperactivity of dorsal horn neurons in both intact and deafferented rats (Lombard and Besson, 1989). These results, however do not totally support the classical clinical claims that morphine is ineffective against all neuropathic pains of peripheral origin. Indeed the interpretation of our data must be extremely cautious for the following reasons.

• As we have shown, even after a large deafferentation lesion, there still remains a reasonable amount of opioid binding sites located postsynaptically in the superficial layers of the dorsal horn and increasing doses of morphine still reduces, although to a lesser extent, the responses of nociceptive neurons.

• The spinal cord, where morphine exerts a direct depressive effect on the transmission of nociceptive information, is not its only site of action. Other sites of action have been clearly identified, for example morphine acts on descending control systems and directly depresses nociceptive signals in various supraspinal structures (see Refs. in Basbaum and Besson, 1991). Thus morphine can still be active at these levels after peripheral injury.

• For theoretical reasons, in our experimental approaches we used a large unilateral dorsal rhizotomy. This lesion aims to mimic, at least in part, the syndromes encountered after brachial plexus avulsions (Wynn-Parry, 1980, 1983). Thus this experimental model is quite different from the various other syndromes due to more restricted lesions and classified under the general term of peripheral neuropathy. Consequently, we looked at the fate of spinal opioid receptors in the rat model of neuropathy described by Bennett and Xie (1988).

In this model, the neuropathy is induced by placing four loose ligatures around one sciatic nerve. This procedure produces a chronic nerve constriction. Behavioral studies performed on this model have described a pain-related behavior, with mainly spontaneous symptoms and both hyperalgesia and allodynia in response to mechanical and thermal stimuli. According to the extensive investigation of Attal et al. (1991), the time courses of pain-related disorders are similar whatever the behavioral test: following an early period of hypoalgesia at 5 days PL, hyperalgesia develops, being maximal at 2 weeks PL, with a recovery occurring around 2 months PL. We studied, in this model, the modification of μ, δ and κ opioid binding sites at the following post-ligation delays : 3 days and 2, 4, 8 and 15 weeks (Besse et al., 1993).

In this model complex regulations of opioid binding sites occurred. Briefly, a significant bilateral up-regulation (30–50%) of μ binding sites occurred in Laminae I–II as early as 5 days PL as compared to intact rats. On the side contralateral to the ligation, this up-regulation was permanent all along the period of observation (until 15 weeks PL). On the ipsilateral side, the up-regulation was also permanent, but it was reduced at 2 weeks when a transient downregulation took place. This transient downregulation corresponds to a decrease in the ipsi/contralateral side binding ratio of 28% ($P < 0.01$). Interestingly, this delay corresponds to the period of maximal hyperalgesia. For δ sites, no significant up-regulation of specific binding could be measured in any side whatever the PL delay, but a 24% ($P < 0.01$) decrease in binding ratio was present at 2 weeks PL. For longer survival delays (4, 8 and 15 weeks PL), μ and δ binding ratios return towards control values. There was no significant modification of κ sites (labelled with [^{3}H]U.69593) whatever the post-lesion delay. These modifications in binding densities reflect changes in the number of binding sites since saturation studies failed to reveal any changes in receptor affinities.

Thus, from these results, there is apparently a relatively good relationship between behavioral observations (maximal hyperalgesia at 2 weeks) and the decrease in μ and δ ipsi/contralateral side binding ratios. Although the bilateral increase in [^{3}H]DAMGO specific binding was unexpected, complex bilateral modifications have also been reported in the same model by Stevens et al. (1991a), in a model of 'unilateral footrot' in the sheep by Brandt and Livingstone (1990a,b) and in a model of monoarthritis in the rat (Besse et al., 1993). We will not go further into details concerning this last point, but to explain this contralateral increase in μ binding one hypothesis can be proposed. It could result from regulation of spinal endogenous opioid systems as a consequence of activation of segmental, heterosegmental and/or supraspinal pain modulating systems in response to peripheral nociceptive input generated at the ligature site.

The decrease in ratio of μ and δ binding sites in the side ipsilateral to the ligature is reminiscent of the results from our restricted rhizotomy studies discussed above. Actually, the sciatic nerve afferents reach the spinal cord mainly via two dorsal roots, L4 and L5, and therefore the ligature procedure is far less damaging than dorsal rhizotomy or even sciatic nerve section. In these conditions, one can expect limited central metabolic alteration and/or degeneration of fine diameter primary afferent fibers. Concerning this point, maximal alteration of unmyelinated primary afferent fibers has been shown to occur around 2 weeks after the ligature in the distal part of the constricted nerve (Bennett et al., 1989; Gautron et al., 1990; Basbaum et al., 1991), while no evident signs of degeneration of these fibers can be observed in the dorsal horn superficial layers (Ralston et al., 1993). However, reduced terminals and synaptic contact are described at this level (Ralston et al., 1993), quite concomitant (20 days) with a depletion of SP (21%) and calcitonin gene-related peptide (19%) (Bennett et al., 1989).

It is clear that, in this animal model of neuropathy, the decrease in opioid binding sites ratio between both sides of the spinal cord is weak and transient. These variations are not likely to account alone for the decreased effect of morphine on neuropathic pains. Similar results were ob-

tained in the case of restricted unilateral dorsal rhizotomies. Moreover, as we have shown, the capacity of adjustment in response to injury (increase in number of opioid binding sites) after long-term delays provides an additional basis for responsiveness to opioids in some particular circumstances of partial deafferentation or peripheral nerve lesions.

From a clinical point of view, it is reasonable to speculate that the decrease in opioid binding sites that occurs in most of the neuropathies of peripheral origin is rather weak and cannot alone account for an eventual lack of effect of opiates on these pain syndromes. Consequently, from a general point of view, our data do not exclude the other two hypotheses: neuropathic pains are so severe that even morphine does not produce sufficient analgesia; Aβ fibers could be responsible for pain in some neuropathic conditions thus resulting in an eventual lack of effect of morphine.

In fact, under the general term of neuropathic pain, different pathologies can be distinguished, in which the spinal opioid binding sites are probably differently regulated. From this assertion, one can expect variable degrees of efficacy for morphine according to the precise physiopathological origin of the pain. In conclusion, the only way to assess the analgesic effects of morphine in neuropathic pain seems largely dependent on the elucidation of the underlying pathophysiological mechanisms with a parallel appraisal of individual pharmacodynamic and pharmacokinetic factors. If all these factors are taken into account, it could undoubtedly clarify some of the apparent interindividual variability of opioid analgesic effects described in the literature.

References

Aanonsen, L.M. and Wilcox, G.L. (1987) Nociceptive action of excitatory amino acids in the mouse: effects of spinally administered opioid, phencyclidine and sigma agonists. *J. Pharmacol. Exp. Ther.*, 243: 9–19.

Abbadie, C. and Besson, J.M. (1993) C-*fos* expression in rat lumbar spinal cord following peripheral stimulation in adjuvant-induced arthritic and normal rats. *Brain Res.*, 607: 195–204.

Abbadie, C., Lombard, M.C., Morain, F. and Besson, J.M. (1992) Fos-like immunoreactivity in the rat superficial dorsal horn induced by formalin injection in the forepaw: effects of dorsal rhizotomies. *Brain Res.*, 578: 17–25.

Ardvidsson, J. and Pfaller, K. (1990) Central projections of C4-C8 dorsal root ganglia in the rat studied by anterograde transport of WGA-HRP. *J. Comp. Neurol.*, 292: 349–362.

Arnèr, S. and Meyerson, B.A. (1991) Opioid sensitivity of neuropathic pain. A controversial issue. In: J.M. Besson and G. Guilbaud (Eds.) *Lesions of Primary Afferent Fibers as a Tool for the Study of Pain*, Elsevier, Amsterdam, pp. 259–276.

Attal, N., Chen, Y.L., Kayser, V. and Guilbaud, G. (1991) Behavioural evidence that systemic morphine may modulate a phasic pain-related behaviour in a rat model of peripheral mononeuropathy, *Pain,* 47: 65–70.

Barker, J.L., Smith, T.G. and Neale, J.H. (1978) Multiple membrane actions of enkephalin revealed using cultured spinal neurons. *Brain Res.,* 154: 153–158.

Barker, J.L., Gruol, D.L., Huang, M., MacDonald, J.F. and Smith, T.G. (1980) Peptide receptor functions on cultured spinal neurons. In: A. Costa and M. Trabucchi (Eds.) *Neural Peptides and Neuronal Communications*, Raven Press, New York, pp. 409–423.

Basbaum, A.I. and Besson, J.M. (1991) Towards a new pharmacotherapy of pain. *Dalhem Workshop Reports. Life Sciences Research Report 49*, Wiley, Chichester, 457 pp.

Basbaum, A.I., Gautron, M., Jazat, F., Mayes, M. and Guilbaud, G. (1991) The spectrum of fiber loss in a model of neuropathic pain in the rat: an electron microscopic study. *Pain*, 47: 247–380.

Bennett, G.J. and Xie, Y.K. (1988) A peripheral mononeuropathy in rat that produces abnormal pain sensation like those seen in man. *Pain*, 33: 87–107.

Bennett, G.J., Kajander, K.C., Sahara, Y., Iadarola, M.J. and Sugimoto, T. (1989) Neurochemical and anatomical changes in the dorsal horn of rats with an experimental painful peripheral neuropathy. In: F. Cervero, G.J. Bennett and P.M. Headley (Eds.) *Processing of Sensory Information in the Superficial Dorsal Horn of the Spinal Cord, NATO Asi Series, Vol. 176*, NATO, New York, pp 463–471.

Besse, D., Lombard, M.C., Zajac, J.M., Roques, B.P. and Besson, J.M. (1990) Pre- and postsynaptic distribution of μ, δ and κ opioid receptors in the superficial layers of the cervical dorsal horn of the spinal cord. *Brain Res.,* 521: 15–22.

Besse, D., Lombard, M.C. and Besson, J.M. (1991a) Autoradiographic distribution of μ, δ and κ opioid binding sites in the superficial dorsal horn over the rostrocaudal axis of the rat spinal cord. *Brain Res.,* 548: 287–291.

Besse, D., Lombard, M.C. and Besson, J.M. (1991b) The distribution of μ and δ opioid binding sites belonging to a single cervical dorsal root in the superficial dorsal horn of the rat spinal cord: a quantitative autoradiographic study. *Eur. J. Neurosci.*, 3: 1343–1352.

Besse, D., Lombard, M.C. and Besson, J.M. (1992) Time-related decreases in μ and δ opioid receptors in the superficial layers of the rat spinal cord following a large unilateral dorsal rhizotomy. *Brain Res.,* 578: 115–121.

Besse, D., Lombard, M.C. and Besson, J.M. (1993) Plasticity of mu and delta opioid receptors in the superficial dorsal horn of the adult rat spinal cord following dorsal rhizotomies: a quantitative autoradiographic study. *Eur. J. Neurosci.*, 4: 954–965.

Besse, D., Lombard, M.C., Perrot, S. and Besson, J.M. (1993) Regulation of opioid binding sites in the superficial dorsal horn of the rat spinal cord following loose ligation of the sciatic nerve; comparison with sciatic nerve section and lumbar dorsal rhizotomy. *Neuroscience*, 50: 921–933.

Besson, J.M. and Chaouch, A. (1987) Peripheral and spinal mechanisms of nociception. *Physiol. Rev.,* 67: 67–186.

Besson, J.M., Lombard, M.C., Zajac, J.M., Besse, D. and Roques, B.P. (1990) Deafferentation, nociceptive dorsal horn neurons and opioids. In: M. Dimitrijevic, P.D. Wall and U. Lindblom (Eds.) *Recent Achievements in Restorative Neurology, Vol. 3: Altered Sensations and Pain*, Karger, Basel, pp. 143–151.

Brandt, S.A. and Livingstone, A. (1990a) Receptor changes in the spinal cord of sheep associated with exposure to chronic pain. *Pain*, 42: 323.

Brandt, S.A. and Livingstone, A. (1990b) An autoradiographic investigation of the distribution of [^{3}H]DAGO and [^{3}H]DPDPE in the spinal cord of sheep and sheep experiencing chronic pain. In: J.M. Van Ree, A.H. Milder, V.M. Wiegant and G. Van Wimersma (Eds.) *New Leads in Opioid Research*, Excerpta Medica, Amsterdam, pp. 51–52.

Campbell, J.N., Raja, S.N., Meyer, R.A. and MacKinnon, S.E. (1988) Myelinated afferents signal the hyperalgesia associated with nerve injury. *Pain*, 32: 89–94.

Czlonkowski, A., Costa, T., Przewlocki, R., Pasi, A. and Herz, A. (1983) Opiate receptor binding sites in human spinal cord. *Brain Res.,* 267: 392–396.

Devor, M., Basbaum, A.I., Bennett, G.J., Blumberg, H., Campbell, J.N., Dembowsky, K.P., Guilbaud, G., Jänig, W., Koltzenburg, M., Levine, J.D. Otten, U.H. and Portenoy, R.K. (1991) Mechanisms of neuropathic pain following peripheral nerve injury. In: A.I. Basbaum and J.M. Besson (Eds.) *Towards a New Pharmacotherapy of Pain: Dalhem Workshop Reports. Life Sciences Research Report 49*, Wiley, Chichester, pp. 417–440.

Dickenson, A.H. (1993) Spinal pharmacology of opiates, adrenergic agonists and their interactions. In: Balagny, Cathelin, Clergue, Conseiller, Coriat, Cousin, Haberer, Lienhart, Motin, Payen, Rouby, Scherpereel, Seebacher and Viars (Eds.), *Analgésie Périopératoire*, Arnette, France, pp 13–25.

Dickenson, A.H., Sullivan, A.F., Knox, R.J., Zajac, J.M. and Roques, BP. (1987) Opioid receptor subtypes in the rat spinal cord: electrophysiological studies with μ and δ opioid receptor agonists in the control of nociception. *Brain Res.*, 413: 36–44.

Duggan, A.W. and Fleetwood-Walker, S.M. (1993) Opioids and sensory processing in the central nervous system. In: A. Herz (Ed.) *Opioids I*, Springer-Verlag, Berlin, Heidelberg, New York, London Paris, Tokyo, Hong Kong, Barcelona, Budapest, pp. 731–771.

Duggan, A.W. and North, R.A. (1984) Electrophysiology of opioids. *Pharmacol. Rev.*, 35: 219–281.

Faull, R.L.M. and Villiger, J.W. (1987) Opiate receptors in the human spinal cord: a detailed anatomical study comparing the autoradiographic localization of [³H]diprenorphine binding sites with the laminar pattern of substance P, myelin and Nissl staining. *Neuroscience*, 20: 295–408.

Fitzgerald, M. (1989) The course and termination of primary afferent fibres. In: P.D. Wall and R. Melzack (Eds:) *Textbook of Pain*, 2nd Edn., Churchill Livingstone, Edingurgh, London, Melbourne and New York, pp 46–62.

Foley, K.M. and Portenoy, R.K. (1991) The role of opioid analgesics in neuropathic pain. In: J.M. Besson and G. Guilbaud (Eds.) *Lesions of Primary Afferent Fibers as a Tool for the Study of Clinical Pain*, Elsevier, Amsterdam, pp. 277–292.

Gamse, R., Holzer, P. and Lembeck, F. (1979) Indirect evidence for presynaptic location of opiate receptors on chemosensitive primary sensory neurones. *Naunyn-Schmiedberg's Arch. Pharmacol.*, 308: 281–285.

Gautron, M,. Jazat, F., Ratinahirana, H., Hauw, J.J. and Guilbaud, G. (190) Alterations in myelinated fibres in the sciatic nerve of rats after constriction: possible relationships between the presence of abnormal small myelinated fibres and pain-related behaviour. *Neurosci. Lett.*, 111: 28–33.

Gouadères, C., Kopp, N., Cros, J. and Quirion, R. (1986) Kappa opioid receptors in human lumbo-sacral spinal cord. *Brain Res. Bull.*, 16: 355–361.

Gouadères, C., Beaudet, A., Zajac, J.M., Cros, J. and Quirion, R (1991) High resolution autoradiographic localization of [¹²⁵I]mu opioid receptors in the spinal cord of normal and deafferented rats. *Neuroscience*, 43: 197–209.

Heimer, L. and Wall, P.D. (1968) The dorsal root distribution to the substancia gelatinosa of the rat with a note on the distribution in the cat. *Exp. Brain Res.*, 6: 89–99.

Hunt, S.P., Pini, A. and Evan, G. (1987) Induction of c-*fos*-like protein in spinal cord neurons following sensory stimulation. *Nature*, 328: 632–634.

Hylden, J.L.K. and Wilcox, G.L. (1983) Pharmacological characterization of substance P-induced nociception in mice: modulation by opioid and noradrenergic agonists at the spinal level. *J. Pharmacol. Exp. Ther.*, 226: 398–404.

Knox, R.J. and Dickenson, A.H. (1987) Effects of selective and non-selective κ opioid receptor agonists on cutaneous C-fibre-evoked responses of rat dorsal horn neurones. *Brain Res.*, 415: 21–29.

Lamotte, C., Pert, C.B. and Snyder, S.H. (1976) Opiate recep-

tor binding in primate spinal cord: distribution and changes after dorsal root section. *Brain Res.*, 112: 407–412.

Le Bars, D., Guilbaud, G., Jurna, I. and Besson, J.M. (1976) Differential effects of morphine on response of dorsal horn lamina V type cells elicited by A and C fibre stimulation on the spinal cat. *Brain Res.*, 115: 518–524.

Leighton, G.E., Rodriguez, R.E., Hill, R.G. and Hughes, J. (1988) κ-Opioid agonists produce antinociception after i.v. and i.c.v. but not intrathecal administration in the rat. *Br .J. Pharmacol.*, 93: 553–560.

Lombard, M.C. and Besson, J.M. (1989) Attempts to gauge the relative importance of pre- and postsynaptic effects of morphine on the transmission of noxious messages in the dorsal horn. *Pain*, 37: 335–345.

McMahon, S.B. and Wall, P.D. (1985) The distribution and central termination of single cutaneous and muscle unmyelinated fibres in the rat spinal cord. *Brain Res.*, 359: 39–48.

McNeill, D.L., Carlton, S.M., Coggeshall, R.E. and Hulsebosch, C.E. (1990) Denervation-induced intraspinal synaptogenesis of calcitonin gene-related peptide containing primary afferent terminals. *J. Comp. Neurol.*, 296: 263–268.

Murray, M. (1993) Plasticity in the spinal cord: the dorsal root connection. *Restor. Neurol. Neurosci.*, 5: 37–45.

Nagy, J.I., Vincent, S.R., Staines, W.M.A., Fibiger, H.C., Reisine, T.D. and Yamamura, H.I. (1980) Neurotoxic action of capsaicin in spinal substance P neurons. *Brain Res.*, 186: 435–444.

Nashold, B.S., Jr. and Ostdahl, R.H. (1979) Dorsal root entry zone lesions for pain relief. *J. Neurosurg.*, 51: 59–69.

Ralston, H.J., III, Ralston, D.D., Desmeules, J. and Guilbaud G. (1993) Changes in synaptic organization of the superficial dorsal horn of the rat after experimental peripheral mononeuropathy. In: *Abstracts, Society for Neuroscience, 23rd Annual Meeting*, Society for Neuroscience, Washington, 575.6

Ray, B.S. (1943) The management of intractable pain by posterior rhizotomy. *Proc. Assoc. Res. Nerv. Ment. Dis.*, 23: 391–407.

Ruda, M.A. (1982) Opiates and pain pathways: demonstration of enkephalin synapses on dorsal horn projection neurones. *Science*, 215: 1523–1525.

Ruda, M.A., Coffield, J. and Dubner, R. (1984) Demonstration of postsynaptic opioid modulation of thalamic projection neurons by the combined techniques of retrograde horseradish peroxidase and enkephalin immunohistochemistry. *J Neurosci.*, 4: 2117–2132.

Sindou, M., Fischer, G. and Mansuy, L. (1976) Posterior spinal rhizotomy and selective posterior rhizidotomy. In: P.E. Maspes and W.H. Sweet (Eds.) *Progress in Neurological Surgery, Vol. 7*, Karger, Munich, pp. 201–250.

Stevens, C.W., Kajander, K.C., Bennett, G.J. and Seybold, V.S. (1991a) Bilateral and differential changes in spinal mu, delta and kappa opioid binding in rats with a painful, unilateral neuropathy. *Pain*, 46: 315–326.

Stevens, C.W., Locey, C.B., Miller, K.E., Elde, R.P. and Seybold, V.S. (1991b) Biochemical characterization and regional quantification of μ, δ and κ opioid binding sites in the rat spinal cord. *Brain Res.*, 550: 77–85.

Sugiura, Y., Lee, C.L. and Perl, E.R. (1986) Central projections of indentified, unmyelinated (C) fibers innervating mammalian skin. *Science*, 234: 358–361.

Sugiura, Y., Terui, N., Hosoya, Y. and Khono, K. (1989) Distribution of unmyelinated primary afferent fibers in the dorsal horn. In: F. Cervero, G.J. Bennett and P.M. Headley (Eds.), *Processing of Sensory Information in the Superficial Dorsal Horn of the Spinal Cord, NATO Asi Series, Vol. 176*, NATO, New York, pp. 15–27.

Traub, R.J. and Mendell, L.M. (1988) The spinal projection of individual identified A-δ and C-fibers. *J. Neurophysiol.*, 59: 41–55.

Traub, R.J., Sedivec, M.J. and Mendell, L.M. (1986) The rostral projection of small diameter primary afferents in Lissauer's tract. *Brain Res.*, 399: 185–189.

White, J.C. and Kjellberg, R.N. (1973) Posterior spinal rhizotomy: a substitute for cordotomy in the relief of localized pain in patients with normal life expectancy. *Neurochirurgia*, 16: 141–170.

Wilcockson, W.S., Kim, J., Shin, H.K., Chung, J.M. and Willis, W.D. (1986) Actions of opioids on primate spinothalamic tract neurones. *J. Neurosci.*, 6: 2509–2520.

Wynn-Parry, C.B. (1980) Pain in avulsion lesions of the brachial plexus. *Pain*, 9: 41–54.

Wynn-Parry, C.B. (1983) Management of pain in avulsion lesions of the brachial plexus. In: J.J. Bonica, U. Lindblom and A. Iggo (Eds.) *Advances in Pain Research and Therapy, Vol. 5.*, Raven Press, New York, pp.751–761.

Yaksh, T.L., Durant, P., Onofrio, B. and Stevens, C.W. (1985) The effects of spinally administered agents on pain transmission in man and animals. In: J.M. Besson and Y. Lazorthes, (Eds.), *Colloque INSERM, Substances opioiädes médullaires et analgésie: Aspects fondamentaux et applications cliniques (Spinal opioids and the relief of pain: Basic mechanisms and clinical applications), Vol. 127*, Les Editions INSERM, Paris, pp 267–306.

Zajac, J.M., Lombard, M.C., Peschanski, M., Besson, J.M. and Roques, B.P. (1989) Autoradiographic study of μ and δ opioid binding sites and neutral endopeptidase 24–11 in rat after dorsal root rhizotomy. *Brain Res.*, 477: 400–403.

Zieglgänsberger, W. (1986) Central control of nociception. In V.B. Mountcastle, F.E. Bloom and S.R. Geiger (Eds.) *Handbook of Physiology, The Nervous System, IV*, William and Wilkins, Baltimore.

Zieglgänsberger, W. and Tulloch, I.F. (1979) The effects of methionine- and leucine-enkephalin on spinal neurones of the cat. *Brain Res.*, 167 :53–64.

F. Nyberg, H.S. Sharma and Z. Wiesenfeld-Hallin (Eds.)
Progress in Brain Research, Vol 104
© 1995 Elsevier Science BV. All rights reserved.

CHAPTER 6

Tachykinin receptors in the spinal cord

V.H. Routh and C.J. Helke

*Department of Pharmacology, Uniformed Services University of the Health Sciences, 4301 Jones Bridge Road,
Bethesda, MD 20814-4799, USA*

Introduction and history

In 1931, von Euler and Gaddum isolated a hypotensive agent from equine brain that they named substance P (SP), due to its powdered form. About 50 years later, two similar peptides were isolated in mammals (Kangawa et al., 1983; Kimura et al., 1983; Maggio et al., 1983; Minamino et al., 1984), and are now known as neurokinin A (NKA) and neurokinin B (NKB) (Henry et al., 1987). All three of these peptides cause a rapid contraction of the smooth muscle of the gut, hence this family of peptides are referred to as 'tachykinins'. They are found extensively in the periphery, where they function as vasodilators and potent constrictors of many smooth muscles, as well as in the brain, where they are involved in neurotransmission. More recently, they have been found in discrete nuclei in the spinal cord, where they modulate many physiological systems via multiple tachykinin receptors. The focus of this chapter is on tachykinin receptors in the spinal cord, however, when relevant information is unavailable from studies of spinal cord, studies using other tissues will be discussed. Erspamer et al. (1981) noted different potencies for substance P and its analogues in different assays. This observation led to the discovery of three tachykinin receptor types, termed NK_1, NK_2 and NK_3. The existence of these receptor subtypes has been confirmed by molecular biology studies in which the genes for these receptors have been isolated (see Nakanishi, 1991, for review). SP binds preferentially to the NK_1 receptor, NKA to the NK_2 receptor and NKB to the NK_3 receptor. Binding characteristics for these receptors have been extensively characterized in tissues containing a single population of tachykinin receptors. For the NK_1 receptor, these include dog carotid artery and guinea pig ileum; for the NK_2 receptor, rabbit pulmonary artery, rat duodenum, rat vas deferens and hamster trachea; and for the NK_3 receptor, the rat portal vein. Although most of the pharmacological work has been done in tissues other than the spinal cord, Charlton and Helke (1985a) have reported that Scatchard analysis of SP binding in the rat spinal cord reveals high and low affinity binding sites (high affinity site: $K_D = 0.162$ nM, $B_{max} = 2.89$ fmol/μg protein; low affinity site: $K_D = 3.69$ nM, $B_{max} = 17.4$ fmol/μg protein). For extensive reviews of binding characteristics see Glowinski et al. (1987), Maggi et al. (1991, 1993), Burcher et al. (1991) and Mussap et al. (1993). The affinities of tachykinin receptors for their endogenous ligands is as follows: NK_1 receptor, SP > NKA > NKB; NK_2 receptor, NKA > NKB > SP; and the NK_3 receptor, NKB > NKA > SP.

Structure of tachykinin receptors

The genes for the tachykinin receptors have been cloned (for review see Nakanishi, 1991). In the human, the NK_1 receptor is on chromosome 2 (Gerard et al., 1991), the NK_2 receptor is on the q23pter portion of chromosome 10 (Gerard et al., 1990), and the chromosomal location of the NK_3 receptor is unknown. All three receptors are encoded in five exons which are very similar between the three genes, however, the introns for NK_1 and NK_3 are larger than those seen for the NK_2 receptor (see review by Gerard, 1993).

The basic structure of the tachykinin receptors is shown in Fig. 1. In the rat, the NK_1 receptor contains 407 amino acid residues, the NK_2 receptor contains 390, and the NK_3 receptor contains 452 (Masu et al., 1987). Tachykinin receptors share significant sequence similarity with receptors in the G-protein coupled receptor family, and like all G-protein coupled receptors have seven α-helical transmembrane domains, three extracellular loops (e1, e2 and e3), three cytoplasmic loops (c1, c2 and c3), and a cytoplasmic C-terminal region (Krause et al., 1990; Nakanishi, 1991). The three receptors share 54–66% homology in their transmembrane and cytoplasmic regions. The transmembrane segment II for the NK_2 and NK_3 receptors contains one aspartate residue, as do other G-protein coupled receptors, however, the NK_1 receptor has a glutamate residue instead. All three tachykinin receptors contain one histidine residue in transmembrane segments V and VI. The third cytoplasmic loop is highly conserved between the NK_1 and NK_3 receptors, however the NK_2 receptor diverges in this region. Finally, the number of serine and threonine residues in the third cytoplasmic loop as well as the carboxyl terminal region differs between the three receptors (Krause et al., 1990; Nakanishi, 1991; Ohkubo and Nakanishi, 1991). This considerable homology between receptor subtypes is consistent with the fact that all three tachykinins are capable of binding each receptor subtype.

The tachykinin receptors have the structural and functional properties of G-protein coupled receptors. Radioligand binding to tachykinin receptors is inhibited by nonhydrolysable G proteins (Nakata et al., 1988; Too and Hanley, 1988; Ingi et al., 1991; Holland et al., 1993). Moreover, activation of all three tachykinin receptors results in hydrolysis of phosphoinositols and increased levels of cAMP (Nakajima et al., 1991). In oocytes, tachykinin receptors cause hydrolysis of phosphoinositols, and increased intracellular Ca^{2+} which activates a Ca^{2+}-dependent Cl^- channel (Nakanishi et al., 1990). The binding of substance P and NKA to rabbit iris sphincter muscle in the presence of lithium increases the levels of inositol triphosphates. This response is attenuated when EGTA is added to the solution, however it persists in a Ca^{2+}-free medium, indicating that the tachykinins cause increased levels of intracellular Ca^{2+} (Taniguchi et al., 1992). Additionally, in neonatal rat spinal cord, the NK_3 agonist, senktide, increased levels of inositol phosphates (Guard et al., 1989). Thus, tachykinin receptors interact with G-proteins, resulting in stimulation of protein kinase C, hydrolysis of phosphoinositols and increased levels of intracellular Ca^{2+}.

The NK_1 and NK_2 receptors have both high- and low-affinity binding sites, however the NK_3 receptor appears to form a single population (Ingi et al., 1991). Binding of GTP-τ-S inhibits binding of radioligands to the high- but not the low-affinity sites in monkey kidney COS cells (Ingi et al., 1991), and Gpp(NH)p decreases binding to the high-affinity site in the dorsal horn of the spinal cord in rats (Holland et al., 1993). The decreased binding seen with Gpp(NH)p is similar to that seen following repeated exposure to substance P, suggesting that desensitization may involve an uncoupling of the receptor and G-protein (Holland et al., 1993).

Aspects of structure conferring specificity

The majority of evidence indicates that the C-terminal portions of the tachykinin peptides interact with tachykinin receptors and are biologically active (Glowinski et al., 1987; Cascieri et al., 1992; Fong et al., 1992a,b). Although the N-terminal region is also biologically active, it is believed to be acting on a non-neurokinin receptor. That is, the N-terminal region of SP potentiated kainic acid-induced behavioral activity in mice (Larson et al., 1992), however [D-Pro² D-Phe⁷]SP(1–7), a

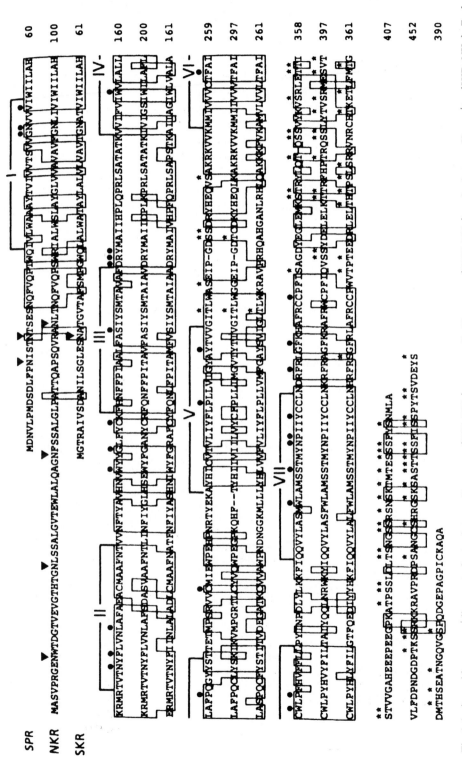

Fig. 1 Amino acid sequence alignment of rat substance P receptor (SPR, NK₁), neuromedin K receptor (NKR, NK₃), and substance K receptor (SKR, NK₂). *Enclosed amino acids,* identical residues in two or all three sequences; *hyphens,* deletions of amino acid residues; *dots,* amino acid residues conserved in the sequences of the tachykinin, adrenergic and muscarinic receptors; *asterisks,* serine and threonine residues as possible phosphorylation sites in the cytoplasmic regions; *triangles,* potential N-glycosylation sites. (Reprinted with permission from Nakanishi, 1991.)

neurokinin antagonist, had no effect on this response (Larson et al., 1992). Moreover, non-neurokinin receptors have been found on mouse brain and spinal cord membranes (Igwe et al., 1990). Since this chapter deals exclusively with tachykinin receptors, the rest of this section will focus on NK_1, NK_2 and NK_3, receptors and on responses mediated by the C-terminal region of the tachykinins and by selective tachykinin receptor agonists and antagonists (Table 1).

All three tachykinins share a common C-terminal hexapeptide: Phe-X-Gly-Leu-Met-NH2, where X = Phe, Tyr, Ile or Val (Nakanishi, 1991; Mussap et al., 1993). Carboxyl-terminal fragments of SP as small as [p-Glu]SP(6–11) show high affinity for the NK_1 receptor, however, fragments smaller than this have equal affinity for all three tachykinin receptors (Cascieri et al., 1992). Primary structure of the tachykinins is necessary for affinity and specificity of the tachykinin receptors. The amino acid tryptophan appears to be especially critical for specificity. D-Tryptophan in positions 6, 8 and 9 dramatically increases the affinity of NKA for the NK_2 receptor, and the further substitution of tyrosine at position 5 and arginine at position 10 produces the highly selective NK_2 antagonist, MEN 10207 (Rovero et al., 1990). Alternately, changing each of these tryptophan

TABLE I

Documentation of the use of tachykinin receptor-specific agonists and antagonists in the spinal cord over 5 years (1989–1993)

NK$_1$ agonists		NK$_1$ antagonists	
[^{125}I]BH-SP	Yashpal et al., 1991; Stucky et al., 1993	RP 67580	Laird et al., 1993; Thompson et al., 1993
Met(OH)-SP	Fleetwood-Walker et al., 1990	CP 96345	Couture et al., 1993;
Glp^{6}LProSP (6–11)	Fleetwood-Walker et al., 1990		Urban et al., 1993;
Physaleamin	Salter et al., 1991		Picard et al., 1993;
SPOMe	Ireland et al., 1992		Lecci et al., 1991;
			Xu et al., 1992;
			Pham et al., 1993;
			Thompson et al., 1993
		Sar^9 Met(O$_2^{11}$)-SP	Couture et al., 1993
		Spantide	Fleetwood-Walker, 1990
		Spantide II	Weisenfeld-Hallin et al., 1991
		SCY I	Raffa et al., 1993
		Acetyl-Arg^6-septide	Suzuki et al., 1993
		DArg^{1}DPro^{2}DTrp^{7,9}Leu^{11}-SP	Kangrga et al., 1990
NK$_2$ agonists		**NK$_2$ antagonists**	
[^{125}I]BH-NKA	Yashpal et al., 1992	SR 48968	Couture et al., 1993; Picard et al., 1993
Kassinin	Fleetwood-Walker et al., 1990		
Glp^{6}DPro^{9}SP (6–11)	Fleetwood-Walker et al., 1990	MEN 10207	Xu et al., 1992
		MEN 10376	Urban et al., 1993; Thompson et al., 1993
		SCY I	Raffa et al., 1993
NK$_3$ agonists		**NK$_3$ antagonists**	
[^{125}I]BH-E	Yashpal et al., 1992; Beresford et al., 1992	R 487	Couture et al., 1993
		MePhe^7 NKB	Couture et al., 1993
Succ[Asp^{6}MePhe^8]-SP (6–11)	Fleetwood-Walker et al., 1990	Senktide	Ireland et al., 1992
		SCY II	Raffa et al., 1993
		NKB-A	Fleetwood-Walker et al., 1990

residues produces distinct changes in affinity for all three receptor types, indicating that all three tryptophan residues are important for affinity and selectivity (Rovero et al., 1991).

More recently, alterations in primary structure have provided evidence for NK_2 subtypes. Specific NK_2 agonists and antagonists have been found to have heterogeneous effects in the rabbit pulmonary artery and hamster trachea (believed to contain NK_2 monoreceptor populations) suggesting the existence of multiple NK_2 receptor subtypes (Pattacchini et al., 1991), and aspartate at position 2 and tryptophan at position 4 (R396) appear to confer specificity for the NK_{2b} receptor subtype (Rovero et al., 1992).

Secondary and tertiary conformation also appear to be involved in binding of the tachykinins to their respective receptors. NMR studies indicate that the conformation of SP is strongly influenced by environment. For example, SP shows different conformations in different solvents (Lembeck et al., 1979). Moreover, physalaemin (which has a similar pharmacological profile to SP) has a similar conformation in methanol, whereas NKA does not. Recent evidence indicates that the degree of conformational constraints in the C-terminal region play a significant role in binding affinity. The cyclic peptides which introduce a carbon bridge between the α-carbon of glycine and the N of leucine yielding a cyclic lactam unit dramatically decrease affinity for NK_1 while increasing it for NK_2 and NK_3 (McKnight et al., 1991). Deal et al. (1992) have shown that replacing the glycine in position 9 of SP with Pro increases NK_1 selectivity, whereas the introduction of an r-γ-lactam unit increases the selectivity for NK_2 receptors. Finally, the γ-lactam-constrained NKA analog, GR 64349, has a similar activity to NKA with greater selectivity (Deal et al., 1992). Thus, decreasing the conformational freedom of the C-terminal end of the tachykinin molecule enhances NK_2 selectivity.

Due to the fact that the three tachykinin receptors share significant homology (see review by Naganishi, 1991), Fong et al. (1992a,b) have investigated the receptor itself (refer to Fig. 1). Deletion of the following residues from the NK_1 re-

ceptor: 2–7 and 14–27 resulted in a 1000-fold decrease in affinity for the wild-type receptor; however substituting glutamate for valine 97 significantly increased affinity of the NK_3 (but not NK_1 or NK_2) receptor. This suggests that the second extracellular domain is important for specificity between the three receptors (Fong et al., 1992a). This was further explored by substituting extracellular loops of human NK_1 with those found in NK_3. Substitution of the second extracellular loop of NK_1 significantly decreased its affinity for SP and NKB, however G-protein activation was normal and the non-peptide antagonist, L 703606, bound similarly to both the wild type and mutant receptor. Substitution of the third extracellular domain abolished binding of both SP and L 703606. Substitution of residues 170–174 causes the following change in the order of affinities: SP > NKB > NKA. Further substitution of residues 176–183 decreased affinities for the endogenous ligands without affecting L 703606, whose affinity was finally decreased by substituting 176–183. Substitution of the fourth extracellular loop had no effect on affinity for SP, but NKA and NKB both exhibited an increase in binding. Furthermore, various transmembrane point mutations also affected the affinity of all three tachykinins. These data indicate that both the extracellular and transmembrane domains of the tachykinin receptors are crucial for affinity and specificity (Fong et al., 1992b).

Thus primary, secondary and tertiary structures of the tachykinin molecule are important for receptor affinity and specificity. Specifically, tryptophan residues, the α-helical conformation and the degree of conformational freedom at the C-terminal end of the tachykinin peptides affects the selectivity for the three receptor subtypes. Finally, both extracellular and transmembrane domains of the receptor itself are important in conferring specificity.

Anatomy of tachykinin receptors in spinal cord

NK_1 binding sites

The regional localization of NK_1 receptors has

been extensively studied in the spinal cord by autoradiography using the ligands, [^{3}H]SP- and [^{125}I]Bolton Hunter-labelled SP (BH-SP), and more recently the very selective NK$_1$ ligand, [Sar^9,Met(O$_2$)^{11}-^{3}H]SP (Charlton and Helke, 1985b; Mantyh and Hunt, 1985; Shults et al., 1985; Buck et al., 1986; Dam et al., 1990b). The reported distributions were similar in each case. Moreover, the autoradiographic studies were recently confirmed and enhanced by studies using in situ hybridization histochemistry for NK$_1$ receptor mRNA and immunocytochemistry with anti-peptide antibodies to the NK$_1$ receptor (Elde et al., 1990; Moussaoui et al., 1992; Brown et al., 1993; Maeno et al., 1993).

The density of NK$_1$ binding sites in the spinal cord is the highest in Laminae I–II of the dorsal horn, intermediolateral cell column and Lamina X ventral horn regions are generally only moderately labelled by receptor autoradiography.

NK$_1$ binding sites in the dorsal horn

The dorsal horn of the spinal cord was extensively labelled with NK$_1$ binding sites throughout the entire length of the spinal cord (Ninkovic et al., 1984; Charlton and Helke, 1985b; Massari et al., 1985; Helke et al., 1986). Laminae I and II were heavily labelled, Laminae III and IV less densely labelled, and Lamina V had a very low concentration of NK$_1$ binding sites. The NK$_1$ binding sites in the dorsal horn appear to be present on perikarya and dendrites. Hosli and Hosli (1985) showed that SP binding in explant cultures of dorsal spinal cord was associated with the soma and processes of groups of small neurons, probably interneurons. NK$_1$ receptor mRNA is expressed in neurons of the dorsal horn (Elde et al., 1990; Maeno et al., 1993). Recent immunocytochemical studies with anti-peptide antibodies raised to the NK$_1$ receptor showed a high density of NK$_1$ receptor-immunoreactivity on dendrites in the superficial dorsal horn and the presence of immunoreactive cell bodies in deeper layers of the dorsal horn (Moussaoui et al., 1992; Brown et al., 1993). Electron microscopic immunocytochemistry with an NK$_1$ antibody showed substance P-containing primary afferent terminals in

synaptic contact with NK$_1$ receptor-laden neurons of the superficial dorsal horn, however many NK$_1$ receptor-containing processes were not associated with SP-containing terminals (Liu et al., 1993).

The NK$_1$ binding sites in the dorsal horn are not located on the primary afferent fibers. Dorsal root ganglion neurons do not contain NK$_1$ receptor immunoreactivity (Brown et al., 1993). In addition, selective removal of the primary sensory innervation of the dorsal horn increased rather than decreased the binding of [^{125}I]BH-SP and the density of NK$_1$-immunoreactivity in the dorsal horn (Mantyh and Hunt, 1985; Massarie et al., 1985; Helke et al., 1986; Yashpal et al., 1991; Brown et al., 1993).

NK$_1$ binding sites in autonomic regions

A very dense labelling of NK$_1$ binding sites is found in the intermediolateral cell column (IML) of the thoracic spinal cord and the sacral preganglionic nucleus of L$_{VI}$–S$_1$ in the rat (Shults et al., 1984; Charlton and Helke, 1985b; Buck et al., 1986; Helke et al., 1986). These regions are sites of origin of sympathetic and parasympathetic preganglionic neurons, respectively. The nucleus intercalatus and central autonomic region of the rat thoracic spinal cord also contained significant NK$_1$ binding (Charlton and Helke, 1985b; Helke et al., 1986).

In the IML, NK$_1$ binding sites appear to be primarily located on preganglionic neurons. The distribution of NK$_1$ binding sites correlates very closely with the distribution of cholinesterase-stained and presumably preganglionic IML neurons (Helke et al., 1986). NK$_1$ receptor immunoreactivity is present in IML neurons (Moussaioui et al., 1992; Brown et al., 1993) and NK$_1$ receptor mRNA is expressed by neurons in the IML (Elde et al., 1990). Moreover, transneuronal degeneration of sympathetic preganglionic neurons reduced the binding of radiolabelled SP in dissected homogenates of IML (Takano and Loewy, 1985). Subsequent studies used injections of the retrogradely-transported cellular toxin, ricin, into the superior cervical ganglion to selectively destroy the cholinesterase-stained preganglionic sympathetic neurons in the IML without altering other cellular elements. This procedure also selectively reduced the density of [^{125}I]BH-SP binding in the relevant levels of the thoracic IML (Helke et al., 1986).

No evidence exists for the presence of presynaptic NK$_1$ binding sites in the IML. Lesions of bulbospinal SP-containing neurons failed to alter the NK$_1$ binding in the IML (Helke et al., 1986). Although numerous noradrenergic and serotonergic neurons project to the IML, neither destruction of noradrenergic terminals nor destruction of serotonergic nerve terminals in the spinal cord reduced the binding of [^{125}I]BH-SP in the IML (Helke et al., 1986).

NK$_1$ binding sites in ventral horn

NK$_1$ binding sites were found in association with motor neurons of the ventral horn at all levels of the spinal cord. However, the density varied considerably both within and throughout various levels of the spinal cord. Laminae VIII–IX generally contained low to moderate levels of NK$_1$ binding (Charlton and Helke, 1985a,b; Buck et al., 1986). However, specific regions of the ventral horn were densely labelled, these included: phrenic motor nucleus in C$_{III-V}$; a ventrolateral region in C$_{VII}$; and Onuf's nucleus and a dorsolateral motor nucleus in L$_{V-VI}$ (Charlton and Helke, 1985b; Charlton and Helke, 1986). Large motoneurons in Lamina IX contained both NK$_1$ receptor immunoreactivity (Moussaoui et al., 1992) and NK$_1$ receptor mRNA (Maeno et al., 1993). In addition, selective destruction of phrenic motoneurons or sciatic motoneurons caused an associated loss of NK$_1$ binding sites in the phrenic motor nucleus or the dorsolateral portion of the L$_{IV-VI}$ ventral horn, respectively (Helke et al., 1986).

NK$_2$ binding sites

Compared to the periphery, where NK$_2$ receptor expression is widespread, the presence and role of NK$_2$ receptors in the CNS is poorly defined. The existence of NK$_2$ receptors in the CNS has been questioned. [^{3}H]NKA or [^{125}I]iodohistidyl NKA, which successfully labelled NK$_2$ sites in peripheral tissues, showed very limited binding in the spinal cord (Buck et al., 1986; Mantyh et al., 1989; Yashpal et al., 1990). Moreover, the lack of specificity of these ligands and their affinities for both NK$_1$ and NK$_3$ sites confuse the interpretation of these studies. The highly selective NK$_2$ ligand, [^{125}I]MEN 10,376, failed to specifically label binding sites in the spinal cord (Humpel and Saria, 1993). Recently, a novel NK$_2$ antagonist radioligand, [^{3}H]GR 100679, was used to demonstrate the presence of NK$_2$ receptors in the developing rat CNS, although similar data could not be obtained with adult CNS (Hagan et al., 1993). These data coupled with the finding that $< 1\%$ of the tachykinin receptor message in the rat brain was NK$_2$ receptor mRNA (Tsuchida et al., 1990; Poosh et al., 1991), suggest that the expression of NK$_2$ receptor mRNA in the rat spinal cord is of a low level.

In contrast, functional studies suggest the presence of NK$_2$-mediated responses in the spinal cord, e.g., modulation of thermal nociceptive inputs and associated changes in preprodynorphin mRNA in the dorsal horn neurons (Fleetwood-Walker et al., 1990; Parker et al., 1993), capsaicin evoked C-fiber excitation of dorsal horn neurons (Urban et al., 1992), and the rat flexor reflex (Xu et al., 1991).

NK$_3$ binding sites

The regional localization of NK$_3$ binding sites in the spinal cord has been autoradiographically studied using [^{125}I]BH-eledoisin (Ninkovic et al., 1984; Buck et al., 1986; Danks et al., 1986; Hunter et al., 1987; Yashpal et al., 1991). Although the selective ligand, [^{3}H]senktide, was used to label brain NK$_3$ binding sites (Dam et al., 1990a; Stoessl and Hill, 1990), similar studies have not been published for spinal cord.

The distribution of NK$_3$ binding sites in the spinal cord is more restricted than that of NK$_1$ binding sites. The NK$_3$ binding sites are restricted to Laminae I and II in all segments of the spinal cord dorsal horn (Ninkovic et al., 1984; Buck et al., 1986; Danks et al., 1986; Hunter et

100

al., 1987). These moderate to densely labelled sites contrasted with the very low levels of NK_3 binding noted in other regions of the spinal cord grey matter (Buck et al., 1986). Whereas the cellular localization of NK_3 binding sites has not been thoroughly studied, the reported increase in the density of dorsal horn NK_3 binding sites after dorsal rhizotomy suggests a localization post-synaptic to the primary afferent fibers (Yashpal et al., 1991; Fig. 2).

Although NK_3 binding sites were not associated with motor neurons in the IML or the ventral horn (Ninkovic et al., 1984; Buck et al., 1986), selective NK_3 agonists elicited depolarizing re-

sponses from ventral horn motoneurons in neonatal rats (Ireland et al., 1992; Fisher and Nistri, 1994)

Physiology

Electrophysiology

In general, activation of tachykinin receptors results in depolarization (Ireland et al., 1992; Konishi et al., 1992; Inokuchi et al., 1993). Using intracellular recordings in the rat coeliac/superior ganglia, Konishi et al. (1992) found two distinct depolarizing responses following injection of

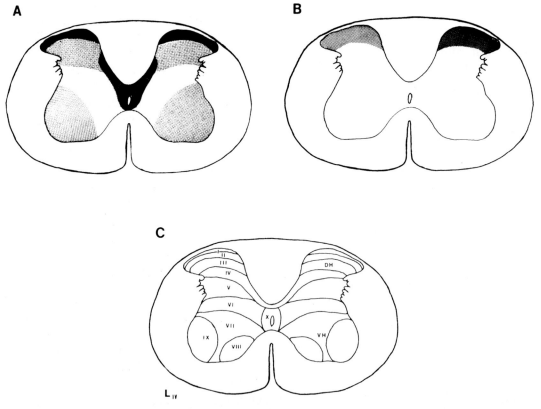

Fig. 2. Changes in NK_1 and NK_3 receptor binding in the adult rat lumbar (L_{IV}) spinal cord following inflammation and injury, respectively. A. NK_1 receptor binding sites. Left side: [^{125}I]BH-SP binding in the intact spinal cord (Charlton and Helke, 1985; Buck et al., 1986; Helke et al., 1986). Right side: [^{125}I]BH-SP binding following unilateral adjuvant-induced inflammation of the ipsilateral hindpaw (Stucky et al., 1993). B. NK_3 receptor binding sites. Left side: [^{125}I]BH-Eledoisin binding in the intact spinal cord (Buck et al., 1986; Beresford et al., 1992). Right side: [^{125}I]BH-Eledoisin binding following dorsal rhizotomy (ipsilateral, L4-L6; Yashpal et al., 1991). C. Spinal cord Laminae I–X.

SP, NKA, and NKB. The first was a fast depolarization that peaked within 1.2 sec, and lasted 5–10 sec. The second was a slow depolarization peaking in 20 sec, and lasting 120–140 sec. The fast response was found to be due to a Ca^{2+}-dependent cation channel, and the slow to a decrease in K^+ conductance. SP and NKA were also shown to decrease a persistent Ca^{2+}-dependent K^+ conductance in sympathetic preganglionic cells in the IML (Inokuchi et al., 1993), as well as lumbar motoneurons in neonatal rat spinal cord (Fisher and Nistri, 1994).

The depolarization induced by the different tachykinin receptors is not identical. In extracellular single unit recordings in cat lumbar spinal cord, NKA caused a delayed, prolonged excitation in both nociceptive and non-nociceptive cells; whereas SP preferentially excited nociceptive cells (Salter et al., 1991). Moreover, in ventral root motoneurons, tetrodotoxin (TTX) and APS-5 (an NMDA antagonist) depressed the depolarizing response to the NK_3 agonist, senktide, while having no effect on the SP-induced depolarization; leading to the conclusion that NK_1 receptors resulted in a direct activation of motoneurons, while the effects of the NK_3 receptor were indirect (Ireland, 1992). Finally, all three tachykinins produced a slow excitation of rat spinal motoneurons, however, while TTX blocked the NKA and NKB response, the response to SP was unaffected by TTX. This suggests that NK_1 receptors are located on motoneurons, while NK_2 and NK_3 receptors are located on interneurons (Fisher and Nistri, 1994)

Functional roles of specific receptor subtypes in the spinal cord

Sensory systems

As mentioned previously, Laminae I and II are extensively labelled with NK_1 receptor binding sites (Ninkovic, et al., 1984; Charlton and Helke, 1985a,b; Massari, et al., 1985; Helke et al., 1986). These NK_1 binding sites are not located on the primary afferent fibers (Brown et al., 1993). As one would expect from these data, the NK_1 re-

ceptor is involved in the processing of sensory information at the level of the spinal cord.

There is evidence for a role for the NK_1 receptor in the mediation of spinal reflexes. Xu et al. (1991) found that intrathecal (i.t.) SP facilitated the hamstring flexor reflex elicited by stimulation of afferent C-fibers. This facilitation is specifically related to the response to a conditioning stimulus. Spantide II, an NK_1 antagonist, blocked the facilitatory response to a conditioning stimulus (Weisenfeld-Hallin et al., 1991). Morever, the NK_1 antagonists, CP 96345 and RP 67580 (the latter being rodent specific), attenuate this response while having no effect on the baseline reflex (Xu et al., 1992; Laird et al., 1993).

The role of the NK_1 receptor in nociception is less clear. NK_1 agonists cause a decrease in latency of the tail flick response to noxious heat (Lecci et al., 1991; Picard et al., 1993). However, the work of Fleetwood-Walker et al. (1993) is not consistent with this. In this study, the NK_1 receptor antagonists, L688169, GR82334 and [D-Pro^4, D-Trp^{7,9,10} Phe^{11}]SP(4–11), inhibit the response to brush, but not noxious heat or pinch (Fleetwood Walker et al., 1993).

In contrast to the situation for the NK_1 receptor, binding sites for the NK_2 receptor in the spinal cord are limited, at best. However, functional studies suggest the presence of NK_2-mediated responses in the spinal cord. NKA also facilitates the hamstring reflex, however, in this case it is the baseline reflex that is enhanced and not the response to a conditioning stimulus (Xu et al., 1991, 1992). MEN 10207, a specific NK_2 antagonist, blocked the NKA, but not SP, response (Xu et al., 1991); and MEN 10207 has no effect on the enhanced response to a conditioning stimulus (Xu et al., 1991). Moreover, CP 96345 did not block NKA facilitation (Xu et al., 1992). These data suggest that the NK_2 receptor may mediate the flexor reflex itself, while the NK_1 receptor mediates the facilatory response to a conditioning stimulus.

The NK_2 receptors are also involved in the nociceptive response. NKA decreased tail flick latency (for a longer duration than that seen with

SP) and, while CP 96345 antagonized the NK_1 response, the NK_2 response was unaffected (Picard et al., 1993). This is consistent with the work of Fleetwood-Walker et al. (1993), showing that the NK_2 receptor antagonist, L 658874, inhibits the response to noxious heat, but not noxious pinch or brush.

In addition to playing a role in the mediation of thermal nociception, the NK_2 receptor may also mediate the response of polymodal nociceptors. Activation of polymodal nociceptors by capsaicin is attenuated by MEN 10376, a selective NK_2 antagonist, while CP 96345 has no effect (Urban et al., 1993). Moreover, mustard oil-induced sustained C-afferent activity is also inhibited by L 659874, a selective NK_2 antagonist, while NK_1 antagonists, L 668169 and GR 82334 have little effect (Munro et al., 1993). The NK_2 antagonist, L 659874, inhibits the carrageenan-induced increase in preprodynorphin while NK_1 antagonists do not (Parker et al., 1993). Thus, while there are a number of studies suggesting a role for the NK_2 receptor in the mediation of nociceptive information, the role of the NK_1 receptor is still unclear.

Finally, consistent with the presence of NK_3 binding sites in the dorsal horn described previously (Ninkovic et al., 1984; Buck et al., 1986; Danks et al., 1986; Hunter et al., 1987), Couture et al. (1993) proposed a role for NK_3 receptors in sensory transduction. Selective antagonists, CP 96345, SR 48968 and R487 (for NK_1, NK_2 and NK_3 receptors, respectively) inhibit only the response for their specific receptors, without affecting the response to any other tachykinin. Interestingly, unlike SP and NKA, NKB increases the latency of tail flick reaction time (Couture et al., 1993). Furthermore, the NK_3 receptor hypoalgesic response is blocked by prior intrathecal injection of naloxone, implicating it in opiate-mediated analgesia (Laneuville et al., 1988).

Autonomic systems

The localization of NK_1 receptor binding sites suggests a role in autonomic neurotransmission. As discussed earlier, NK_1 receptor binding sites are found in high concentrations in the au-

tonomic regions of the spinal cord (Shults et al., 1984; Charlton and Helke, 1985b; Buck et al., 1986; Helke et al., 1986). These sites appear to be located on sympathetic preganglionic neurons (Helke et al., 1986; Elde et al., 1990; Moussaioui et al., 1992; Brown et al., 1993). Intrathecal administration of SP and an agonist, $[pGlu^5MePhe^8MeGly^9]$-SP_{5-11}, into the IML excited sympathetic preganglionic neurons (presumably by the decreased K^+ conductance discussed earlier; Backman et al., 1984) and caused an increase in mean arterial pressure (Helke et al., 1987; Pham et al., 1993a). The NK_1 receptor antagonist, $[D-Arg^1,D-Pro^2,D-Trp^{7,9},Leu^{11}]$-SP, reduced stroke volume, resulting in decreased mean arterial pressure and cardiac output (Helke et al., 1987). Moreover, intrathecal (T_{IX}) injection of the more selective antagonist, CP 96345, blocks the increase in blood pressure and tachycardia resulting from injection of substance P (Pham et al., 1993a). These data indicate that activation of the NK_1 receptor has an excitatory effect on sympathetic preganglionic neurons in the IML.

NK_2 binding sites have not been found in autonomic sites in the spinal cord and, although intrathecal administration of NKA has been shown to increase heart rate and mean arterial pressure in some studies (Pham et al., 1993a,b), this is not always the case (Hassessian et al., 1988). Thus, the involvement of the NK_2 receptor in spinal autonomic systems is highly questionable. Intrathecal injection of CP 96345 at T_{IX} blocks the increase in blood pressure and tachycardia resulting from both NKA and SP, indicating that the NK_1 receptor mediates the cardiovascular response to both SP and NKA in the spinal cord (Pham et al., 1993a). In a companion paper, activation of the NK_2 receptor by intrathecal NKA resulted in increased plasma levels of norepinephrine, epinephrine and neuropeptide Y (NPY), in addition to its cardiovascular function. This was attenuated by both adrenalectomy and sympathectomy (Pham et al., 1993b). Although this would appear to indicate that the NK_2 receptor stimulates the sympathoadrenal system, the NK_1 antagonist CP 96345 was not used in this study. Thus, in light of the previous study, it is unclear whether this response is mediated by the NK_1 or NK_2 receptors.

Motor systems

Although NK_1 receptors are the only tachykinin receptors present in the adult rat ventral horn, both NK_1 and NK_3 receptors have been demonstrated in neonatal rat ventral horns (Charlton and Helke, 1985b; Buck et al., 1986; Beresford et al., 1992). Moreover, as discussed previously, all three tachykinin receptors have been shown to depolarize ventral horn motoneurons, suggesting a role for tachykinins in motor systems as well (Ireland et al., 1993; Fisher and Nistri, 1994). However, all of these studies have been done in neonates, leaving the function of NK_3 receptors in the adult unclear.

Modulation of the release of the other transmitters

Tachykinin receptors have been shown to interact with other neurotransmitter systems in the spinal cord. All three tachykinin receptors appear to play a role in the modulation of acetylcholine (ACh) release. SP, NKA, NKB, the NK_1 agonist, acetyl-Arg[6]-septide, and the NK_3 agonist, senktide, all dose-dependently increase Ach release in isolated spinal cord from neonatal rats (Kobayashi et al., 1991). More recent evidence, also in isolated spinal cord from neonatal rats, shows that the Ach release evoked by NKA and acetyl-Arg[6]-septide is decreased by the NK_1 antagonists, spantide and GR71251, however these agents have no effect on release evoked by SP and NKB. In this study, polymerized chain reaction amplification and subsequent DNA sequencing revealed DNA fragments in rat spinal cord with sequences identical to those contained in NK_1 and NK_3, but not NK_2 receptors (Suzuki et al., 1993). Thus, the effects of NKA appear to be mediated, not by a classical NK_2 receptor, but by a receptor that binds the above NK_1 antagonists. These data suggest that the NK_1 and NK_3 receptors, as well as a novel NK_1 receptor, may be involved in Ach release in the spinal cord.

Tachykinins not only affect the release of Ach, but are involved in other transmitter systems as well. SP, but not NKA or NKB, has been shown to dose dependently decrease central [^{3}H]MeTRH binding, suggesting that the NK_1 receptor is negatively coupled to the TRH receptor (Sharif et al., 1990). Moreover, in spinal cord motoneurons, both SP and TRH cause a slowly developing, persistent depolarization accompanied by increased membrane resistance (Fisher and Nistri, 1993). This suggests that SP and TRH share a common effector pathway.

Finally, there is evidence that tachykinin receptors interact with excitatory amino acids. Both the NK_2 receptor antagonist, MEN 10376, and the NMDA antagonist DAPS5, given singly, decrease the area and duration of the C fiber-evoked ventral root potential. This response is significantly greater when the two antagonists are combined (Thompson et al., 1993). Although the NK_1 antagonists, CP 96345 and RP 67580, had no effect in the previous study, both SP and NKA potentiated the NMDA-induced current in isolated rat dorsal horn neurons (Randić et al., 1993).

These studies provide evidence that the tachykinin peptides interact with other neurotransmitter systems. The NK_1 receptor modulates the response to ACh, TRH and excitatory amino acids. The NK_2 receptor modulates the response to excitatory amino acids, while the NK_3 receptor modulates ACh release.

Plasticity

Tachykinin receptors have been shown to exhibit developmental changes. In 3-day-old rats, high levels of [^{125}I]BH-E binding is seen in the whole spinal cord (in both dorsal and ventral horns) the majority of which resemble NK_3 sites. However, at 35 days of age [^{125}I]BH-E binding is found primarily in Laminae I and II of the dorsal horn, and exclusively represents NK_3 sites (Beresford et al., 1992). Similarly, [^{125}I]BH-SP binding is distributed over the entire spinal cord gray matter up to about 15 days postnatally, at which point binding becomes defined in specific nuclei (Charlton and Helke, 1986). Thus, tachykinin receptors show changes with development, and might play a role in the development of the spinal cord. Alternatively, the factors regulating tachykinin receptor binding might show developmental alterations.

In addition to developmental changes, the tachykinin receptor system shows significant plasticity following inflammation. Unilateral adjuvant-induced inflammation in the hindpaw of the rat resulting in edema and hyperalgesia, causes an increase in $[^{125}I]BH$-SP binding in Laminae I and II, ipsilateral to the injury (Stucky et al., 1993; Fig. 2). Moreover, this same treatment resulted in a doubling of NK_1 receptor mRNA in Laminae I and II ipsilateral to the inflammation (Shafer et al., 1993). Chronic constriction of the sciatic nerve has also been shown to increase $[^{125}I]BH$-SP binding in Laminae I and II, ipsilateral to the constriction, 5 days after surgery. Binding returned to control levels 20 days after surgery. This increased binding was due to an increase in affinity of the receptor (Aanonsen et al., 1992).

As seen in the response to peripheral injury, spinal cord injury will also cause alterations in tachykinin receptors. Transection of L_{IV-VI} dorsal roots resulted in the following changes in tachykinin receptor binding: $[^{125}I]BH$-SP, $[^{125}I]BH$-NKA and $[^{125}I]BH$-E binding increased in the superficial laminae of the dorsal horn. The greatest increase was seen for eledoisin binding sites. Binding of $[^{125}I]BH$-NKA was also increased in the ventromedial portion of the cord. Binding of $[^{125}I]BH$-SP and $[^{125}I]BH$-NKA recovered after 28 days post surgery, however the altered $[^{125}I]BH$-E binding persisted (Yashpal et al., 1991; Fig. 2). When the dorsolateral funiculus is lesioned unilaterally, substance P binding is increased in Laminae II and III, ipsilateral to the lesion. This recovered after 28 days. Binding of SP was also elevated in Lamina X at 7 and 14 days, but not at 28 days (Bernau et al., 1993). One week after transection of the spinal cord between $T_{VIII-VIX}$ substance P receptors were upregulated in the dorsal horn and central canal in the lumbar region, as well as Laminae III, IV and V, and the ventral horn of the cervical region. The up-regulation returned to normal after 3 weeks in all of these regions except the cervical ventral horn (Vita et al., 1990).

Injection of capsaicin into neonatal rats increased SP, but not SP receptor mRNA in the spinal cord, indicating that the transmitter and receptor can be controlled independently in the spinal cord (Sivam et al., 1992). Finally, in cases of human amyotrophic lateral sclerosis, substance P binding was reduced in the ventral horn of the spinal cord (Dietl et al., 1989). Changes in NK_1 and NK_3 binding in the rat lumbar spinal cord in response to injury or inflammation are illustrated in Fig. 2.

The developmental changes in tachykinin receptor binding may reflect a trophic role for the tachykinin peptides during development. Alternatively, tachykinin receptor systems may be affected by other changes occurring during development. The up-regulation seen following injury may also be trophic in nature; however since up-regulation also follows inflammation, it seems likely that tachykinin receptors may play a role in the mediation of chronic nociception.

Summary

In summary, all three tachykinin receptors appear to be important modulators of physiological systems in the spinal cord. However, although there is a good deal of data concerning binding characteristics in peripheral tissues, work done in the spinal cord is scanty, leading to a number of unanswered questions. Firstly, Lui et al. (1993) have suggested a discrepancy between the location of SP binding sites and SP containing terminals. This might explain the conflicting evidence on the role of NK_1 receptors in the dorsal horn. Furthermore, evidence that NK_2 receptors are involved in nociception is increasing, however binding sites for these receptors in the spinal cord have not been demonstrated. This appears to be due to the difficulty in locating an ideal receptor specific ligand. The role of NK_2 receptors in autonomic function is also unclear, perhaps for the same reason. Finally, there is evidence indicating that NK_3 binding sites are increased following transection of the L_{IV-VI} dorsal roots, however, studies on the effects of inflammation have not been done, as they have with the NK_1 and NK_2 receptors. All of these and many more unanswered questions require further investigation.

References

Aanonsen, L.M., Kajander, K.C., Bennett, G.J. and Seybold, V.S. (1992) Autoradiographic analysis of ^{125}I-substance P binding in rat spinal cord following chronic constriction injury of the sciatic nerve. Brain Res., 596: 259–268.

Backman, S.B. and Henry, J.L. (1984) Physiological properties of sympathetic preganglionic neurones in the thoracic intermediolateral nucleus of the cat. Can. J. Physiol. Pharmacol., 62: 1183–1193.

Beresford, I.J.M., Ireland, S.J., Staples, J. and Hagan, R.M. (1992) Ontogeny and characterization of [^{125}I]bolton hunter-eledoisin binding sites in rat spinal cord by quantitative autoradiography. Neuroscience, 46(1): 225–232.

Bernau, N.A., Dawson, S.D., Kane, L.A. and Pubols, L.M. (1993) Changes in substance P and 5-HT binding in the spinal cord dorsal horn and lamina X after dorsolateral funiculus lesions. Brain Res., 613: 106–114.

Brown, J., Jasmin, L., Mantyh, P.W., Heinricher, M.M., Vigna, S.P. and Basbaum, A.L. (1993) Immunocytochemical localization of NK_1 receptor in the spinal cord of the rat. Soc. Neurosci. Abstr., 19: 298.7.

Buck, S.H., Helke, C.J., Burcher, E., Shults, C.W. and O'Donohue, T.L. (1986) Pharmacologic characterization and autoradiographic distribution of binding sites for iodinated tachykinins in the rat central nervous system. Peptides, 7: 1109–1120.

Burcher, E., Mussap, C.J., Geraghty, D.P., McClure-Sharp, J.M. and Watkins, D.J. (1991) Concepts in characterization of tachykinin receptors. Ann. NY Acad. Sci., 632: 123–136.

Cascieri, M.A., Huang, R.C., Fong, T.M., Cheung, A.H., Sadowski, S., Ber, E. and Strader, C.D. (1992) Determination of the amino acid residues in substance conferring selectivity and specificity for the rat neurokinin receptors. Mol. Pharmacol., 41: 1096–1099.

Charlton, C.G. and Helke, C.J. (1985a) Characterization and segmental distribution of ^{125}I-Bolton-Hunter labeled substance P binding sites in rat spinal cord. J. Neurosci., 5: 1293–1299.

Charlton, C.G. and Helke, C.J. (1985b) Autoradiographic localization and characterization of spinal cord substance P binding sites: High densities in sensory, autonomic, phrenic, and Onuf's motor nuclei. J. Neurosci., 5: 1653–1661.

Charlton, C.G. and Helke, C.J. (1986) Ontogeny of substance P receptors in rat spinal cord: Quantitative changes in

receptor number and differential expression in specific loci. Dev. Brain Res., 29: 81–91.

Couture, R., Boucher, S., Picard, P. and Regoli, D. (1993) Receptor characterization of the spinal action of neurokinins on nociception: a three receptor hypothesis. Regul. Peptides, 46: 426–429.

Dam, T.V., Escher, E. and Quirion, R. (1990a) Visualization of neurokinin-3 receptor sites in rat brain using the highly selective ligand [^{3}H]senktide. Brain Res., 506: 175–179.

Dam, T., Martinelli, B. and Quirion, R. (1990b) Autoradiographic distribution of brain neurokinin-1/substance P receptors using a highly selective ligand [^{3}H]-[Sar^9,Met(O$_2$)^{11}]-Substance P. Brain Res., 531: 333–337.

Danks, J.A., Rothman, R.B., Cascieri, M.A., Chicchi, G.G., Liang, T. and Herkenham, M. (1986) A comparative autoradiographic study of the distributions of substance P and eledoisin binding sites in the rat. Brain Res., 385: 273–281.

Deal, M.J., Hagan, R.M., Ireland, S.J., Jordan, C.C., McElroy, A.B., Porter, B., Ross, B.C., Stephens-Smith, M. and Ward, P. (1992) Conformationally constrained tachykinin analogues: potent and highly selective neurokinin NK_2 receptor antagonists. J. Med. Chem., 35: 4195–4204.

Dietl, M.M., Sanchez, M., Probst, A. and Palacios, J.M. (1989) Substance P receptors in the human spinal cord: decrease in amyotrophic lateral sclerosis. Brain Res., 483: 39–49.

Elde, R., Schalling, M., Ceccatelli, S., Nakanishi, S. and Hökfelt, T. (1990) Localization of neuropeptide receptor mRNA in rat brain: initial observations using probes for neurotensin and substance P receptors. Neurosci. Lett., 120: 134–138.

Erspamer, V. (1981) The tachykinin peptide family. Trends Neurosci. (TINS), 5: 269–297.

Fisher, N.D. and Nistri, A. (1993) Substance P and TRH share a common effector pathway in rat spinal motoneurons: an in vitro electrophysiological investigation. Neurosci. Lett., 153: 115–119.

Fisher, N.D., Baranauskas, G. and Nistri, A. (1994) Multiple types of tachykinin receptor mediate a slow excitation of rat spinal motoneurones in vitro. Neurosci. Lett., 165(1–2): 84–88.

Fleetwood-Walker, S.M., Mitchell, R., Hope, P.J., El-Yassir, N., Molony, V. and Bladon, C.M. (1990) The involvement of neurokinin receptor subtypes in somatosensory processing in the superficial dorsal horn of the cat. Brain Res., 519: 169–182.

Fleetwood-Walker, S.M., Parker, R.M.C., Munro, F.E., Young, M.R., Hope, P.J. and Mitchell, R. (1993) Evidence for a role of tachykinin NK_2 receptors in mediating brief nociceptive inputs to rat dorsal horn (laminae III–V) neurons. Eur. J. Pharmacol., 242: 173–181.

Fong, T.M., Huang, R.C. and Strader, C.D. (1992a) Localization of agonist and antagonist binding domains of the human neurokinin-1 receptor. J. Biol. Chem., 267(36): 25664–25667.

Fong, T.M., Yu, H., Huang, R.C. and Strader, C.D. (1992b) The extracellular domain of the neurokinin-1 receptor is required for high-affinity binding of peptides. *Biochem.*, 31(47): 11806–11811.

Gerard, N.P., Eddy, R.L., Jr., Shows, T.C. and Gerard, C. (1990) The human neurokinin A (substance K) receptor: molecular cloning of the gene, chromosome localization, and isolation of cDNA from tracheal and gastric tissues. *J. Biol. Chem.*, 265: 20455–20462.

Gerard, N.P., Garaway, L.A., Eddy, R.L.Jr., Shows, T.B., Iijima, H., Paquet, J.L. and Gerard, C. (1991) Human substance P receptor (NK$_1$): organization of the gene, chromosomal localization and functional expression of cDNA clones. *Biochemistry*, 30: 10640–10646.

Gerard, N.P., Bao, L., Xiao-Ping, H. and Gerard, C. (1993) Molecular aspects of the tachykinin receptors. *Regul. Peptides*, 43: 21–35.

Guard, S., Watling, K.J. and Watson, S.P. (1989) NK$_3$ tachykinin receptors are coupled to inositol phospholipid hydrolysis in neonatal rat spinal cord. *Br. J. Pharmacol.*, 98: 908P.

Glowinski, J., Torrens, Y., Saffroy, M., Bergstrom, L., Beaujouan, J.C., Lavielle, S., Ploux, O., Chassaing, G. and Marquet, A. (1987) Tachykinin receptors in the CNS. *Progr. Brain Res.*, 72: 197–203.

Hagan, R.M., Beresford, I.J.M., Stables, J., Dupere, J., Stubbs, C., Elliot, P.J., Sheldrick, R.L.G., Chollet, A., Kawashima, E., McElroy, A.B. and Ward, P. (1993) Characterization, CNS distribution and function of NK$_2$ receptors studied using potent NK$_2$ receptor antagonists. *Regul. Peptides*, 46: 9–19.

Hassessian, H., Drapeau, G. and Couture, R. (1988) Spinal actions of neurokinins producing cardiovascular responses in the conscious freely moving rat: evidence for a NK$_1$ receptor mechanism. *Naunyn-Schmiedebergs Arch. Pharmacol.*, 338: 649–654.

Helke, C.J., Charlton, C.G. and Wiley, R.G. (1986) Studies on the cellular localization of spinal cord substance P receptors. *Neuroscience*, 19: 523–533.

Helke, C.J., Phillips, E.T. and O'Neill, J.T. (1987) Intrathecal administration of a substance P receptor antagonist: studies on peripheral and central nervous system hemodynamics and on specificity of action. *J. Pharmacol. Exp. Ther.*, 242: 131–136.

Henry, J.L. (1987) Discussion of nomenclature for tachykinins and tachykinin receptors. *Substance P Neurokinins*, 17–18.

Holland, L.N., Goldstein, B.D. and Aronstam, R.S. (1993) Substance P receptor desensitization in the dorsal horn: possible involvement of receptor-G protein complexes. *Brain Res.*, 600: 89–96.

Hosli, E. and Hosli, L. (1985) Binding sites for [^{3}H]substance P on neurons of cultured rat spinal cord and brainstem: an autoradiographic study. *Neurosci. Lett.*, 56: 199–203.

Humpel, C. and Saria, A. (1993) Characterization of neurokinin binding sites in rat brain membranes using highly selective ligands. *Neuropeptides*, 25: 65–71.

Hunter, J.C., Kilpatrick, G.J. and Brown, J.R. (1987) Pharmacological analysis of ^{125}I-bolton and hunter labelled eledoisin binding sites in rat spinal cord by quantitative autoradiography. *Neurosci. Lett.*, 78: 12–16.

Igwe, O.J., Kim, D.C., Seybold, V.S. and Larson, A.A. (1990) Specific binding of substance P aminoterminal heptapeptide [SP(1–7)] to mouse brain and spinal cord membranes. *J. Neurosci.*, 10: 3653–3663.

Ingi, T., Kitajima, Y., Minamitaki, Y. and Nakanishi, S. (1991) Characterization of ligand-binding properties and selectivities of three rat tachykinin receptors by transfection and functional expression of their clone cDNAs in mammalian cells. *J. Pharmacol. Exp. Ther.*, 259(3): 968–975.

Inokuchi, H., Yoshimura, M., Polosa, C. and Nishi, S. (1993) Tachykinins depress a calcium-dependent potassium conductance in sympathetic preganglionic neurons. *Regul. Peptides*, 46: 367–369.

Ireland, S.J., Wright, I.K. and Jordan, C.C. (1992) Characterization of tachykinin-induced ventral root depolarization in the neonatal rat isolated spinal cord. *Neuroscience*, 46(1): 217–223.

Kangawa, H., Minamino, N., Fukuda, A. and Matsuo, H. (1983) Neuromedin K: a novel mammalian tachykinin identified in porcine spinal cord. *Biochem. Biophys. Res. Commun.*, 114: 533–540.

Kangrga, I. and Randić, M. (1990) Tachykinins and calcitonin gene-related peptide enhanced release of endogenous glutamate and aspartate from the rat spinal dorsal horn slice. *J. Neurosci.*, 10(6): 2026–2038.

Kimura, S., Okada, M., Sugita, Y., Kanazawa, I. and Munekata, E. (1983) Novel neuropeptides, neurokinin A and B, isolated from porcine spinal cord. *Proc. Jpn. Acad.*, 59B: 101–104.

Kobayashi, N., Sakuma, M., Yoshioka, K., Onishi, Y., Yanigisawa, M., Kawashima, K. and Otsuka, M. (1991) Substance P-evoked release of acetylcholine from isolated spinal cord of the newborn rat. *Neuroscience*, 45(2): 331–337.

Konishi, S., Song, S., Ogawa, T. and Kanazawa, I. (1992) Fast and slow depolarization produced by substance P and other tachykinins in sympathetic neurons of rat prevertebral ganglia. *Neurosci. Res.*, 14: 81–95.

Krause, J.E., Hershey, A.D., Dykema, P.E. and Takeda, Y. (1990) Molecular biological studies on the diversity of chemical signalling in tachykinin peptidergic neurons. *Ann. NY Acad. Sci.*, 579: 254–272.

Laird, J.M.A., Hargreaves, R.J. and Hill, R.G. (1993) Effect of RP 67580, a non-peptide neurokinin 1 receptor antagonist, on facilitation of a nociceptive spinal flexion reflex in the rat. *Br. J. Pharmacol.*, 109(3): 713–718.

Laneuville, O., Dorais, J. and Couture, R. (1988) Characterization of the effects produced by neurokinins and three agonists selective for neurokinin receptor subtypes in a spinal nociceptive reflex of the rat. *Life Sci.*, 42: 1295–1305.

Larson, A. and Sun, X. (1992) Amino terminus of substance P potentiates kainic acid-induced activity in the mouse spinal cord. *J. Neurosci.*, 12(12): 4905–4910.

Lecci, A., Giuliani, S., Patacchini, R., Vita, G. and Maggi, C.A. (1991) Role of NK$_1$ tachykinin receptors in thermonociception: effect of (+/-)-CP 96,345, a non-peptide substance P antagonist, on the hot plate test in mice. *Neurosci. Lett.*, 129: 299–302.

Lembeck, F., Saria, A. and Mayer, N. (1979) Substance P: model studies of its binding to phospholipids. *Naunyn-Schmiedebergs Arch. Pharmacol.*, 306: 189–194.

Lui, H., Brown, J., Jasmin, L., Maggio, J., Vigna, S., Mantyh, P. and Basbaum, A. (1994) Synaptic relationship between substance P and the substance P receptor: light and electron microscope characterization of the mismatch between neuropeptides and their receptors. *Proc. Natl. Acad. Sci. USA*, 91: 91(18): 8383–8387.

Maeno, H., Kiyama, H. and Tohyma, M. (1993) Distribution of the substance P receptor (NK$_1$ receptor) in the central nervous system. *Mol. Brain Res.*, 18: 4358.

Maggi, C.A., Patacchini, R., Astolfi, M., Rovero, P., Giuliani, S. and Giachetti, A. (1991) NK$_2$ receptor agonist and antagonists. *Ann. NY Acad. Sci.*, 632: 184–191.

Maggi, C.A., Patacchini, R., Rovero, P. and Giachetti, A. (1993) Tachykinin receptors and tachykinin receptor antagonists. *J. Autonom. Pharmacol.*, 13: 23–93.

Maggio, J.E., Bradley, C.V., Iversen, L.L., Santikarn, S., Williams, B.H., Hunter, J.C. and Hanley, M.R. (1983) Substance K: a novel tachykinin in rat spinal cord. In: P. Skrabanck and D. Powell (Eds.), *Substance P—Dublin 1983*, Boule Press, Dublin, pp. 20–21.

Mantyh, P.W. and Hunt, S.P. (1985) The autoradiographic localization of substance P receptors in the rat and bovine spinal cord and the rat and cat trigeminal nucleus pars caudalis and the effect neonatal capsaicin. *Brain Res.*, 332: 315–324.

Mantyh, P.W., Gates, T.S., Mantyh, C.R. and Maggio, J.E. (1989) Autoradiographic localization and characterization of tachykinin receptor binding sites in the rat brain and peripheral tissues. *J. Neurosci.*, 9: 258–279.

Massari, V.J., Shults, C.W., Park, C.H., Tizabi, Y., Moody, T.W., Chromwall, B.M., Colver, M. and Chase, T.N. (1985) Deafferentation causes a loss of presynaptic bombesin receptors and supersensitivity of substance P receptors in the dorsal horn of the cat spinal cord. *Brain Res.*, 343: 268–274.

Masu, Y., Nakayama, K., Tamaki, H., Harada, Y., Kuno, M. and Nakanishi, S. (1987) cDNA cloning of bovine substance-K receptor through oocyte expression system. *Nature*, 329: 836–838.

McKnight, A.T., Maquier, J.J., Elliot, N.J., Fletcher, A.E., Foster, A.C., Tridgett, R., Williams, B.J., Longmore, I. and Iversen, L.L. (1991) Pharmacological specificity of novel, synthetic, cyclic peptides as antagonists at tachykinin receptors. *Br. J. Pharmacol.*, 140(2): 355–360.

Minamino, N., Kangawa, H., Fukuda, A. and Matsuo, H. (1984) Neuromedin K: a novel mammalian peptide identified in porcine spinal cord. *Neuropeptides*, 4: 157–166.

Moussaoui, S.M., Hermans, E., Mathieu, A.M., Bonici, B., Clerc, F., Guinet, F., Garret, C. and Laduron, P.M. (1992) Polyclonal antibodies against the rat NK$_1$ receptor:char-

acterization and localization in the spinal cord. *NeuroReport*, 3: 1073–1076.

Munro, F.E., Fleetwood-Walker, S.M., Parker, R.M.C. and Mitchell, R. (1993) The effects of neurokinin receptor antagonists on mustard oil-evoked activation of rat dorsal horn neurons. *Neuropeptides*, 25: 299–305.

Mussap, C.J., Geraghty, D.P. and Burcher, E. (1993) Tachykinin receptors: a radioligand binding perspective. *J. Neurochem.*, 60(6): 1987–2009.

Nakajima, Y., Tsuchida, K., Negishi, M., Ito, S. and Nakanishi, S. (1991) Direct linkage of three tachykinin receptors to stimulation of both phosphatidyl inositol hydrolysis and cyclic cAMP cascades in chinese hamster ovary cells. *J. Biol. Chem.*, 267: 2437–2442.

Nakanishi, S. (1991) Mammalian Tachykinin Receptors. *Annu. Rev. Neurosci.*, 14: 123–136.

Nakanishi, S., Ohkubo, H., Kakizuka, A., Yokota, Y., Shigemoto, R., Sasai, Y. and Takumi, T. (1990) Molecular characterization of mammalian tachykinin receptors and a possible epithelial potassium channel. *Recent Progr. Hormone Res.*, 46: 59–84.

Nakata, Y., Tanaka, H., Morishma, Y. and Segawa, T. (1988) Solubilization and characterization of substance P binding protein from bovine brainstem. *J. Neurochem.*, 50: 522–527.

Ninkovic, M., Beajouan, Y., Torrens, Y., Saffroy M., Hall, M.D. and Glowinski, J. (1984) Differential localization of tachykinin receptors in rat spinal cord. *Eur. J. Pharmacol.*, 106: 463–464.

Ohkubo, H. and Nakanishi, S. (1991) Molecular characterization of the three tachykinin receptors. *Ann. NY Acad. Sci.*, 632: 53–62.

Parker, R.M.C., Fleetwood-Walker, S.M., Rosie, R., Munro, F.E. and Mitchell, R. (1993) Inhibition by NK$_2$ but not NK$_1$ antagonists of carrageenan-induced preprodynorphin mRNA expression in rat dorsal horn lamina I neurons. *Neuropeptides*, 25: 213–222.

Patacchini, R., Astolfi, M., Quartara, L., Rovero, P., Giachetti, A. and Maggi, C.A. (1991) Further evidence for the existence of NK$_2$ tachykinin receptor subtypes. *Br. J. Pharmacol.*, 104: 91–96.

Pham, T., De Champlain, J. and Couture, R. (1993a) Inhibitory action of (+/-) CP-96,345 on the cardiovascular responses to intrathecal substance P and neuropeptide K in the conscious freely moving rat. *Naunyn-Schmiedebergs Arch. Pharmacol.*, 347: 34–41.

Pham, T., De Champlain, J. and Couture, R. (1993b) Cardiovascular and sympathoadrenal responses to intrathecal injection of neuropeptide K in the conscious rat. *Naunyn-Schmiedebergs Arch. Pharmacol.*, 347: 42–49.

Poosh, M.S., Goebel, D.J. and Bannon, M.J. (1991) Distribution of neurokinin receptor gene expression in the rat brain. *Soc. Neurosci. Abstr.*, 17: 806.

Picard, P., Boucher, S., Regoli, D., Gitter, B., Howbert, J. and Couture, R. (1993) Use of non-peptide tachykinin receptor antagonists to substantiate the involvement of NK$_1$ and

NK$_2$ receptors in a spinal nociceptive reflex in the rat. *Eur. J. Pharmacol.*, 232(2–3): 255–261.

Raffa, R.B., Martinez, R.P. and Connelly, C.D. (1993) Scyliorhinin-I and -II induce reciprocal hindlimb scratching in mice: differentiation of spinal and supraspinal neurokinin receptors in vivo. *Neurosci. Lett.*, 158: 87–91.

Randić, M., Jiang, M.C., Rusin, K.I., Cerne, R. and Kolaj, M. (1993) Interactions between excitatory amino acids and tachykinins and long-term changes of synaptic responses in the rat spinal dorsal horn. *Regul. Peptides*, 46: 418–420.

Rovero, P., Pestellini, V., Maggi, C.A., Patacchini, R., Regoli, D. and Giachetti, A. (1990) A highly selective NK$_2$ tachykinin receptor antagonist containing D-tryptophan. *Eur. J. Pharmacol.*, 175: 113–115.

Rovero, P., Astolfi, M., Renzetti, A.R., Patacchini, R., Giachetti, A. and Maggi, C.A. (1991) Role of D-tryptophan for affinity of MEN 10207 tachykinin antagonist at NK$_2$ receptors. *Peptides*, 12: 1015–1018.

Rovero, P., Astolfi, M., Manzinin, S., Jukic, D., Rouissi, N., Maggi, C.A. and Regoli, D. (1992) Structure-activity relationship study of R396, an NK$_2$ tachykinin antagonist selective for the NK$_2$B receptor subtype. *Neuropeptides*, 23: 143–145.

Salter, M.W. and Henry, J.L. (1991) Responses of functionally identified neurones in the dorsal horn of the cat spinal cord to substance P, neurokinin A and physalaemin. *Neuroscience*, 43(2/3): 601–610.

Shafer, M.K.H., Nohr, D., Krause, J.E. and Weihe, E. (1993) Inflammation-induced upregulation of NK$_1$ receptor mRNA in dorsal horn neurons. *NeuroReport*, 4: 1007–1010.

Sharif, N.A. (1990) A novel substance P binding site in rat brain regions modulates TRH receptor binding. *Neurochem. Res.*, 15(10): 1045–1049.

Shults, C.W., Quirion, R., Chronwall, B., Chase, T.N. and O'Donohue, T.L. (1984) A comparison of the anatomical distribution of substance P and substance P receptors in the rat central nervous system. *Peptides*, 5: 1097–1128.

Shults, C.W., Yajima, H., Gullner, H.G., Chase, T.N. and O'Donohue, T.L. (1985) Demonstration and distribution of kassinin-like material (substance K) in the rat central nervous system. *J. Neurochem.*, 45: 552–558.

Sivam, S.P. and Krause, J.E. (1992) Tachykinin systems in the spinal cord and basal ganglia: influence of neonatal capsaicin treatment or dopaminergic intervention on levels of peptides, substance P-encoding mRNAs, and substance P receptor mRNA. *J. Neurochem.*, 59: 2278–2284.

Stoessl, A.J. and Hill, D.R. (1990) Autoradiographic visualization of NK$_3$ tachykinin binding sites in the rat brain, utilizing [^{3}H]senktide. *Brain Res.*, 534: 1–7.

Stucky, C.L., Galeazza, M.T. and Seybold, V.S. (1993) Time-dependent changes in Bolton-Hunter labeled ^{125}I-substance P binding in rat spinal cord following unilateral adjuvant-induced peripheral inflammation. *Neuroscience*, 57(2): 397–409.

Suzuki, H., Yoshioka, K., Maehara, T., Hagan, R.M., Nakan-ishi, S. and Otsuka, M. (1993) Pharmacological characteristics of tachykinin receptors mediating acetylcholine release from neonatal rat spinal cord. *Eur. J. Pharmacol.*, 241: 105–110.

Takano, Y. and Loewy, A.D. (1985) Reduction of [^{3}H]substance P binding in the intermediolateral cell column after sympathectomy. *Brain Res.*, 333: 193–196.

Taniguchi, T., Ninomiya, H., Fukanaga, R., Ebii, K., Yamamoto, M. and Fujiwara, M. (1992) Neurokinin A stimulated phosphoinositide breakdown in rabbit iris sphincter muscle. *Jpn. J. Pharmacol.*, 59(2): 213–220.

Thompson, S.W.N., Urban, L. and Dray, A. (1993) Contribution of NK$_1$ and NK$_2$ receptor activation to high threshold afferent fibre ventral root responses in the rat spinal cord in vitro. *Brain Res.*, 625: 100–108.

Too, H.P. and Hanley, M.R. (1988) Solubilization and characterization of substance P binding sites from chick brain membranes. *Biochem. J.*, 252: 947–951.

Tsuchida, I., Shigemoto, R., Yokota, Y. and Nakanishi, S. (1990) Tissue distribution and quantification of the mRNAs for three tachykinin receptors. *J. Biochem.*, 193: 751–757.

Urban, L., Maggi, C.A., Nagy, I. and Dray, A. (1992) The selective NK$_2$ receptor antagonist MEN 10376 inhibits synaptic excitation of dorsal horn neurones evoked by c-fibre activation in the in vitro rat spinal cord. *Neuropeptides*, 22: 68–75.

Urban, L., Dray, I. and Maggi, C.A. (1993) The effects of NK$_1$ and NK$_2$ receptor antagonists on the capsaicin evoked synaptic response in the rat spinal cord in vitro. *Regul. Peptides*, 46: 413–414.

Vita, G., Haun, C.K., Hawkins, E.F. and Engel, W.K. (1990) Effects of experimental spinal cord transection on substance P receptors: a quantitative autoradiography. *Neuropeptides*, 17: 147–153.

Von Euler, U.S. and Gaddum, J.H. (1931) An unidentified depressor substance in certain tissue extracts. *J. Physiol. (London)*, 72: 74–87.

Wiesenfeld-Hallin, Z., Xu, X., Hakanson, R., Feng, D. and Folkers, K. (1991) Tachykinins mediate changes in spinal reflexes after activation of unmyelinated muscle afferents in the rat. *Acta Physiol. Scand.*, 141: 57–61.

Xu, X.J., Maggi, C.A. and Wiesenfeld-Hallin, Z. (1991) On the role of NK$_2$ tachykinin receptors in the mediation of spinal reflex excitability in the rat. *Neuroscience*, 44(2): 483–490.

Xu, X.J., Dalsgaard, C.J. and Wiesenfeld-Hallin, Z. (1992) Intrathecal CP-96,345 blocks reflex facilitation induced in rats by substance P and c-fiber conditioning stimulation. *Eur. J. Pharmacol.*, 216: 337–344.

Yashpal, K., Dam, T.V. and Quirion, R. (1990) Quantitative autoradiographic distribution of multiple neurokinin binding sites in rat spinal cord. *Brain Res.*, 506: 259–266.

Yashpal, K., Dam, T.V. and Quirion R. (1991) Effects of dorsal rhizotomy on neurokinin receptor subtypes in the rat spinal cord: a quantitative autoradiographic study. *Brain Res.*, 552: 240–247.

SECTION III

Neuropeptide Processing and Degrading Enzymes

F. Nyberg, H.S. Sharma and Z. Wiesenfeld-Hallin (Eds.)
Progress in Brain Research, Vol 104
© 1995 Elsevier Science BV. All rights reserved.

CHAPTER 7

Neuropeptide converting and processing enzymes in the spinal cord and cerebrospinal fluid

Stefan Persson[1,2], Pierre Le Grevés[1], Madeleine Thörnwall[1], Ulrica Eriksson[1], Jerzy Silberring[3] and Fred Nyberg[1]

[1]*Department of Pharmaceutical Biosciences, Division of Biological Research on Drug Dependence, University of Uppsala, Sweden,* [2]*Department of Cell and Molecular Biology, Unit of Medical Inflammation Research, Lund University, Lund, Sweden, and* [3]*Department of Clinical Neurosciences, Karolinska Institute, Stockholm, Sweden*

Introduction

Neuropeptides comprise a large class of neuroactive substances suggested to act as neurotransmittors or/and neuromodulators. Many of these compounds have been identified and characterized only during the last decade (for review, see Hökfelt, 1991). By the application of immunohistochemical and molecular biological techniques a great variety of neuropeptides has been localized in the spinal cord. Among them are, e.g., calcitonin gene-related peptide (CGRP) (Gibson et al., 1984), galanin (Melander et al., 1986) neurokinin A (Brodin et al., 1986), opioid peptides (Botticelli et al., 1981; Vincent et al., 1982; Cruz and Basbaum, 1985; Sasek and Elde, 1986; Harlan et al., 1987; Ruda et al., 1988; Weihe, 1992) and substance P (Hökfelt et al., 1977). The opioid peptides, CGRP and the tachykinins substance P/neurokinin A (see Table I) are present at high concentrations in the dorsal horn of the spinal cord, particularly in the superficial laminae. This anatomical area of the central nervous system (CNS) is known to be a relay for peripheral nociceptive signalling and these peptides are likely to be involved in the modulation and transmission of pain at this site (Besson and Chaouch, 1987; Duggan and Weihe, 1991; Weihe, 1992; Millan, 1993).

Studies on the biosynthesis of many neuropeptides have shown that these compounds are derived from the enzymatic cleavage of larger, and generally inactive, prepropeptides which are synthesized under the direction of mRNA on membrane-bound ribosomes in the cell body of the peptidergic neuron. Following enzymatic removal of the hydrophobic N-terminal signal peptide and protein folding (Gething and Sambrook, 1992) in the lumen of the endoplasmic reticulum, the propeptide is packed into secretory vesicles in the Golgi apparatus (Sossin et al., 1989). These vesicles are transported along the axon to the nerve terminal. Sequential cleavage (processing) of the propeptide is likely to take place within the secretory granules or vesicles, yielding one or more biologically active peptides that are available for secretion (cf. Hökfelt et al., 1980; Hughes, 1983; Loh, 1987; Sossin et al., 1989). Due to their size and hydrophilic nature, neuropeptides have a poor ability to cross biological membranes and therefore their release from the nerve ending is believed to occur via exocytosis. Following release, the neuroactive peptides may act on pre- or postsynaptically located receptors. Peptides almost invariably produce their actions through activation of a second messenger system. The inactivation process of neuropeptides involves more-or-less specific proteases which hydrolyse the active peptide (for reviews, see Lynch and Snyder, 1986; McKelvy and Blumberg, 1986; Skidgel et al., 1987; Nyberg and Terenius, 1991). In addition to this degrading process the active peptide may also be converted by specific proteases into products with retained or changed biological activity. Several neuropeptide converting enzymes capable of releasing bioactive fragments from their substrate peptides have been identified in various CNS tissues (Fricker and Snyder, 1983; Benuck et al., 1984; Devi and Goldstein, 1984, 1986; Acker et al., 1987; Camargo et al., 1987; Skidgel et al., 1987).

In this chapter we will focus on some of our recent studies on converting activities specifically acting on the opioid peptide dynorphin and substance P. These enzymes were previously isolated from human and bovine spinal cord, but have also been identified in human and rat cerebrospinal fluid (Nyberg et al., 1984, 1985; Silberring and Nyberg, 1989; Nyberg and Silberring, 1990; Persson et al., 1992a; Silberring et al., 1992a). The dynorphin converting enzyme (DCE) recognizes its substrate principally at the Arg^6-Arg^7 sequence, whereas substance P endopeptidase (SPE) cleaves in between or at the carboxylic side of the Phe^7-Phe^8 bond of its substrate (Table I). This review will consider the biochemical properties of the above convertases but also measurement of their activity in various experimental models to investigate their possible function in the regulation of peptide levels.

Dynorphin converting enzymes and substance P endopeptidase

Dynorphins and dynorphin converting enzymes

Opioid peptides belonging to the dynorphin family are based on the Leu-enkephalin unit, which constitute their N-terminal sequence (Table I). They are all derived from a common precursor prodynorphin (Kakidani et al., 1982; Civelli et al., 1985; Horikawa et al., 1983). Among these peptides are dynorphin A (Dyn A) and its fragments Dyn A(1–8) and Dyn A(1–13), all of them with potent opioid activity. Other prodynorphin-derived opioid peptides are dynorphin B (Dyn B) and α-neoendorphin (Table I). All the above-mentioned peptides (including the Dyn A fragments) exhibit binding affinity preferentially for κ-opioid receptors (Chavkin and Goldstein, 1981; Corbett et al., 1982; Kosterlitz, 1985).

The prodynorphin-derived peptides are widely distributed through most levels of the CNS (cf. Goldstein and Ghazarossian, 1980; Zamir et al., 1983; Civelli et al., 1985; Khachaturian et al., 1985). They are found within the dorsal horn of the spinal cord, with especially dense concentrations in Laminae I–II and IV/V (Botticelli et al.,

TABLE I

Structure of dynorphins and substance P and their bioactive fragments generated by dynorphin-converting enzyme (DCE) and substance P endopeptidase (SPE)

Peptide	Structure	Receptor selectivity
Dyn A	Tyr-Gly-Gly-Phe-Leu-Arg-Arg-Ile-Arg-Pro-Lys-Leu-Lys-Trp-Asp-Asn-Gln	κ
Dyn B	Tyr-Gly-Gly-Phe-Leu-Arg-Arg-Gln-Phe-Lys-Val-Val-Thr	κ
Leu-enk-Arg^6	Tyr-Gly-Gly-Phe-Leu-Arg	δ
SP	Arg-Pro-Lys-Pro-Gln-Gln-Phe-Phe-Gly-Leu-Met-NH$_2$	NK$_1$
SP (1–7)	Arg-Pro-Lys-Pro-Gln-Gln-Phe	NK$_L^a$

[a] See Igwe et al., 1990

Dyn, dynorphin; enk, enkephalin; SP, substance P.

1981; Vincent et al., 1982, Cruz and Basbaum, 1985; Sasek and Elde, 1986; Ruda et al., 1988; Weihe, 1992). Due to their location in the spinal cord and to their opioid activity dynorphins are believed to have a modulatory function in pain processing pathways (Millan, 1993; Yaksh, 1993).

The mechanism responsible for the inactivation of the dynorphins is likely to involve several proteases. Different enzymes acting on dynorphin and dynorphin-derived peptides have been described in the CNS (Stewart et al., 1981; Fricker and Snyder, 1982, 1983; Benuck et al., 1984; Nyberg et al., 1985, 1987; Acker et al., 1987; Inaoka and Tamaoki, 1987; Malfroy et al., 1989; Silberring and Nyberg, 1989; Healy and Orlowski, 1992; Nyberg and Silberring, 1990; Silberring et al., 1992a). Some of these activities may not only terminate their activity, known to be mediated through κ-receptors, but also release a product with changed bioactivity. For example, with regard to dynorphin A both its N-terminal (Leu-enkephalin) and C-terminal sequences are known to produce biological effects (Chavkin and Goldstein, 1981; Corbett et al., 1982; Herrera-Marschitz et al., 1984; Kosterlitz, 1985; Fujimoto et al., 1990). Peptidases capable of releasing active products from their substrates are known as converting enzymes. In recent years we have identified several convertases with high specificity towards the dynorphins (Nyberg et al., 1985, 1991; Silberring and Nyberg, 1989; Nyberg and Silberring, 1990; Silberring et al., 1992a; Persson et al., 1993).

Dynorphin converting enzyme (DCE) in human CSF

Measurements of opioid peptides in CSF have a long tradition in clinical research focused on the endogenous opioids. Actually, even before the structure of the endorphins was elucidated, their presence in human CSF was known (Terenius and Wahlström, 1974, 1975). Today, 20 years later, a number of clinical studies dealing with CSF measurements of opioid peptides in various diseases have been reported (for reviews, see Nyberg et al., 1987a, 1988; Terenius, 1987, 1988; Nyberg 1993). Chemical characterization of the opioid active material in human CSF has revealed that the various peptides in this fluid display molecular heterogeneity (Nyberg et al., 1983). For instance, dynorphin as measured by radioimmunoassay (RIA) was found to be present in three separable forms: the heptadecapeptide itself, a prestage (molecular weight, 5 kDa) and a fragment thereof (Nyberg and Nylander, 1987). The fragment was tentatively identified as Dyn A(7–17). Other Dyn A fragments (N-terminal fragments) identified in human CSF are Leu-enkephalin and Leu-enkephalin-Arg[6] (Nyberg et al., 1983; Terenius et al., 1984). The latter fragment and the above C-terminal portion of Dyn A seem to represent products from a single cleavage of the heptadecapeptide. In fact, about 10 years ago we were able to identify and partially purify, from human CSF, an enzyme capable of releasing these two fragments from Dyn A (Nyberg et al., 1985). The enzyme was classified as a serine protease and appeared to be very specific for cleaving the Arg[6]-Arg[7] bond of its substrate (Nyberg et al., 1985; Demuth and Nyberg, 1991). It has a molecular weight of approximately 40 kDa and exhibits a very high specificity towards prodynorphin-derived opioid peptides (Dyn A, Dyn B and α-neoendorphin), and it was therefore named dynorphin converting enzyme or DCE (Nyberg, 1987). However, it was also shown that DCE may hydrolyse other neuropeptide structures with somewhat different specificity and at a lower rate (Gluschankof et al., 1988). In human CSF the DCE-activity appears at comparatively high concentrations and, furthermore, a significantly negative correlation between the level of DCE and the concentration of prodynorphin-derived opioid peptides has been observed (Thörnwall et al., 1994). Due to limited amounts of CSF, it has not yet been possible to isolate DCE to homogeneity but for that purpose other sources have been considered. However, the actual origin of the CSF enzyme is so far not known.

Studies on the rat CSF have revealed that DCE-like activity is also present in this fluid

(Persson et al., 1989, 1992a,b, 1993, 1994). However, the rat enzyme differs from the human variant of DCE with regard to several properties. For instance, while the human enzyme was classified as a serine protease the rat analogue was considered rather as a thiol-dependent enzyme (Persson et al., 1993). Furthermore, it also appears to be more selective for Dyn B than Dyn A and α-neoendorphin. Altogether, the DCE activity found in rat CSF exhibits close similary to DCE-B identified in the spinal cord (see below).

DCE activities in the spinal cord

Since the CSF is in direct contact with the extracellular fluid of the CNS, and as it is assumed that neuropeptides present in CSF may have neuronal origin, we have hypothesed that DCE-activity detected in the fluid is likely to reflect proteolytic actions taking place in the CNS. In our search for DCE in CNS tissues we have mainly focused on the spinal cord. In our first attempt we were able to identify and purify a DCE-like enzyme from bovine spinal cord to homogeneity (Silberring and Nyberg, 1989). This enzyme, however, seemed to differ from the one in human CSF with regard to several properties. Firstly, it appeared to cleave Dyn B at a higher rate than that of Dyn A or α-neoendorphin. Secondly, its specificity was not found to be unique for the Arg^6-Arg^7 bond. It was found to hydrolyse its substrate also at the amino- and the carboxylic side of the dibasic stretch. It also showed a different inhibition profile as compared to the CSF enzyme and differed with regard to molecular size (Table II).

Using spinal cord tissue collected from humans we were able to identify and recover three separate enzymes with specificity towards the dynorphins (Nyberg and Silberring, 1990). All these convertases were capable of releasing the N-terminal sequence Leu-enkephalin-Arg^6 from the substrate peptide. However, they differed with respect to several properties including the cleavage specificity (Table II). One of these enzymes (named DCE-B) appeared to be highly specific

for dynorphin B and showed close similarity to the above-mentioned bovine endopeptidase (Silberring et al., 1993). Among the other two, the most acidic protease was purified to homogeneity (Silberring et al., 1992a). It showed activity optimum at pH 5.6 and exhibited high specificity for Dyn A. The other prodynorphin-derived opioids Dyn B and α-neoendorphin were also cleaved but at a much lower rate. However, it was shown that Dyn B is a potent inhibitor towards the actual enzyme. Due to its unique cleavage specificity towards Dyn A the enzyme was named DCE-A. In contrast to the other DCE activities identified in spinal cord, DCE-A has its optimal activity at pH 5.6. This property, suggesting a possible localization within secretory granules, and the observed specificity could be indicative of Dyn A being a natural substrate of DCE-A. The third human spinal cord enzyme was found to hydrolyse both Dyn A and Dyn B at similar rates. It seems to be a protein of less acidic nature than DCE-A and DCE-B and, with respect to its inhibition profile and pH optimum, it appears to be similar to the human CSF convertase. However, the estimated molecular size of this enzyme highly exceeds that of DCE in human CSF (see Table II). On the other hand, this size difference could be indicative of the CSF entity being a degradation product of its congener in the spinal cord. It should be emphasized here that all dynorphin converting enzymes identified in bovine, human as well as rat (see below) spinal cord are extracted and purified from the soluble fraction of the spinal cord homogenates.

In the rat spinal cord, as well as in the human spinal cord, three different DCE activities have been identified (unpublished observations). The biochemical and kinetic properties of one of the convertases in the rat spinal cord are in agreement with those found for both the bovine and human DCE-B enzyme (see above). From studies of rat DCE-B it was evident that the enzyme level in the dorsal part of the spinal cord highly exceeds that of the ventral part (Silberring et al., 1992b). The other two convertases hydrolysing dynorphin in the rat spinal cord resemble the

TABLE II

Properties of dynorphin converting enzymes (DCE) and substance P endopeptidase (SPE) in human spinal cord and cerebrospinal fluid

	Spinal cord		Cerebrospinal fluid	
	DCE-A	DCE-B	DCE	SPE
Apparent molecular weight (kDa)	50 000	55 000	40 000	43 000
Sensitive to EDTA	–	–	–	+
Sensitive to thiol group sensitive inhibitors	+	+	–	+
Sensitive to serine protease inhibitors	–	–	+	–
Cleavage sites of substrate	$\downarrow$ $\downarrow$ $\downarrow$ - Arg - Arg -	$\downarrow$ $\downarrow$ $\downarrow$ - Arg - Arg -	$\downarrow$ -Arg - Arg-	$\downarrow$ $\downarrow$ -Phe - Phe - Gly
K_m for the release of Leu-enkephalin-Arg[6] from dyn A (μM)	7.3[a]	–	130[b]	–
K_m for the release of Leu-enkephalin-Arg[6] from dyn B (μM)	–	12.6[a]	159[b]	–
K_m for the release of substance P (1–7) from substance P (μM)	–	–	–	19[c]

[a] See Silberring et al., 1993.
[b] See Demuth and Nyberg, 1991.
[c] See Nyberg et al., 1984.
Dyn, dynorphin; enk, enkephalin; SP, substance P.

human spinal cord enzymes in that one enzyme has an acidic pH optimum (pH 5.6), and the second enzyme active at neutral pH shows broader substrate specificity for the dynorphins. The distribution of these two latter enzymes in the spinal cord is unclear, although the neutral enzyme shows equal activities in the dorsal and ventral rat spinal cord (unpublished observations).

At this stage it is relevant to raise the question about the function of these enzymes and whether they are identical to any other proteases described in the literature. The functional significance of DCE will be discussed in a following section. With regard to the question of a possible identity between DCE and other proteases, it is evident that several enzymes with specificity to-

wards paired basic amino acids have been described (e.g., Goldstein, 1982; Mizuno and Matsuo, 1984; Acker et al., 1987; Camargo et al., 1987; Gluschankof et al., 1988; Berman et al., 1994). We have compared DCE-A, DCE-B and DCE in human spinal cord with several proteases with similar activity but, although some properties seemed to be common, no obvious identity could be seen. Very recently, Cohen and co-workers reported an arginine-specific dibasic convertase which was isolated from rat testis (Chesneau et al., 1994). By using an oligonucleotide probe and antibodies to screen a rat testis cDNA library they succeeded in isolating a full-length cDNA of the enzyme (Pierotti et al., 1994). Although this enzyme is also present in the CNS, and seems to be a prototype of a class of processing enzymes, it differs from the CSF and spinal cord DCE activities as its major cleavage is found to occur N-terminally of the Arg-Arg bond. Another family of propeptide-cleaving enzymes is that of subtilisin/kexin-like convertase (for reviews, see Steiner et al., 1992; Seidah et al., 1991a, 1994). Among these are furin (Fuller et al., 1989; Van de Ven et al., 1991), PC-1 (Seidah et al., 1990, 1991b) or PC-3 (Smeekens et al., 1991), PC-2 (Seidah et al., 1990; Smeekens and Steiner, 1990), PACE-4 (Kiefer et al., 1991), PC-4 (Nakayama et al., 1992; Seidah et al., 1992), and PC-5 or PC-6. Analysis of the mRNA pattern of these enzymes (Schäfer et al., 1993; Seidah et al., 1994) has revealed an almost unique distribution pattern of each of these enzymes. However, most of these proteases are acting on dibasic amino acid pairs (including Lys-Arg and Lys-Lys) in the prohormone sequence and do not recognize the matured product (e.g., the dynorphin) sequence as its major substrate. An additional group of neuropeptide processing endopeptidases are those capable of releasing a matured peptide by a cleavage at a single basic amino acid residue (for review, see Schwartz, 1986; Berman et al., 1994). One of these enzymes, also designated 'dynorphin converting enzyme' is known to release Dyn B from a prestage (Dyn B − 29) by a monobasic cleavage at the N-terminal side of a single arginine (Berman et al., 1994; Devi and Goldstein, 1984, 1986). The tissue distribution of this enzyme activity in the rat was reported to be high in the brain, ileum, neurointermediate pituitary and adrenal (Devi, 1993). Lower activity was found in the anterior pituitary, inner organs and serum.

The group of DCE-like activities present in CSF and the spinal cord of human, bovine and rat origin also appears to constitute a family of neuropeptide convertases. A major difference between this group of enzymes and others known to act on the dynorphins seems to be that all DCE-like activities release Leu-enkephalin-Arg[6] as a major product, thus hydrolysing their substrate within its dibasic stretch. The distribution of each DCE within the CNS has not yet been established.

In line with the increasing number of newly discovered peptides, an apparent increase in the discovery of new enzymes responsible for peptide processing, conversion and inactivation seems to have occurred. The progress in identifying DCE-like activities is probably due to the very specific tool available for their detection. In all these cases the enzyme activity has been identified and probed by a radioimmunoassay very specific for the product formed from the particular dynorphin substrate (Nyberg et al., 1985; Persson et al., 1992a). This procedure has allowed us to identify and purify a specific protease from a pool of one hundred (perhaps even more) other enzymes present in the particular fluid or extract under consideration. As soon as the enzyme was recovered in a purified fraction, free from contaminating proteases, it was possible to apply HPLC, sometimes combined with mass spectrometry, for product identification (Silberring et al., 1991).

Many studies on proteases and peptidases have utilized chromogenic substrates based on two or three amino acids. Such methods should have failed to detect DCE, as it appears that the complete N-terminal hexapeptide sequence is required. Also the C-terminal sequence beyond the actual cleavage site seems to be of importance.

Substance P and substance P converting enzymes

The undecapeptide substance P (SP) is one of the most extensively studied peptides with regard to its various biological or clinical aspects (Pernow, 1983; Watling and Krause, 1993). It has a widespread distribution throughout the CNS, but is also present in the peripheral nervous system (PNS), indicating a function in a variety of physiological processes (Lembeck and Gamse, 1982; Pernow, 1983; Warden and Young, 1988). Since immunohistochemical analysis showed substance P to be present in primary afferents (Hökfelt et al., 1975, 1977; Otzuka et al., 1982), presumably pain fibers, particular interest has been focused on substance P in its relation to nociception.

Substance P belongs to the tachykinin family of neuropeptides. Members of this family share a common C-terminal sequence, Phe-X-Gly-Leu-Met-NH_2 (Erspamer, 1981; Maggio, 1988). The C-terminal amino acid is amidated. The phenylalanine residue at the beginning of the common sequence (position 7 in SP) is conserved in all tachykinins and appears to be essential for the biological activity. The N-terminal sequence is unique for each peptide and accounts for its specific action. Substance P could be released from three different precursors (preprotachykinins, PPT), all of which originating from one distinct gene (Nawa et al., 1983; Krause et al., 1987). Three different mRNAs are thus produced from this gene (α-PPT, β-PPT and γ-PPT) as a result of alternative splicing. Each of these mRNAs gives rise to a prepropeptide containing the substance P sequence. Other tachykinins are limited to one or two precursors. For instance, the neurokinin A sequence resides in β-PPT and γ-PPT but not in α-PPT, whereas neuropeptide K only resides in β-PPT. Substance P or rather a C-terminal extension of it (SP-Gly^{12}-Lys^{13}) is excised from its precursor by trypsin-like cleavage, probably through the action of one of the abovementioned PC activities. The released tridecapeptide is further modified by the action of an α-amidating monooxygenase (EC 1.14.17.3) to yield the final active peptide (Bradbury et al., 1982; Eipper et al., 1992). Following release and exertion of its effect, substance P is likely to be inactivated by various proteases. Although no specific peptidase has yet been attributed to be the single one responsible for substance P inactivation, several enzymes capable of hydrolysing the peptide have been described. Some of these enzymes, e.g., dipeptidylaminopeptidase IV (DAP-IV) degrade the peptide sequentially from the N-terminal side (Kato et al., 1978), whereas others, e.g., angiotensin converting enzyme (ACE), hydrolyse substance P from its C-terminal part (Skidgel et al., 1984, 1987). Other proteases have been shown to hydrolyse substance P by an endopeptidase action (Blumberg et al., 1980; Matsas et al., 1984; Oblin et al., 1989; Katayama et al.,

1991; Mauborgne et al., 1991). Most of these enzymes, however, are known to potently act on several other peptides. However, there is one enzyme originally isolated from human brain which seemed to be specific for substance P (Lee et al., 1981). We have previously reported a similar enzyme in human CSF (Nyberg et al., 1984, 1986). The CSF enzyme appeared to be very specific for the undecapeptide, and was found to release products with retained biological activity; we named this enzyme substance P endopeptidase (SPE).

Substance P converting enzymes in CSF

A limited number of studies focused on substance P analysis of CSF samples originating from human subjects (Almay et al., 1988; Nyberg et al., 1988; Rimón et al., 1984; Russell et al., 1994; Tam et al., 1985) and in rats (Calvino et al., 1991) have been reported. All these studies have utilized RIA procedures to quantify the undecapeptide. However, it was found that the immunoreactivity detected was not only due to substance P, but also to its fragments (Rimón et al., 1984) and an N-terminal elongation (Toresson et al., 1988). We were able to identify the presence in human CSF of the N-terminal fragment substance P (1–7) using a specific RIA for this peptide. This finding prompted us to search for an enzyme in human CSF yielding that product. We subsequently were able to identify and partially purify an endoprotease capable of releasing both substance P (1–7) and (1–8) fragments from the parent peptide (Nyberg et al., 1984). Interestingly, both these fragments have been found to possess biological activity (Stewart et al., 1982; Hall and Stewart, 1983, 1984, 1991; Sakurada et al., 1988; Hasenöhrl et al., 1990; Herrera-Marschitz et al., 1990; Reid et al., 1990; Budai et al., 1992; Larson and Sun, 1992, 1993; Kreeger and Larson, 1993). The enzyme (named, by us, SPE) thus hydrolyses the undecapeptide within and at the carboxylic side of the double-Phe bond. It has a molecular weight of around 40 kDa and was characterized as a metal-dependent thiol-sensitive endoprotease

(Nyberg et al., 1984, 1986; Nyberg, 1987). It showed optimum activity at neutral pH and was inhibited by bacitracin. However, the most profound feature concerns its specificity. SPE shows a surprisingly high preference for substance P. It also cleaves its C-terminal fragments substance P (3–11) and (5–11) but at a much lower rate. Other tachykinins, lacking the double-Phe residues, such as neurokinin A and neurokinin B, were almost unaffected. Studies also revealed that SPE was strongly inhibited by calcitonin gene-related peptide (CGRP) (Le Grevés et al., 1985). CGRP is colocalized with substance P in many primary sensory neurons. It has also been demonstrated that CGRP potentiates the action of substance P in several ways (Wiesenfeld-Hallin et al., 1984; Woolf and Wiesenfeld-Hallin, 1986). Recently, we observed that CGRP is also cleaved by SPE (Le Grevés et al., 1989). The enzyme was found to hydrolyse the Leu-Leu bond residing in CGRP, however, at a significantly lower rate than that observed for substance P. With regard to substance P, it thus seems that SPE releases products with potent activity, i.e., it terminates the action of substance P by releasing a second signal from its structure.

Attempts to characterize SPE in the rat CSF have indicated that the major activity capable of releasing fragment 1–7 from SP present in the fluid is not identical with that of the enzyme found in human CSF (unpublished observations). By ion exchange chromatography (DEAE-Sepharose CL-6B), at least three different SPE-like activities have been detected. Two of these activities are inhibited by captopril (an inhibitor of angiotensin converting enzyme, ACE) and one by phosphoramidon (an inhibitor of neutral endopeptidase 24.11, NEP). The third SPE-like activity, representing a minor pool of the substance P (1–7)-generating activity in the rat CSF, was not affected by any of these inhibitors and could perhaps be identical to the human CSF variant of the enzyme. The presence of ACE in rat CSF has indeed been reported by others, and this enzyme may represent the major part of the SPE-like activity detected in CSF samples from this species

(Yoshida and Nosaka, 1990). However, in CSF collected from polyarthritic rats, where we see a change in substance P (1–7) -generating activity (see below) the level of ACE remained invariant and therefore it is possible that the observed alteration is due to SPE.

Substance P endopeptidase (SPE) in the spinal cord

The observation that the substance P fragment (1–7) is present in the dorsal spinal cord (Sakurada et al., 1985) has challenged us to search for SPE-like activity in this area of the CNS. However, so far we have only focused on the tissues from the whole cord. In the rat we examined homogenates, where the major part of substance P (1–7)-generating activity appeared to be due to proteases other than SPE. Thus, in accordance with the finding in rat CSF, the major activity responsible for the release of the heptapeptide was sensitive towards the ACE inhibitor captopril and to some extent also, phosphoramidon, the above-mentioned inhibitor of neutral endopeptidase 24.11 (NEP). Immunohistochemical and autoradiography studies have revealed that both ACE and NEP are also distributed throughout the CNS and PNS (Delay-Goyet et al., 1989; Pollard et al., 1989; Healy and Orlowski, 1992). Both enzymes are known to act on a number of neuroactive peptides. For instance, NEP is considered to be one of the major peptidases involved in the physiological termination of the enkephalinergic signal, whereas ACE is known to hydrolyse both the enkephalins and substance P (Skidgel et al., 1984, 1987). However, a recent study reported a membrane-bound substance P endopeptidase in the rat brain (Bergmann and Bauer, 1986). Except for a larger molecular weight this activity shows close similarity to the human SPE.

Our attempts to isolate SPE from human spinal cord are still in progress. Our current data indicate that SPE-like activity could be recovered both from the soluble and the membrane-bound fraction. From both fractions we were able to purify activity releasing substance P (1–7) from substance P which exhibited biochemical and kinetic properties in close similarity to SPE present in human CSF. Also, it seems that the relative abundance of SPE in human tissue or CSF highly exceeds that of the rat.

Functional studies of dynorphin converting enzyme and substance P endopeptidase

DCE- and SPE-like activities in chronic pain

In the acute phase of collagen-induced arthritis (CIA) the activity of both DCE and SPE in the female rat CSF is significantly reduced (Persson et al., 1992a). The acute phase of arthritis is characterized by swelling of the paws, soft-tissue edema and infiltration of inflammatory cells. In a parallel study of DCE and SPE, in a model of monoarthritis developed and characterized by Butler et al. (1990), where the inflammation is anatomically largly confined to one joint, a similar observation was made (Persson et al., 1992b). In both models of arthritis, the activity of the two enzymes was restored to control levels at more advanced stages of the disease ('chronic state'). There are reasons to believe that the acute phase of both these models is more painful than the chronic phase. For instance, the edematous process is more pronounced in the acute phase and, furthermore, sustained arthritis gradually leads to erosion of the cartilage and bone tissue with a subsequent fibrous or cartilaginous ankylosis with new bone formation of the joint (Holmdahl et al., 1990; Butler et al., 1992), which may reduce the sensation of pain.

With regard to peptide levels, it has been shown that both substance P (Schoenen et al., 1985) and the dynorphins (Millan et al., 1985; Iadarola et al., 1988; Ruda et al., 1988; Weihe et al., 1988a,b,c, 1989; Nahin et al., 1989; Noguchi et al., 1991; Przewlocka et al., 1992) are elevated in the dorsal spinal cord at the acute phase of peripheral inflammation, i.e., from a few hours up to one week after the induction of inflammation. Increased substance P levels were also observed in CSF as determined by radioimmunoassay (Calvino et al.,

1991). The time-course of DCE and SPE seems to follow that of dynorphin and substance P during polyarthritis. In a few studies, repeated measurements of substance P and dynorphin have been performed showing that the peptide levels in CSF and dorsal spinal cord normalize to control levels 6–10 weeks after induction with Freund's complete adjuvant (Millan et al., 1985, 1986; Calvino et al., 1991). Thus, in the acute phase, the peptide levels seem to increase at the expense of the activity of the enzymes, i.e., there appears to be an inverse relationship between the particular enzyme and its substrate. This observation may be indicative that the enzyme activities have a regulatory function in the respective peptide system. However, whether this is correct or not, the peptide levels may also be regulated at the level of mRNA expression. In the acute phase of arthritis or peripheral inflammation, the expressions of mRNA for prodynorphin (Iadarola et al., 1988; Ruda et al., 1988; Draisci and Iadarola, 1989; Weihe et al., 1989; Noguchi et al., 1991; Przewlocka et al., 1992; Ji et al., 1994; Persson et al., 1994) and preprotachykinin A gene (Minami et al., 1989) were seen to increase in the dorsal spinal cord. Also, the expression of mRNA for PC was found to be significantly enhanced (Weihe et al., 1994).

Among other enzymes known to act on substance P, ACE was found not to be affected in the CSF of polyarthritic rats during the edematous process in the acute phase (unpublished observations). A similar observation has previously been reported for NEP in the spinal cord (Delay-Goyet et al., 1989). Therefore, it is likely that the observed alteration in substance P (1–7)-generating activity relates to changes in the activity of the enzyme, which appears to be similar to the human SPE.

Analysis of DCE in spinal cord tissue of rats with Freund's adjuvant-induced polyarthritis indicated that the enzyme activity in the acute phase was significantly decreased in the dorsal part of the spinal cord, whereas its level in the ventral part remained unchanged (Silberring et al., 1992b). Measurements of the DCE product Leu-enkephalin-Arg[6] showed that the level of this peptide also was significantly altered in the dorsal spinal cord during the acute phase of arthritis. This finding was considered to indicate a clear relationship between the enzyme and its putative product. Moreover, it also gives support to the idea that the DCE activity observed in the CSF originates from a pain-processing area in the spinal cord.

Whether the reduced converting activity reflects a decrease in the concentration of DCE or SPE, or a reduced ability to convert the substrate, is not known. However, preliminary results suggest that DCE is inhibited by an unknown factor in CSF (unpublished results). The reduction seen in SPE activity could be due to an interaction between the enzyme and CGRP. Both CGRP and substance P coexist in primary afferent neurons and are likely to be co-released from the terminals of these nerves (cf. Saria et al., 1986). As mentioned above, CGRP is shown to inhibit SPE and to prolong and potentiate several of the biological actions of substance P (Le Grevés et al., 1985; Wiesenfeld-Hallin et al., 1984; Woolf and Wiesenfeld-Hallin, 1986). In this context it should be stressed that the procedures used to probe the CSF enzymes in these studies measure their activity and not their actual concentration.

DCE- and SPE-like activities in opioid tolerance and dependence

Chronic treatment of mammals with opioids is shown to induce adaptive changes in the CNS leading to the development of tolerance and dependence. While tolerance is characterized as a consequence of chronic opiate administration linked to changes in receptor coupling, the mechanism behind the development of opiate dependence is not clear. Many studies have been carried out in order to elucidate the possible role of opioid peptides and substance P in opiate tolerance and addiction. However, so far it has been hard to identify any marked changes in the CNS levels of these peptides. In a recent study, a reduction in the level of dynorphin A and substance P in the rat spinal cord at 24 h following cessation of chronic administration of morphine was observed (Nylander et al., 1991). Furthermore, a study where dynorphin A1–13 was decreased in the spinal cord, but increased in the pituitary and hypothalamus, 18 h after removal of implanted morphine pellets in morphine-tolerant rats was also reported (Rattan et al., 1992). A more recent study indicated a reduction in dynorphin A in nucleus accumbens at the abstinence phase in morphine-tolerant rats (Yukhananov et al., 1993). Thus, there is some data available in the literature indicating alterations in the CNS levels of dynorphin A and substance P, as well in animals exposed to opiates. Both peptides have also been shown to modify tolerance development to opiates and abstinence reactions (Chahl, 1983; Jones and Olpe, 1984; Green and Lee, 1988; Smith and Lee, 1988).

We recently observed changes in the CSF activities in DCE and SPE in opiate tolerant rats (Persson et al., 1989). The animals rendered tolerant to the mixed opioid agonist/antagonist, dezocine morphine and, by continuous subcutaneous infusion at a constant rate by miniosmotic pumps showed an increased activity of both DCE and SPE in their CSF. The significance of this increase is not clear and may only be speculated upon. Increased DCE activity may, of course, affect the levels of dynorphin A and would be in agreement with reduced concentrations of this peptide as found in the spinal cord in the above-mentioned study. Dynorphin peptides are shown to have morphine antagonistic properties and attenuate the rate of tolerance development to opiates (Green and Lee, 1988; Smith and Lee, 1988). Provided that the increased DCE activity reflects an enhanced conversion of dynorphin to enkephalin, chronic opiate treatment would appear to reduce the modulatory action of dynorphins. The elevation of SPE activity would have consequences for the level of substance P. Thus, the concentration of the fragment substance P (1–7) may increase at the expense of the parent peptide. This would be in agreement with decreased levels of substance P in the spinal cord as observed in morphine tolerant rats (Nylander et al., 1991). Both substance P and its fragment substance P (1–7) are shown to attenuate morphine withdrawal reactions (Stern and Hadzovic, 1973; Kreeger and Larson, 1993), the effect of substance P may be produced after a prior conversion to its N-terminal fragment. Moreover, N-terminal metabolites of substance P enhance the binding of μ-opiate-selected agonists to μ-opioid receptors (Krumins et al., 1993). Therefore, the interaction between substance P (1–7) and the endogenous opioid system together with the ability of the substance P fragment to modulate withdrawal behaviours in opiate-dependent animals suggests a functional role of SPE in states of morphine tolerance.

Effects of glucocorticosteroids on DCE activity in rat CSF

Corticosteroids are known to influence the biogenic amine systems as well as neuropeptides (Harlan, 1988; McEwen, 1987; Chalmers et al., 1993). The effect of corticosteroids on the dynorphin system is well documented (Persson et al., 1994a; Thai et al., 1992). For instance, in control rats the glucocorticosteroid budesonide was found to increase the expression of preprodynorphin mRNA in Laminae I/II of the dorsal spinal cord, whereas an opposite effect, i.e., down-regulation of the inflammation-induced increase in preprodynorphin mRNA expression, was produced in Laminae I/II and IV/V of collagen-induced arthritic rats treated with budesonide (Persson et al., 1994a). Preliminary evidence also indicates that this steroid can down-regulate the up-regulated CGRP expression in primary afferents of collagen-induced arthritic rats (Nohr et al., 1993). However, in the CSF, a significant reduction of DCE activity was observed following budesonide and prednisolone treatment (Persson et al., 1994b). This decrease was first observed 48 h after the steroid injection. After 24 h, the DCE activity was still unaffected. A glucocorticosteroid-mediated reduction of DCE suggests a possible increase of dynorphin level and, thereby,

an enhanced signalling on κ-receptors; as mentioned above, dynorphins are believed to be endogenous ligands at the κ-receptor (Chavkin and Goldstein, 1981; Corbett et al., 1982, Kosterlitz, 1985). Under stress conditions, the endogenous secretion of glucocorticosteroids may be greatly enhanced, and in stress states related to chronic pain (e.g., arthritis) the activity of DCE is highly reduced (see above). It is therefore tempting to speculate whether the mechanism behind the down-regulation of DCE seen in arthritic rats is similar to that observed in animals treated with glucocorticosteroids. At the molecular level, the mechanism underlying the alteration in DCE activity is not clear and may only be speculated upon. The observation that DCE was unaffected 24 h following steroid injection, but reduced after 48 h, favours a genomic regulation of DCE activity. This could possibly occur directly on the enzyme synthesis or indirectly through the action of a possible endogenous inhibitor.

Clinical studies of DCE activity in CSF

A few studies of DCE in CSF samples of clinical origin have been performed. The enzyme activity was found to be reduced in CSF collected from women at term pregnancy (Lyrenäs et al., 1988). This reduction was paralleled by an increase in levels of prodynorphin-derived opioid peptides. A negative correlation between prodynorphin-derived opioids and DCE activity was also seen in CSF from chronic pain patients (Thörnwall et al., 1994). Moreover, CSF analysis of patients with fibromyalgia indicated elevated levels of dynorphin A at the expense of a decrease in DCE activity (Thörnwall et al., 1994). It thus seems that the CSF level of prodynorphin-derived opioids is inversely correlated to DCE activity suggesting a possible role of the enzyme in the regulation of the peptide concentration. From this observation it was proposed that DCE may be a good marker for activity in the prodynorphin system. The mechanism by which the DCE activity could be altered is, however, not yet clear. One possibility is that the rate of enzyme biosynthesis is altered and another is that the enzyme activity is reduced or regulated by the release of an endogenous inhibitor.

Studies on DCE in CSF from patients with ischialgia (a kind of neurogenic pain due to herniated discs) showed elevated activity of the enzyme, whereas in patients with coxarthrosis the DCE activity remained unaltered (unpublished observations). These findings were considered to indicate that measurements of DCE activity in CSF of chronic pain patients could be helpful in the diagnosis of these patients. However, also in connection with this, it should be stressed that before the question about the origin of DCE in human CSF is finally settled it will be difficult to come to any firm conclusions about its function.

DCE and SPE inactivators

Access to specific inhibitors of DCE and SPE would facilitate the functional studies of these enzymes. Therefore, in recent years our studies have been directed towards the design of irreversible acting inhibitors for both DCE and SPE.

Inhibitors of DCE

With regard to DCE from human CSF we used peptidyl methylketone derivatives and N-peptidyl-O-acyl hydroxylamines, which have previously been shown to be specific inhibitors of several serine and cysteine proteinases (Demuth and Nyberg, 1991). Preincubation of the enzyme with these compounds resulted in substantial loss of the DCE activity, using both dynorphin A and B as substrates and the RIA-method for activity determination (Table III). It was further observed that compounds containing phenylalanine (Z-Phe-Phe-NHO-Ma) induced the strongest inhibition of the enzyme.

The N-peptidyl-O-acyl hydroxylamines were also used in studies on DCE-A and DCE-B from human spinal cord (Silberring et al., 1993). Z-Phe-Phe-NHO-Ma was also found to be the most potent inhibitor for these enzymes. However, according to the calculated values for the inhibitory constants, this compound was about 5-times more potent against DCE-A (K_i 3.2 μM), when compared to DCE-B (K_i 16.9 μM). Moreover, the N-terminal protected peptide Boc-Phe-Gly-NHO-Bz (Table III) was also documented as having a higher inhibitory potency against DCE-A compared to DCE-B. The difference observed in the inhibition of the two proteinases by these compounds might be of use in further searches for

TABLE III

Effects of several peptide inhibitors on the activity of human cerebrospinal fluid DCE towards Dyn A and Dyn B

Inhibitor	DCE activity[a] on Dyn A (% of control)	DCE activcity[a] on Dyn B (% of control)
Boc-Ala-Ala-NHO-Nb	72	79
Boc-Ala-Ala-Ch$_2$-Cl	80	56
Boc-Ala-Pro-Val-NHO-Nb	87	59
Z-Ala-Ala-Phe-CH2-Cl	52	29
Z-Ala-Ala-Phe-CH$_3$	51	7.6
Z-Phe-Phe-NHO-Nb	18	1.0
Boc-Phe-Gly-NHO-Bz	76	39
PMSF	19	14

(Data from Demuth and Nyberg, 1991.)
[a] The enzyme activity was monitored by following the conversion of the substrate peptide using radioimmunoassay specific for the hexapeptide (Leu-enkephalin-Arg[6]) product.

inhibitors allowing discrimination between the two enzymes.

In additional work we have designed appropriate enkephalin-analogue structures as potential inactivators of enzymes exhibiting trypsin-like substrate specificity, including DCE from human CSF (Demuth et al., 1991). It was found that trypsin and papain were inactivated by the enkephalin analogue, diacyl hydroxylamine (Leu-enkephalin-Lys-NHO-Bz), in a time-dependent and irreversible manner, whereas DCE was only moderately inhibited by this compound. From these results it was concluded that the reaction mechanism of DCE is different from the catalytic mechanism of the 'classical' serine proteases.

The access of specific DCE inhibitors may be of importance for the development of drugs to be used as pain modulators. In fact, several strategies have been developed to obtain new potent analgesic compounds by protecting the endogenous opioid peptides from enzymatic inactivation. For instance, it was recently shown that a mixed inhibitor prodrug (RB 101) which prevents degradation of the enkephalins by aminopeptidase and NEP, has a potent analgetic effect (Noble et al., 1992; Roques et al., 1993). Furthermore, this compound only induces weak tolerance and was not seen to induce physical dependence. The idea of developing inhibitors to DCE as possible analgesics is, besides the promising results with NEP inhibitors, also supported by the finding that inhibition of metalloendopeptidase 24.15 produces antinociception (Kest et al., 1991). This latter enzyme transforms dynorphins, particular dynorphin A(1–8) into Leu-enkephalin. This is essentially a similar enzymatic conversion as compared to DCE. Both enzymes attenuate a κ-opioid signal (dynorphins) and increase the δ-opioid message (enkephalins).

Inhibitors of SPE

In our attempts to develop specific inhibitors against human SPE we have substituted the bis-phenyl-alanine moiety in substance P with a non-peptidergic fragment (Jenmalm et al., 1992). This change in the structure of the undecapeptide yielded a product which potently inhibited the endopeptidase. However, the modified compound retained recognition of, and binding to, the substance P receptor (NK_1-receptor).

In further studies, a series of benzyl- or aryl-substituted 1,2,4-oxadiazole derivatives of phenylalanine was synthesized (Borg et al., 1993). Some of these compounds exhibited weak inhibitory activity towards SPE, but all of them lacked appreciable affinity for the NK_1-receptor. It was thus found that a 2-pyridyl oxadiazole derivative, as well as compounds with an electron-deficient aromatic ring, produced an inhibitory action on the enzyme. Additional studies focused on evaluation of the selectivity of these inhibitors and on the synthesis of more potent compounds are in progress.

Concluding remarks

Most enzymes so far identified in spinal cord tissue show broad substrate specificity and are likely to function in the general protein/peptide catabolism within this part of the CNS. However, there are also other enzymes present in this region with a more defined specificity. This chapter has attempted to describe the characteristics of some neuropeptide convertases specifically acting on dynorphins and substance P. It is obvious that these enzymes do not only act as inactivators of the actual peptides, but are also capable of releasing a second signal from the parent compound. From functional and clinical studies, it seems that both DCE and SPE may have a regulatory role in the respective neuropeptide system. Evidently, the activity of these convertases appears to be related to a variety of pathophysiological conditions. Therefore, both DCE and SPE could be considered as highly relevant targets for the development of specific inhibitors. Potent inhibitors of DCE and SPE would be of use in further attempts to define the functional relevance of the actual substrates and their products, but could also serve as leads for the rational design of drugs which can act as inactivators of these enzymes.

Acknowledgements

This work is supported by the Swedish Medical Research Council (Grant 9459) and by the Swedish National Board for Industrial and Technical Development (NUTEC).

The skilful secretarial assistance of Agneta Bergström is gratefully acknowledged.

References

Acker, G., Molineaux, Ch. and Orlowski, M. (1987) Synaptosomal membrane-bound form of endopeptidase 24.15 generates Leu-enkephalin from dynorphin A_{1-8}, α- and β-neoendorphin and Met-enkephalin from Met-enkephalin-Arg^6-Gly^7-Leu^8. *J. Neurochem.*, 48: 284–292.

Almay, B.G.L., Johansson, F., Von Knorring, L., Le Grevés, P. and Terenius, L. (1988) Substance P in CSF of patients with chronic pain syndromes. *Pain*, 33: 3–9.

Benuck, M., Berg, M.J. and Marks, N. (1984) Membrane-bound enzymes and their role in processing of the dynorphins and of the proenkephalin octapeptide Met-enkephalin-Arg-Gly-Leu. *Neurochem. Res.* 9: 733–749.

Bergmann, A. and Bauer, K. (1986) A membrane-bound substance P degrading endopeptidase from rat brain. *Natl. Inst. Drug Abuse Res. Monogr. Ser.*, 75: 283–286.

Berman, Y.L., Rattan, A.K., Carr, K. and Devi, L. (1994) Regional distribution of neuropeptide processing endopeptidases in adult rat brain. *Biochimie*, 76: 245–250.

Besson, J. and Chaouch, A. (1987) Peripheral and spinal mechanisms of nociception. *Physiol. Rev.*, 67: 67–186.

Blumberg, S., Teichberg, V.I., Charli, J.L., Hersh, L.B. and McKelvy, J.F. (1980) Cleavage of substance P to an N-terminal tetrapeptide and a C-terminal heptapeptide by a post-proline cleaving enzyme from bovine brain. *Brain Res.*, 192: 477–486.

Borg, S., Luthman, K., Nyberg, F., Terenius, L. and Hacksell, U. (1993) 1,2,4-Oxadiazole derivatives of phenylalanine; potential inhibitors of substance P endopeptidase. *Eur. J. Med. Chem.*, 28: 801–810.

Botticelli, L.J., Cox, B.M. and Goldstein, A. (1981) Immunoreactive dynorphin in mammalian spinal cord and dorsal root ganglia. *Proc. Natl. Acad. Sci. USA*, 78: 7783–7786.

Bradbury, A.F., Finnie, M.D.A. and Smyth, D.G. (1982) Mechanism of C-terminal amide formation by pituitary enzymes. *Nature*, 298: 686–688.

Brodin, E., Lindefors, N., Dalsgaard, C.J., Theodorsson-Norheim, E. and S. Rosell (1986) Tachykinin multiplicity in rat central nervous system as studied using antisera raised against substance P and neurokinin A. *Regul. Peptides*, 13: 252–272.

Budai, D., Wilcox, G.L. and Larson, A.A. (1992) Modulation of *N*-methyl-D-aspartate and (R,S)-α-amino-3-hydroxy-5-methylisoxazole-4-propionate (AMPA) responses of spinal nociceptive neurons by a N-terminal fragment of substance P. *Eur. J. Pharmacol.*, 216: 441–444.

Butler, S.H., Godefroy, F., Besson, J. and Weil-Fugazza, J. (1990) Production of a limited arthritic model for chronic pain and inflammation studies in rats. *Eur. J. Pharmacol.*, 183: 2275–2276.

Butler, S.H., Godefroy, F., Besson, J.-M. and Weil-Fugazza, J. (1992) A limited arthritic model for chronic pain studies in the rat. *Pain*, 48: 73–81.

Calvino, B., Maillet, S., Pradelles, P., Besson, J.-M. and Couraud, J.-Y. (1991) Levels of substance P-like immunoreactivity in plasma and cerebrospinal fluid during the course of Freund adjuvant-induced arthritis, a chronic pain model. *CR Acad. Sci. Paris Sér. III*, 312: 427–432.

Camargo, A.C.M., Olivera, E.G., Toffoletto, O., Metters, K.M. and Rossier, J. (1987) Brain endooligopeptidase A, a putative enkephalin converting enzyme. *J. Neurochem.*, 48: 1258–1263.

Chahl, L.A. (1983) Contracture of guinea-pig ileum on withdrawal of methionine^5-enkephalin is mediated by substance P. *Br. J. Pharmacol.*, 80: 741–749.

Chalmers, D.T., Kwak, S.P., Mansour, A., Akil, H. and Watson, S.J. (1993) Corticosteroids regulate brain hippocampal 5-HT$_{1A}$ receptor mRNA expression. *J. Neurosci.*, 13: 914–923.

Chavkin, C. and Goldstein, A. (1981) Specific receptor for the opioid peptide dynorphin: structure-activity relationships. *Proc. Natl. Acad. Sci. USA*, 78: 6543–6547.

Chesneau, V., Pierotti, A.R., Barré, N., Créminon, Ch., Toagard, C. and Cohen, P. (1994) Isolation and characterization of a dibasic selective metalloendopeptidase from rat testes that cleaves at the amino terminus of arginine residues. *J. Biol. Chem.*, 269(3): 2056.

Civelli, O., Douglass, J., Goldstein, A. and Herbert, E. (1985), Sequence and expression of the rat prodynorphin gene. *Proc. Natl. Acad. Sci. USA*, 82: 4291–4295.

Corbett, A.D., Paterson, S.J., McKnight, A.T., Magnan, J. and Kosterlitz, H.W. (1982) Dynorphin$_{1-8}$ and dynorphin$_{1-9}$ are ligands for the κ-subtype of opiate receptor. *Nature*, 299: 79–81.

Cruz, L. and Basbaum, A.I. (1985) Multiple opioid peptides and the modulation of pain: immunohistochemical analysis of dynorphin and enkephalin in the trigeminal nucleus caudalis and spinal cord of the cat. *J. Comp. Neurol.*, 240: 331–348.

Delay-Goyet, P., Kayser, V., Zajac, J., Guilbaud, G., Besson, J. and Roques, B.P. (1989) Lack of significant changes in μ, δ opioid binding sites and neutral endopeptidase EC 3.4.24.11 in the brain and spinal cord of arthritic rats. *Neuropharmacology*, 28: 1341–1348.

Demuth, H. and Nyberg, F. (1991) Studies of specificity and inhibition of human cerebrospinal fluid dynorphin converting enzyme. *J. Enz. Inhibit.*, 4: 299–306.

Demuth, H., Silberring, J. and Nyberg, F. (1991) Inhibition of proteases with enkephalin analogue inhibitors. *J. Enz. Inhibit.*, 4: 289–298.

Devi, L. (1993) Tissue distribution of a dynorphin-processing endopeptidase. *Endocrinology*, 132: 1139–1144.

Devi, L. and Goldstein, A. (1984) Dynorphin converting enzyme with unusual specificity from rat brain. *Proc. Natl. Acad. Sci. USA*, 81: 1892–1896.

Devi, L. and Goldstein, A. (1986) Conversion of Leumorphin (dynorphin B-29) to dynorphin B and dynorphin B-14 by thiol protease activity. *J. Neurochem.*, 47: 154–157.

Draisci, G. and Iadarola, M.J. (1989) Temporal analysis of increases in c-fos, preprodynorphin and preproenkephalin mRNAs in rat spinal cord. *Mol. Brain Res.*, 6: 31–37.

Duggan, A.W. and Weihe, E. (1991) Central transmission of impulses in nociceptors: events in the superficial dorsal horn, In: A.I. Basbaum and J. Besson (Eds.), *Towards a New Pharmacotherapy of Pain*, John Wiley & Sons Ltd, Chichester, pp. 35–67.

Eipper, B.A., Stoffers, D.A. and Mains, R.E. (1992) The biosynthesis of neuropeptides: peptide α-amidation. *Annu. Rev. Neurosci.*, 15: 57–85.

Erspamer, V. (1981) The tachykinin peptide family. *Trends Neurosci.*, 4: 267–269.

Fricker, L.D. and Snyder, S.H. (1982) Enkephalin convertase: purification and characterization of a specific enkephalin-synthesizing carboxypeptidase localized to adrenal chromaffin granules. *Proc. Natl. Acad. Sci. USA*, 79: 3886–3890.

Fricker, L.D. and Snyder, S.H. (1983) Purification and characterization of enkephalin convertase, an enkephalin-synthesizing carboxypeptidase. *J. Biol. Chem.*, 258: 10950–10955.

Fujimoto, J.M., Arts, K.S., Rady, J.J. and Tseng, L.F. (1990) Spinal dynorphin $A_{(1-17)}$: possible mediator of antianalgesic action. *Neuropharmacology*, 29: 609–617.

Fuller, R.S., Brake, A.J. and Thorner, J. (1989) Intracellular targeting and structural conservation of a prohormone-processing endoprotease. *Science*, 246: 482–486.

Gething, M. and Sambrook, J. (1992) Protein folding in the cell. *Nature*, 355: 33–45.

Gibson, S.J., Polak, J.M., Bloom, S.R., Sabate, I.M., Mulderry, P.M., Ghatei, M.A., McGregor, G.P., Morison, J.F.B., Kelly, J.S., Evans, R.M. and Rosenfeld, M.G. (1984) Calcitonin gene related peptide immunoreactivity in the spinal cord of man and eight other species. *J. Neurosci.*, 4: 3101–3111.

Gluschankof, P., Gomez, S., Lepage, A., Créminon, C., Nyberg, F., Terenius, L. and Cohen, P. (1988) Role of substrate structure in selective processing of peptide hormones at basic amino acid pairs by endopeptidases. *FEBS Lett.*, 234: 149–152.

Goldstein, A. (1982) Immunoreactive dynorphin in *Escherichia coli*: tracer degradation by a heat-stable endopeptidase. *Life Sci.*, 31: 2267–2270.

Goldstein, A. and Ghazarossian, V.E. (1980) Immunoreactive dynorphin in pituitary and brain. *Proc. Natl. Acad. Sci. USA*, 77: 6207–6210.

Green, P.G. and Lee, N.M. (1988) Dynorphin A-(1–13) attenuates withdrawal in morphine-dependent rats: effect of route of administration. *Eur. J. Pharmacol.*, 145: 267–272.

Hall, M.E. and Stewart, J.M. (1983) Substance P and behavior: opposite effects of N-terminal and C-terminal fragments. *Peptides*, 4: 763–768.

Hall, M.E. and Stewart, J.M. (1984) Modulation of isolation-induced fighting by N- and C-terminal analogs of substance P: evidence for multiple recognition sites. *Peptides*, 5: 85–89.

Hall, M.E. and Stewart, J.M. (1991) The substance P fragment SP(1–7) stimulates motor behavior and nigral dopamine release. *Pharmacol. Biochem. Behav.*, 41: 75–78.

Harlan, R.E. (1988) Regulation of neuropeptide gene expression by steroid hormones. *Mol. Neurobiol.*, 2: 183–200.

Harlan, R.E., Shivers, B.D., Romano, G.J., Howells, R.D. and Pfaff, D.W. (1987) Localization of preproenkephalin mRNA in the rat brain and spinal cord by in situ hybridization. *J. Comp. Neurol.*, 258: 159–184.

Hasenöhrl, R.U., Gerhardt, P. and Huston, J.P. (1990) Substance P enhancement of inhibitory avoidance learning: mediation by the N-terminal sequence. *Peptides*, 11: 163–167.

Healy, D.P. and Orlowski, M. (1992) Immunocytochemical localization of endopeptidase 24.15 in rat brain. *Brain Res.*, 571: 121–128.

Herrera-Marschitz, M., Hökfelt, T., Ungerstedt, U., Terenius, L., and Goldstein, M. (1984) Effect of intranigral injections of dynorphin, dynorphin fragments and alfa-neoendorphin on rotational behaviour in rat. *Eur. J. Pharmacol.*, 102: 213–227.

Herrera-Marschitz, M., Terenius, L., Sakurada, T., Reid, M.S. and Ungerstedt, U. (1990) The substance P(1–7) fragment is a potent modulator of substance P actions in the brain. *Brain Res.*, 521: 316–320.

Holmdahl, R., Andersson, M., Goldschmidt, T.J., Gustafsson, K., Jansson, L. and Mo, J.A. (1990) Type II collagen autoimmunity in animals and provocations leading to arthritis. *Immunol. Rev.*, 118: 193–232.

Horikawa, S., Takai, T., Toyosato, M., Takahashi, H., Noda, M., Kakidani, H., Kubo, T., Hirose, T., Inayama, S., Hayashida, H., Miyata, T. and Numa, S. (1983) Isolation and structural organization of the human preproenkephalin B gene. *Nature*, 306: 611–614.

Hughes, J. (1983) Biogenesis, release and inactivation of enkephalins and dynorphins. *Br. Med. Bull.*, 39: 17–24.

Hökfelt, T. (1991) Neuropeptides in perspective: the last ten years. *Neuron*, 7: 867–879.

Hökfelt, T., Kellerth, J., Nilsson, G. and Pernow, B. (1975), Experimental immunohistochemical studies on the localiza-

126

tion and distribution of substance P in cat primary sensory neurons. *Brain Res.*, 100: 235–252.

Hökfelt, T., Ljungdahl, L.A., Terenius, L., Elde, R.P. and Nilsson, G. (1977) Immunohistochemical analysis of peptide pathways related to pain and analgesia: enkephalin and substance P. *Proc. Natl. Acad. Sci. USA*, 74: 3081–3085.

Hökfelt, T., Johansson, O., Ljungdahl, Ä., Lundberg, J.M. and Schultzberg, M. (1980) Peptidergic neurones. *Nature*, 284: 515–521.

Iadarola, M.J., Douglass, J., Civelli, O. and Naranjo, J.R. (1988) Differential activation of spinal cord dynorphin and enkephalin neurons during hyperalgesia: evidence using cDNA hybridization. *Brain Res.*, 455: 205–212.

Igwe, O.J., Kim, D.C., Seybold, V.S., Larson, A.A. (1990) Specific binding of substance P aminoterminal heptapeptide [SP(1–7)] to mouse brain and spinal cord membranes. *J. Neurosci.*, 10: 3653–3663.

Inaoka, Y. and Tamaoki, H. (1987) Purification and characterization of enkephalinase B from rat brain membrane. *Biochim. Biophys. Acta*, 925: 27–35.

Jenmalm, A., Luthman, K., Lindberg, G., Nyberg, F., Terenius, L. and Hacksell, U. (1992) Novel peptidomimetics: inhibitors of substance P endopeptidase. *Bioorg. Med. Chem. Lett.*, 2(12): 1693–1698.

Ji, R.-R., Zhang, X., Wiesenfeld-Hallin, Z. and Hökfelt, T. (1994) Expression of neuropeptide Y and neuropeptide Y (Y1) receptor mRNA in rat spinal cord and dorsal root ganglia following peripheral tissue inflammation. *J. Neurosci.*, 14: 6423–6434.

Jones, R.S.G. and Olpe, H. (1984) An increase in sensitivity of rat cingulate cortical neurones to substance P occurs following withdrawal of chronic administration of antidepressant drugs. *Br. J. Pharmacol.*, 81: 659–664.

Kakidani, H., Furutani, Y., Takahashi, H., Noda, M., Morimoto, Y., Hirose, T., Asai, M., Inayama, S., Nakanishi, S. and Numa, S. (1982) Cloning and sequence analysis of cDNA for porcine β-neo-endorphin/dynorphin precursor. *Nature*, 298: 245–249.

Khachaturian, H., Lewis, M.E., Schäfer, M.K. and Watson, S.J. (1985) Anatomy of the CNS opioid systems. *Trends Neurosci.*, 8: 111–119.

Katayama, M., Nadel, J.A., Bunnett, N.W., Di Maria, G.U., Haxhiu, M. and Borson, D.B. (1991) Catabolism of calcitonin gene-related peptide and substance P by neutral endopeptidase. *Peptides*, 12: 563–567.

Kato, T., Nagatsu, T., Fukasawa, K., Harada, M., Nagatsu, I. and Sakakibara, S. (1978) Successive cleavage of N-terminal Arg^1-Pro^2 and Lys^3-Pro^4 from substance P but no release of Arg^1-Pro^2 from bradykinin, by X-Pro dipeptidyl-aminopeptidase. *Biochim. Biophys. Acta*, 525: 417–422.

Kest, B., Orlowski, M., Molineaux, C.J. and Bodnar, R.J. (1991) Antinociceptive properties of inhibitors of endopeptidase 24.15. *Int. J. Neurosci.*, 56: 141–149.

Kiefer, M.C., Tucker, J.E., Joh, R., Landsberg, K.E., Saltman, D. and Barr, P.J. (1991) Identification of a second human subtilisin-like protease gene in the *fes/fps* region of chromosome 15. *DNA Cell Biol.*, 10: 757–769.

Kosterlitz, H.W. (1985) The Welcome Foundation lecture, 1982. Opioid peptides and their receptors. *Proc. R. Soc. London (Biol.)*, 225: 27–40.

Krause, J.E., Chirgwin, J.M., Carter, M.S., Xu, Z.S. and Hershey, A.D. (1987) Three rat preprotachykinin mRNAs encode the neuropeptides substance P and neurokinin A. *Proc. Natl. Acad. Sci. USA*, 84: 881–885.

Kreeger, J.S. and Larson, A.A. (1993) Substance P-(1–7), a substance P metabolite, inhibits withdrawal jumping in morphine-dependent mice. *Eur. J. Pharmacol.*, 238: 111–115.

Krumins, S.A., Kim, D.C., Igwe, O.J. and Larson, A.A. (1993) DAMGO binding to mouse brain membranes: influence of salts, guanine nucleotides, substance P, and substance P fragments. *Peptides*, 14: 309–314.

Larson, A.A. and Sun, X. (1992) Amino terminus of substance P potentiates kainic acid-induced activity in the mouse spinal cord. *J. Neurosci.*, 12: 4905–4910.

Larson, A. and Sun, X. (1993) Modulation of kainic acid-induced activity in the mouse spinal cord by amino terminus of substance P: sensitivity to opioid antagonists. *J. Pharmacol. Exp. Ther.*, 265: 159–165.

Le Grevés, P., Nyberg, F., Terenius, L. and Hökfelt, T. (1985) Calcitonin gene-related peptide is a potent inhibitor of substance P degradation. *Eur. J. Pharmacol.*, 115: 309–311.

Le Grevés, P., Nyberg, F., Hökfelt, T. and Terenius, L. (1989) Calcitonin gene related peptide is metabolized by an endopeptidase hydrolyzing substance P. *Regul. Peptides*, 25: 277–286.

Lee, C., Sandberg, B.E.B., Hanley, M.R. and Iversen, L.L. (1981) Purification and characterisation of a membrane-bound substance-P-degrading enzyme from human brain. *Eur. J. Biochem.*, 114: 315–327.

Lembeck, F. and Gamse, R. (1982) Substance P in peripheral sensory processes, In: R. Porter and M. O'Connor (Eds.), *Substance P in the Nervous System*, Pitman, London, pp. 35–48.

Loh, Y.P. (1987) Peptide precursor processing enzymes within secretory vesicles. *Ann. NY Acad. Sci.*, 493: 292–307.

Lynch, D.R. and Snyder, S.H. (1986) Neuropeptides: multiple molecular forms, metabolic pathways, and receptors. *Annu. Rev. Biochem.*, 55: 773–799.

Lyrenäs, S., Nyberg, F., Lindberg, B. and Terenius, L. (1988) Cerebrospinal fluid activity of dynorphin-converting enzyme at term pregnancy. *Obstet. Gynecol.*, 72: 54–58.

Maggio, J.E. (1988) Tachykinins. *Annu. Rev. Neurosci.*, 11: 13–28.

Malfroy, B., Kado-Fong, H., Gros, C., Giros, B., Schwartz, J. and Hellmiss, R. (1989) Molecular cloning and amino acid sequence of rat kidney aminopeptidase M: a member of a super family of zinc-metallohydrolases. *Biochem. Biophys. Res. Commun.*, 161: 236–241.

Matsas, R., Fulcher, I.S., Kenny, A.J. and Turner, A.J. (1984) Substance P and (Leu) enkephalin are hydrolyzed by an enzyme in pig caudate synaptic membranes that is identical with the endopeptidase of kidney microvilli. *Proc. Natl. Acad. Sci. USA*, 80: 3111–3115.

Mauborgne, A., Bourgoin, S., Benoliel, J.J., Hamon, M. and Cesselin, F. (1991) Is substance P released from slices of the rat spinal cord inactivated by peptidase(s) distinct from both 'enkephalinase' and 'angiotensin-converting enzyme'?. *Neurosci. Lett.*, 123: 221–225.

McEwen, B.S. (1987) Glucocorticoid-biogenic amine interactions in relation to mood and behavior. *Biochem. Pharmacol.*, 36: 1755–1763.

McKelvy, J.F. and Blumberg, S. (1986) Inactivation and metabolism of neuropeptides. *Annu. Rev. Neurosci.*, 9: 415–434.

Melander, T., Hökfelt, T. and Rokaeus, A. (1986) Distribution of galanin-like immunoreactivity in the rat central nervous system. *J. Comp. Neurol.*, 248: 475–517.

Millan, M.J. (1993) Multiple opioid systems and chronic pain, In: A. Herz, H. Akil and E.J. Simon (Eds.) *Handbook of Experimental Pharmacology*, Springer-Verlag, Berlin, vol. 104/II, pp. 127–162.

Millan, M.J., Millan, M.H., Pilcher, C.W.T., Czlonkowski, A., Herz, A. and Colpaert, F.C. (1985) Spinal cord dynorphin may modulate nociception via a κ-opioid receptor in chronic arthritic rats. *Brain Res.*, 340: 156–159.

Millan, M.J., Millan, M.H., Czlonkowski, A., Höllt, V., Pilcher, C.W.T., Herz, A. and Colpaert, F.C. (1986) A model of chronic pain in the rat: response of multiple opioid systems to adjuvant-induced arthritis. *J. Neurosci.*, 6: 899–906.

Minami, M., Kuraishi, Y., Kawamura, M., Yamaguchi, T., Masu, Y., Nakanishi, S. and Satoh, M. (1989) Enhancement of preprotachykinin A gene expression by adjuvant-induced inflammation in the rat spinal cord: possible involvement of substance P-containing spinal neurons in nociception. *Neurosci. Lett.*, 98: 105–110.

Mizuno, K. and Matsuo, H. (1984) A novel protease from yeast with specificity towards paired basic residues. *Nature*, 309: 558–560.

Nahin, R.L., Hylden, J.L.K., Iadarola, M.J. and Dubner, R. (1989) Peripheral inflammation is associated with increased dynorphin immunoreactivity in both projection and local circuit neurons in the superficial dorsal horn of the rat lumbar spinal cord. *Neurosci. Lett.*, 96: 247–252.

Nakayama, K., Kim, W., Torii, S., Hosaka, M., Nakagawa, T., Ikemizu, J., Baba, T. and Murakami, K. (1992) Identification of the fourth member of the mammalian endoprotease family homologous to the yeast Kex2 protease. *J. Biol. Chem.*, 267: 5897–5900.

Nawa, H., Hirose, T., Takashima, H., Inayama, S. and Nakanishi, S. (1983) Nucleotide sequence of cloned cDNAs for two types of bovine brain substance P precursor. *Nature*, 306: 32–36.

Noble, F., Ceric, P., Fournié-Zaluski, M.C. and Roques, B. (1992) Lack of physical dependence in mice after repeated systemic administration of the mixed inhibitor prodrug of enkephalin-degrading enzyme, RB 101. *Eur. J. Pharmacol.*, 223: 91–96.

Noguchi, K., Kowalski, K., Traub, R., Solodkin, A., Iadarola, M.J. and Ruda, M.A. (1991) Dynorphin expression and Fos-like immunoreactivity following inflammation induced hyperalgesia are colocalized in spinal cord neurons. *Mol. Brain Res.*, 10: 227–233.

Nohr, D., Stark, R., Källström, J., Persson, S., Romeo, H., Schäfer, M.K. and Weihe, E. (1993) Reaktion von CGRP primärafferenzen auf entzündung: corticosteroidsensitive hochregulierung der genexpression und topospezifisches peripheres sprouting. *Schmerz*, 7(Suppl. 1): 40.

Nyberg, F. (1987) Peptidases in human cerebrospinal fluid converting dynorphin and substance P to bioactive fragments. *Adv. Biosci.*, 65: 65–72.

Nyberg, F. (1993) CSF opioids in pathophysiology, In: A. Herz, H. Akil and E. Simon (Eds), *Handbook of Experimental Pharmacology*, Springer-Verlag, Berlin, Heidelberg, vol. 104/II, pp. 653–672.

Nyberg, F. and Nylander, I. (1987) Characterization of dynorphin immunoreactivity in human cerebrospinal fluid. *Regul. Peptides*, 17: 159–166.

Nyberg, F. and Silberring, J. (1990), Conversion of the dynorphins to Leu-enkephalin in human spinal cord, In: C. Quirion, K. Jhamandas and C. Gianoulakis (Eds.), *The International Narcotics Research Conference (INRC) 89*, Alan R. Liss Inc., New York, pp. 261–265.

Nyberg, F. and Terenius, L. (1991) Enzymatic inactivation of neuropeptides, In: J.H. Henriksen (Ed.), *Degradation of Bioactive Substances: Physiology and Pathophysiology*, CRC Press Inc., New York, pp. 189–200.

Nyberg, F., Le Grevés, P., Sundqvist, C. and Terenius, L. (1984) Characterization of substance P (1–7) and (1–8) generating enzyme in human cerebrospinal fluid. *Biochem. Biophys. Res. Commun.*, 125: 244–250.

Nyberg, F., Nordström, K. and Terenius, L. (1985) Endopeptidase in human cerebrospinal fluid which cleaves proenkephalin B opioid peptides at consecutive basic amino acids. *Biochem. Biophys. Res. Commun.*, 131: 1069–1074.

Nyberg, F., Sundqvist, C. and Le Gréves, P. (1986) Substance P converting endopeptidase in human cerebrospinal fluid. *Protides Biol. Fluids*, 34: 181–185.

Nyberg, F., Christensson-Nylander, I. and Terenius, L. (1987a) Measurement of opioid peptides in biologic fluids by radioimmunoassay, In: C. Patrono and B.A. Peskar, *Handbook of Experimental Pharmacology*, Springer-Verlag, Berlin, Heidelberg, pp. 227–253.

Nyberg, F., Bålöw, R., Tomkinson, B. and Zetterquist, Ö. (1987b) Degradation of Leu- and Met-enkephalin and their C-terminal extensions by tripeptidyl peptidase II. *Protides Biol. Fluids*, 35: 193–196.

Nyberg, F., Vaeroy, H. and Terenius, L. (1988) Opioid peptides and substance P in cerebrospinal fluid: regulation and significance to pain. In: J. Olesen, J. and L. Edvinson, *Basic Mechanism of Headache*, Elsevier Science Publishers B.V., Amsterdam, pp. 311–325.

Nyberg, F., Kankaanranta, S., Brostedt, P. and Silberring, J. (1991) Purification and characterization of endoproteases from human choroid plexus cleaving prodynorphin-derived opioid peptides. *Brain Res.*, 552: 129–135.

Nylander, I., Sakurada, T., Le Gréves, P. and Terenius, L. (1991) Levels of dynorphin peptides, substance P and CGRP in the spinal cord after subchronic administration of morphine in the rat. *Neuropharmacology*, 30: 1219–1223.

Oblin, A., Danse, M.J. and Zivkovic, B. (1989) Metalloendopeptidase (EC 3.4.24.11) but not angiotensin converting enzyme is involved in the inactivation of substance P by synaptic membranes of the rat substantia nigra. *Life Sci.*, 44: 1467–1474.

Otsuka, M., Konishi, M., Yanayisawa, A., Tsunoo, A. and Akayi, H. (1982) Role of substance P as a sensory transmitter in spinal cord and sympathetic ganglia. In: *Substance P in the Nervous System, Ciba Foundation Symposium*, Pitman Medical, London pp. 13–34.

Pernow, B. (1983) Substance P. *Pharmacol. Rev.*, 35: 85–141.

Persson, S., Post, C., Alari, L., Nyberg, F. and Terenius, L. (1989) Increased neuropeptide-converting enzyme activities in cerebrospinal fluid of opiate-tolerant rats. *Neurosci. Lett.*, 107: 318–322.

Persson, S., Post, C., Holmdahl, R. and Nyberg, F. (1992a) Decreased neuropeptide-converting enzyme activities in cerebrospinal fluid during acute but not chronic phases of collagen induced arthritis in rats. *Brain Res.*, 581: 273–282.

Persson, S., Post, C., Weil-Fugazza, J., Butler, S.H. and Nyberg, F. (1992b) Decreased cerebrospinal fluid neuropeptide-converting enzyme activity in monoarthritic rats. *Neurosci. Lett.*, 143: 247–250.

Persson, S., Jónsdóttir, I., Thorén, P., Post, C., Nyberg, F. and Hoffmann, P. (1993) Cerebrospinal fluid dynorphin-converting enzyme activity is increased by voluntary exercise in the spontaneously hypertensive rat. *Life Sci.*, 53: 643–652.

Persson, S., Schäfer, M.K., Nohr, D., Ekström, G., Post, C., Nyberg, F. and Weihe, E. (1994a) Spinal prodynorphin gene expression in collagen-induced arthritis: influence of the glucocorticosteroid budesonide. *Neuroscience*, 63: 313–326.

Persson, S., Malmberg, A., Post, C. and Nyberg, F. (1994b) Glucocorticosteroids decrease the activity of a dynorphin-converting endopeptidase in rat cerebrospinal fluid. *Regul. Peptides* Suppl. I: S157-S160.

Pierotti, A.R., Prat, A., Chesneau, V., Gaudoux, F., Leseney,

A.M., Foulon, T. and Cohen, P. (1994) *N*-Arginine dibasic convertase, a metalloendopeptidase as a prototype of a class of processing enzymes. *Proc. Natl. Acad. Sci. USA*, 92: 6078–6082.

Pollard, H., Bouthenet, M.L., Moreau, J., Souil, E., Verroust, P., Ronco, P. and Schwartz, J.C. (1989) Detailed immunoautoradiographic mapping of enkephalinase (EC 3.4.24.11) in rat central nervous system: comparision with enkephalins and substance P. *Neuroscience*, 30: 339–376.

Przewlocka, B., Lason, W. and Przewlocki, R. (1992) Time-dependent changes in the activity of opioid systems in the spinal cord of monoarthritic rats: a release and in situ hybridization study. *Neuroscience*, 46: 209–216.

Rattan, A.K., Kao, K.L., Tejwani, G.A. and Bhargava, H. (1992) The effect of morphine tolerance, dependence, and abstinence on immunoreactive dynorphin (1–13) levels in discrete brain regions, spinal cord, pituitary gland and peripheral tissue in the rat. *Brain Res.*, 584: 207–212.

Reid, M.S., Herrera-Marschitz, M., Terenius, L. and Ungerstedt, U. (1990) Intranigral substance P modulation of striatal dopamine: interaction with N-terminal and C-terminal substance P fragments. *Brain Res.*, 526: 228–234.

Rimón, R., Le Gревés, P., Nyberg, F., Heikkiló, L., Salmela, L. and Terenius, L. (1984) Elevation of substance P-like peptides in the CSF of psychiatric patients. *Biol. Psychiat.*, 19: 509–516.

Roques, B.P., Noble, F., Daugé, V., Fournie-Zaluski, M. and Beaumont, A. (1993) Neutral endopeptidase 24.11; structure, inhibition, and experimental and clinical pharmacology. *Pharmacol. Rev.*, 45: 87–146.

Ruda, M.A., Iadarola, M.J., Cohen, L.V. and Young, W.S. III (1988) In situ hybridization histochemistry and immunocytochemistry reveal an increase in spinal dynorphin biosynthesis in a rat model of peripheral inflammation and hyperalgesia. *Proc. Natl. Acad. Sci. USA*, 85: 622–626.

Russell, I.J., Orr, M.D., Littman, B., Vipraio, G.A., Alboukrek, D., Michalek, J.E., Lopez, Y. and McKillip, F. (1994) Elevated cerebrospinal fluid levels of substance P in patients with fibromyalgia syndrome. *Arthr. Rheum.*, 37: 1593–1601.

Sakurada, T., Le Gревés, P., Stewart, J. and Terenius, L. (1985) Measurement of substance P metabolites in rat CNS. *J. Neurochem.*, 44: 718–722.

Sakurada, T., Kuwahara, H., Takahashi, K., Sakurada, S., Kisara, K. and Terenius, L. (1988) Substance P (1–7) antagonizes substance P-induced aversive behavior in mice. *Neurosci. Lett.*, 95: 281–285.

Saria, A., Gamse, R., Petermann, J., Fischer, J.A., Theodorsson-Norheim, E. and Lundberg, J.M. (1986) Simultaneous release of several tachykinins and calcitonin gene-related peptide from rat spinal cord slices. *Neurosci. Lett.*, 63: 310–314.

Sasek, C.A. and Elde, R.P. (1986) Coexistence of enkephalin and dynorphin immunoreactivities in neurons in the dorsal gray commissure of the sixth lumbar and first sacral spinal cord segments in rat. *Brain Res.*, 381: 8–14.

Schoenen, J., Van Hees, J., Gybels, J., de Castro Costa, M. and Vanderhaeghen, J.J. (1985) Histochemical changes of substance P, FRAP, serotonin and succinic dehydrogenase in the spinal cord of rats with adjuvant arthritis. *Life Sci.*, 36: 1247–1254.

Schwartz, T.W. (1986) The processing of peptide precursors: 'proline-directed arginyl cleavage' and other monobasic processing mechanisms. *FEBS Lett.*, 200: 1–10.

Schäfer, M.K., Day, R., Cullinan, W.E., Chrétien, M., Seidah, N.G. and Watson, S.J. (1993) Gene expression of prohormone and proprotein convertases in the rat CNS: a comparative in situ hybridization analysis. *J. Neurosci.*, 13: 1258–1279.

Seidah, N.G., Gaspar, L., Mion, P., Marcinkiewicz, M., Mbikay, M. and Chrétien, M. (1990) cDNA sequence of two distinct pituitary proteins homologous to Kex2 and Furin gene products: tissue-specific mRNAs encoding candidates for pro-hormone processing proteinases. *DNA Cell Biol.*, 9: 415–424.

Seidah, N.G., Day, R., Marcinkiewicz, M., Benjannet, S. and Chrétien, M. (1991a) Mammalian neural and endocrine pro-protein and pro-hormone convertases belonging to the subtilisin family of serine proteinases. *Enzyme*, 45: 271–284.

Seidah, N.G., Marcinkiewicz, M., Benjannet, S., Gaspar, L., Beaubien, G., Mattei, M.G., Lazure, C., Mbikay, M. and Chrétien, M. (1991b) Cloning and primary sequence of a mouse candidate prohormone convertase PC1 homologous to PC2, Furin and Kex2: distinct chromosomal localization and messenger RNA distribution in brain and pituitary compared to PC2. *Mol. Endocrinol.*, 5: 111–122.

Seidah, N.G., Day, R., Hamelin, J., Gaspar, A., Collard, M.W. and Chrétien, M. (1992) Testicular expression of PC4 in the rat: molecular diversity of a novel germ cell-specific kex2/subtilisin-like proprotein convertase. *Mol. Endocrinol.*, 6: 1559–1569.

Seidah, N.G., Chrétien, M. and Day, R (1994) The family of subtilisin/kexin like pro-protein and pro-hormone convertases: divergent or shared functions. *Biochimie*, 76: 197–209.

Silberring, J. and Nyberg, F. (1989) A novel bovine spinal cord endoprotease with high specificity for dynorphin B. *J. Biol. Chem.*, 264: 11082–11086.

Silberring, J., Brostedt, P., Thörnwall, M. and Nyberg, F. (1991) Approach to studying proteinase specificity by continuous-flow fast atom bombardment mass spectrometry and high-performance liquid chromatography combined with photodiode-array ultraviolet detection. *J. Chromatogr.*, 554: 83–90.

Silberring, J., Castello, M. and Nyberg, F. (1992a) Characterization of dynorphin A-converting enzyme in human spinal cord. *J. Biol. Chem.*, 267: 21324–21328.

Silberring, J., Sakurada, T. and Nyberg, F. (1992b) Dynorphin converting enzyme in the rat spinal cord: decreased activities during acute phase of adjuvant induced arthritis. *Life Sci.*, 50: 839–847.

Silberring, J., Demuth, H.U., Brostedt, P and Nyberg, F. (1993) Inhibition of dynorphin converting enzymes from human spinal cord by N-peptidyl-O-acyl hydroxylamines. *J. Biochem.*, 114: 648–651.

Skidgel, R.A., Engelbrecht, S., Johnson, A.R. and Erdös, E.G. (1984) Hydrolysis of substance P and neurotensin by converting enzyme and neutral endopeptidase. *Peptides*, 5: 769–776.

Skidgel, R.A., Defendini, R. and Erdös, E.G. (1987) Angiotensin I converting enzyme and its role in neuropeptide metabolism, In: A.J. Turner (Ed.), *Neuropeptides and their Peptidases*, Ellis Horwood, Chichester, England, pp. 165–182.

Smeekens, S.P. and Steiner, D.F. (1990) Identification of a human insulinoma cDNA encoding a novel mammalian protein structurally related to the yeast dibasic processing protease Kex2. *J. Biol. Chem.*, 265: 2997–3000.

Smeekens, S.P., Avruch, A.S., LaMendola, J., Chan, S.J. and Steiner, D.F. (1991) Identification of a cDNA encoding a second putative prohormone convertase related to PC2 in AtT20 cells and islet of Langerhans. *Proc. Natl. Acad. Sci. USA*, 88: 340–344.

Smith, A.P. and Lee, N.M. (1988) Pharmacology of dynorphin. *Annu. Rev. Pharmacol. Toxicol.*, 28: 123–140.

Sossin, W.S., Fisher, J.M. and Scheller, R.H. (1989) Cellular and molecular biology of neuropeptide processing and packaging. *Neuron*, 2: 1407–1417.

Steiner, D.F., Smeekens, S.P., Ohagi, S. and Chan, S.J. (1992) The new enzymology of precursor processing endoproteases. *J. Biol. Chem.*, 267: 23435–23438.

Stern, P. and Hadzovic, J. (1973) Pharmacological analysis of central actions of synthetic substance P. *Arch. Int. Pharmacodyn.*, 202: 259–262.

Stewart, T.A., Weare, J.A. and Erdös, E. (1981) Purification and characterization of human converting enzyme (kininase II). *Peptides*, 2: 145–152.

Stewart, J.M., Hall, M.E., Harkins, J., Frederickson, R.C.A., Terenius, L., Hökfelt, T. and Krivoy, W.A. (1982) A fragment of substance P with specific central activity: SP (1–7). *Peptides*, 3: 851–857.

Tam, P.K.H., Dockray, G.J. and Lister, J. (1985) Substance P concentrations in human cerebrospinal fluid vary inversely with age. *Neurosci. Lett.*, 54: 327–332.

Terenius, L. (1987) Endorphins and substance P in chronic pain. *Adv. Pain. Res. Ther.*, 10: 9–15.

Terenius, L. (1988) Significance of opiod peptides and other potential markers of neuropeptide systems in cerebrospinal fluid. In: H.L. Fields, and J.M. Besson (Eds.), *Progress in Brain Research, Vol. 77*, Elsevier Science Publishers, Amsterdam, pp. 419–429.

Terenius, L. and Wahlström, A. (1974) Inhibitor(s) of narcotic receptor binding in brain extracts and cerebrospinal fluid. *Acta Pharmacol. Toxicol.*, 35(Suppl.): 55.

Terenius, L. and Wahlström, A. (1975) Morphine-like ligand for opiate receptors in human CSF. *Life Sci.*, 16: 1759–1764.

Terenius, L., Nyberg, F. and Wahlström, A. (1984) Opioid peptides in human cerebrospinal fluid. In: J. Hughes, H.O.J. Collier, M.J. Rance and M.B. Tyers (Eds.), *Opioids, Past, Present and Future*, Taylor & Francis, London and Philadelphia, pp. 179–191.

Thai, L., Lee, P.H.K., Ho, J., Suh, H. and Hong, J.S. (1992) Regulation of prodynorphin gene expression in the hippocampus by glucocorticoids. *Mol. Brain Res.*, 16: 150–157.

Thörnwall, M., Schwartzmayer, S., Almay, B., Post, C., Vaerøy, H. and Nyberg, F. (1994) Dynorphin converting enzyme in human cerebrospinal fluid. A negative correlation between activity and levels of prodynorphin derived opioid peptides. *Regul Peptides*, suppl. 1, 235–236.

Toresson, G., Brodin, E., Wahlström, A. and Bertilsson, L. (1988) Detection of N-terminally extended substance P but not of substance P in human cerebrospinal fluid: quantitation with HPLC-Radioimmunoassay. *J. Neurochem.*, 50: 1701–1707.

Van de Ven, W.J.M., Creemers, J.W.M. and Roebroek, A.J.M. (1991) Furin: the prototype mammalian subtilisin-like proprotein-processing enzyme. Endoproteolytic cleavage at paired basic residues of proproteins of the eukaryotic secretory pathway. *Enzyme*, 45: 257–270.

Vincent, S.R., Hökfelt, T., Christensson, I. and Terenius, L. (1982) Dynorphin-immunoreactive neurons in the central nervous system of the rat. *Neurosci. Lett.*, 33: 185–190.

Warden, M.K. and Young, W.S. (1988) Distribution of cells containing mRNAs encoding substance P and neurokinin B in the rat central nervous system. *J. Comp. Neurol.*, 272: 90–113.

Watling, K.J. and Krause, J.E. (1993) The rising sun shines on substance P and related peptides. *Trends Pharmacol. Sci.*, 14: 81–84.

Weihe, E. (1992) Neurochemical anatomy of the mammalian spinal cord: functional implications. *Ann. Anat.*, 174: 89–118.

Weihe, E., Millan, M.J., Leibold, A., Nohr, D. and Herz, A. (1988a) Co-localization of proenkephalin- and prodynorphin-derived opioid peptides in laminae IV/V spinal neurons revealed in arthritic rats. *Neurosci. Lett.*, 85: 187–192.

Weihe, E., Nohr, D., Millan, M.J., Stein, C., Gramsch, C.,

Höllt, V. and Herz, A. (1988b) Experimental mono- and polyarthritis differentially intensify immunostaining of multiple proenkephalin- and prodynorphin-opioid peptides in rat lumbosacral neurons. *Adv. Biosci.*, 75: 359–362.

Weihe, E., Nohr, D., Millan, M.J., Stein, C., Müller, S., Gramsch, C. and Herz, A. (1988c) Peptide neuroanatomy of adjuvant-induced arthritic inflammation in rat. *Agents Actions*, 25: 255–259.

Weihe, E., Millan, M.J., Höllt, V., Nohr, D. and Herz, A. (1989) Induction of the gene encoding pro-dynorphin by experimentally induced arthritis enhances staining for dynorphin in the spinal cord of rats. *Neuroscience*, 31: 77–95.

Weihe, E., Schäfer, M.K., Nohr, D. and Persson, S. (1994) Expression of neuropeptides, neuropeptide receptors and neuropeptide processing enzymes in spinal neurons and peripheral non-neural cells and plasticity in models of inflammatory pain, In: T. Hökfelt, H.-G. Schaible and R.F. Schmidt (Eds), *Neuropeptides, Nociception and Pain*, Chapman & Hall GmbH, Weinheim, pp. 43–69.

Wiesenfeld-Hallin, Z., Hökfelt, T., Lundberg, J.M., Forssmann, W.G., Reinecke, M., Tschopp, F.A. and Fischer, J.A. (1984) Immunoreactive calcitonin gene-related peptide and substance P coexist in sensory neurons to the spinal cord and interact in spinal behavioral responses of the rat. *Neurosci. Lett.*, 52: 199–204.

Woolf, C. and Wiesenfeld-Hallin, Z. (1986) Substance P and calcitonin gene-related peptide synergistically modulate the gain of the nociceptive flexor withdrawal reflex in the rat. *Neurosci. Lett.*, 66: 226–230.

Yaksh, T.L. (1993) The spinal actions of opioids, In: A. Herz, H. Akil and E.J. Simon (Eds.), *Handbook of Experimental Pharmacology*, Springer-Verlag, Berlin, vol. 104/II, pp. 53–90.

Yoshida, T. and Nosaka, S. (1990) Some characteristics of a peptidyl dipeptidase (kininase II) from rat CSF: differential effects of NaCl on the sequential degradation steps of bradykinin. *J. Neurochem.*, 55: 1861–1869.

Yukhananov, R.Y., Zhai, Q.Z., Persson, S., Post, C. and Nyberg, F. (1993) Chronic administration of morphine decreases level of dynorphin A in the rat nucleus accumbens. *Neuropharmacology*, 32: 703–709.

Zamir, N., Palkovits, M. and Brownstein, M.J. (1983) Distribution of immunoreactive dynorphin in the central nervous system of the rat. *Brain Res.*, 280: 81–93.

F. Nyberg, H.S. Sharma and Z. Wiesenfeld-Hallin (Eds.)
Progress in Brain Research, Vol 104
© 1995 Elsevier Science BV. All rights reserved.

CHAPTER 8

Inactivation of neuropeptides

E. Csuhai, S.S. Little and L.B. Hersh

Department of Biochemistry, University of Kentucky, Chandler Medical Center, 800 Rose Street,
Lexington, KY 40536-0084, USA

Introduction

Neuropeptides (Moore and Black, 1991) are biologically potent molecules of 2–40 amino acids, with physiological activity ranging from their acting as neurotransmitters (Kondo et al., 1993), local hormones or, more generally, as neuromodulators (Brownstein, 1989). The number of identified neuropeptides in the mammalian nervous system is now over 50 and new potential members of the neuropeptide family are being described and evaluated continuously (Nishimura and Hazato, 1993).

For a list of selected neuropeptides considered in this chapter see Table I.

Neuropeptides fulfill their physiological role acting in the extracellular space transmitting chemical messages by binding to specific receptors on the cell surface. Because of their crucial role in neuronal information processing, the regulation of the activity of neuropeptides is of utmost importance. Since there is only very limited evidence for the uptake of neuropeptide ligands by the cell following receptor binding in vivo (which would allow for intracellular processing) (Morel, 1994; Beudet et al., 1994), their levels and thus their action must be controlled by the regulation of their equilibrium concentrations in the extracellular space. Therefore, it is generally believed that neuropeptide inactivation is carried out by peptidases anchored to the cell membrane, with their active sites facing the extracellular space.

Such enzymes have been termed ectoenzymes. For an overview of ectoenzyme classification and functions see Kenny and Turner (1987).

According to this assumption, an enzyme can be classified as a neuropeptidase in vivo if it can be shown that it fulfills the requirements of being an ectoenzyme, it is co-localized with its presumed target and it is capable of degrading relevant peptides.

Neuropeptide-degrading enzymes

The enzymes capable of degrading peptides in the nervous system are generally characterized by broad substrate specificity, and it is accepted that a few general peptidases act as inactivators for all neuropeptides instead of each peptide having its corresponding specific peptidase. The in vivo specificity of these peptidases is governed by a range of factors including the localization of the enzymes and that of their potential substrates in the tissue of interest (Turner et al., 1985). Individual enzymes usually show a preference for a particular type of peptide bond, or certain concensus sequences of the peptide substrate involved in cleavage (e.g., N-terminal amino acids, proline residues, after mono- or dibasic sequences, etc.), but sometimes this specificity can vary even between similar peptides (Devi, 1991).

Although the number of neuropeptides and peptidases reported to have been found in the

TABLE I

Peptides	Amino acid sequence
Opioid peptides:	
Leu-enkephalin	Tyr-Gly-Gly-Phe-Leu
Met-enkephalin	Tyr-Gly-Gly-Phe-Met
Dynorphin A	Tyr-Gly-Gly-Phe-Leu-Arg-Arg-Ile-Arg-Pro-Lys-Leu-Lys-Trp-Asp-Asn-Gln
Dynorphin B	Tyr-Gly-Gly-Phe-Leu-Arg-Arg-Gln-Phe-Lys-Val-Val-Thr
α-Neo-endorphin	Tyr-Gly-Gly-Phe-Leu-Arg-Lys-Tyr-Pro-Lys
β-Neo-endorphin	Tyr-Gly-Gly-Phe-Leu-Arg-Lys-Tyr-Pro
γ-Endorphin	Tyr-Gly-Gly-Phe-Met-Thr-Ser-Glu-Lys-Ser-Gln-Thr-Pr -Leu-Val-Thr-Leu
β-Endorphin	Tyr-Gly-Gly-Phe-Met-Thr-Ser-Glu-Lys-Ser-Gln-Thr-Pr-Leu-Val-Thr-Leu-Phe-Lys-Asn-Ile-Ile-Lys-Asn-Ala-Tyr-Lys-Lys-Gl-Glu
Tachykinin family:	
Substance P	Arg-Pro-Lys-Pro-Gln-Gln-Phe-Phe-Gly-Leu-Met-NH_2
Neurokinin A	His-Lys-Thr-Asp-Ser-Phe-Val-Gly-Leu-Met-NH_2
Neurokinin B	Asp-Met-His-Asp-Phe-Phe-Val-Gly-Leu-Met-NH_2
Neuropeptide K	< Ser-His-Lys-Arg-His-Lys-Thr-Asp-Ser-Phe-Val-Gly-Leu-Met-NH^2
Other neuropeptides:	
Bradykinin	Arg-Pro-Pro-Gly-Phe-Ser-Pro-Phe-Arg
Neurotensin	< Glu-Leu-Tyr-Glu-Asn-Lys-Pro-Arg-Arg-Pro-Tyr-Ile-eu
Cholecystokinin octapeptide	Asp-Tyr-Met-Gly-Trp-Met-Asp-Phe-NH_2
Angiotensin I	Asp-Arg-Val-Tyr-Ile-His-Pro-Phe-His-Leu
Angiotensin II	Asp-Arg-Val-Tyr-Ile-His-Pro-Phe
Angiotensin III	Arg-Val-Tyr-Ile-His-Pro-Phe
Oxytocin	Cys-Tyr-Ile-Gln-Asn-Cys-Pro-Leu-Gly-NH_2
Vasopressin	Cys-Tyr-Ile-Gln-Asn-Cys-Pro-Arg-Gly-NH_2
Thyrotropin-releasing hormone	pGlu-His-Pro-NH_2
Luteinizing hormone-releasing hormone	pGlu-His-Trp-Ser-Tyr-Gly-Leu-Arg-Pro-Gly-NH_2
Somatostatin	Ala-Gly-Cys-Lys-Asn-Phe-Phe-Trp-Lys-Thr-Phe-Thr-Ser-Dys

spinal cord is continually increasing (e.g., Zhu et al., 1992; Rowan et al., 1993) — due largely to the development of sensitive immunochemical methods — most of our knowledge of the mechanism of neuropeptide inactivation has been based on in vivo and in vitro studies of enzymes in the brain. The material presented here clearly emphasizes the need for the isolation, characterization and comparison of the corresponding enzymes from the spinal cord (Nishimura, 1993).

A large number of exo- and endopeptidases have been identified in various tissues (e.g., Marks et al., 1988; Yaron and Naider, 1993), but to date only the following enzymes have been shown to be ectoenzymes with neuropeptide-degrading capability:

- neprilysin ('enkephalinase', neutral endopeptidase 24.11, NEP; EC 3.4.24.11) (Roques et al., 1993)

- angiotensin converting enzyme (ACE, kininase II, peptidyl dipeptidase A; EC 3.4.15.1) (Jaspard et al., 1992; Welches et al., 1993)
- aminopeptidase M (aminopeptidase N; EC 3.4.11.2) (Gros et al., 1985; Taylor, 1993)
- pyroglutamyl peptidase II (EC 3.4.11.8) (Charli et al., 1988)
- dipeptidyl peptidase IV (EC 3.4.14.5) (Yaron and Naider, 1993).

In addition, other enzymes potentially involved in neuropeptide inactivation are: prolyl endopeptidase (EC 3.4.21.26) (Kalwant and Porter, 1991); calpain (Ca^{2+}-activated neutral protease) (Murachi et al., 1987); endopeptidase 24.15 (EC 3.4.24.15) (Tisljar, 1993); endopeptidase 24.16 (EC 3.4.24.16) (Checler et al., 1993); aminopeptidase A (EC 3.4.11.7) aminopeptidase B (EC 3.4.11.6) (Dauch et al., 1993); and puromycin sensitive aminopeptidase (Hersh, 1985; Dyer et al., 1990). Although these enzymes cleave a number of neuropeptides in vitro, their precise location and orientation needs to be ascertained to allow for the characterization of these enzymes as neuropeptide-degrading or -inactivating enzymes in vivo (e.g., Mentlein, 1988).

Inhibition of neuropeptide-degrading enzymes by specific inhibitors

In vivo studies on the degradation of neuropeptides have been aided by the development of selective mechanism-based inhibitors for many peptidases (Bateman and Hersh, 1987). With the use of selective inhibitors, measurements of changes in the levels of any given neuropeptide in vivo provide information regarding the existence and characteristics of potential peptidases involved in the inactivation of that neuropeptide (Skidgel, 1993). A neuropeptide can generally be a substrate for more than one peptidase and, to prevent cleavage, either a combination of specific inhibitors or inhibitors with specificity toward more than one enzyme are employed (e.g., Roques, 1993). A list of the most frequently used inhibitors is illustrated in Table II.

In addition to the mechanism-based inhibitors specific for each enzyme, the activity of peptidases can be blocked by group-specific reagents, depending on the chemical characteristics of the enzyme. Some frequently used group-specific reagents that cause inactivation of different kinds of enzymes are shown in Table III.

For a review of some applications of peptidase inhibitors see, e.g., Skidgel (1993).

In the following sections the specificity and enzymological properties of the most important neuropeptide-degrading enzymes will be discussed. Since the specific enzymes responsible for the conversion of a particular biologically active neuropeptide into a second neuropeptide with different biological activity/receptor preference will be discussed elsewhere in this volume (see also, e.g., Borg et al., 1993; Persson et al., 1993), here we only consider the enzymes involved in the final inactivation of peptides.

Neprilysin

Neprilysin (EC 3.4.24.11), also known as 'enkephalinase', or neutral endopeptidase (NEP), is probably the major neuropeptide-degrading peptidase. It is a glycosylated membrane-bound ectoenzyme, containing a Zn^{2+} atom necessary for catalytic activity (Kerr and Kenny, 1974a,b), with a molecular weight of 87 000 Da. NEP is widely distributed in the body, having been detected in brain (Sullivan et al., 1978), spinal cord (Waksman et al., 1986), intestine (Danielsen et al., 1980), kidney (Wong-Leung and Kenny, 1968; Kerr and Kenny, 1974a) and a number of other tissues (Gee et al., 1985). The enzyme cleaves a variety of substrates, including the enkephalins (Malfroy et al., 1978), atrial natriuretic factor (Koehn et al., 1987; Stephenson and Kenny, 1987), substance P and the neurokinins (Matsas et al., 1983, 1984), neurotensin (Checler et al., 1983) and the endothelins (Vijayaraghavan and Hersh, 1990). NEP preferentially cleaves substrates on the amino side of hydrophobic residues (e.g., Met, Leu, Phe) (Kerr and Kenny, 1974a), with Phe-Phe-Ala-Phe-Leu-Ala as the optimal substrate se-

TABLE II

Enzyme	Inhibitor	K_i (nM)	Reference
Endopeptidase 24.11	phosphoramidon	3	Almenoff et al., 1983
	Thiorphan	2	Soleilhac et al., 1992
	RB 104	0.03	Roques, 1993
NEP 24.11/ACE	ES 34	4.5/55	Roques, 1993
	PC 57	1.4/0.2	Roques, 1993
ACE	captopril	0.33	Goli and Galardy, 1986
	enalapril	2–8	Wei et al., 1992
Aminopeptidase M	amastatin	20	Rich et al., 1984
	bestatin	1400	Taylor, 1993
	actinonin	170	Umezawa et al., 1985
Pyroglutamyl peptidase II	benarthin	1200	Aoyagi et al., 1992
Dipeptidyl peptidase IV	diprotin A	(subst)	Rahfeld et al., 1991
	Pro-boroPro	2	Yaron and Naider, 1993
	H-Glu(NHO-Bz)-pyrrolidide·HCl		Demuth et al., 1993
Prolyl endopeptidase	BOC-Glu(NHO-Bz)-pyrrolidide	30	Demuth et al., 1993
	Z-Pro-Prolinal	1000	Welches et al., 1991
Endopeptidase 24.15	carboxyphenylethyl-Ala-Ala-Phe-*p*-aminobenzoate	50000	McDermott et al., 1987
24.15/24.16	phosphodiepryl	5/0.3	Barelli et al., 1992
Endopeptidase 24.16	Pro-Ile	90000	Dauch et al., 1991

quence (from P_3–P_3') (Hersh and Morihara, 1986). See Turner (1987) for a summary of the major cleavage sites of neprilysin substrates.

Specific inhibitors of NEP have been developed: thiorphan, a synthetic thiol inhibitor, and phosphoramidon, a phosphorus-containing dipeptide produced by *Streptomyces tanashiensis* (Umezawa, 1972; Roques et al., 1993). Thiorphan, especially the R-isomer, is highly specific for NEP ($K_i = 2$ nM), having only minor inhibitory activity for ACE ($K_i = 860$ nM), however, variants of thiorphan, such as ES37 (NEP, $K_i = 5.2$ nM; ACE, $K_i = 12$ nM) and ES34 (NEP, $K_i = 4.5$ nM; ACE, $K_i = 55$ nM) (Roques et al., 1980, 1982 1993; Fournié-Zaluski et al., 1984) are potent mixed inhibitors of NEP and ACE.

The primary amino acid sequence of NEP from rabbit, mouse, rat and human (Devault et al., 1987; Malfroy et al., 1987, 1988) have been deduced from cDNA clones. The enzymes from these species are 740–750 amino acids in length and share $> 90\%$ homology. The only major difference between them is the number of potential N-glycosylation sites, with rabbit NEP containing five and rat and human NEP containing six sites. The sequence of NEP shows little homology to other Zn metallopeptidases, but does show conservation of some of the catalytic residues of the active site, including the consensus sequence VxxHExxH (Benchetrit et al., 1988).

Current studies of the NEP enzyme are focusing on determination of the tertiary structure of the active site, through crystallographic studies and computer modelling, so that more specific inhibitors with fewer side effects may be developed for clinical use (Roques et al., 1993).

TABLE III

Enzymes	Inactivating reagents
Metalloenzymes	EDTA 1,10-phenanthroline other chelating agents
Cysteine proteases	N-ethyl maleimide iodoacetamide iodoacetate organomercurials
Serine peptidases	diisopropylfluorophosphate phenylmethylsulfonyl fluoride
Enzymes containing essential disulfide bonds	2-mercaptoethanol dithiothreitol

Angiotensin converting enzyme

Angiotensin converting enzyme has been purified in various forms from human lung, kidney and brain. It also has been found in the intestine, blood vessels, placenta, lymph nodes, retina (Kenny et al., 1987) and in the spinal cord (Santos et al., 1988). ACE cDNA has been cloned and the tissue-specific expression of the enzyme examined (Bernstein et al., 1992). It is a Zn^{2+} metallopeptidase of molecular weight $\approx 150-180$ kDa that is bound to the outer surface of the plasma membrane (Erdös and Skidgel, 1985). ACE was originally characterized as the enzyme cleaving the C-terminal dipeptide of angiotensin I, thus converting it to angiotensin II. The enzyme, however, has a much broader substrate specificity, and will cleave bradykinin, neurotensin, substance P, luteinizing hormone-releasing hormone (LHRH), dynorphin(1–6), dynorphin(1–8), Leu-enkephalin, Met-enkephelin, β-neo-endorphin, etc. (Turner et al., 1987).

The predominant mode of cleavage is characterized by the generation of the C-terminal dipeptide (hence the name peptidyl dipeptidase A) (Turner et al., 1987), but endopeptidase activity has also been observed, for example, in the case of the amidated peptide LHRH (Skidgel and Erdös, 1985) or amidated substance P (Skidgel et al., 1984), where C-terminal tripeptides are the products of cleavage from the blocked peptides. Minor cleavage sites include Phe^4-Leu^5 of dynorphin(1–8), Gly^3-Phe^4 and Leu^5-Arg^6 of β-neoendorphin and Phe^5-Ser^6 of bradykinin (Turner et al., 1987). Peptides with a proline, glutamate or aspartate residue on the C-terminal inhibit ACE-activity (Cheung et al., 1980), and neurokinin A and B are not hydrolysed by angiotensin converting enzyme (Hooper et al., 1985).

Aminopeptidase M

Membrane-associated aminopeptidase M has been purified and characterized as the enzyme responsible for the cleavage of the Tyr^1-Gly^2 bond of enkephalins (Gros et al., 1985). This enzyme appears to be identical with the independently described aminopeptidase N (Matsas et al., 1985), but is different from the cytosolic 'puromycin-sensitive aminopeptidase' (Hersh, 1985). Aminopeptidases by their nature are generally acceptant of many amino acid residues on the N-terminal, but they are inactive toward proline-containing N-terminal sequences and blocked N-termini (Wang et al., 1991).

Aminopeptidase M is also a Zn^{2+}-metalloenzyme with a molecular weight of approximately 160 kDa, anchored to the cell membrane (Hussain et al., 1981). It has been found in the brain, intestine, placenta, lymph nodes, lung, liver and blood vessels (Kenny et al., 1987).

Neuropeptide substrates of aminopeptidase M include the enkephalins (as shown by the potentiation of their biological action by bestatin, an in vivo aminopeptidase M inhibitor), neurokinins, somatostatin, angiotensin III (Ward et al., 1990) and many others. It has been suggested that a substrate-specific aminopeptidase also plays a role in dynorphin A(1–17) degradation to dynorphin A(2–17) (Young et al., 1987), but further studies are needed to substantiate such a possibility.

Pyroglutamyl peptidase II

A neutral ectoenzyme, pyroglutamyl peptidase II (an enzyme distinct from the cytosolic pyroglutamyl peptidase I) demonstrates high specificity for the cleavage of thyrotropin-releasing hormone (TRH) by cleaving the N-terminal pyroglutamic acid of TRH (Charli et al., 1989). Bacterial pyroglutamyl peptidase has been cloned and expressed in *E. coli* (Yoshimoto et al., 1993). The enzyme has been found in the brain, liver, spinal cord, kidney and adrenal gland (Prasad, 1987; Vargas et al., 1992).

Inactivation has been observed with heavy metals, EDTA and dithiothreitol, but phenylmethylsulfonyl fluoride and iodoacetamide had little effect on peptidase activity (Prasad and Jayaraman, 1986). A selective inhibitor for the enzyme, the natural product benarthin, has been recently reported (Aoyagi et al., 1992).

Dipeptidyl peptidase IV

Dipeptidyl peptidase IV, purified from kidney microvillar membrane, is a two subunit glycoprotein with a molecular weight of approximately 260 kDa. It is a serine peptidase which can be liberated from the cell membrane by treatment with papain (Abbs and Kenny, 1983). Dipeptidyl peptidase IV has been found in the intestine, placenta, lymph nodes, liver, blood vessels and pancreas (Kenny et al., 1987), with the highest activity in the kidney and in the intestinal brush-border membrane (Macnair and Kenny, 1979). The liver enzyme has been recently cloned (Misumi et al., 1992).

Dipeptidyl peptidase IV generates Xaa-Pro(Ala) dipeptides through cleavage at the N-terminal peptide fragments. It is a proline (or alanine)-specific ectoenzyme (proline-containing sequences being better substrates than alanine-containing ones), and its in vivo activity has recently been confirmed by the report that rats deficient in this enzyme excrete more proline-containing peptides than control animals (Watanabe et al., 1993).

Since dipeptidyl peptidase IV was presumed to be the only serine peptidase on the cell surface, diisopropylfluorophosphate, a serine-reagent has been used as a specific inhibitor for studies of this enzyme's action (Kenny et al., 1987). The findings of membrane-bound prolyl endopeptidase, another serine peptidase, however, make this method questionable (Sudo and Tanabe, 1985). A specific inhibitor, diprotin A has also been employed in in vivo studies (Wang et al., 1991), however, this method will also need re-evaluation in light of the fact that the enzyme cleaves diprotin A as a substrate (Rahfeld et al., 1991). Dipeptidyl peptidase IV is the main enzyme of substance P hydrolysis generating the N-terminal dipeptide Arg-Pro (Wang et al., 1991).

Other potential neuropeptide-degrading enzymes

Endopeptidase 24.15

Endopeptidase 24.15, also known as thimet oligopeptidase, Pz-peptidase and endo-oligopeptidase A, is a metallopeptidase (70 kDa) that has been isolated from rat, rabbit and human tissues, and has been shown to be active in the brain, pituitary and testis (Carvalho and Camargo, 1981; Orlowski et al., 1983, 1989; Acker et al., 1987; Dando et al., 1993). The enzyme exists in both a soluble (80%) and a membrane-bound (20%) form and therefore may not be a true neuropeptidase (ectoenzyme) (Kenny and Turner, 1987).

Endopeptidase 24.15 cleaves peptides of between five and 20 amino acids, and is known to act on bradykinin, neurotensin, the angiotensins, LHRH, substance P, VIP, α-endorphin, β-neo-endorphin and somatostatin (Molineaux et al., 1988; Orlowski et al., 1989; Lasdun et al., 1989; Dahms and Mentlein, 1992; Dando et al., 1993). The specificity of the enzyme is thought to be influenced by aromatic amino acid residues in the P_1, P_1' and P_3' positions of the substrate (Orlowski et al., 1983) and also by the presence of three residues C-terminal to the scissile bond, a free C-terminus and the location of a proline residue in certain positions near the scissile bond (Dando et al., 1993).

This enzyme is also thought to be a Zn^{2+} metallopeptidase (Orlowski et al., 1989). Specific inhibitors of 24.15 include the synthetic peptide analogs Cpp-Ala-Ala-Phe-pAb and Cpp-Ala-Pro-Phe-pAb (Dando et al., 1993).

Endopeptidase 24.16

Endopeptidase 24.16, or prolyl oligopeptidase, is an oligopeptidase that exists in both soluble (80%) and membrane-bound (20%) forms (Barelli et al., 1993). It was originally isolated from rat brain synaptic membranes as a neurotensin-degrading activity (Checler et al., 1986) and has since been purified from rat kidney, rat intestine and pig brain (Barelli et al., 1993, 1988; Millican et al., 1991). Endopeptidase 24.16 is another Zn^{2+} metallopeptidase with a molecular weight of 70 kDa and a pI of 6.0 (Checler et al., 1986). In addition to neurotensin, it has been shown to cleave neuromedin N, dynorphin A(1-7), dynorphin A(1-8) and substance P (Checler et al., 1986; Barelli et al., 1993). The specificity of the enzyme is not clearly understood but it seems likely that a C-terminal extension of at least three residues from the scissile bond is necessary (Barelli et al., 1993).

Few natural inhibitors of endopeptidase 24.16 are known (Barrett and Rawlings, 1992). However, there are several effective chemical and synthetic inhibitors, including o-phenanthroline, EDTA, Cpe-Ala-Ala-Phe-Abz, Cpp-Ala-Ala-Tyr-Abz, Cpp-Ala-Ala-Phe-pAB and Pro-Ile (Checler et al., 1986; Barelli et al., 1993; Mentlein and Dahms, 1994).

Prolyl endopeptidase

Also known as post-proline cleaving enzyme and endo oligopeptidase B, prolyl endopeptidase is an $\approx$ 70 kDa serine peptidase with specificity toward peptide-bond cleavage after Pro residues (but not between Pro-Pro) (Mentlein, 1988). The enzyme was found to be similar to dipeptidyl peptidase IV, with conserved sequences including the pro-

posed catalytic sites (Barrett and Rawlings, 1992; Polgár and Szabó, 1992). Neither prolyl endopeptidase nor dipeptidyl peptidase IV belongs to the trypsin/chymotrypsin or the subtilisin families of serine proteases. It is, however, also inactivated by thiol reagents (p-chloromercuribenzoate, N-ethylmaleimide), signalling the possible existence of a catalytically active cysteine residue as well (Welches et al., 1993).

In vitro substrates of prolyl endopeptidase include substance P, neurotensin, luteinizing hormone-releasing hormone, thyrotropin-releasing hormone, bradykinin, dynorphin, angiotensin I, oxytocin and vasopressin (Wilk, 1983; Yaron and Naider, 1993). By the use of Z-Pro-Prolinal as a specific inhibitor, the in vivo cleavage of angiotensin I by prolyl endopeptidase has been proposed in canine brain.

The enzyme has been found in the testis, liver, skeletal muscle, lung, brain and kidney (Yaron and Naider, 1993). The cytoplasmic enzyme was cloned, and the peptide including the active site serine labelled with ^{3}H-diisopropylfluorophosphate (Rennex et al., 1991). Although prolyl endopeptidase activity has been found in brush-border membranes of the rat kidney (Sudo and Tanabe, 1985), additional evidence is needed to classify this peptidase as an in vivo neuropeptide inactivator.

Puromycin sensitive aminopeptidase

In addition to the cytosolic form of puromycin-sensitive aminopeptidase (Hersh and McKelvy, 1981), a membrane bound form was also isolated from rat brain, and was shown to be responsible for most of the degradation of enkephalins in the brain (Hersh, 1985). The membrane-bound and cytosolic forms were found to have identical N-terminal sequences and peptide maps, and show similar behaviour toward substrates and inhibitors (Dyer et al., 1990). Both have a molecular weight of around 100 kDa. The membrane form could be solubilized not only by the addition of detergent, but also in the presence of thiols (Hersh, 1985). This enzyme shows a behaviour

138

different from aminopeptidase M in the respect that it is profoundly affected by the presence of puromycin ($K_i = 0.24$ μM) as opposed to aminopeptidase M ($K_i = 925$ μM).

References

Abbs, M.T. and Kenny, A.J. (1983) Proteins of the kidney microvillar membrane: analysis by sodium dodecyl sulphate-polyacrylamide gel electrophoresis and cross immunoelectrophoresis. *Clin. Sci.*, 65: 551–559.

Acker, G.R., Molineaux, C.J. and Orlowski, M. (1987) Synaptosomal membrane-bound form of endopeptidase 24.15 generates Leu-enkephalin from dynorphin$_{1-8}$, α- and β-neoendorphin, and Met-enkephalin from Met-enkephalin-Arg[6]-Gly[7]-Leu [8]. *J. Neurochem.*, 48: 284–292.

Almenoff, J. and Orlowski, M. (1983) Membrane bound kidney metalloendopeptidase: interaction with synthetic substrates, natural peptides and inhibitors. *Biochemistry*, 22: 590–599.

Aoyagi, T., Hatsu, F., Kojima, F., Hayashi, C., Hamada, M. and Takeuchi, T. (1992) Benarthin: a new inhibitor of pyroglutamyl peptidase. I. Taxonomy, fermentation, isolation and biological activities. *J. Antibiot.*, 45: 1079–1083.

Barelli, H., Vincent, J.P. and Checler, F. (1988) Peripheral inactivation of neurotensin: Isolation and characterization of a metallopeptidase from rat ileum. *Eur. J. Biochem.*, 175: 481–489.

Barelli, H., Dive, V., Yiotakis, A., Vincent, J.P. and Checler, F. (1992) Potent inhibition of endopeptidase 24.16 and endopeptidase 24.15 by the phosphonamide peptide *N*-(phenylethylphosphonyl)-Gly-L-Pro-L-aminohexanoic acid. *Biochem. J.*, 287: 621–625.

Barelli, H., Vincent, J.P. and Checler, F. (1993) Rat kidney endopeptidase 24.16: Purification, physico-chemical characteristics and differential specificity towards opiates, tachykinins and neurotensin-related peptides. *Eur. J. Biochem.* 211: 79–90.

Barrett, A.J. and Rawlings, N.D. (1992) Oligopeptidases, and the emergence of the prolyl oligopeptidase family. *Biol. Chem. Hoppe-Seyler*, 373: 353–360.

Bateman, R.C. and Hersh, L.B. (1987) Mechanism based design of inhibitors of neuropeptide degrading enzymes. *Drug Design Delivery*, 2: 55–68.

Benchetrit, T., Bissery, V., Mornon, J.P., Devault, A., Crine, P. and Roques, B.P. (1988) Primary structure homologies between two Zn-metallopeptidases, the neutral endopeptidase 24.11 'enkephalinase' and the thermolysin through clustering. *Biochemistry*, 27: 592–597.

Bernstein, K.E., Howard, T.E., Shai, S.-Y., Langford, K.G. and Balogh, R. (1992) Tissue specific expression of angiotensin converting enzyme. *Agents Actions*, 38/I(Suppl.): 376–383.

Beudet, A., Mazella, J., Nouel, D., Chabry, J., Castel, M.-N.,

Laduron, P., Kitabgi, P. and Faure, M.-P. (1994) Internalization and intracellular mobilization of neurotensin in neuronal cells. *Biochem. Pharmacol.*, 47:43–52.

Borg, S., Luthman, K., Nyberg, F., Terenius, L. and Hacksell, U. (1993) 1,2,4-Oxadiazole derivatives of phenylalanine: potential inhibitors of substance P endopeptidase. *Eur. J. Med. Chem.*, 28: 801–810.

Brownstein, M.J. (1989) Neuropeptides. In G. Siegel, B. Agranoff, R.W. Albers and P. Molinoff (Eds.). *Basic Neurochemistry*, Raven Press, New York, pp. 287–309.

Carvalho, K.M. and Camargo, A.C.M. (1983) Purification of rabbit brain endooligopeptidases and preparation of antienzyme antibodies. *Biochem. Biophys. Res. Commun.*, 116: 1151–1159.

Charli, J.-L., Cruz, C., Vargas, M.A. and Joseph-Bravo, P. (1988) The narrow specificity pyroglutamate aminopeptidase degrading TRH in rat brain is an ectoenzyme. *Neurochem. Int.*, 13: 237–242.

Charli, J.-L., Cruz, C., Vargas, M.A., Cisneros, M., Assai, M., Joseph-Bravo, P. and Wilk, S. (1989) Pyroglutamyl peptidase II inhibition specifically increases recovery of TRH released from rat brain slices. *Neuropeptides*, 14: 191–196.

Checler, F., Vincent, J.P. and Kitabgi, P. (1983) Degradation of neurotensin by rat brain synaptic membranes: involvement of a thermolysin like metalloendopeptidase (enkephalinase), angiotensin converting enzyme, and other unidentified peptidases. *J. Neurochem,.* 41: 375–384.

Checler, F., Vincent, J.P. and Kitabgi, P. (1986) Purification and characterization of a novel neurotensin-degrading peptidase from rat brain synaptic membranes. *J. Biol. Chem.*, 261: 11274–11281.

Checler, F., Barelli, H., Dauch, P., Vincent, B., Dive, V., Beudet, A., Daniel, E.E., Fox-Threlkeld, J.E.T., Masuo, Y. and Vincent, J.P. (1993) Recent advances on endopeptidase 24.16. *Biochem. Soc. Trans.*, 21: 692–697.

Cheung, H.-S., Wang, F.-L., Ondetti, M.A., Sabo, E.F. and Cushman, D.W. (1980) Binding of peptide substrates and inhibitors of angiotensin-converting enzyme. *J. Biol. Chem.*, 255: 401–407.

Dahms, P. and Mentlein, R. (1992) Purification of the main somatostatin-degrading proteases from rat and pig brains, their action on other neuropeptides, and their identification as endopeptidases 24.15 and 24.16. *Eur. J. Biochem.*, 208: 145–154.

Dando, P.M., Brown, M.A. and Barrett, A.J. (1993) Human thimet oligopeptidase. *Biochem. J.*, 294: 451–457.

Danielsen, E.M., Vyas, J.B. and Kenny, A.J. (1980) A neutral endopeptidase in the microvillar membrane of pig intestine: partial purification and properties. *Biochem. J.*, 191: 645–648.

Dauch, P., Vincent, J.-P. and Checler, F. (1991) Specific inhibition of endopeptidase 24.16 by dipeptides. *Eur. J. Biochem.*, 202: 269–276.

Dauch, P., Masuo, Y., Vincent, J.-P. and Checler, F. (1993) A survey of the cerebral regionalization and onthogeny of eight exo- and endopeptidases in murines. *Peptides*, 14: 593–599.

Demuth, H.-U., Schlenzig, D., Schierhorn, A., Grosche, G., Chapot-Chartier, M.-P. and Gripon, J.-C. (1993) Design of (ω-N-(O-acyl)hydroxyamid)aminodicarboxylic acid pyrrolidides as potent inhibitors of proline-specific peptidases. *FEBS Lett.*, 320:23–27.

Devault, A., Lazure, C., Nault, C., Le Moual, H., Seidah, N.G., Chretien, M., Kahn, P., Powell, J., Mallet, J., Beaumont, A., Roques, B.P., Crine, P. and Boileau, C. (1987) Amino acid sequence of rabbit kidney neutral endopeptidase 24.11 (enkephalinase) deduced from a complimentary DNA. *EMBO J.*, 6: 1317–1322.

Devi, L. (1991) Concensus sequence for processing of peptide precursors at monobasic sites. *FEBS Lett.*, 280: 189–194.

Dyer, S.H., Slaughter, C.A., Orth, K., Moomaw, C.R. and Hersh, L.B. (1990) Comparison of the soluble and membrane bound forms of the puromycin-sensitive enkephalin-degrading aminopeptidases from rat. *J. Neurochem.*, 54: 547–554.

Erdös, E.G., and Skidgel, R.A. (1985) Structure and functions of human angiotensin I converting enzyme (kininase II). *Biochem. Soc. Trans.*, 13: 42–44.

Fournié-Zaluski, M.C., Soroca-Lucas, E., Waksman, G., Llornes, C., Schwartz, J.C. and Roques, B.P. (1982) Differential recognition of 'enkephalinase' and angiotensin converting enzyme by new carboxyalkyl inhibitors. *Life Sci.*, 31: 2947–2954.

Fournié-Zaluski, M.C., Soroca-Lucas, E., Waksman, G. and Roques, B.P. (1984) Differences in the structural requirements for selective interaction with neutral metalloendopeptidase (enkephalinase) or angiotensin converting enzyme: molecular investigation by use of new thiol inhibitors. *Eur. J. Biochem.*, 139: 267–274.

Gee, N.S., Bowes, M.A. Buck, P. and Kenny A.J. (1985) An immunoradiometric assay for endopeptidase 24.11 shows it to be a widely distributed enzyme in pig tissues. *Biochem. J.*, 228: 119–126.

Goli, U.B. and Galardy, R.E. (1986) Kinetics of slow, tight binding inhibitors of angiotensin converting enzyme. *Biochemistry*, 25: 7136–7142.

Gros, C., Giros, B. and Schwartz, J.-C. (1985) Identification of aminopeptidase M as an enkephalin-inactivating enzyme in rat cerebral membrane. *Biochemistry*, 24: 2179–2185.

Hersh, L.B. (1981) Solubilization and characterization of two rat brain membrane-bound aminopeptidases active on Met-enkephalin. *Biochemistry*, 20: 2345–2350.

Hersh, L.B. (1985) Characterization of membrane-bound aminopeptidases from rat brain: identification of the enkephalin-degrading aminopeptidase. *J. Neurochem.*, 44: 1427–1435.

Hersh, L.B. and McKelvy, J.F. (1981) An aminopeptidase from bovine brain which catalyses the hydrolysis of enkephalin. *J. Neurochem.*, 36: 171–178.

Hersh, L.B. and Morihara, K. (1986) Comparison of the subsite specificity of the mammalian neutral endopeptidase 24.11 (enkephalinase) to the bacterial neutral endopeptidase thermolysin. *J. Biol. Chem.*, 261: 6433–6437.

Hooper, N.M., Kenny, A.J. and Turner, A.J. (1985) The metabolism of neuropeptides: neurokinin A (substance K) is a substrate for endopeptidase 24.11 but not for peptidyl dipeptidase A (angiotensin converting enzyme). *Biochem. J.*, 231: 357–361.

Hussain, M.M., Tranum-Jensen, J., Norén, O., Sjöström, H. and Christiansen, K. (1981) Reconstitution of purified amphiphilic pig intestinal microvillus aminopeptidase. *Biochem. J.*, 199: 179–186.

Jaspard, E., Costerousse, O., Wei, L., Corvol, P. and Alhenc-Gelas, F. (1992) The angiotensin I-converting enzyme (kininase II): molecular and regulatory aspects. *Agents Actions*, 38/I (Suppl.): 349–358.

Kalwant, S. and Porter, A.G. (1991) Purification and characterization of human brain prolyl endopeptidase. *Biochem. Int.*, 276: 237–244.

Kenny, A.J. and Turner, A.J. (1987) What are ectoenzymes? In: A.J. Kenny and A.J. Turner (Eds.) *Mammalian Ectoenzymes*, Elsevier, Amsterdam, pp. 1–13.

Kenny, A.J., Stephenson, S.L. and Turner, A.J. (1987) Cell surface peptidases. In: A.J. Kenny and A.J. Turner (Eds.) *Mammalian Ectoenzymes*, Elsevier, Amsterdam, pp. 169–210.

Kerr, M.A. and Kenny, A.J. (1974a) The purification and specificity of a neutral endopeptidase from rabbit kidney brush border. *Biochem. J.*, 137: 477–488.

Kerr, M.A. and Kenny, A.J. (1974b) The molecular weight and properties of a neutral metallo-endopeptidase from rabbit kidney brush border. *Biochem. J.*, 137: 489–495.

Koehn, J.A., Norman, J.A., Jones, B.N., Le Sueur, L., Sakane, Y. and Ghai, R.D. (1987) Degradation of atrial natriuretic factor by kidney cortex membranes. *J. Biol. Chem.*, 262: 11623–11627.

Kondo, Y., Ogawa, N., Asanuma, M., Hirata, H., Tanaka, K., Kawada, Y. and Mori, A. (1993) Regional changes in neuropeptide levels after 5,7-dihydroxytryptamine-induced serotonin depletion in the brain. *J. Neural. Transm.*, 92: 151–157.

Lasdun, A., Reznik, S., Molineaux, C.J. and Orlowski, M. (1989) Inhibition of endopeptidase 24.15 slows the in vivo degradation of luteinizing hormone-releasing hormone. *J. Pharmacol. Exp. Ther.*, 251(2): 439–447.

McDermott, J.R., Gibson, A.M. and Turner, J.D. (1987) Involvement of endopeptidase 24.15 in the inactivation of bradykinin by rat brain slices. *Biochem. Biophys. Res. Commun.*, 146: 154–158.

Macnair, R.D.C. and Kenny, A.J. (1979) Proteins of kidney

microvillar membrane: the amphipathic form of dipeptidyl peptidase IV. *Biochem. J.*, 179: 379–395.

Malfroy, B., Swerts, J.P., Guyon, A., Roques, B.P. and Schwartz, J.C. (1978) High-affinity enkephalin-degrading peptidase in mouse brain and its enhanced activity following morphine. *Nature (London)*, 276: 523–526.

Malfroy, B., Schofield, P.R., Kuang, W.J., Seeburg, P.H., Mason, A.J. and Henzel, W.J. (1987) Molecular cloning and amino acid sequence of rat enkephalinase. *Biochem. Biophys. Res. Commun.*, 144: 59–66.

Malfroy, B., Kuang, W.J., Seeburg, P.H., Mason, A.J. and Schofield, P.R. (1988) Molecular cloning and amino acid sequence of human enkephalinase (neutral endopeptidase). *FEBS Lett.*, 229: 206–210.

Marks, N., Terenius, L. and Nyberg, F. (1988) Neuropeptide-processing, -converting and -inactivating enzymes in human cerebrospinal fluid. *Int. Rev. Neurobiol.*, 30: 101–121.

Matsas, R., Fulcher, I.S., Kenny, A.J. and Turner, A.J. (1983) Substance P and Leu-enkephalin are hydrolyzed by an enzyme in pig caudate synaptic membranes that is identical with the endopeptidase of kidney microvilli. *Proc. Natl. Acad. Sci. USA*, 80: 3111–3114.

Matsas, R., Kenny, A.J. and Turner, A.J. (1984) The metabolism of neuropeptides: the hydrolysis of peptides including enkephalins, tachykinins and their analogues, by endopeptidase 24.11. *Biochem. J.*, 223: 433–440.

Matsas, R., Stephenson, S.L., Hryszko, J., Kenny, A.J. and Turner, A.J. (1985) The metabolism of neuropeptides: phase separation of synaptic membrane preparations with Triton X-114 reveals the presence of aminopeptidase N. *Biochem. J.*, 231: 445–449.

Mentlein, R. (1988) Proline residues in the maturation and degradation of peptide hormones and neuropeptides. *FEBS Lett.*, 234:251–256.

Mentlein, R. and Dahms, P. (1994) Endopeptidases 24.16 and 24.15 are responsible for the degradation of somatostatin, neurotensin, and other neuropeptides by cultivated rat cortical astrocytes. *J. Neurochem.*, 62(1): 27–36.

Millican, P.E., Kenny, A.J. and Turner, A.J. (1991) Purification and properties of a neurotensin-degrading endopeptidase from pig brain. *Biochem J.*, 276: 583–591.

Misumi, Y., Hayashi, Y., Arakawa, F. and Ikehara, Y. (1992) Molecular cloning and sequence analysis of human dipeptidyl peptidase IV, a serine protease on the cell surface. *Biochim. Biophys. Acta*, 1131: 333–336.

Molineaux, C.J., Lasdun, A., Michaud, C. and Orlowski, M. (1988) Endopeptidase-24.15 is the primary enzyme that degrades luteinizing hormone releasing hormone both in vitro, and in vivo. *J. Neurochem.*, 51(2): 624–633.

Morel, G. (1994) Internalization and nuclear localization of peptide hormones. *Biochem. Pharmacol.*, 47:63–76.

Moore, M.R. and Black, P.McL. (1991) Neuropeptides *Neurosurg. Rev.*, 14: 97–110.

Murachi, T., Hatanaka, M. and Hamakubo, T. (1987) Calpains and neuropeptide metabolism. In: A.J. Turner (Ed.) *Neuropeptides and their Peptidases*, Horwood, Chichester, pp. 202–228.

Nishimura, K. and Hazato, T. (1993) Isolation and identification of an endogenous inhibitor of enkephalin-degrading enzymes from bovine spinal cord. *Biochem. Biophys. Res. Commun.*, 194: 713–719.

Orlowski, M., Michaud, C. and Chu, T.G (1983) A soluble metalloendopeptidase from rat brain: Purification of the enzyme and determination of specificity with synthetic and natural peptides. *J. Biochem.*, 135: 81–88.

Orlowski, M., Reznik, S., Ayala, J. and Pierotti, A.R. (1989) Endopeptidase 24.15 from rat testes: isolation of the enzyme and its specificity toward synthetic and natural peptides, including enkephalin-containing peptides. *Biochem. J.*, 261: 951–958.

Persson, S., Jónsdóttir, I., Thorén, P., Post, C., Nyberg, F. and Hoffmann, P. (1993) Cerebrospinal fluid dynorphin-converting enzyme activity is increased by voluntary exercise in the spontaneously hypertensive rat. *Life Sci.*, 53: 643–652.

Polgár, L. and Szabó, E. (1992) Prolyl endopeptidase and dipeptidyl peptidase IV are distantly related members of the same family of serine proteases. *Biol. Chem. Hoppe-Seyler*, 373: 361–366.

Prasad, C. (1987) Activation/inactivation of rat tissue pyroglutamate aminopeptidase by disulfide bond-reducing agents. *Neuropeptides*, 9: 211–215.

Prasad, C. and Jayaraman, A. (1986) Metabolism of thyrotropin-releasing hormone in human cerebrospinal fluid. Isolation and characterization of pyroglutamate aminopeptidase activity. *Brain Res.*, 364: 331–337.

Rahfeld, J., Schierhorn, M., Hartrodt, B., Neubert, K. and Heins, J. (1991) Are diprotin A (Ile-Pro-Ilr) and diprotin B (Val-Pro-Leu) inhibitors or substrates of dipeptidyl peptidase IV? *Biochim. Biophys. Acta*, 1076: 314–316.

Rennex, D., Hemmings, B.A., Hofsteenge, J. and Stone, S.R. (1991) cDNA cloning of porcine brain prolyl endopeptidase and identification of the active-site seryl residue. *Biochemistry*, 30: 2195–2203.

Rich, D.H., Moon, B.J. and Harbeson, S. (1984) Inhibition of aminopeptidases by amastatin and bestatin derivatives. Effect of inhibitor structure on slow-binding processes. *J. Med. Chem.*, 27: 417–422.

Roques, B.P. (1993) Active site structure and design of selective and mixed inhibitors: new approaches in the search for analgesics and anti-hypertensives. *Biochem. Soc. Trans.*, 21: 678–685.

Roques, B.P., Fournié-Zaluski, M.C., Soroca, E., Lecomte, J.M., Malfroy, B., Llorens, C. and Schwartz, J.C. (1980) The enkephalinase inhibitor thiorphan shows antinociceptive activity in mice. *Nature (London)*, 288: 286–288.

Roques, B.P., Fournié-Zaluski, M.C., Florentin, D., Waksman, G., Sassi, A., Chaillet, P., Collado, H. and Costentin, J. (1982) New enkephalinase inhibitors as probes to differentiate 'enkephalinase' and angiotensin-converting-enzyme active sites. *Life Sci.*, 31: 1749–1752.

Roques, B.P., Noble, F., Daugé, V., Fournié-Zaluski, M.-C. and Beaumont, A. (1993) Neutral endopeptidase 24.11: structure, inhibition and experimental and clinical pharmacology. *Pharmacol. Rev.*, 45: 87–146.

Rowan, S., Todd, A.J. and Spike, R.C. (1993) Evidence that neuropeptide Y is present in GABAergic neurons in the superficial dorsal horn of the rat spinal cord. *Neuroscience*, 53: 537–545.

Santos, R.A.S., Brosnihan, K.B., Chappall, M.C., Pesquero, J., Chernicky, C.L., Greene, L.J. and Ferrario, C.M. (1988) Converting enzyme activity and angiotensin metabolism in the dog brainstem. *Hypertension*, 11: 1153–1157.

Skidgel, R.A. (1993) Bradykinin-degrading enzymes: structures, function, distribution, and potential roles in cardiovascular pharmacology. *J. Cardiovasc. Pharmacol.*, 20(Suppl. 9): S4–S9.

Skidgel, R.A. and Erdös, E.G. (1985) Novel activity of human angiotensin converting enzyme: release of the NH_2- and COOH-terminal tripeptides from the luteinizing hormone-releasing hormone. *Proc. Natl. Acad. Sci. USA*, 82: 1025–1029.

Skidgel, R.A., Engelbrecht, S., Johnson, A.R. and Erdös, E.G. (1984) Hydrolysis of substance P and neurotensin by converting enzyme and neutral endopeptidase. *Peptides*, 5: 769–776.

Soleilhac, J.M., Lucas, E., Beaumont, A., Turcand, S., Michel, J.B., Ficheux, D., Fournié-Zaluski, M.-C. and Roques, B.P. (1992) A 94-kDa protein, identified as neutral endopeptidase-24.11 can inactivate atrial natriuretic peptide in the vascular endothelium. *Mol. Pharmacol.*, 41: 609–614.

Stephenson, S.L. and Kenny, A.J. (1987) The hydrolysis of a human atrial natriuretic peptide by pig kidney microvillar membranes is initiated by endopeptidase 24.11. *Biochem J.*, 243: 183–187.

Sudo, J.-I. and Tanabe, T. (1985) Distributions of post-proline cleaving enzyme-, converting enzyme-, trypsin- and chymotrypsin-like activities in various nephron segments and in brush border membranes isolated from rat kidney. *Chem. Pharm. Bull.*, 33: 1694–1702.

Sullivan, A.F., Akil, H. and Barchas. J.D. (1978) In vitro degradation of enkephalin: evidence for cleavage at the Gly-Phe bond. *Psychopharmacology*, 2: 525–531.

Taylor, A. (1993) Aminopeptidases: structure and function. *FASEB J.*, 7: 290–298.

Tisljar, U. (1993) Thimet oligopeptidase: a review of a thiol dependent metallo-endopeptidase also known as Pz-peptidase, endopeptidase 24.15 and endo-oligopeptidase. *Biol. Chem. Hoppe-Seyler*, 374: 91–100.

Turner, A.J. (1987) Endopeptidase-24.11 and neuropeptide metabolism. In: A.J. Turner (Ed.) *Neuropeptides and Their Peptidases*, Horwood, Chichester, pp. 183–201.

Turner, A.J., Matsas, R. and Kenny, A.J. (1985) Are there neuropeptide-specific peptidases? *Biochem. Pharmacol.*, 34: 1347–1356.

Turner, A.J., Hooper, N.M. and Kenny, A.J. (1987) Metabolism of neuropeptides. In: A.J. Kenny and A.J. Turner (Eds.) *Mammalian Ectoenzymes*, Elsevier, Amsterdam, pp. 211–248.

Umezawa, S. (1972) A new microbial metabolite phosphoramidon (isolation and structure). *Tetrahedron Lett.*, 1: 97–100.

Umezawa, H., Aoyagi, T., Tanake, T., Suda, H., Okuyama, A., Naganawa, H., Hamada, M. and Takeuchi, T. (1985) Production of actinonin, inhibitor of aminopeptidase M, by *Actinomycetes*. *J. Antibiot.*, 38: 1629–1630.

Vargas, M.A., Cisneros, M., Herrera, J., Joseph-Bravo, P. and Charli, J.-L. (1992) Regional distribution of pyroglutamyl peptidase II in rabbit brain, spinal cord and organs. *Peptides*, 13: 255–260.

Vijayaraghavan, J., Scicli, A.G., Carretero, O.A., Slaughter, C., Moomaw, C. and Hersh, L.B. (1990) The hydrolysis of endothelins by neutral endopeptidase 24.11 (enkephalinase). *J. Biol. Chem.*, 265: 14150–14155.

Waksman, G., Hamel, E., Fournié-Zaluski, M.C. and Roques, B.P. (1986) Autoradiographic comparison of the distribution of the neutral endopeptidase 'enkephalinase' and of mu and delta opioid receptors in rat brain. *Proc. Natl. Acad. Sci USA*, 83: 1523–1527.

Wang, L., Ahmad, S., Benter, I.F., Chow, A., Mizutani, S. and Ward, P.E. (1991) Differential processing of substance P and neurokinin A by plasma dipeptidyl (amino)peptidase IV, aminopeptidase M and angiotensin converting enzyme. *Peptides*, 12: 1357–1364.

Ward, P.E., Benter, I.F., Dick, L. and Wilk, S. (1990) Metabolism of vasoactive peptides by plasma and purified renal aminopeptidase M. *Biochem. Pharmacol.*, 40: 1725–1732.

Watanabe, Y., Kojima-Komatsu, T., Iwaki-Egawa, S. and Fujimoto, Y. (1993) Increased excretion of proline-containing peptides in dipeptidyl peptidase IV-deficient rats. *Res. Commun. Chem. Pathol. Pharmacol.*, 81: 323–330.

Wei, L., Clauser, E., Alhenc-Gelas, F. and Corvol, P. (1992) The two homologous domains of human angiotensin I-converting enzyme interact differently with competitive inhibitors. *J. Biol. Chem.*, 267: 13398–13405.

Welches, W.R., Santos, R.A.S., Chappell, M.C., Brosnihan, K.B., Greene, L.J. and Ferrario, C.M. (1991) Evidence that prolyl endopeptidase participates in the processing of brain angiotensin. *J. Hypertension*, 9: 631–638.

Welches, W.R., Brodnihan, K.B. and Ferrario, C.M. (1993) A comparison of the properties and enzymatic activities of three angiotensin processing enzymes: angiotensin converting enzyme, prolyl endopeptidase and neutral endopeptidase 24.11. *Life Sci.*, 52: 1461–1480.

Wilk, S. (1983) Minireview: prolyl endopeptidase. *Life Sci.*, 33: 2149–2157.

142

Wong-Leung, Y.L. and Kenny, A.J. (1968) Some properties of a microsomal peptidase in rat kidney. *Biochem. J.,* 110: 5P.

Yaron, A. and Naider, F. (1993) Proline-dependent structural and biological properties of peptides and proteins. *Crit. Rev. Biochem. Mol. Biol.*, 28: 31–81.

Yoshimoto, T., Shimada, T., Kitazono, A., Kabashima, T., Ito, K. and Tsaru, D. (1993) Pyroglutamyl peptidase gene from *Bacillus amyloliquefaciens*: cloning, sequencing, expression and crystallization of the expressed enzyme. *J. Biochem.,* 113: 67–73.

Young, E.A., Walker,J.M., Houghten, R. and Akil, H. (1987) The degradation of dynorphin A in brain tissue in vivo and in vitro. *Peptides*, 8: 701–707.

Zhu, J., Jhamandas, K. and Yang, H.-Y.T. (1992) Release of neuropeptide FF (FLFQPQRF-NH$_2$) from rat spinal cord. *Brain Res.*, 592: 326–332.

SECTION IV

Physiology and Pharmacology in the Spinal Cord

F. Nyberg, H.S. Sharma and Z. Wiesenfeld-Hallin (Eds.)
Progress in Brain Research, Vol 104

CHAPTER 9

Spinal cord tachykinins in the micturition reflex

A. Lecci and C.A. Maggi

Pharmacology Department, A. Menarini Pharmaceuticals, Via Sette Santi 3, 50131 Florence, Italy

Introduction

Tachykinins (TKs) are a family of peptides which share the common C-terminal sequence Phe-Xaa-Gly-Leu-MetNH$_2$. The first member of this family, substance P (SP) was discovered in the 1930s (Von Euler and Gaddum, 1931) and its aminoacid sequence was identified about 40 years later (Chang et al., 1971). In the past 10 years, other members of the TK family have been identified in mammals; at the present time, two other tachykinins, neurokinin A (NKA) and neurokinin B (NKB) have an established status of neurotransmitters in mammals (for review, see Otsuka and Yoshioka, 1993). TKs produce a wide range of biological effects: these are mediated by the activation of three different receptor types, termed NK$_1$, NK$_2$ and NK$_3$, for which SP, NKA and NKB have preferential but not exclusive affinity, respectively (for review, see Maggi et al., 1993). Since the early discovery that SP is more concentrated in the dorsal than in the ventral half of the spinal cord (Lembeck, 1953), a role for this peptide in sensory processing was proposed, and this idea has been extended to include the other members of this family. Especially relevant in this context was the demonstration that SP is one of the neuropeptides actively synthesized and released from a class of primary afferent neurons (Hökfelt et al., 1975; Gamse et al., 1981) which are identified, from a purely pharmacological point of view, by their sensitivity to capsaicin (for review, see Maggi and Meli, 1988). On this ground,

a role of SP and TKs as primary afferent transmitters has been speculated; this idea has received strong support, in recent years, following the development of potent and selective TK receptor antagonists: the use of these ligands has enabled to prove unequivocally the concept that a release of endogenous TKs and activation of TK receptors takes place at the spinal cord level following peripheral noxious stimulation (e.g., De Koninck and Henry, 1991). While the major part of studies on the role of TKs as primary afferent transmitters has been focussed on their possible role as pain transmitters from the somatic domain, several lines of evidence have also indicated an involvement of TKs in the regulation of visceral primary afferent input to the spinal cord. Our group has been involved in studying the latter issue, especially in relation to the primary afferent input regulating the micturition reflex (for reviews, see Maggi and Meli, 1986a; Maggi, 1993). In this chapter we will outline some of the recent findings, indicating a role for TKs as modulators of the micturition reflex at the spinal cord level, which have emerged from studies in which potent and selective receptor antagonists have been used to unravel the role of TKs in the spinal pharmacology of micturition.

Anatomical background

Spinal cord distribution of urinary bladder afferents

Afferent nerves arising from the urinary bladder reach the spinal cord through the pelvic and hypogastric nerves. Two main areas of projection of bladder afferents thus exists in mammals: pelvic afferents project to the lumbosacral spinal cord (at the S1–S3 level in most species; at the L6–S1 level in rats) and hypogastric afferents project to the thoracolumbar spinal cord (mostly at the T11–L2 level): a large proportion of bladder afferents contains neuropeptides (Keast and De Groat, 1992). Pelvic afferents enter Lissauer's tract and the ipsilateral dorsal columns projecting to the nucleus gracilis: at the lumbosacral level, the afferent fibers enter into the dorsal horns via a lateral and a medial collateral pathway (for reviews, see De Groat, 1986, 1987; Maggi, 1991). The lateral collateral pathway terminates in the junction between Laminae I and V, in the outer Lamina II, in Lamina VII close to the lumbosacral parasympathetic nucleus, and in the ventral portion of the dorsal gray commissure (Lamina X). The medial collateral pathway projects to the ipsi- and contralateral dorsal portion of the dorsal gray commissure and to Lamina V. No fibers project to Lamina II, which is known to receive only somatic afferent projections. The terminal fields of projection of the lateral and of the medial collateral pathways largely overlap with the somatic projections originating from pudendal nerves; however somatic afferents also terminate in Laminae II, III and IV, where no bladder projections were found.

The hypogastric bladder afferents enter Lissauer's tract and project to Laminae I, II and X ventral to the central canal, in the dorsolateral funiculus and in its nucleus. As will be discussed below, the capsaicin-sensitive primary afferent neurons are a source of sensory SP innervation to the dorsal half of the spinal cord: accordingly, neonatal capsaicin pretreatment, producing a neurotoxic effect on these afferent neurons, greatly reduces the projections of bladder afferents at both the lumbosacral and the thoracolumbar level of the rat spinal cord. In the lumbosacral spinal cord, the capsaicin-sensitive bladder afferents terminate in Laminae I, V, VII and X (Jancso and Maggi, 1987).

Spinal cord distribution of tachykinin-like immunoreactivity and tachykinin receptors

A large amount of nerve fibres containing SP-like immunoreactivity (SP-LI) observed in the dorsal half of the spinal cord at immunohistochemistry are of primary afferent origin: these are the central projections of sensory neurons located in dorsal root ganglia (DRG). The subset of DRG neurons expressing SP-LI in mammals (15–20% of total DRG neuron population in various species) is characterized by their sensitivity to the stimulant and neurotoxic action of capsaicin, mediated through the expression of a specific 'vanilloid' receptor (Szallasi and Blumberg, 1990). These primary afferent neurons express the preprotachykinin I gene, leading to the synthesis of both SP and NKA (Nakanishi, 1987); accordingly, the co-release of SP and NKA occurs from the central endings of these primary afferent neurons upon application of depolarizing stimuli to the dorsal half of the spinal cord (e.g., Hua et al., 1986; Saria et al., 1986), or following stimulation of their peripheral receptive field (Duggan et al., 1987). Since these afferent neurons innervate both the somatic and visceral domains, the distribution of SP-LI-positive fibres in the dorsal half of the spinal cord overlaps with the areas of distribution of urinary bladder afferents, but SP-LI-fibers are also present in other regions of the spinal cord which do not receive visceral afferent input (e.g., Laminae II and III). To further complicate the issue, part of the SP-LI present in the the spinal cord is present in fibers descending from supraspinal centers, and intrinsic SP-LI neurons are also present in the dorsal horns. The relative contribution of primary afferent neurons to the total population of SP-LI-positive fibers in the dorsal half of the spinal cord can be shown by studying the effect of dorsal rhizotomy or capsaicin-pretreatment both of which selectively eliminate this source of innervation. In the human sacral spinal cord, SP-LI has been detected in the lateral marginal area of the dorsal horns and in the area of the sacral autonomic nucleus, which provide most of the efferent input to the urinary bladder (De Groat et al., 1986).

Autoradiographic binding studies have identified SP-binding sites (NK_1 receptor) in the dorsal spinal cord with higher densities of binding in the proximity of cholinesterase-stained neurons at the lumbosacral level in Laminae I, II, V, VI, VII and X and in Onuf's nucleus, which regulates urethral sphincter activity (Charlton and Helke, 1985a,b; Yashpal et al., 1990). Recently, the mRNA encoding the synthesis of NK_1 receptors has been localized in cells around the central canal and in Laminae III, IV and V, and only sparse labelling was found in the substantia gelatinosa (Lamina II) (Maeno et al., 1993). Only a few studies have detected NK_2 receptors in the spinal cord (e.g., Yashpal et al., 1990): the maximal density has been reported at the lumbar level in the dorsal part of the dorsal horns and near the central canal. NK_3 receptors are also present in the dorsal horns of the spinal cord, however the preferred natural ligand for these receptors (NKB) is not expressed by DRG neurons (e.g., Moussaui et al., 1992). Capsaicin-pretreatment increases the density of SP (NK_1)-binding sites by 20% in Laminae I, II and III, and by 100% in Lamina X; this increase has been interpreted as a consequence of denervation supersensitivity (Helke et al., 1986; Rossler et al., 1993).

In summary, the tachykininergic sensory input to the dorsal half of the spinal cord originates from both somatic and visceral afferent pathways, and TK receptors have been localized in projection areas of these afferent neurons; however, part of the contents of the TK originates from neurons localized inside the central nervous system.

Primary afferent input and the micturition reflex

Vesicourethral afferents encode a number of sensory modalities which provide the background for the co-ordination of reflexes which regulate urine storage and voiding (for reviews, see De Groat et al., 1993; Janig and Koltzenburg, 1993). In both rats and cats, urinary bladder afferents are either thinly myelinated (A δ-fibers) or unmyelinated (C-fibers). The mechanosensitive input from the lower urinary tract which signals, e.g., the degree of filling/distension of the urinary bladder, is chiefly, if not exclusively, mediated through A δ-fibers; most of the urinary bladder unmyelinated afferents are either poorly sensitive to mechanical stimuli or totally unexcitable by this sensory modality. On the other hand, unmyelinated afferents exhibit a pronounced chemosensitivity: following application of chemical irritants into the bladder lumen, they display an ongoing activity and a novel mechanosensitivity, thus generating a powerful afferent barrage to the spinal cord even at low degrees of bladder filling (Habler et al., 1990). This class of bladder afferents has been termed 'silent nociceptors' and, while playing virtually no role in the normal storage-voiding cycle of the vesicourethral complex, they may become active during pathophysiological events, e.g., cystitis. Although this point has not yet been verified experimentally, there is a high a likelihood that the C-fiber 'silent nociceptors' overlap with the capsaicin-sensitive population of primary afferent neurons innervating the urinary bladder. The latter are also known to produce an 'efferent' function on their target tissues, by releasing sensory neuropeptides (TKs and CGRP) following application of stimuli which produce calcium entry into the sensory nerve terminals. In turn, the released neuropeptides produce a plethora of local effects (changes in muscle tone, vasodilation, increase in vascular permeability, etc.) collectively known as 'neurogenic inflammation' (Maggi, 1993). There is no evidence that 'neurogenic inflammation' occurs during the normal micturition cycle (Koltzenburg and McMahon, 1986; Lecci et al., 1993c) which activates distension-sensitive bladder afferents. Again, this process could be important during bladder irritation/cystitis, by providing a neural contribution to the overall inflammatory process and possibly reinforcing the afferent barrage to the spinal cord. The capsaicin-sensitive afferents also play an important role in mediating pain arising from the urinary bladder/urethra, as judged from the abolition of the aversive behaviour evoked by bladder noxious stimulation in capsaicin-pretreated rats (Abelli et al., 1988).

The existence of functionally and anatomically distinct sources of bladder afferent input, signalling physiological bladder distension vs. irritation/noxious events, is further supported by the results of experiments determining c-*fos* expression into the spinal cord after various peripheral experimental manipulations (distension/irritation) (Birder and De Groat, 1992). In general, a wide overlap of labelling of spinal cord areas showing c-*fos* expression was observed in response to different kinds of stimuli, but quantitative differences were observed at the lumbosacral level. In fact, vesical irritation greatly increased c-*fos* expression in the lumbosacral segments of the spinal cord, whereas no consistent response was observed at the upper levels. After bladder irritation, the number of c-*fos*-positive neurons was increased in the medial and the lateral portions of the dorsal horns and in the dorsal gray commissure. In the latter area, and at the level of the sacral parasympathetic nucleus, c-*fos* expression was also increased by repeated micturition cycles. Therefore, the spinal cord areas which show a differential activation in response to physiological and pathophysiological (bladder irritation) stimuli are the parasymphathetic nucleus, and the medial and the dorsal parts of the dorsal horns, respectively. Also interesting was the comparison of c-*fos* expression in response to irritation after transection of the pelvic or pudendal nerves, which innervate the bladder and the urethra, respectively (a portion of the urethral afferents also travels within the pelvic nerve). Pelvic nerve transection reduced the irritation-induced c-*fos* labelling to 39% of control, the greatest reduction being observed at the level of parasympathetic nucleus and in the lateral dorsal horn, where labelling was almost abolished. On the contrary, section of the pudendal nerves caused the greatest reduction of c-*fos*-labelled cells in the medial and lateral areas of dorsal horns.

From the above, a quite simple scheme could be outlined: A δ fiber mechanosensitive afferents signalling bladder distension and subserving normal micturition, and C fiber afferents signalling noxious events and participating in the genesis of symptoms of urgency and frequency during cystitis. However, additional elements which complicate the issue should be considered: (a) although most of the SP-positive DRG neurons give rise to C fiber afferents, a fraction of them also has fibers with conduction velocity in the A δ range (McCarthy and Lawson, 1989); (b) while most of the capsaicin-sensitive afferents have conduction velocity in the C fiber range, some of them are also thinly myelinated (A δ-fibers) (e.g., Szolcsanyi et al., 1988); (c) myelinated afferents, which are silent when the bladder is empty, respond vigorously after intravesical application of irritants (Habler et al., 1993a,b), indicating that, either directly or indirectly, at least some of them are also chemosensitive; (d) under certain experimental conditions, a modulatory influence of capsaicin-sensitive afferents on the distension-induced micturition reflex can be demonstrated (e.g., Maggi et al., 1986a), suggesting that this class of sensory nerves may exert an influence also on 'normal' micturition.

Since the mechanosensitivity of electrophysiologically characterized bladder afferents responding to the acute application of capsaicin has not been probed yet, it is not possible to simply equate the TK-containing, capsaicin-sensitive afferents innervating the urinary bladder to the afferent neurons responding exclusively or chiefly to irritation rather than to distension. In particular, it not possible to exclude, at present, that a portion of the A δ-fibers which mediate the distension-induced micturition reflex are also capsaicin-sensitive. Thus, while the role of TK-containing afferents in mediating bladder pain and inflammation seems to be well established, if not proven, the significance of TK release during normal micturition is more elusive. As discussed below, experiments with TK receptor antagonists could help in solving the issue.

Pharmacological studies

The evidence summarized in the previous sections strongly supports a role of TK-containing primary afferent neurons in the transmission of sensory modalities from the bladder and urethra to the spinal cord, thereby influencing micturition and mediating bladder pain/irritation. The anatomical and neurophysiological evidence outlined above has been integrated by the results of functional studies investigating either the effect of capsaicin to produce stimulation/inactivation of TK-containing afferent nerves and, more recently, of TK receptor ligands (agonists and antagonists).

Studies with capsaicin

In urethane-anaesthetized rats, the topical application of low doses of capsaicin onto the serosal surface of the urinary bladder induces two distinct motor responses: (a) a low-amplitude, tonic-type bladder contraction ascribable to local release of TKs within the bladder wall; and (b) a series of high-amplitude phasic contractions which are sustained through the activation of a supraspinal chemoceptive micturition reflex (Maggi et al., 1984, 1986a,c). Systemic pretreatment with large doses of capsaicin produces a total depletion of the urinary bladder content of TKs, prevents the acute stimulant effect of capsaicin on bladder motility, and also increases the threshold volume of infused fluid required for eliciting the micturition reflex (Santicioli et al., 1985; Maggi et al., 1984, 1989b). The latter result is of special interest because it implies a certain degree of mechanosensitivity of capsaicin-sensitive bladder afferents (as discussed previously, this postulate has not yet been verified experimentally). It is also possible that the capsaicin-sensitive afferents, which modulate the afferent arm of the distension-induced micturition reflex in anaesthetized rats, are not intrinsically mechanosensitive but are excited by chemicals produced in the bladder during fluid-induced distension, especially by prostanoids (Maggi, 1992).

Since the increase in bladder capacity produced by capsaicin pretreatment in adult rats is accompanied by a total depletion of the TK content of the urinary bladder, it may be speculated that the release of TKs from either the central or peripheral endings of afferent nerves mediates part of the distension-induced sensory discharge. The peripheral administration of TK receptor antagonists blocks the tonic-type bladder contractions without affecting the reflex response induced by topical application of capsaicin (Lecci et al., 1993c). Therefore, a peripheral release of TKs is not a determinant for the sensory stimulant action of capsaicin. Furthermore, peripherally administered TK receptor antagonists have no effect on the distension-induced micturition reflex in urethane-anaesthetized rats; since the peripheral blockade of TK receptors does not reproduce the increase in bladder capacity observed following systemic pretreatment with capsaicin, TKs could have a role as spinal cord modulators of the micturition reflex (Lecci et al., 1993a).

Therefore, studies in *anaesthetized* rats indicate a modulatory role of capsaicin-sensitive, TK-containing sensory neurons on the afferent arm of the distension-induced micturition reflex: since the peripheral blockade of TK receptors does not modulate this reflex, a role of TKs at spinal cord level may be postulated.

In *unanaesthetized* rats, however, the picture appears quite different, since capsaicin pretreatment had no effect on bladder capacity (Maggi and Conte, 1990). Therefore, the modulatory effect of capsaicin pretreatment on bladder capacity during a physiological-like vesical filling can be evidenced only under urethane anaesthesia. These results have led to the speculation that the afferent pathways mediating 'reflex' and 'conscious' micturition are different (Maggi and Meli, 1986b). The modifications of afferent pathways of the micturition reflex occurring under anaesthesia are not necessarily related to the activity of primary afferent neurons but could involve spinal or supraspinal neuronal networks involved in processing afferent input from the urinary tract. Despite the fact that the effect of systemic capsaicin pretreatment on bladder capacity is evident in anaesthetized animals only, the acute intravesical infusion of capsaicin in awake rats still induces bladder hyperreflexia and increases the amplitude of micturition contractions (Ishizuka, Igawa, Lecci, Maggi, Mattiasson and Andersson, submitted), indicating that capsaicin-sensitive bladder afferents are able to modulate bladder motility even in unanaesthetized animals. Similar results have been obtained in humans at cystometry: the intravesical instillation of capsaicin produced a concentration-dependent decrease of bladder capacity and a painful sensation (Maggi et al., 1989a), indicating that capsaicin-sensitive afferents mediate pain and modulate bladder capacity in the human bladder.

The contribution of the capsaicin-sensitive fibers in the distension-induced micturition reflex becomes more important after spinal cord injury. In anaesthetized rats, the hexamethonium-sensitive distension-induced bladder-to-bladder reflex contractions, emerging after spinal cord transection, are totally abolished by capsaicin pretreatment (Maggi et al., 1987). Similar results have been obtained in cats, where systemic capsaicin pretreatment had no effect on the micturition pattern in normal animals; however, in chronic spinal cats, systemic capsaicin treatment abolished the distension-evoked micturition reflex. The altered sensitivity to capsaicin treatment is accompanied by electrophysiological modifications of the afferent limb of the reflex, which is signalled by $A\delta$ and by C-fibers before and after chronic spinal cord transection, respectively (De Groat et al., 1990).

Studies with tachykinin receptor agonists

If TKs act as primary afferent transmitters in the micturition reflex pathway, it may be expected that the intrathecal (i.t.) administration of natural TKs or of TK receptor agonists will influence

bladder motility. However, only a few studies have investigated this aspect, and the results have not been univocal.

In urethane-anaesthetized rats, low doses of i.t. SP elicited contractions of the empty bladder and increased the frequency of ongoing micturition contractions. At high doses, a mixed excitatory-inhibitory activity, or a pure inhibitory effect, was observed (Mallory and De Groat, 1987). In about 50% of barbiturate-anaesthetized rats, i.t. SP was found to evoke and/or enhance bladder contractions. The electromyographic activity of the external urethral sphincter was consistently increased in all animals (Mersdorf et al., 1992). However, since similar effects were induced by i.v. SP, and peripheral signs of activation of TK receptors (e.g., salivation) were also observed after i.t. administration of the peptide, it was unclear which part of the bladder effects may be ascribed to leakage of SP outside of the central nervous system. In addition, as barbiturates at anaesthetic doses produced a significant inhibition or abolishment of the micturition reflex (Morikawa et al., 1989), and reduce the SP-induced phosphatidylinositol hydrolysis at the spinal cord level (Hassessian et al., 1992), the effects of i.t. substance P on the micturition reflex could have been dampened by barbiturates.

In urethane-anaesthetized rats, with urinary bladders filled with a subthreshold volume of saline, the i.t. administration of NKA (1–10 nmol) produced a tonic-type detrusor contraction with micturition contractions superimposed (Table Ia). This kind of response was qualitatively similar to that observed after topical application of NKA or other TKs onto the bladder (Maggi et al., 1986b). Various elements indicate that the effects of i.t. administration of NKA are actually due to a peripheral leakage of the peptide. First, the reflex but not the tonic contraction was blocked by i.v. hexamethonium (Table Ib); second, both the tonic and reflex urinary bladder contractions were reduced by i.v. administration of the peptide NK_2 receptor antagonist L 659,877 (Table Ic); third, a tonic-type detrusor contraction produced by i.t. NKA was still present after bilateral ablation of

TABLE I

Effect of i.t. administration (L1–L2 segments) of neurokinin A on urinary bladder motility (transurethral recording) in urethane-anaesthetized rats

Treatment and dose/rat	Rhythmic contractions			Tonic contraction		
	Incidence of rhythmic contractions	Amplitude (mmHg)	Duration (min)	Amplitude (mmHg)	Duration (min)	AUC (% of baseline)
A: Saline	0/7	0	0	0	0	109 ± 5
NKA 1 nmol	2/7	29 ± 4	9 ± 3	3 ± 1	13 ± 2	140 ± 18
NKA 10 nmol	5/7*	32 ± 2	22 ± 11	21 ± 4	31 ± 5	315 ± 84**
B: NKA 10 nmol	8/8	35 ± 3	13 ± 2	10 ± 2	17 ± 2	199 ± 16
NKA 10 nmol + hexamethazone 30 mg/kg, i.v.	3/8*	26 ± 2*	16 ± 3	13 ± 2	23 ± 2	207 ± 10
C: NKA 10 nmol	6/9	29 ± 1	9 ± 1	14 ± 1	21 ± 3	196 ± 12
NKA 10 nmol + L 659,877 0.3 μmol/kg, i.v.	1/9*	30	18	8 ± 1*	15 ± 1*	138 ± 11**
D: NKA 10 nmol	6/8	28 ± 2	6 ± 2	13 ± 1	20 ± 2	188 ± 18
NKA 10 nmol + ganglionect.	0/8*	0	0	8 ± 2	24 ± 2	153 ± 15

*,** $P < 0.05$ and 0.01 vs control, respectively.

pelvic ganglia (Table Id). Intrathecal administration of the selective NK$_1$ receptor agonist [Sar^9]SP sulfone induced effects similar to those observed with NKA (Table II).

In summary, spinally-administered TKs facilitate the micturition reflex by modulating bladder contractions and urethral sphincter activity; however, some of these effects are due to the leakage of the peptide in the bloodstream and activation of peripheral TK receptors. Although the results of the above mentioned and of similar studies (Kawatani et al., 1987; Tiseo and Yaksh, 1990) have been disappointing, there are theoretical reasons whereby it may not be easy to demonstrate an excitatory effect of spinally applied TKs on the micturition reflex. In fact, if TKs are general transmitters of primary afferent input, especially for the signalling of painful or noxious

sensory modalities, it would appears quite logical to expect that TK receptors accessible to i.t. administered agonists were expressed in a variety of neuronal pathways at the spinal cord level, and that their concomitant activation during application of exogenous agonists may exert mixed and partially counteracting effects on bladder motility. This general point is in keeping with the physiological knowledge that noxious mechanical (Sato et al., 1975; Maggi and Meli, 1986c) or chemical stimuli (Sato et al., 1979; Conte et al., 1989; Palea et al., 1993) applied to visceral or somatic structures can produce both excitatory or inhibitory influences on bladder motility; dependent especially on the physiological state (degree of filling) of the viscus. In general, noxious stimulation activates bladder motility when the bladder contains a subthreshold amount of fluid for activation of the micturition reflex, while the same stimuli exert an inhibitory effect on the ongoing reflex contractions activated by bladder distension.

Studies with tachykinin receptor antagonists

The recent availability of potent and selective TK receptor antagonists, including various ligands of nonpeptide nature (for review, see Maggi et al., 1993) has represented a major advance in studies aiming to elucidate the role of these peptides in the spinal regulation of vesicourethral function.

Distension-induced micturition reflex

With regard to the distension-induced micturition reflex in normal rats, various non-peptide NK_1 receptor antagonists tested so far, have proven to be effective in increasing bladder capacity after i.t. administration in *anaesthetized* animals, documenting a modulatory role of spinal cord NK_1 receptors in this response. In urethane-anaesthetized rats, the nonpeptide NK_1 receptor antagonist CP 96,345 decreases the amplitude of distension-induced bladder contractions at low i.t. doses (10–25 nmol) and completely abolished the micturition reflex at high doses (100–400 nmol) (Kawatani et al., 1993; Lecci et al., 1993a). However, since CP 96,345 possesses

calcium and sodium channels blocking activity at high concentrations (Schmidt et al., 1992; Caeser et al., 1993), and in view of its relatively poor affinity for the rat NK_1 receptor (Gitter et al., 1991; Barr and Watson, 1993), the results obtained with CP 96,345 in rats cannot be regarded as conclusive. The problem has been circumvented by using other compounds, especially the nonpeptide antagonist RP 67,580, which possesses a high affinity for rat NK_1 receptors (Fong et al., 1992) and has a greater 'selectivity window' between specific effects (on NK_1 receptor) vs. nonspecific effects in rats (Rupniak et al., 1993). Similar to CP 96,345, RP 67,580 was also found to block the distension-induced micturition contractions and to increase the bladder capacity and residual volume at cystometry after i.t. administration in rats (Table III): in both respects, RP 67,580 is about 10-times more potent than CP 96,345. Evidence that these effects are indeed related to blockade of NK_1 receptors came from the demonstration that RP 68,651, the inactive enantiomer of RP 67,580, had no effect (Lecci et al., 1993a).

The effects produced by i.t. RP 67,580 on the distension-induced micturition reflex in anaesthetized rats are qualitatively and quantitatively similar to those observed after partial sensory

TABLE II

Effect of i.t. administration of [Sar9] SP sulfone on urinary bladder motility in urethane-anaesthetized rats

Treatment and dose/rat	Rhythmic contractions			Tonic contraction		
	Incidence of rhythmic contractions	Amplitude (mmHg)	Duration (min)	Amplitude (mmHg)	Duration (min)	AUC (% of baseline)
A: Saline	0/7	0	0	0	0	106 ± 5
[Sar9] SP 1 nmol	4/12	26 ± 5	10 ± 8	4 ± 1	10 ± 3	119 ± 5
[Sar9] SP 10 nmol	10/12**	30 ± 2	13 ± 6	14 ± 3	15 ± 1	174 ± 16**
B: [Sar9] SP 10 nmol	8/9	37 ± 6	17 ± 8	11 ± 3	16 ± 2	144 ± 6
[Sar9] SP 10 nmol + hexameth., 30 mg/kg, i.v.	2/9*	22 ± 3*	2 ± 1*	10 ± 2	16 ± 2	154 ± 11

*,** $P < 0.05$ and 0.01 vs control, respectively.

denervation produced by capsaicin-pretreatment in adult rats. Moreover, when i.t. RP 67,580 was administered to capsaicin-pretreated rats, its modulatory effect on the distension-induced micturition reflex was no longer evident (Fig. 1). Therefore, the non-additivity of the effect of i.t. RP 67,580 and systemic capsaicin pretreatment indicates that NK_1 receptor antagonists modulate the afferent limb of the micturition reflex through the blockade of the effects of TKs released from primary afferent neurons; the participation of NK_2 receptors was excluded because various NK_2 receptor-selective antagonists (MEN 10,376, L 659,877, GR 94,800 and SR 48,968) had no effect on the distension-induced bladder contractions (Lecci et al., 1993a; Maggi et al., 1993b; Magnan et al., 1993).

Interestingly, the peptide-based NK_1 receptor antagonist GR 82,334, up to doses producing a neurotoxic effect after i.t. administration, had no effect on the distension-evoked micturition reflex in rats (Table III) (Lecci et al., 1992, 1993a; Magnan et al., 1993). On the other hand, both GR 82,334 and RP 67,580 effectively block the bladder hyperreflexia induced by irritants (see below), further indicating that the spinal pathways conveying sensory information during normal micturition could be different from those activated during noxious stimulation of the urinary bladder (discussed above). A different degree of penetration in deeper laminae of the dorsal horns may account for the different pharmacological profiles of GR 82,334 and RP 67,580 in blocking the mechanosensitive (distension-induced) and chemosensitive (capsaicin-induced) micturition reflex in anaesthetized rats. Alternatively, the existence of NK_1 receptor subtypes in the spinal cord (Sakurada et al., 1991) may be involved.

A few studies have investigated the effect of i.t. administration of tachykinin receptor antagonists on the distension-induced micturition reflex in *unanaesthetized* rats. In one early study, however, the weak TK antagonist, spantide I, produced a blockade of urethral sphincter function which was associated with hindlimb paralysis (Tiseo and

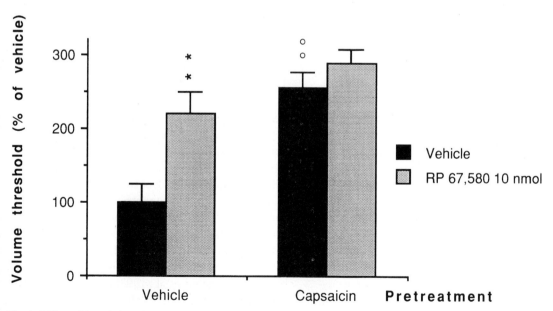

Fig. 1. Effect of i.t. administration of RP 67,580 on bladder capacity in vehicle- and capsaicin-pretreated (50 mg/kg, s.c., 4 days previously) urethane-anaesthetized rats. ** and °° = $P < 0.01$ vs. vehicle (Tukey test).

TABLE III

Effect of i.t. administration of tachykinin receptor antagonists on various cytometric parameters (46 μl/min) in urethane-anaesthetized rats

Treatment	(dose/rat)	B.C. (μl)	R.V. (% of B.C.)	M.A.C. (mmHg)
Saline	10 μl	586 ± 99	53 ± 7	26.9 ± 0.8
GR 82,334	1 nmol	722 ± 123	58 ± 8	25.1 ± 1.0
RP 67,580	1 nmol	665 ± 115	56 ± 10	28.7 ± 1.7
RP 67,580	10 nmol	1287 ± 155**	86 ± 4*	23.8 ± 1.2
RP 68,658	10 nmol	502 ± 80	57 ± 6	29.8 ± 1.3
CP 96,345	100 nmol	1189 ± 182**	85 ± 9*	24.5 ± 1.6
SR 48,968	10 nmol	615 ± 108	57 ± 6	25.6 ± 0.9

B.C., bladder capacity (volume of fluid determining the first micturition, μl); R.V., the residual volume (% of B.C.); M.A.C., mean amplitude of micturition contractions (mmHg).
*,**$P < 0.05$ and $P < 0.01$ vs saline, respectively (Dunnett's test).

Yaksh, 1990). In a more recent study, the effect of two non-peptide tachykinin receptor antagonists has been investigated in rats with bladder hypertrophy induced by urethral obstruction. It was found that the NK_1 receptor antagonist RP 67,580 induces overflow incontinence in rats with bladder hypertrophy, while it only reduces the amplitude of urinary bladder contractions in control animals. The NK_2 receptor antagonist SR 48,968 had no effect on cystometries either in controls or in rats with bladder hypertrophia. However, SR 48,968 significantly reduced detrusor hyperreflexia induced by intravesical infusion of capsaicin (Ishizuka, Igawa, Lecci, Maggi, Mattiasson and Andersson, submitted).

Similar to the effect observed with systemic capsaicin pretreatment, the effect of i.t. TK receptor antagonists is profoundly influenced by anaesthesia: in anaesthetized rats the NK_1 receptor antagonists exert an inhibitory influence on micturition reflex, whereas in unanaesthetized rats a marked inhibitory effect is observed only in models simulating pathological conditions. Although the possibility of a specific pharmacodynamic interaction between the anaesthetic and capsaicin pretreatment or between anaesthetic and acute i.t. administration of TK receptor an-

tagonists cannot be totally excluded at present, it appears more likely that the interaction occurs because anaesthesia induces a change in the activity of specific neural pathways involved in regulating vesicourethral function. In this respect, it is noteworthy that anaesthesia not only influences the supraspinal excitatory input to the spinal cord but could also modify the activity of descending inhibitory pathways: for istance, bladder capacity is larger in conscious rats than in decerebrate or in urethane-anaesthetized rats (Morikawa et al., 1989; Yoshiyama et al., 1993).

Animal models of cystitis / bladder irritation

Several models have been developed to induce bladder irritation and to mimic the symptoms of cystitis. The intravesical infusion of 1% acetic acid induced bladder hyperreflexia and increased a vesico-anal reflex (contraction of the anal sphincter coordinated with micturition contractions) in rats sensitive to capsaicin pretreatment (Muhlhauser and Thor, 1992). Intrathecal CP 96,345 inhibited the contractility of the irritated bladder (Kawatani et al., 1993) and decreased the vesico-anal reflex, wheras the activity of the urethral sphincter was unaffected (Iyengar et al., 1992). The infusion of acetic acid into the urinary bladder also increased c-*fos* expression in the dorsal horn superficial laminae, the dorsal gray commissure and in the sacral parasympathetic nucleus, and i.t. administration of CP 96,345 reduced the irritant-induced c-*fos* expression in all these areas of the lumbosacral spinal cord (Kawatani et al., 1993). Since low pH is an adequate stimulus for activation of capsaicin-sensitive afferents in the urinary bladder (Geppetti et al., 1990), and capsaicin pretreatment prevents spinal cord c-*fos* expression following irritation of the bladder (Birder et al., 1990), the above mentioned results are fully consistent with the idea that spinal cord NK_1 receptors are activated during bladder irritation by chemicals. In addition to CP 96,345, a number of other intrathecally administered NK_1 receptor antagonists, such as GR 82,334, RP 67,580 (Lecci et al., 1993a) and SR 140,333 (Lecci, Giuliani, Meini and Maggi, submitted), block the micturition contractions induced by topical application of capsaicin or bradykinin onto the serosal surface of the urinary bladder (chemoceptive reflex). Further evidence for activation of spinal NK_1 receptors following application of noxious stimuli to the urinary bladder comes from the study of Cutrufo et al. (1993), showing that the electroencephalographic desynchronization produced by noxious mechanical (overdistension) or chemical stimulation of the urinary bladder in rats is prevented by either capsaicin pretreatment or by i.t. GR 82,334 and RP 67,580.

Intrathecally administered GR 82,334 antagonizes the hyperreflexic response, induced by bladder filling, in anaesthetized rats which had been pretreated with intravesical xylene 30 min before cystometry. The effect of GR 82,334 was prevented by the coadministration of the selective NK_1 receptor agonist GR 73,632 (Magnan et al., 1993). The intrathecal administration of NK_1 receptor antagonists (GR 82,334 and RP 67,580) also reverted detrusor hyperreflexia associated with cyclophosphamide-induced cystitis (Lecci et al., 1993b). In the latter model, cystitis is caused by a metabolite of cyclophosphamide, acrolein, which accumulates in the urine and stimulates capsaicin-sensitive afferents at the urinary bladder level (Ahluwalia et al., 1994). Cyclophosphamide-induced bladder hyperreflexia was also prevented by systemic capsaicin pretreatment (Maggi et al., 1992), but not by the intravenous administration of NK_1 or NK_2 receptor antagonists; therefore, the blockade of the efferent function of capsaicin-sensitive fibers does not impair their ability to stimulate reflex responses induced by compounds which directly activate the sensory nerves. It is interesting to observe that, in this model of subacute cystitis (cystometries were performed 48 h after cyclophosphamide administration), the blockade of spinal NK_2 receptors by the selective antagonist SR 48,968 also became effective in modulating the detrusor hyperreflexia (Lecci, Giuliani, Santicioli and Maggi, submitted). These results clearly differentiated cyclophosphamide- from xylene-induced cystitis where NK_2 receptor antagonists had no effect (Magnan et al., 1993).

Summarizing, the results obtained in anaesthetized rats combine to indicate that the activation of capsaicin-sensitive bladder afferents through various noxious modalities (capsaicin, bradykinin, low pH, xylene, acrolein or overdistension) induces the release of TKs at the spinal cord level which facilitate micturition contractions by the stimulation of NK_1 receptors, whereas NK_2 receptors seem to become important only after a persistent inflammation.

Other studies

At present, only one study has investigated the effect of i.t. administration of TK receptor antagonists on cystometry in urethane-anaesthetized guinea pigs. This study was conducted in animals subjected to spinal cord transection; the intravesical infusion of capsaicin caused an inhibition of the ongoing micturition contractions which, in this species, are mediated through a spinal reflex. This inhibition, which was naloxone-sensitive, was also prevented by the i.t. administration of GR 82,334, but not of the NK_2 receptor antagonist GR 94,800, suggesting the involvement of spinal cord NK_1 receptors. However it must be pointed out that another NK_1 receptor antagonist, CP 96,345, did not modify the inhibitory effect of capsaicin (Palea et al., 1993).

The effect of spinally administered TK receptor antagonists has been investigated with regard to the somatovesical excitatory reflex evoked by noxious pinching of the perineal skin. This reflex has a different anatomical organization from the chemoceptive reflex or the distension-induced micturition reflex. In fact, the pinch-evoked bladder contraction is a spinal reflex (Maggi et al., 1986b), and its afferent arm is capsaicin-resistant (Maggi et al., 1986c). Accordingly, NK_2 or NK_1 receptor antagonists, at i.t. doses which effectively block the reflex response evoked by capsaicin or by irritants, had no effect on this model (Lecci et al., 1993a).

In conclusion, the i.t. administration of NK_1 receptor antagonists increases bladder capacity and delays the distension-induced micturition reflex in urethane-anaesthetized rats. This inhibitory effect appears to be due to the blockade of afferent input from capsaicin-sensitive fibers. NK_1 receptor antagonists, including GR 82,334, also reduce the bladder hyperreflexia caused by vesical irritation. Spinal NK_2 receptors, which are not normally involved in the distension-induced micturition reflex, could have a role in the hyperreflexia caused by prolonged or intense activation of capsaicin-sensitive fibers.

Conclusions

The anatomical, physiological and pharmacological evidence reviewed in this chapter combine to implicate TKs, released from central endings of capsaicin-sensitive primary afferent neurons, to be excitatory transmitters in the micturition reflex pathway. A role of these mediators in signalling bladder irritation/inflammation to the spinal cord seems well defined, while their significance in the modulation of normal urine storage and voiding is less well understood. Since capsaicin-sensitive nerves appear to innervate the human urinary bladder and subserve a sensory function (Maggi et al., 1989; Fowler et al., 1992; Barbanti et al.,

1993), and that changes in bladder and spinal cord SP levels occur during human diseases associated with bladder disfunction (Crowe et al., 1991; Tomokane et al., 1991), the hypothesis may be advanced that the manipulation of spinal cord TK receptors could be used to either stimulate (agonists) or inhibit (antagonists) bladder voiding during pathological conditions in humans.

Acknowledgements

Dr. A. Lecci acknowledges the collaboration of Dr. Stefania Meini, his wife, who quietly accepted to delay the honeymoon until completion of the writing of this manuscript. Dr. C.A. Maggi acknowledges the collaboration of Dr. Stefania Meini for keeping quiet Dr. A. Lecci.

References

Abelli, L., Conte, B., Somma, V., Maggi, C.A., Giuliani, S., Geppetti, P., Alessandri, M., Theodorsson, E. and Meli, A. (1988) The contribution of capsaicin-sensitive sensory nerves to xylene-induced visceral pain in conscious, freely moving rats. *Naunyn-Schmiedeberg's Arch. Pharmacol.*, 337: 545–551.

Ahluwalia, A., Maggi, C.A., Santicioli, P., Lecci, A. and Giuliani, S. (1994) Characterization of the capsaicin-sensitive component of cyclophosphamide-induced inflammation in the rat urinary bladder. *Br. J. Pharmacol.*, 111: 1017–1022.

Barbanti, G., Maggi, C.A., Beneforti, P., Baroldi, P. and Turini, D. (1993) Relief of pain following intravesical capsaicin in patients with hypersensitive disorders of the lower urinary tract. *Br. J. Urol.*, 71: 686–691.

Barr, A.J. and Watson, S.P. (1993) Non-peptide antagonists, CP 96,345 and RP 67,580, distinguish species variants in tachykinin NK_1 receptors. *Br. J. Pharmacol.*, 108: 223–227.

Birder, L.A. and De Groat, W.C. (1992) Increased c-fos expression in spinal neurons after irritation of the lower urinary tract in the rat. *J. Neurosci.*, 12: 4878–4889.

Birder, L.A., Roppolo, J.R., Iadarola, M.J. and De Groat, W.C. (1990) C-fos as a marker for subsets of visceral second order neurons in the rat lumbosacral spinal cord. *Soc. Neurosci. Abstr.*, 16: 703.

Caeser, M., Seabrook, G.R. and Kemp, J.A. (1993) Block of voltage-dependent sodium currents by the substance P receptor antagonist ($\pm$)-CP 96,345 in neurones cultured from rat cortex. *Br. J. Pharmacol.*, 109: 918–924.

Chang, M.M., Leeman, S.E. and Niall, H.D. (1971) Aminoacid sequence of substance P. *Nature*, 232: 86–87.

Charlton, C.G. and Helke, C.J. (1985 a) Characterization and segmental distribution of ^{125}I-Bolton-Hunter labeled substance P binding sites in rat spinal cord. *J. Neurosci.*, 5: 1293-1299.

Charlton, C.G. and Helke, C.J. (1985 b) Autoradiographic localization and characterization of spinal cord substance P binding sites: high densities in sensory, autonomic, phrenic, and Onuf's motor nuclei. *J. Neurosci.*, 5: 1653-1661.

Conte, B., Maggi, C.A. and Meli, A. (1989) Vesico-inhibitory responses and capsaicin-sensitive afferents in rats. *Naunyn-Schmiedeberg's Arch. Pharmacol.*, 339: 178-183.

Crowe, R., Moss, H.E., Chapple, C.R., Light, J.K. and Burnstock, G. (1991) Patients with lower motor spinal cord lesion: a decrease of vasoactive intestinal peptide, calcitonin gene-related peptide and substance P, but not neuropeptide Y and somatostatin-immunoreactive nerves in the detrusor muscle of the bladder. *J. Urol.*, 145: 600-604.

Cutrufo, C., Conte, B. and Manzini, S. (1993) EEG arousal following application of noxious stimuli on the urinary bladder of anaesthetized rats: effects of intrathecal administration of NK$_1$ antagonists. *Neuropeptides*, 24: 220.

De Groat, W.C. (1986) Spinal cord projections and neuropeptides in visceral afferent neurons. In F. Cervero and J.F.B. Morrison (Eds.), *Progress in Brain Research*, Vol. 67, Elsevier, Amsterdam, pp. 165-185.

De Groat, W.C. (1987) Neuropeptides in pelvic afferent pathways. *Experientia*, 43: 801-813.

De Groat, W.C., Kawatani, Hisamitsu, T., Booth, A.M., Roppolo, J.R., Thor, K., Tuttle, P. and Nagel, J. (1986) Neural control of micturition: the role of neuropeptides. *J. Autonom. Nerv. Syst.*, 6(Suppl.): 361-368.

De Groat, W.C., Kawatani, M., Hisamitsu, T., Cheng, C.L., Ma, C.P., Thor, K., Steers, W. and Roppolo, J.R. (1990) Mechanisms underlying the recovery of urinary bladder function following spinal cord injury. *J. Autonom. Nerv. Syst.*, 30 Suppl: 571-577.

De Groat, W.C., Booth, A.M. and Yoshimura, N. (1993) Neurophysiology of micturition and its modification in animal models of human disease. In: C.A. Maggi (Ed.) *The Nervous Control of the Urogenital System, The Autonomic Nervous System, Vol. 3*, Harwood, Chur, pp. 227-290.

De Koninck, Y. and Henry, J.L. (1991) Substance P-mediated slow excitatory postsynaptic potential elicited in dorsal horn neurons in vivo by noxious stimulation. *Proc. Natl. Acad. Sci. USA*, 88: 11,344-11,348.

Duggan, A.W., Morton, C.R., Zhao, Z.Q. and Hendry, I.A. (1987) Noxious heating of skin releases immunoreactive substance P in the substantia gelatinosa of the cat: a study with antibody microprobes. *Brain Res.*, 403, 345-349.

Fong, T.M., Yu, H. and Strader, C.D. (1992) Molecular basis for the species selectivity of neurokinin-1 receptor antagonists CP 96,345 and RP 67,580. *J. Biol. Chem.*, 267: 25668-25671.

Fowler, C.J., Jewkes, D., McDonald, W.I., Lynn, B. and De

Groat, W.C. (1992) Intravesical capsaicin for neurogenic bladder dysfunction. *Lancet*, 339: 1239.

Gamse, R., Lackner, D., Gamse, G. and Leeman, S.E. (1981) Effect of capsaicin pretreatment on capsaicin-evoked release of immunoreactive somatostatin and substance P from primary sensory neurons. *Naunyn-Schmiedeberg's Arch. Pharmacol.*, 316: 38-41.

Geppetti, P., Tramontana, M., Patacchini, R., Del Bianco, E., Santicioli, P. and Maggi, C.A. (1990) Neurochemical evidence for the activation of the efferent function of capsaicin-sensitive nerves by lowering of the pH in the guinea-pig urinary bladder. *Neurosci. Lett.*, 114: 101-106.

Gitter, B.D., Waters, D.C., Bruns, R.F., Mason, N.R., Nixon, J.A. and Howbert, J.J. (1991) Species differences in affinities of non peptide antagonists for substance P receptors. *Eur. J. Pharmacol.*, 197: 237-238.

Habler, H.-J., Janig, W. and Koltzenburg, M. (1990) Activation of unmyelinated afferent fibers by mechanical stimuli and inflammation of the urinary bladder in the cat. *J. Physiol.*, 425: 545-562.

Habler, H.-J., Janig, W. and Koltzenburg, M. (1993a) Myelinated primary afferents of the sacral spinal cord responding to slow filling and distension of the cat urinary bladder. *J. Physiol.*, 463: 449-460.

Habler, H.-J., Janig, W. and Koltzenburg, M. (1993b) Receptive properties of myelinated primary afferents innervating the inflamed urinary bladder of the cat. *J. Neurophysiol.*, 69: 395-405.

Hassessian, H., Prat, A. and Couture, R. (1992) Anaesthetic doses of pentobarbital antagonize phosphatidylinositol hydrolysis induced by substance P or carbachol in the spinal cord and cerebral cortex of the rat. *Eur. J. Pharmacol.*, 227: 103-107.

Hökfelt, T., Kellerth, J.-O., Nilsson, G. and Pernow, B. (1975) Substance P: localization in the central nervous system and in some primary sensory neurons. *Science*, 190: 889-890.

Helke, C.J., Charlton, C.G. and Wiley, R.G. (1986) Studies on the cellular localization of spinal cord substance P receptors. *Neuroscience*, 19: 523-533.

Hua, X.-Y., Saria, A., Gamse, R., Theodorsson-Norheim, E., Brodin, E. and Lundberg, J.M. (1986) Capsaicin induced release of multiple tachykinins (substance P, neurokinin A and eledoisin-like material) from guinea-pig spinal cord and ureter. *Neuroscience*, 19: 313-319.

Iyengar, S., Muhlhhauser, M.A., Howbert, J.J. and Thor, K.B. (1992) Inhibitory effect of a NK − 1 antagonist, CP 96,345, on visceral nociceptive activity and non-nociceptive bladder activity in rats. *Regul. Peptides*, Suppl. 1: S80.

Jancso, G. and Maggi, C.A. (1987) Distribution of capsaicin-sensitive urinary bladder afferents in the rat spinal cord. *Brain Res.*, 418: 371-376.

Janig, W. and Koltzenburg, M. (1993) Pain arising from the urogenital tract. In: C.A. Maggi (Ed.), *The Nervous Control* of the Urogenital System: The Autonomic Nervous System, Vol. 3, Harwood, Chur, pp. 525–567.

Kawatani, M., Takeshige, C. and De Groat, W.C. (1987) Effects of intrathecal administration of VIP, substance P, and CGRP on the micturition reflex of the cat. Soc. Neurosci. Abstr., 13: 269.

Kawatani, M., Matsumoto, G., Birder, L.A., Fukuoka, H., Yoshiyama, M., Misaki, A. and Suzuki, S. (1993) Intrathecal administration of NK$_1$ receptor antagonist, CP 96,345, inhibits the micturition reflex in the rat. Regul. Peptides, 46: 392–395.

Keast, J.R. and De Groat, W.C. (1992) Segmental distribution and peptide content of primary afferent neurons innervating the urogenital organs and colon of male rats. J. Comp. Neurol., 319: 615–623.

Koltzenburgh, M. and McMaon, S.B. (1986) Plasma extravasation in the rat urinary bladder following mechanical, electrical and chemical stimuli: evidence for a new population of chemosensitive primary sensory neurons. Neurosci. Lett., 72: 352–356.

Lecci, A., Giuliani, S. and Maggi, C.A. (1992) Effect of the NK-1 receptor antagonist GR 82,334 on reflexly-induced bladder contractions. Life Sci., 51: PL277–280.

Lecci, A., Giuliani, S., Garret, C. and Maggi, C.A. (1993a) Evidence for a role of tachykinins as sensory transmitters in the activation of micturition reflex. Neuroscience, 54: 827–837.

Lecci, A., Giuliani, S. and Maggi, C.A. (1993b) Spinal tachykinin NK$_1$ receptors modulate the afferent arm of the micturition reflex through capsaicin-sensitive primary afferent neurons. J. Autonom. Nerv. Syst., 43(Suppl.): 90.

Lecci, A., Giuliani, S., Patacchini, R. and Maggi, C.A. (1993c) Evidence against a peripheral role of tachykinins as sensory transmitters in the initiation of micturition reflex in rats. J. Pharmacol. Exp. Ther., 264: 1327–1332.

Lembeck, F. (1953) Zur frage der zentralen Übertragung afferenter impulse. III. Mitteilung. das Vorkommen und die Bedeutung der Substanz P in den dorsalen Wurzeln des Rückenmarks. Arch. Exp. Pathol. Pharmacol., 219: 197–213.

Maeno, H., Kiyama, H. and Tohyama, M. (1993) Distribution of the substance P receptor (NK$_1$ receptor) in the central nervous system. Mol. Brain Res., 18: 43–58.

Maggi, C.A. (1991) The role of peptides in the regulation of the micturition reflex, an update. Gen. Pharmacol., 22: 1–24.

Maggi, C.A. (1992) Prostanoids as local modulators of reflex micturition. Pharmacol. Res., 25: 13–20.

Maggi, C.A. (1993) The dual, sensory and 'efferent' function of the capsaicin-sensitive primary sensory neurons in the urinary bladder and urethra. In: C.A. Maggi (Ed.) The Nervous Control of the Urogenital System: The Autonomic Nervous System, Vol. 3, Harwood, Chur, pp. 383–422.

Maggi, C.A. and Conte, B. (1990) Effect of urethane anesthesia on micturition reflex in capsaicin-treated rats. J. Autonom. Nerv. Syst., 30: 247–252.

Maggi, C.A. and Meli, A. (1986a) The role of neuropeptides in the regulation of the micturition reflex. J. Autonom. Pharmacol., 6: 133–162.

Maggi, C.A. and Meli, A. (1986b) Do 'conscious' and 'reflex' micturition have a separate sensory input? Neurourol. Urodyn., 5: 563–571.

Maggi, C.A. and Meli, A. (1986c) Suitability of urethane anaesthesia for physiopharmacological investigations. Part 3: Other systems and conclusions. Experientia, 42: 531–537.

Maggi, C.A. and Meli, A. (1988) The sensory-efferent function of capsaicin-sensitive nerves. Gen. Pharmacol., 19: 1–43.

Maggi, C.A., Santicioli, P. and Meli, A. (1984) The effects of topical capsaicin on rat urinary bladder motility in vivo. Eur. J. Pharmacol., 103: 41–50.

Maggi, C.A., Santicioli, P., Borsini, F., Giuliani, S. and Meli, A. (1986a) The role of capsaicin-sensitve innervation of the activation of micturition reflex. Naunyn-Schmiedeberg's Arch. Pharmacol., 332: 276–283.

Maggi, C.A., Santicioli, P., Giuliani, S., Regoli, D. and Meli, A. (1986b) Activation of micturition reflex by substance P, substance K: indirect evidence for the existance of multiple tachykinin receptors in the rat urinary bladder. J. Pharmacol. Exp. Ther., 238; 259–266.

Maggi, C.A., Santicioli, P. and Meli, A. (1986c) Somatovesical and vesicovesical excitatory reflexes in urethane-anaesthetized rats. Brain Res., 380: 83–93.

Maggi, C.A., Santicioli, P., Geppetti, P., Furio, M., Frilli, S., Conte, B., Fanciullacci, M., Giuliani, S. and Meli, A. (1987) The contribution of capsaicin-sensitive innervation to activation of the spinal vesico-vesical reflex in rats: relationship between substance P levels in the urinary bladder and the sensory-efferent function of capsaicin-sensitive sensory neurons. Brain Res., 415: 1–13.

Maggi, C.A., Barbanti, G., Santicioli, P., Beneforti, P., Misuri, D., Meli, A. and Turini, D. (1989a) Cystometric evidence that capsaicin-sensitive nerves modulate the afferent branch of micturition reflex in humans. J. Urol., 142: 150–154.

Maggi, C.A., Lippe, I.T., Giuliani, S., Abelli, L., Somma, V., Geppetti, P., Jancso, G., Santicioli, P. and Meli, A. (1989b) Topical versus systemic capsaicin desensitization: specific and unspecific effects as indicated by modification of reflex micturition in rats. Neuroscience, 31: 745–756.

Maggi, C.A., Lecci, A., Santicioli, P., Del Bianco, E. and Giuliani, S. (1992) Cyclophosphamide cystitis in rats: involvement of capsaicin-sensitive primary afferents. J. Autonom. Nerv. Syst., 38: 201–206.

Maggi, C.A., Patacchini, R., Rovero, P. and Giachetti, A. (1993a) Tachykinin receptors and tachykinin receptor antagonists. J. Autonom. Pharmacol., 13: 23–93.

Maggi, C.A., Lecci, A. and Giuliani, S. (1993b) Spinal effects of selective NK$_1$ and NK$_2$ receptor antagonists on bladder motility in anaesthetized rats. Regul. Peptides, 46: 389–391.

Magnan, A.L., Bettelini, L., Hagan, R.M. and Pietra, C. (1993) Effects of intrathecal NK − 1 and NK − 2 antagonists on xylene-induced cystitis in rat. Neuropeptides, 24: 199.

Mallory, B. and De Groat, W.C. (1987) Effect of intrathecal substance P on micturition contractions in the urethane anaesthetized rats. *Soc. Neurosci. Abstr.*, 13: 270.

McCarthy, P.W. and Lawson, S.N. (1989) Cell type and conduction velocity of rat primary sensory neurons with substance P-like immunoreactivity. *Neuroscience*, 28: 745–753.

Mersdorf, A., Schmidt, R.A., Kaula, N. and Tanagho, E.A. (1992) Intrathecal administration of substance P in the rat: the effect on bladder and urethral sphincter activity. *Urology*, 40: 87–96.

Morikawa, K., Ichihashi, M., Kakiuchi, M., Yamauchi, T., Kato, H., Ito, Y., Gomi, Y. (1989) Effects of various drugs on bladder function in conscious rats. *Jpn. J. Pharmacol.*, 50: 369–376.

Moussaui, S.M., Le Prado, N., Bonici, D., Faucher, D.C., Cuiné, F., Laduron, P.M. and Garret, C. (1992) Distribution of neurokinin B in rat spinal cord and peripheral tissues: comparison with neurokinin A and substance P and effects of neonatal capsaicin treatment. *Neuroscience*, 48: 969–978.

Muhlhauser, M.A. and Thor, K. (1992) Vesicoanal reflex activity in the rat: a model of urinary bladder irritation. *Soc. Neurosci. Abstr.*, 18: 500.

Nakanishi, S. (1987) Substance P precursor and kininogen: their structures, gene organizations and regulation. *Physiol. Rev.*, 67: 1117–1142.

Otsuka, M. and Yoshioka, K. (1993) Neurotransmitter functions of mammalian tachykinins. *Physiol. Rev.*, 73: 229–308.

Palea, S., Ziviani, L. and Pietra, C. (1993) Characterization of the inhibitory response to intravesical capsaicin during cystometry in guinea-pig with spinal cord transection. *Neuropeptides*, 24: 199.

Rossler, W., Gerstberger, R., Sann, H. and Pierau, F-K. (1993) Distribution and binding sites of substance P and calcitonin gene-related peptide and their capsaicin-sensitivity in the spinal cord of rats and chicken: a comparative study. *Neuropeptides*, 25: 241–253.

Rupniak, N.M.J., Boyce, S., Williams, A.R., Cook, G., Longmore, J., Seabrook, G.R., Caeser, M., Iversen, S.D. and Hill, R.G. (1993) Antinociceptive activity of NK$_1$ receptor antagonists: non-specific effects of racemic RP 67,580. *Br. J. Pharmacol.*, 110: 1607–1613.

Sakurada, T., Yamada, T., Tan-No, K., Manome, Y., Sakurada, S., Kisara, K. and Ohba, M. (1991) Differential effects of substance P analogs on neurokinin-1 receptor agonists in the mouse spinal cord. *J. Pharmacol. Exp. Ther.*, 259: 205–210.

Santicioli, P., Maggi, C.A. and Meli, A. (1985) The effect of capsaicin pretreatment on the cystometograms of urethane-anaesthetized rats. *J. Urol.*, 133: 700–703.

Saria, A., Gamse, R., Petermann, J., Fischer, A., Theodorsson-Norheim, E. and Lundberg, J.M. (1986) Simultaneous release of several tachykinins and calcitonin gene-related peptide from rat spinal cord slices. *Neurosci. Lett.*, 63: 310–314.

Sato, A., Sato, Y., Shimada, F. and Torigata, Y. (1975) Changes in vesical function produced by cutaneous stimulation in rats. *Brain Res.*, 94: 465–474.

Sato, A., Sato, Y. and Schmidt, P.F. (1979) Effects on reflex bladder activity of chemical stimulation of small diameter afferents from skeletal muscle in the cat. *Neurosci. Lett.*, 11: 13–17.

Schmidt, A.W., McLean, S. and Heym, J. (1992) The substance P receptor antagonist CP 96,345 interacts with Ca^{2+} channels. *Eur. J. Pharmacol.*, 219: 491–492.

Szallasi, A. and Blumberg, P.M. (1990) Specific binding of resiniferatoxin, an ultrapotent capsaicin analog, by dorsal root ganglion membranes. *Brain Res.*, 524: 106–111.

Szolcsany, J., Anton, F., Reeh, P.W. and Handwerker, H.O. (1988) Selective excitation by capsaicin of mechano-heat sensitive nociceptors in rat skin. *Brain Res.*, 446: 262–268.

Tiseo, P.J. and Yaksh, T.L. (1990) The spinal pharmacology of urinary function: studies on urinary continence in the unaesthetized rat. In: Greg Book and Julie Whelan (Eds), *Neurobiology of Incontinence*, Wiley, Chichester (Chiba Foundation Symposium 151), pp. 91–109.

Tomokane, N., Kitamoto, T., Tateishi, J. and Sato, Y. (1991) Immunohistochemical quantification of substance P in spinal dorsal horns of patients with multiple system atrophy. *J. Neurol. Neurosurg. Psychiat.*, 54: 535–541.

Von Euler, U.S. and Gaddum, J.H. (1931) An unidentified depressor substance in certain tissue extracts. *J. Physiol.*, 72: 74–86.

Yashpal, K., Dam, T-V. and Quiron, R. (1990) Quantitative autoradiographic distribution of multiple tachykinin binding sites in rat spinal cord. *Brain Res.*, 506: 259–266.

Yoshiyama, M., Roppolo, J.R. and De Groat, W.C. (1993) Comparison of micturition reflexes in urethane-anesthetized and unanesthetized decerebrate rats. *Soc. Neurosci. Abstr.*, 19: 510.

F. Nyberg, H.S. Sharma and Z. Wiesenfeld-Hallin (Eds.)
Progress in Brain Research, Vol 104
© 1995 Elsevier Science BV. All rights reserved.

CHAPTER 10

Neuropeptides in morphologically and functionally identified primary afferent neurons in dorsal root ganglia: substance P, CGRP and somatostatin

S.N. Lawson

Department of Physiology, School of Medical Sciences, University Walk, Bristol BS8 1TD, UK

Introduction

Peptides can be released from the central and/or peripheral terminals of primary afferent neurons and can have important effects on the functioning of spinal neurons and/or peripheral tissues. For a full understanding of the functional significance of the peptides including the circumstances of their release, information about the types and properties of primary afferent neurons which secrete and release these peptides is essential. Dorsal root ganglion (DRG) neurons can be categorised by their features including morphology, cell size, conduction velocity and sensory receptor type. These categories and the way in which they relate to each other will first be introduced in order to examine the relationship between them and peptide content. Many different neuropeptides are expressed in these neurons, including substance P (SP), neurokinin A, calcitonin gene-related peptide (CGRP), somatostatin (SOM), vasoactive intestinal peptide (VIP), galanin, opioid peptides, and atrial natriuretic peptide. In this chapter, the properties of DRG neurons expressing substance P, CGRP and SOM will be examined.

Cell size and type in dorsal root ganglia

Perhaps the simplest and most easily accessible properties of sensory neurons to examine in relation to peptide content are cell size and cell 'type' defined by morphological criteria. These two properties are closely connected, and their backgrounds will therefore be introduced together. DRG neurons have been divided, on the basis of their morphological appearance into subpopulations, for nearly 100 years. Two main subgroups have stood out in all these studies (e.g., Andres, 1961; Duce and Keen, 1977; Lawson, 1979; Rambourg et al., 1983). With conventional (Nissl) stains the L neurons (also called light, large light or A neurons) are characterised by patchy cytoplasmic staining due to aggregations of ribosomes and rough endoplasmic reticulum (Nissl substance), between which are unstained regions with microtubules and large amounts of neurofilament (e.g., Duce and Keen, 1977). The SD neurons (also called small dark, or B neurons) have a cytoplasm with a more even and a denser distribution of organelles, few neurofilaments and a greater number of Golgi bodies, leading to a more even and intense staining with Nissl stains.

Cell size analysis of the L and SD populations with such stains has shown that, in mouse, rat and cat DRGs (Lawson, 1979; Lawson et al., 1984; Perry and Lawson, 1993), the L and SD neurons each have a normal distribution of cell size, and these two distributions overlap, such that the L neuron distribution extends over the entire size range of the ganglion, while that of the SD neurons is limited to the lower end of the distribution. Immunocytochemical studies have shown that the L neuronal population in rat DRGs have neurofilament-rich somata while the SD neurons have neurofilament-poor somata. The L and SD populations can be distinguished with antibodies against all three NF subunits (Perry et al., 1991), and in rat the distinction is particularly clear with an antibody RT97 against a highly phosphorylated epitope on the 200-kDa protein subunit. Figure 1 shows the size distribution of the neurofilament-rich, L neuronal population in rat lumbar DRGs. The greater amount of neurofilament in the somata of L neurons than SD neurons is a pattern which is well conserved across the species, e.g., in chick, rat, cat and human DRGs (Lawson et al., 1993b; Holford et al., 1994), and this pattern can therefore be used to define morphological cell type in a number of species.

Morphological correlates of conduction velocity

Both size and cell type (L or SD) of the somata in these ganglia are related to fibre conduction velocity. Harper and Lawson (1985) found that cell sizes of somata with C-fibres were in the range of the SD neurons, while those of fast conducting A-fibres, like those of the L cell population, spanned the entire size range of cells in the DRG. Like the SD and L populations, the size distributions of the C- and A-fibre neurons overlapped each other. In rat DRG neurons (see Methods), neurofilament-rich L neuronal somata have A-fibres, while those with C-fibres are gen-

erally neurofilament-poor SD neurons (Lawson and Waddell, 1991) see Table II. In rat, therefore, double labelling to show peptides and neurofilament can provide an indication of whether the peptide-containing neurons have myelinated or unmyelinated fibres.

Subpopulations of DRG neurons defined by their electrophysiological properties

Intracellular voltage recordings in DRG neurons of several species have shown two main types of action potential. These are (a) fast, without inflections on the falling phase, with a TTX sensitive Na^+ inward current, found in a proportion of A-fibre neurons of all conduction velocities, and (b) slower, with inflections on the falling phase, with an inward current carried by both a TTX-insensitive Na^+ current and a Ca^{2+} current, found in C cells (very broad action potentials) and in some A cells (less broad action potentials) (Matsuda et al., 1978; Görke and Pierau, 1980; Koerber et al., 1988; Waddell and Lawson, 1990). In rat DRGs, neurons that have action potentials with inflections comprise all C-fibre cells, 60% Aδ- and 20% Aα/β-fibre cells; also, neurons with long-duration action potentials with inflections tend to have longer duration after-hyperpolarisations (Waddell and Lawson, 1990).

Electrophysiological properties in relation to sensory receptor type

These properties have been shown to be related to the sensory receptor properties of cutaneous A-fibre afferent neurons in cat and rat DRGs (Koerber et al., 1988; Ritter and Mendell, 1992). High-threshold mechanoreceptor neurons have long-duration somatic action potentials with inflections while low-threshold mechanoreceptor neurons have faster action potentials with no inflections. Furthermore, within the Aδ conduction velocity range, D hair units (low-threshold mechanoreceptors) have fast action potentials and very fast after-hyperpolarisations, while high-threshold mechanoreceptor units have longer action potentials and longer after-hyperpolarisations. Thus, studies of these electrophysiological properties of DRG neurons expressing peptides may give some indication of whether the peptide content is related to the sensory receptor type of the neurons.

Studies of peptide release in the dorsal horn

Peptides are released in the dorsal horn (presumably at least partly from primary afferent neurons) in response to particular types of sensory stimulus. SP release was evoked by noxious but not non-noxious mechanical stimuli (Kuraishi et al., 1985; Duggan et al., 1988). Results were more variable with other types of stimulus such as noxious heat (possibly due to species differences or to the type, intensity and location of the stimulus used (Kuraishi et al., 1985; Duggan et al., 1988; Tiseo et al., 1990). In rat, noxious cold but not noxious heat stimuli caused SP release (Tiseo et al., 1990), while in cat, noxious mechanical, noxious chemical and strong noxious thermal stimuli evoked SP release (Duggan et al., 1988). SOM was released in rabbit and rat during noxious heat but not noxious mechanical stimulation (Kuraishi et al., 1985; Tiseo et al., 1990). These results seem to indicate that cutaneous noxious mechanical stimuli and strong noxious thermal stimuli evoke SP release and noxious thermal stimuli evoke SOM release, and they provide circumstantial evidence in favour of peptide synthesis being related to sensory receptor type in these neurons. However, this approach, while extremely valuable, gives no information about (a) whether molecules are released from primary afferents or postsynaptic elements of the CNS and, if they are, (b) whether all neurons of a particular sensory receptor type contain or can release these pep-

tides. Direct studies of primary afferent neurons are required to answer these questions.

Sensory receptor types of peptide-containing neurons

Peptides that are important in central signalling of particular types of sensory information might be expected to be preferentially expressed in the primary afferent neurons responsible for signalling that type of information. The most direct way of testing this hypothesis is, in concept, very simple. Intracellular recordings from the neuronal somata of neurons with identified sensory receptor type are followed by dye injection allowing subsequent immunocytochemistry of the identified neuron. Despite the importance and directness of such an approach, there have been few full papers (Leah et al., 1985; Hoheisel et al., 1994) or abstracts (Zhang and Hoffert, 1986; Lawson et al., 1993a, 1994) directly concerning this question. This is probably due to technical difficulties and the very time consuming nature of such studies. The papers by Leah et al. (SP, SOM, VIP) and Hoheisel et al. (CGRP) have provided little or no evidence for any correlation of peptide content and sensory function of the neuron. However, this may to some extent result from the technical problems associated with such studies (see Methods and Discussion).

Peripheral effector functions of peptide-containing neurons

Both substance P and CGRP are released at peripheral terminals of sensory neurons and cause a number of effects in the periphery, including the neurogenic inflammatory response for which both peptides are mediators, affecting small blood vessels in skin and other tissues. Both peptides cause increased blood flow while only substance P causes increased permeability leading to plasma extravasation from these small vessels (e.g., Brain and Williams, 1989). A recent study of single

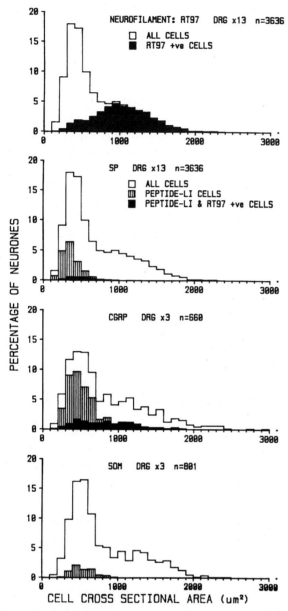

C-fibre recording and stimulation confirmed earlier findings that neurogenic plasma extravasation resulted from stimulation of 70% of polymodal C-fibres in the rat (Bharali and Lisney, 1992).

In this paper, the evidence for any correlation of peptide content with morphological, electrophysiological or functional properties of DRG neurons is re-examined for normal neurons, by comparing the properties of peptide-containing neurons with the patterns of neuronal properties already known to exist in these ganglia.

Methods

Cell counting and measuring, and its problems

Cell measurements (e.g., Fig. 1) are made by drawing the outline of all neurons with a clear nuclear profile in a series of sections taken at regular intervals (400 μm) throughout the DRG. This method eliminates sampling bias resulting from any non-homogeneous distribution of neuronal types throughout the ganglion, but retains any bias due to the greater probability of multiple nuclear sections through large than small neuronal nuclei. Where percentages are referred to from the literature, the majority contain the same bias. Where percentages of neurons from electrophysiological recordings are made, the above bias is not a problem, but is replaced by a bias due to the greater ease of penetrating larger neurons, and the difficulty of making stable penetrations in C cells in these ganglia.

Electrophysiological recording methods

Most of the electrophysiological studies described were in rat DRG neurons in vitro. For more

Fig. 1. Size distribution histograms of cross-sectional areas of lumbar DRG neurons in 10–12-week-old rats. X13 means 13 DRGs included; n, number of cells measured. L5 ganglia were used throughout, except for the CGRP plot which includes two L4 DRGs and one L5 DRG. Open histograms, all cells measured; solid histograms, RT97-positive (neurofilament-rich) neurons in the whole population (top histogram) and in the population of neurons with peptide-LI (lower histograms). Top histogram, neurofilament-rich (L) neurons (solid bars) and neurofilament-poor (SD) neurons (open histogram). Lower histograms: co-localisation of peptide and neurofilament-rich somata by dual label indirect immunofluorescence. The hatched areas show neurofilament-poor neurons with peptide-LI; the neurofilament-rich neurons with peptide-LI are shown in black; and the open regions show neurons without peptide-LI. Neurones with peptide-LI which are neurofilament-rich are likely to have A-fibres (see text). Note that these are evident for neurons with SP-LI and CGRP-LI but not for SOM-LI. (From Lawson et al., 1993b.)

details see McCarthy and Lawson (1989) and Mc-Carthy and Lawson (1990). The methods in brief are as follows. L4–L6 DRGs were dissected from anaesthetised rats (sodium pentobarbitone 50 mg/kg) with their attached peripheral nerves and dorsal roots. The tissue was superfused with oxygenated balanced salt solution and intracellular voltage recordings were made with electrodes filled with 3 M KCl (for recording only) or with Lucifer Yellow in 0.1 M LiCl, or ethidium bromide in 1 M KCl (for dye injection; for methods see McCarthy and Lawson (1988). The peripheral nerve or dorsal root was stimulated electrically and the conduction velocity measured from the latency to the rise of the intracellularly evoked action potential. Conduction velocities in these young rats (6–8-week-old females) were divided on the basis of the frequency distributions of their velocities into C (< 1.3 m/s), Aδ (2–12 m/s), or Aα/β (> 12 m/s) groups. The waveform of the action potential and after-potential evoked by nerve stimulation was recorded, and dye was electrophoretically injected with low currents (< 2 nA.min) into the soma. Only neurons with membrane potentials of > 40 mV and overshooting action potentials were used for waveform analysis. Recordings were made within about 8 h of dissecting out the DRGs. Immunocytochemistry was later carried out on sections of the dye-filled neurons with indirect immunoperoxidase (Lawson and Waddell, 1991), indirect immunofluorescence (McCarthy and Lawson, 1989, 1990), or ABC (avidin biotin complex) techniques (Lawson et al., 1994).

Problems include possible effects of intracellular dye on peptide immunocytochemistry as well as, in the in vitro preparation, possible effects of nerve section on peptide content. Controls for such changes include examination of size distributions and percentages of positive neurons in similar ganglia comparing normal ganglia with (a) DRGs with all cells retrogradely labelled by the intracellular dye, and (b) DRGs after the experimental surgery. Such controls need to be carried out for each peptide and for each set of experimental conditions used. Controls of this type

TABLE I

Neurofilament content (%) of rat DRG neuronal somata with peptide-LI

	NF-poor	NF-rich	All
SP-LI	27	6.1	18
CGRP-LI	66	28	46
SOM-LI	13	0	7.3

This table shows the percentages of neurofilament (NF)-poor neurons, neurofilament-rich neurons and all neurons in lumbar DRGs which have peptide-like immunoreactivity (LI). Data are derived from those plotted in Fig. 1. (From Lawson et al., 1993b.)

showed that, in our in vitro rat DRG preparation, despite occasional reduction in staining intensity, the proportions and size distributions of neurons labelled by RT97, SP, CGRP and SOM (McCarthy and Lawson, 1989, 1990; Lawson and Waddell, 1991) were not altered by either the experimental procedures or the intracellular dye. The only aspect which we cannot test directly is the effect of passing current into the cell. Scharfman et al. (1989) found that intracellular dye injections (mid range 30–50 nA.min) into CA1

TABLE II

Neurofilament and neuropeptide content (%) of rat DRG neuronal somata with C-, Aδ- or Aα/β-fibres

CV range	C	Aδ	Aα/β	n
NF-rich	9	98	100	108
SP-LI	44	20	0	81
CGRP-LI	50	33	22	107

This table shows the percentages of neurons with neurofilament (NF)-rich somata, or with peptide-LI in the different CV groups. The data are from in vitro intracellular recordings in rat DRG (L4–L6) neurons followed by dye injection and immunocytochemistry. n = the total numbers of cells examined. (Data are from McCarthy and Lawson (1989), McCarthy and Lawson (1990), Lawson and Waddell (1991), and McCarthy and Lawson, unpublished.)

neurons in the hippocampus led to false-negative immunocytochemical results for peptides. It therefore seems that high intracellular injection currents may abolish peptide immunoreactivity. However, (a) we use low current (0.5–2 nA.min) and (b) comparison of sizes and percentages of neurons labelled and unlabelled by the markers after intracellular dye injections are similar to those in normal ganglia (compare Tables I and II). The latter is important to establish, since low percentages of labelled neurons (e.g., in Hoheisel et al., 1994) in the experimental population will result in false negatives, especially in cells which normally have lower intensity labelling such as the larger A-cells with CGRP-like immunoreactivity (LI).

Antibodies

RT97 is a mouse monoclonal antibody against a highly phosphorylated epitope on the 200-kDa neurofilament subunit (Wood and Anderton, 1981), donated by J. Wood. The anti-peptide antibodies were all rabbit polyclonal antibodies. Those for substance P had a low affinity for NKA: for the rat studies the antibody was from P. Keen (Harmar and Keen, 1986) and for the guinea pig studies it was from Incstar. The anti-CGRP antibody was from J. Polak (Gibson et al., 1984). The anti-somatostatin antibodies were from P. Keen (Harmar and Keen, 1986) and from J. Winter.

Results and discussion

The tachykinins

Perhaps the most widely studied peptide in DRG neurons is substance P, one of the tachykinins. Neurokinin A, another tachykinin, is also found in these neurons but has been less well studied. The preprotachykinin A gene in sensory neurons gives rise to three types of mRNA and hence three different tachykinin precursors (Boehmer et

al., 1989; MacDonald et al., 1989; Helke et al., 1990). Since SP is contained in all three but neurokinin A in only two, it seems unlikely that SP could be expressed without NKA expression in the same cell. Immunocytochemical studies found that all neurons with neurokinin A-LI also showed SP-LI, while not all SP-LI neurons displayed neurokinin A-LI (Dalsgaard et al., 1985). Therefore, although anti-substance P antibodies may differ in their cross-reactivity with neurokinin A, any such cross-reactivity should not cause an overestimate of neurons with SP-LI. In many papers, especially the earlier ones, the extent of this cross reactivity was not known and/or is not stated for the particular antibodies used.

Substance P (SP)

Substance P-LI is found in 18–20% of rat lumbar DRG neurons when no colchicine treatment is used (e.g., McCarthy and Lawson, 1989; for review, see Lawson, 1992), although a higher percentage has been reported after colchicine treatment (for review, see Lawson, 1992), which may reflect the finding that 28% of neurons express the mRNA in these ganglia (Boehmer et al., 1989). Similar percentages of SP-LI neurons have been described in mouse, guinea pig and cat DRGs (for review, see Lawson, 1992). It is consistently found in small DRG neurons with few medium sized positive neurons (see Fig. 1).

Co-localisation of SP-LI with other peptides

SP coexists with a number of other peptides (for review, see Lawson, 1992). Virtually all neurons with SP-LI in rat also express CGRP-LI (Wiesenfeld-Hallin et al., 1984; Ju et al., 1987), while in cat and guinea pig about 80% express CGRP-LI (Gibbins et al., 1987; Garry et al., 1989). The extent of co-localisation of SP-LI with SOM-LI and VIP-LI is species dependent. There is virtually no coexistence of SP-LI with these peptides in rat and guinea pig in contrast with substantial coexistence in cat (30–40% of SP-LI neurons in cat normally express these two peptides, see review by Lawson, 1992). In guinea pig, 50% of SP-LI neurons show dynorphin-LI (Gibbins et al., 1987).

Soma neurofilament content and conduction velocity of SP-LI neurons

In rat lumbar DRGs about 30% of the neurofilament-poor and 6% of the neurofilament-rich somata showed detectable SP-LI (Lawson et al., 1993b) (see Fig. 1 and Table I). Twenty to thirty percent of SP-LI neurons in these rat DRG neurons are L neurons with neurofilament-rich somata (McCarthy and Lawson, 1989). These data predict that most SP-LI neurons should have C-fibres, and a small proportion should have A-fibres (Lawson and Waddell, 1991). The small cell sizes of even the neurofilament-rich neurons with SP-LI made it likely that only $A\delta$ and no faster conducting A-fibre neurons should display SP-LI. Intracellular electrophysiological recordings from rat lumbar DRG neurons in vitro confirmed these predictions (see Table II), since in these ganglia about 45% of C-fibre cells, 20% of $A\delta$-cells and no fast-conducting A-fibre cells showed SP-LI.

Electrophysiological properties of SP-LI neurons

Analysis of the active membrane properties of rat DRG neurons in vitro showed differences between neurons with and without SP-LI that conduct within the $A\delta$-fibre range. The main difference was a significantly longer mean after-hyperpolarisation duration to 80% recovery in neurons with SP-LI than in those without (McCarthy and Lawson, in preparation). Since D hair neuronal somata have very short after-hyperpolarisation durations both in cat and rat DRG neurons (Koerber et al., 1988; Ritter and Mendell, 1992), while high-threshold mechanoreceptor neurons have much longer duration after-hyperpolarisations, these data are indicative of detectable SP-LI in some $A\delta$ high-threshold mechanoreceptor neurons and of its probable absence from most D hair neuronal somata in rat DRGs.

Sensory receptor types of neurons with SP-LI

C-fibre neurons. A current study (Lawson and Perl) is underway on the relationship of detectable SP-LI in guinea pig DRG neurons to a more detailed characterisation of sensory receptor type than previously reported (see Lawson et al., 1993a; Lawson et al., 1994). Of 48 identified C-fibre neurons, 19 showed SP-LI, a similar proportion to that of rat C-fibre neurons in lumbar DRGs (Table II). Those with detectable SP-LI included some of the C high-threshold mechanoreceptor units in skin and subcutaneous tissue, and some of the C mechano-heat units in skin or subcutaneous tissue. It was not detectable in cold nociceptor units. These findings are compatible with the data on SP release due to noxious mechanical and noxious cold stimuli (see Introduction), and with the more variable data (see Introduction) on SP-LI release with noxious heat stimuli. At first sight, these results are at variance with the findings of Leah et al. (1985), who concluded that "there is no apparent correlation between the peptide content of a sensory cell and its modality". They examined SP-LI in colchicine-treated DRGs of cat. Of 16 C-fibre cells with identified receptor types, five were positive. Three of these responded to innocuous cutaneous mechanical stimuli/cooling while two out of five responded to either noxious mechanical or to noxious mechanical and noxious heat stimuli. Broader categories of receptor type were used than in our study. For instance, no distinction was made between hairy or glabrous skin, or between cutaneous and subcutaneous units. The lack of a clear pattern in the Leah et al. study may have resulted from the broad receptor categories used and the relatively small number of units. However, other differences between the study of Leah et al. and our experiments include their use of cat DRGs, their use of colchicine treatment of the ganglia, and their much higher dye ejection currents.

A-fibre neurons. We also studied A-fibre units (Lawson et al. 1994), and found that of 42 neurons with identified receptor types tested, seven showed SP-LI. The positive neurons included some of the slowly conducting A-fibre nociceptive neurons but no low-threshold mechanoreceptor units of either the D hair type or those with faster conducting fibres. This latter result is consistent with that of Zhang and Hoffert (1986), who examined SP-LI in cat DRGs in a small number (8) of identified neurons with A-fibres. They found SP-LI in two out of three myelinated mechanical nociceptors and in none of five myelinated low-threshold mechanoreceptor units. Leah et al. studied only four A-fibre units in the cat, two nociceptive and two non-nociceptive units. All of these, unlike the results of Zhang and Hoffert, were negative. However, this is not surprising with such small numbers, given that the majority of A-fibre neurons in rat (McCarthy and Lawson, 1989) and guinea pig (see above) are SP-LI negative. Thus, our data and those of Zhang and Hoffert show that SP-LI is expressed in certain myelinated nociceptor units and not in myelinated low-threshold units. This is supported by the prolonged after-hyperpolarisation of A δ-fibre neurons with SP-LI in rat DRGs (see above), indicating a greater likelihood of SP-LI in A δ-fibre high-threshold mechanoreceptor units than in low-threshold D hair units.

SP-LI in primary afferent neuronal somata can therefore be correlated with cell size, morphological cell type, conduction velocity of the axon and also with the sensory receptor type. The sensory receptor types of the SP-LI-positive neurons include mainly or exclusively nociceptors but some nociceptive units are negative. The absence of immunocytochemically detectable SP-LI in the somata does not, however, preclude the possible presence of low, immunocytochemically undetectable, levels of SP and furthermore it is not yet clear whether all neurons with SP-LI in their cell bodies transport it in significant amounts to their central terminals. It is known that much more SP is transported peripherally than centrally from rat DRG neurons, indicating a major role for this peptide in the periphery (Harmar and Keen, 1982).

Calcitonin gene-related peptide (CGRP)

CGRP-LI is found in 30–60% of DRG neurons in rat and chick DRGs, but in only 10–20% in guinea pig DRGs (for review, see Lawson, 1992). In rat, the DRG neurons with CGRP-LI are mainly small intensely labelled neurons, as well as some medium and large neurons with less intense coarse granular immunoreactivity. The predominant form of CGRP is αCGRP found in small, medium and large DRG neurons, while the β form is found only in small and medium sized neurons in rat lumbar DRGs (Mulderry et al., 1988; Noguchi et al., 1990).

Co-localisation of CGRP-LI with other peptides

SP-LI is found in about 50% of rat DRG neurons with CGRP-LI, but in a higher proportion of guinea pig DRG neurons with SP-LI due to the lower overall percentage of neurons with CGRP-LI in the guinea pig. The percentage of all DRG neurons with both peptides may therefore be similar in the two species.

Soma neurofilament content and conduction velocity of neurons with CGRP-LI

CGRP-LI was found in 66% of the neurofilament-poor (SD) neuronal somata and in nearly 30% of the neurofilament-rich (L) somata (see Table I) in rat lumbar DRG neurons. This, together with the cell size distribution of the neurofilament-rich neurons (Fig. 1), is a clear indication that about a third of rat lumbar DRG neurons with A-fibres should have myelinated fibres, and the large size of some of these is an indication that some may conduct in the faster $A\alpha/\beta$ range. That this is the case can be seen in Table II, since 50% of somata with C-fibres, 33% of somata with $A\delta$-fibres and 22% of the somata with fast-conducting A-fibres showed CGRP-LI.

Electrophysiological properties of neurons with CGRP-LI

The active membrane properties of rat DRG neurons with CGRP-LI were also studied (Lawson and Mccarthy, submitted). There were significant differences between properties of DRG neurons with and without CGRP-LI within the A-fibre group, and particularly within the $A\delta$ population. The $A\delta$ cells with CGRP-LI had longer after-potential durations than those without, and within the whole group of A-fibre neurons studied, both the action potential and after potential durations were significantly longer in neurons with CGRP-LI than in those without (McCarthy and Lawson, unpublished).

Sensory receptor types of neurons with CGRP-LI

Since CGRP-LI is found in almost all DRG neurons in the rat with SP-LI, sensory receptor type characteristics of CGRP-LI neurons should include those of SP-LI neurons in both species. However, in the rat, since CGRP is in more than twice as many neurons as SP-LI, a wider range of receptor types is to be expected in positive neurons. Such a high proportion of neurons with CGRP-LI in rat may mean that a correlation with receptor type will be hard to find. For instance, in splanchnic visceral afferent neurons, virtually all neurons showed CGRP-LI, while 70% of muscle afferent neurons express detectable SP-LI (for

review, see Lawson, 1992). Despite this, comparison of the above electrophysiological properties of CGRP-LI-containing rat DRG neurons with the known electrophysiological properties of neurons with identified cutaneous sensory receptor types (see Introduction and Ritter and Mendell, 1992), does appear to predict some correlation in A-fibre neurons. It seems that, within the $A\delta$-fibre group, it may be more likely for CGRP-LI to be detectable in high-threshold mechanoreceptor units than in D hair (low-threshold mechanoreceptor) neurons, and also that there may be a greater likelihood of finding CGRP-LI in high- than in low-mechanical threshold units in A-fibre neurons as a whole. Hoheisel et al. (1994) have examined CGRP-LI in rat DRG neurons with identified sensory receptor types, and found it in only 8/44 dye-injected neurons; in five out of six C-fibre cells and in 3/36 A-fibre cells. This was a rather unexpectedly low percentage of positive A-fibre cells (for possible causes see Methods). Both high- and low-threshold mechanoreceptor units in both the A- and C-fibre categories were labelled, providing negative evidence for a strict correlation between receptor type and CGRP-LI in these neurons. However, in view of the patterns seen in the electrophysiological data above, more data is needed, particularly on A-fibre cells.

Somatostatin (SOM)

In rat DRGs, somatostatin is found exclusively in small neurons, with no positive medium or large neurons. Five to 15% of neurons in rat DRGs show SOM-LI, with the highest percentage being in the lumbar region (for review, see Lawson, 1992). SOM-LI has also been described in other species including guinea pig (Gibbins et al., 1987) and cat.

Co-localisation of SOM-LI with other peptides

The extent of co-localisation of SOM and other peptides is dependent upon the species (for review, see Lawson, 1992). In DRG neurons of rat and guinea pig, there is little or no colocalisation of SOM-LI and SP-LI. In contrast, in cat lumbosacral DRGs (Garry et al., 1989), up to 80% of neurons with SOM-LI also showed SP-LI. In rat, all SOM-LI cells also show CGRP-LI, while in cat only about 20% show CGRP-LI.

Conduction velocity and neurofilament content of neurons with SOM-LI

Co-localisation studies with RT97 have shown that no SOM-LI cells in rat lumbar DRGs have neurofilament like-immunoreactivity (Lawson et al., 1993b). From this and from the neuronal sizes, it therefore seems likely that all SOM-LI DRG neurons in the rat have C-fibres. A limited study of SOM-LI, in 38 rat DRG neurons with identified conduction velocity, yielded only eight C-fibre cells one of which was SOM-LI positive. None of the 30 A-fibre cells was positive. There is, therefore, no evidence yet for SOM-LI in cells other than SD neurons with C-fibres.

Electrophysiology and sensory receptor type of neurons with SOM-LI

No studies have yet been carried out with regard to SOM-LI in neurons with known sensory receptor type and, since we have only one positive neuron with electrophysiological data, it is premature to make predictions from these studies. However, it is released, possibly from primary afferent neurons, in rabbit and rat spinal dorsal horn during heat- but not mechano-nociception (Kuraishi et al., 1985; Tiseo et al., 1990).

Conclusions

These studies provide evidence for a relationship in normal DRG neurons between soma peptide content and the following: DRG cell morphology, cell size, conduction velocity, electrophysiological properties of the soma (CGRP and substance P),

and even sensory receptor types (substance P and possibly CGRP) in normal cells. Further data is needed to establish the relationship between somatostatin content of the soma and receptor type and it would also be useful to establish this relationship for a number of other peptides expressed by these neurons. These studies, in combination with studies on receptor subtypes in the spinal cord and with studies on release in spinal cord, should help establish the function of these peptides in transmission/modulation of the afferent signal from primary afferent neurons.

There are several types of situation in which neuropeptide expression is altered. The peptides discussed in the present paper, namely substance P, CGRP and somatostatin, are all down-regulated after peripheral nerve axotomy (Hökfelt et al., 1994). Normally NGF (nerve growth factor) is taken up by nerve fibres from the periphery, and transported to the somata where it up-regulates both SP and CGRP expression. Therefore nerve section, by preventing NGF transport to the soma, can cause down regulation of these peptides. (In contrast the peptides VIP and galanin are up-regulated after peripheral axotomy (Hökfelt et al., 1994.) NGF is apparently necessary for normal development of A-fibre high-threshold mechanoreceptor units in young rats; its absence leading to more D hair units at their expense and increased NGF leading to a decreased mechanical threshold in these high-threshold mechanoreceptor neurons (Lewin and Mendell, 1993). It is therefore possible that correlations between expression of these peptides and cell properties, such as receptor type, are retained even with these manipulations of NGF levels. During adjuvant-induced arthritis in the rat both SP and CGRP are up-regulated, possibly due to up-regulation of NGF in the tissues (see review by Lewin and Mendell, 1993). However, despite an increase in the amount of preprotachykinin A and αCGRP mRNAs, the percentage of DRG neurons expressing these mRNAs was not increased

(Donaldson et al., 1992), i.e., presumably the same neurons were producing more peptide, rather than de novo synthesis in cells previously not expressing the peptides. It is therefore possible that the relationship between the presence of SP and CGRP, and at least some of the neuronal properties, remain essentially the same in this arthritic model. Further studies are required, however, to establish the extent to which these relationships are maintained or altered in such pathological situations.

Acknowledgements

This work was supported by Grants from the Medical Research Council, UK. Thanks go Barbara Carruthers for technical assistance and to E.R. Perl and P.W. McCarthy for useful comments on the manuscript.

References

Andres, K.H. (1961) Untersuchungen der Feinbau von Spinal Ganglien. *Z. Zellforsch. Mikrosk. Anat.*, 55: 1–48.

Bharali, L.A.M. and Lisney, S.J.W. (1992) The relationship between unmyelinated afferent type and neurogenic plasma extravasation in normal and reinnervated rat skin. *Neuroscience*, 47: 703–712.

Boehmer, C.G., Norman, J., Catton, M., Fine, L.G. and Mantyh, P.W. (1989) High levels of mRNA coding for substance P, somatostatin and alpha-tubulin are expressed by rat and rabbit dorsal root ganglia neurons. *Peptides*, 10: 1179–1194.

Brain, S.D. and Williams, T.J. (1989) Interactions between the tachykinins and calcitonin gene-related peptide lead to the modulation of oedema formation and blood flow in rat skin. *Br. J. Pharmacol.*, 97: 77–82.

Dalsgaard, C.-J., Haegerstrand, A., Theodorrson-Norheim, E., Brodin, E. and Hökfelt, T. (1985) Neurokinin A-like immunoreactivity in rat primary sensory neurons: coexistance with substance P. *Histochemistry*, 83: 37–39.

Donaldson, L.F., Harmar, A.J., McQueen, D.S. and Seckl, J.R. (1992) Increased expression of preprotachykinin, calcitonin gene-related peptide, but not vasoactive intestinal peptide messenger RNA in dorsal root ganglia during the development of adjuvant monoarthritis in the rat. *Mol. Brain Res.*, 16: 143–149.

Duce, I. and Keen, P. (1977) An ultrastructural classification of the neuronal cell bodies of the rat dorsal root ganglion using zinc iodide-osmium impregnation. *Cell Tissue Res.*, 185: 263–277.

Duggan, A.W., Hendry, I.A., Morton, C.R., Hutchison, W.D. and Zhao, Z.O. (1988) Cutaneous stimuli releasing immunoreactive Substance P in the dorsal horn of the cat. *Brain Res.*, 451: 261–273.

Garry, M.G., Miller, K.E. and Seybold, V.S. (1989) Lumbar dorsal root ganglia of the cat: A quantitative study of peptide immunoreactivity and cell size. *J. Comp. Neurol.*, 284: 36–47.

Gibbins, L.L., Furness, J.B. and Costa, M. (1987) Pathway-specific patterns of the co-existence of substance P, calcitonin gene-related peptide, cholecystokinin and dynorphin in neurons of the dorsal root ganglion of the guinea-pig. *Cell Tissue Res.*, 248: 417–437.

Gibson, S.J., Polak, J.M., Bloom, S.R., Sabate, I.M., Mulderry, P.M., Ghatei, M.A., McGregor, G.P., Morrison, J.F.B., Kelly, J.S., Evans, R.M. and Rosenfeld, M.G. (1984) Calcitonin gene-related peptide immunoreactivity in the spinal cord of man and eight other species. *J. Neurosci.*, 4: 3101–3111.

Görke, K. and Pierau, F-K. (1980) Spike potentials and membrane properties of dorsal root ganglion cells in pigeons. *Pflügers Arch. Eur. J. Physiol.*, 386: 21–28.

Harmar, A. and Keen, P. (1982) Synthesis and central and peripheral axonal transport of substance P in a dorsal root ganglion-nerve preparation in vitro. *Brain Res.* 231: 379–385.

Harmar, A. and Keen, P. (1986) Methods for the identification of neuropeptide processing products: somatostatin and the kinins. *Methods Enzymol.*, 124: 335–348.

Harper, A.A. and Lawson, S.N. (1985) Conduction velocity is related to morphological cell type in rat dorsal root ganglia. *J. Physiol. (London)*, 359: 31–46.

Helke, C.J., Krause, J.E., Mantyh, P.W., Couture, R. and Bannon, M.J. (1990) Diversity in mammalian tachykinin peptidergic neurons: Multiple peptides, receptors, and regulatory mechanisms. *FASEB J.*, 4: 1606–1615.

Hoheisel, U., Mense, S. and Scherotzke, R. (1994) Calcitonin gene-related peptide immunoreactivity in functionally identified primary afferent neurons in the rat. *Anat. Embryol.*, 189: 41–49.

Holford, L., Case, P. and Lawson, S.N. (1994) Substance P, neurofilament, peripherin and SSEA4 immunocytochemistry of human dorsal root ganglion neurons obtained from post-mortem tissue: a quantitative analysis. *J. Neurocytol.*, 23: 577–589.

Hökfelt, T., Zhang, X. and Wiesenfeld-Hallin, Z. (1994) Messenger plasticity in primary sensory neurons following axotomy and its functional implications. *Trends Neurosci.*, 17: 22–30.

Ju, G., Hökfelt, T., Brodin, E., Fahrenkrug, J., Fischer, J.A., Frey, P., Elde, R.P. and Brown, J.C. (1987) Primary sensory neurons of the rat showing calcitonin gene-related peptide immunoreactivity and their relation to substance P-, and somatostatin-, galanin-, vasoactive intestinal polypeptide-, and cholecystokinin-immunoreactive ganglion cells. *Cell Tissue Res.*, 247: 417–431.

Koerber, H.R., Druzinsky, R.E. and Mendell, L.M. (1988) Properties of somata of spinal dorsal root ganglion cells differ according to peripheral receptor innervated. *J. Neurophysiol.*, 60: 1584–1596.

Kuraishi, Y., Hiroto, N., Sato, Y., Hino, Y., Satoh, M. and Takagi, H. (1985) Evidence that substance P and somatostatin transmit separate information related to pain in the spinal dorsal horn. *Brain Res.*, 325: 294–298.

Lawson, S.N. (1979) The postnatal development of large light and small dark neurons in mouse dorsal root ganglia: a statistical analysis of cell numbers and size. *J. Neurocytol.*, 8: 275–294.

Lawson, S.N. (1992) Morphological and biochemical cell types of sensory neurons. In: S.A. Scott (Ed.) *Sensory Neurones: Diversity, Development and Plasticity.* Oxford University Press, New York, pp. 27–59.

Lawson, S.N. and Waddell, P.J. (1991) Soma neurofilament immunoreactivity is related to cell size and fibre conduction velocity in rat primary sensory neurons. *J. Physiol. (London)*, 435: 41–63.

Lawson, S.N., Harper, A.A., Harper, E.I., Garson, J.A. and Anderton, B.H. (1984) A monoclonal antibody against neurofilament protein specifically labels a subpopulation of rat sensory neurons. *J. Comp. Neurol.*, 228: 263–272.

Lawson, S.N., Crepps, B., Bao, J., Brighton, B.W. and Perl, E.R. (1993a) Differential correlation of substance P-like immunoreactivity (SP-LI) with the type of C-fiber sensory receptor. *Soc. Neurosci. Abstr.*, 19: 136.6.

Lawson, S.N., Perry, M.J., Prabhakar, E. and McCarthy, P.W. (1993b) Primary sensory neurons: neurofilament, neuropeptides, and conduction velocity. *Brain Res. Bull.*, 30: 239–243.

Lawson, S.N., Crepps, B.A., Bao, J., Brighton, B.W. and Perl, E.R. (1994) Substance P-like immunoreactivity (SP-LI) in guinea pig dorsal root ganglia (DRGs) is related to sensory receptor type in A and C fibre neurons. *J. Physiol. (London)*, Abstr., 476P : 39P.

Leah, J.D., Cameron, A.A. and Snow, P.J. (1985) Neuropeptides in physiologically identified mammalian sensory neurons. *Neurosci. Lett.*, 56: 257–263.

Lewin, G.R. and Mendell, L.M. (1993) Nerve growth factor and nociception. *TINS*, 16: 353–359.

MacDonald, M.R., Takeda, J., Rice, C.M. and Krause, J.E. (1989) Multiple tachykinins are produced and secreted upon post-translational processing of the three substance P precursor proteins, alpha-, beta-, and gamma-prepro-

tachykinin. Expression of the preprotachykinins in AtT-20 cells infected with vaccinia virus recombinants. *J. Biol. Chem.*, 264: 15578–15592.

Matsuda, Y., Yoshida, S. and Yonezawa, T. (1978) Tetrodotoxin sensitivity and Ca component of action potentials of mouse dorsal root ganglion cells cultured in vitro. *Brain Res.*, 154: 69–82.

McCarthy, P.W. and Lawson, S.N. (1988) Differential intracellular labelling of identified neurones with two fluorescent dyes. *Brain Res. Bull.*, 20: 261–265.

McCarthy, P.W. and Lawson, S.N. (1989) Cell type and conduction velocity of rat primary sensory neurons with Substance P-like immunoreactivity. *Neuroscience*, 28: 745–753.

McCarthy, P.W. and Lawson, S.N. (1990) Cell type and conduction velocity of rat primary sensory neurons with calcitonin gene-related peptide-like immunoreactivity. *Neuroscience*, 34: 623–632.

Mulderry, P.K., Ghatei, M.A., Spokes, R.A., Jones, P.M., Pierson, A.M., Hamid, Q.A., Kanse, S., Amara, S.G., Burrin, J.M., Legon, S., Polak, J.M. and Bloom, S.R. (1988) Differential expression of alpha-CGRP and beta-CGRP by primary sensory neurons and enteric autonomic neurons of the rat. *Neuroscience*, 25: 195–205.

Noguchi, K., Senba, E., Morita, Y., Sato, M. and Tohyama, M. (1990) Co-expression of α-CGRP and β-CGRP mRNAs in the rat dorsal root ganglion cells. *Neurosci. Lett.*, 108: 1–5.

Perl, E.R. (1991) Specificity in characteristics of fine primary afferent fibers. In: O. Franzén and J.Westman (Eds.) *Information Processing in the Somatosensory System*, Macmillan Academic and Professional Ltd., Basingstoke, London, pp. 383–398.

Perry, M.J. and Lawson, S.N. (1993) Neurofilament in feline primary afferent neurons: a quantitative immunocytochemical study. *Brain Res.*, 607: 307–313.

Perry, M.J., Lawson, S.N. and Robertson, J. (1991) Neurofilament immunoreactivity in populations of rat primary afferent neurons: a quantitative study of phosphorylated and non-phosphorylated subunits. *J. Neurocytol.*, 20: 746–758.

Rambourg, A., Clermont, Y. and Beaudet, A. (1983) Ultrastructural features of six types of neurons in rat dorsal root ganglia. *J. Neurocytol.*, 12: 47–66.

Ritter, A.M. and Mendell, L.M. (1992) Somal membrane properties of physiologically identified sensory neurons in the rat: Effects of nerve growth factor. *J. Neurophysiol.*, 68: 2033–2041.

Scharfman, H.E., Kunkel, D.D. and Schwartzkroin, P.A. (1989) Intracellular dyes mask immunoreactivity of hippocampal interneurons. *Neurosci. Lett.*, 96: 23–28.

Tiseo, P.J., Adler, M.W. and Liu-chen, L.-Y. (1990) Differential release of substance P and somatostatin in the rat spinal cord in response to noxious cold and heat; effect of dynorphin A (1–17). *J. Pharmacol. Exp. Ther.*, 252: 539–545.

Waddell, P.J. and Lawson, S.N. (1990) Electrophysiological properties of subpopulations of rat dorsal root ganglion neurones in vitro. *Neuroscience*, 36: 811–822.

Wiesenfeld-Hallin, Z., Hökfelt, T., Lundberg, J.M., Forssmann, W.G., Reinecke, M., Tschopp, F.A. and Fischer, J.A. (1984) Immunoreactive calcitonin gene-related peptide and substance P coexist in sensory neurons to the spinal cord and interact in spinal behavioural responses of the rat. *Neurosci. Lett.*, 52: 199–204.

Wood, J.W. and Anderton, B.H. (1981) Monoclonal antibodies to mammalian neurofilaments. *Biosci. Rep.*, 1: 263–268.

Zhang, S. and Hoffert, M. (1986) Substance P is contained in myelinated mechanical nociceptors. *Soc. Neurosci. Abstr.*, 538P.

F. Nyberg, H.S. Sharma and Z. Wiesenfeld-Hallin (Eds.)
Progress in Brain Research, Vol 104

CHAPTER 11

Electrophysiology of neuropeptides in the sensory spinal cord

V. Radhakrishnan and J.L. Henry

Departments of Physiology and Psychiatry, McGill University, 3655 Drummond Street, Montreal, Quebec, Canada H3G 1Y6

Introduction

The dorsal horn has historically been viewed as an important site of integration of sensory information from the periphery. Included in dorsal horn circuitry is not only the primary afferent synapse on to the second order neuron, but also significant regulatory mechanisms, expressed at presynaptic and postsynaptic levels, from feedback and feedforward local inhibitory and, perhaps, even some excitatory neurons, from largely inhibitory propriospinal neurons arising from extrasegmental levels, and from descending fibers arising from neurons in supraspinal levels. A large variety of chemicals has been implicated as chemical mediators of synaptic transmission and modulation in this complex organization of mechanisms involved in integration of sensory information including, most notably, excitatory and inhibitory amino acids, neuropeptides, catecholamines and purines. All classes appear to play critical roles in the overall regulation. This survey focuses on some of the neuropeptides implicated in this regulation, but this should not be construed to reflect in any way a diminution of the importance which must be attributed to the other chemicals implicated.

Considerable advancement in our knowledge of primary afferent sensory transmission, especially of nociceptive signals, has been made as a result of the discovery of endogenous neuropeptides in the spinal cord. These have been found in at least some primary afferents projecting to the spinal cord, in neurons intrinsic to the spinal cord, and in spinal and descending fibers. In fact, the dorsal horn, especially the superficial layers, contains a particularly high concentration and abundance of neuropeptides shared only with such other notable structures as the hypothalamus, the nucleus of the tractus solitarius and the intermediolateral nucleus of the spinal cord. Much of the important and relevant information linking neuropeptides to the sensory spinal cord has arisen from anatomical, biochemical and molecular biological studies. These are dealt with in other chapters of this treatise. In this chapter we shall attempt a survey of electrophysiological evidence implicating neuropeptides in somatosensory processing, stressing extra- and intracellular recordings from single neurons in the dorsal horn in vivo, although evidence from other approaches will be cited in some cases to support the concepts put forward.

The tachykinin, substance P, has probably been the best characterized neuropeptide in the spinal cord and this will be discussed as the prototypic neuropeptide. Early on, a higher level of substance P-like biological activity was found in the dorsal than the ventral spinal roots and this prompted the suggestion that the peptide is *the primary afferent transmitter* (Lembeck, 1953; Pernow, 1953). While this suggestion has not been strictly supported by subsequent evidence, this peptide remains perhaps the most well under-

176

stood of the neuropeptides, at least with regard to its role in sensory function in the dorsal horn.

Classification of dorsal horn neurons

Before discussing the effects of peptides on dorsal horn neurons, the types of neurons found, as well as the strategies used for peripheral stimulation of the cutaneous receptive field and the identification/classification of these neurons will be described. As this is primarily a survey of electrophysiological evidence, a physiological classification will be followed. In our own laboratory the experiments are done in anesthetized or decerebrated cats. The neurons are initially identified by probe stimuli of touch and/or movement of hairs applied to the cutaneous receptive field in the hind limb. Once a neuron responding to the probe stimulus is encountered, it is then subjected to a rigorous testing using a variety of noxious and non-noxious stimuli applied to the

receptive field. The stimuli applied are: (i) light touch; (ii) moderate pressure; (iii) noxious pinch of the skin manually; (iv) low velocity air jet passed over the receptive field just sufficient to move the hairs; and (v) noxious thermal (48–49°C) stimulation of the skin using controlled radiant heat (Radhakrishnan and Henry, 1993a,b). Care is taken to maintain uniformity in applying the pinch stimuli in terms of pressure, duration and the area of the receptive field stimulated. The response to pinch is considered to be nociceptive if it includes a slow, prolonged after-discharge following an initial fast, peak response. The heat stimulus is applied for 10–12 s, and repeated at a constant rate of one per minute by an automatic timer. Neurons thus studied are classified, on the basis of their responses to the natural stimuli (Radhakrishnan and Henry, 1993a), as *non-nociceptive* (responding only to innocuous stimuli), *nociceptive-specific* (responding only to noxious stimuli) or *wide dynamic range* (responding to

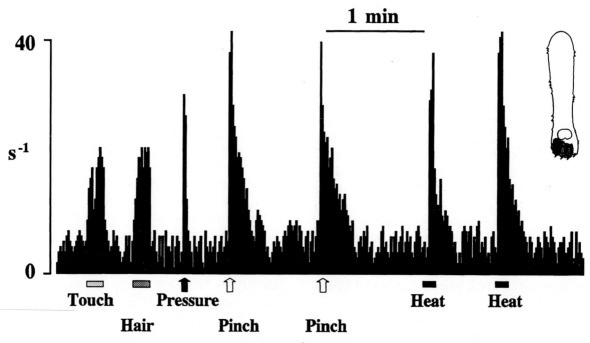

Fig. 1. Ratemeter record showing the firing frequency (impulses·s⁻¹) of a wide dynamic range neuron in the dorsal horn to noxious and non-noxious stimulation of the receptive field in the ipsilateral hind paw of the cat (inset).

both noxious and non-noxious stimuli). Figure 1 illustrates the typical responses of one wide dynamic range neuron to noxious and innocuous natural stimulation of the skin.

Substance P

The presence of substance P in primary afferent terminals in the superficial layers of the dorsal horn, in dorsal root ganglion cells and in dorsal roots has been demonstrated in many species, using chemical (Takahashi and Otsuka, 1975), immunohistochemical (Hökfelt et al., 1975b; Pickel et al., 1977; Barber et al., 1979) and in situ hybridization techniques (Warden and Young, 1988). A high concentration of substance P occurs in dense-core synaptic vesicles (Cuello et al., 1977; Cuello and Kanazawa, 1978) in the terminals of fine diameter primary afferents (Hökfelt et al., 1975a,b) located in the area of the dorsal horn where nociception is integrated (Light and Perl, 1979; Sugiura et al., 1986). Noxious stimulation of the skin by thermal (Duggan et al., 1987, 1988; Go and Yaksh, 1987; Tiseo et al., 1990), mechanical (Duggan et al., 1988) and chemical (Kuraishi et al., 1985; Duggan et al., 1988; Watling, 1992) stimuli, electrical stimulation of unmyelinated afferent fibers (Brodin et al., 1987; Go et al., 1987; Klein et al., 1992) and administration of capsaicin (Go and Yaksh, 1987; Aimone and Yaksh, 1989; Takano et al., 1993) have each been shown to release substance P in the spinal cord, especially in the substantia gelatinosa (Duggan et al., 1987, 1988). Substance P (NK-1) receptors have also been localized in the dorsal horn (Ninkovic et al., 1984; Vita et al., 1990; Yashpal et al., 1990; Aanonsen et al., 1992; Bernau et al., 1993; Gouarderes et al., 1993). The first electrophysiological evidence to indicate that substance P may play a role in nociception was provided by iontophoretic studies in which application of this peptide on to dorsal horn neurons specifically excited nociceptive neurons (Henry, 1976). Studies described below, wherein the effects of antagonists to substance P receptors were tested against the response of dorsal horn neurons to noxious

cutaneous stimuli, lend support to such an involvement. A number of recent reviews have appeared on this topic (Nicoll et al., 1980; Cuello, 1987; Otsuka and Yanagisawa, 1990; Henry, 1993).

Effect of substance P on dorsal horn neurons

Iontophoretic application of substance P in the dorsal horn specifically excites nociceptive (i.e., nociceptive-specific and wide dynamic range) neurons, the response of the non-nociceptive cells, being unaffected (Henry, 1976; Radhakrishnan and Henry, 1991; Salter and Henry, 1991). A fraction of wide dynamic range neurons, however, is insensitive to substance P (Radhakrishnan and Henry, 1991). The excitation induced by substance P is characterized by a delayed onset, normally about 20–40 s, and a slow, prolonged response lasting 30–90 s (Fig. 2). This is in contrast to the fast responses produced by some other chemical mediators such as glutamate, whose effects usually begin within 1–3 s of the onset of application (Radhakrishnan and Henry, 1993a). The slow time course of the response to substance P, also seen in other studies (Randić and Miletić, 1977; Nowak and Macdonald, 1982; Urban and Randić, 1984), indicates that substance P may not be acting as a chemical mediator of fast synaptic responses (Henry et al., 1975). A selective enhancement of C-, but not A-fiber-evoked firing of dorsal horn neurons (Kellstein et al., 1990), and of the response to noxious cutaneous stimuli (Henry and Ben Ari, 1976) by locally applied substance P, has also been reported (Kellstein et al., 1990).

The first demonstration that the response of dorsal horn neurons to substance P application is abolished by an NK-1 receptor antagonist in an in vivo paradigm (Radhakrishnan and Henry, 1991), involved the use of the novel, nonpeptide antagonist, CP-96,345, a $2S3S$ isomer (McLean et al., 1991; Snider et al., 1991) (Fig. 2). Though earlier in vitro studies had shown that the effect of bath application of substance P on dorsal horn neurons could be abolished by peptide antagonists of NK-1 receptors (Urban and Randić, 1984), these could not be confirmed in vivo, owing to the instability of peptide antagonists. The discovery of nonpeptide antagonists to NK-1 receptors, starting with CP-96,345 and followed by CP-99,994 (McLean et al., 1993) and others, has opened up new vistas in understanding the role of substance P in a number of physiological systems (Maggi et al., 1993). One of our recent studies has shown that the effects of substance P on dorsal horn neurons are abolished by CP-96,345 and CP-99,994, but not by CP-96,344, the $2R3R$-inactive enantiomer of CP-96,345 (Radhakrishnan and Henry, 1995). Thus the blockade of the responses to substance P appears to be stereospecific and also to be independent of other non-specific effects attributed to both isomers (McLean et al., 1991; Snider et al., 1991; Schmidt et al., 1992; Guard et al., 1993).

Substance P may be acting directly or indirectly on dorsal horn neurons, as there is evidence to indicate that bath application of substance P induces the release of glutamate and aspartate in spinal cord in vivo (Kawagoe et al., 1986; Skilling et al., 1992; Sluka and Westlund, 1993) and in vitro (Kawagoe et al., 1986; Kangrga and Randić, 1990; Maehara et al., 1993). Substance P has also been shown to coexist with glutamate in primary afferent terminals and in dorsal root ganglion cells (Battaglia and Rustioni, 1988; De Biasi and Rustioni, 1988; Merighi et al., 1991). There appears to be an interaction of substance P with glutamate receptor-mediated responses in the dorsal horn. Combined application of excitatory amino acids such as N-methyl-D-aspartate (NMDA) and substance P to spinothalamic dorsal horn neurons has been shown to induce long-last-

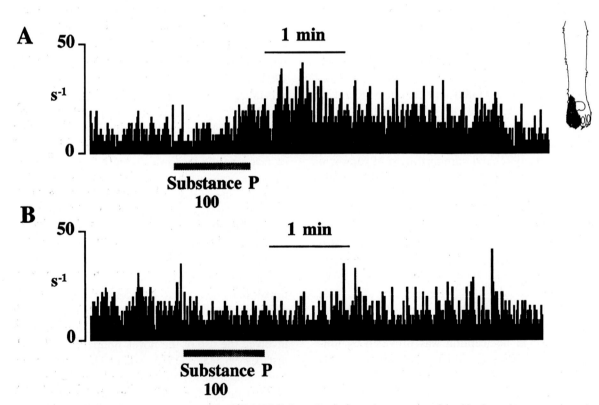

Fig. 2. Effect of the NK-1 receptor antagonist CP-96,345 (0.5 mg/kg, i.v.) on the response of a wide dynamic range neuron to iontophoretic application of substance P (100 nA). A. The response of the neuron to substance P before the administration of CP-96,345. B. Response of the same neuron to substance P after the administration of CP-96,345.

ing responses (Dougherty and Willis, 1991; Dougherty et al., 1993). Both substance P and glutamate elevate intracellular calcium in the same dorsal horn neurons, and this elevation is blocked by the glutamate receptor antagonist, kynurenate (Womack et al., 1988). Supportive evidence of such interactions of substance P with excitatory amino acids is shown by the blockade of substance P-induced facilitation of a spinal nociceptive reflex by intrathecal administration of the specific NMDA-receptor antagonist 2-amino-5-phosphonovaleric acid (APV) (Yashpal et al., 1991), and the enhancement by substance P of ionic currents induced in vitro by the activation of NMDA, and α-amino-3-hydroxy-5-methyl-4-isoxazolepropionic acid (AMPA), but not of kainate receptors (Randić et al., 1990, 1993; Rusin et al., 1992, 1993a,b).

Substance P also appears to enhance at least some inhibitory inputs to dorsal horn neurons. Earlier reports from our laboratory have shown that application of adenosine 5′-triphosphate (ATP) or adenosine 5′-monophosphate (AMP) to dorsal horn neurons (Salter and Henry, 1985), or of a vibratory stimulus to skin (Salter and Henry, 1987a), inhibits the responses of dorsal horn nociceptive neurons via P_1-purinergic receptor stimulation. Application of substance P enhances this adenosine receptor-mediated inhibition (Salter and Henry, 1987b, 1988).

Effect of substance P antagonists on the response of dorsal horn neurons to cutaneous stimulation

An important step in our understanding of the role of substance P in primary afferent transmission is whether selective antagonists alter synaptically-elicited nociceptive responses. This type of evidence has been provided from in vivo experiments. Noxious cutaneous stimulation (thermal or mechanical) of the skin, elicits an initial fast response in the responding dorsal horn neurons, followed by a slow, prolonged after-discharge which outlasts the period of application, as described above. The NK-1 receptor antagonists, CP-96,345 and CP-99,994, consistently inhibit the after-discharge phase of the response, suggesting the involvement of NK-1 receptors in this late, prolonged response (Radhakrishnan and Henry, 1991, 1995). In most of the neurons studied, the initial component of the response remains unaffected. The on-going or baseline firing also is unaffected by these antagonists (Fig. 3). The inactive isomer, CP-96,344, does not affect any component of the responses to noxious cutaneous stimulation (Fig. 3), indicating that the blockade seen after CP-96,345 is actually due to a blockade of NK-1 receptors (Radhakrishnan and Henry, 1995), rather than to any non-specific effects. These data suggest that the spontaneous baseline discharge, as well as the fast component of the nociceptive responses in at least some of the cells, may not involve an activation of NK-1 receptors. A corollary is that substance P may not be released under resting conditions, and that prolonged activation of nociceptive primary afferents may be necessary to elicit the release of substance P in the dorsal horn (Duggan et al., 1987, 1988; Duggan, 1992). Substance P, in turn, by virtue of its slow, prolonged nature of activation of the cells, may play a role primarily in the after-discharge seen after sustained noxious stimulation.

Studies pertaining to spinal reflex activation following noxious stimuli have also indicated that substance P is involved only in the response to a strong noxious stimulus (Cridland and Henry, 1988a; Henry, 1993; Laird et al., 1993; Yashpal et al., 1993), but not in the response to a brief noxious stimulus.

Importantly, the excitatory effects of noxious cutaneous stimulation can be mimicked by a train of high intensity electrical stimulation of sensory afferents. Intracellular recordings from dorsal horn neurons in vivo have shown that such stimulation at intensities sufficient to recruit C-fiber afferents, produces an initial fast EPSP during the phase of stimulation, followed by a late, prolonged depolarization associated with an after-discharge (De Koninck and Henry, 1991; Radhakrishnan and Henry, 1995). CP-96,345 (De Koninck and Henry, 1991) and CP-99,994

180

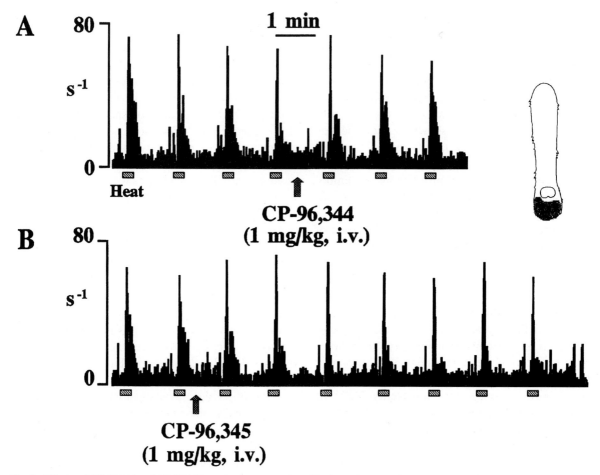

Fig. 3. Effects of CP-96,344 and CP-96,345 on the response of a wide dynamic range neuron to controlled application of noxious radiant heat to the receptive field. Records in A and B are continuous. Note the persistent inhibition of the after-discharge following the administration of CP-96,345 and the lack of any effect of CP-96,344. Also note that the baseline discharge is unaffected by both the compounds.

(Radhakrishnan and Henry, 1995) selectively block the late depolarization without affecting the initial fast EPSP, further supporting the contention that NK-1 receptor activation plays a role in these late events. Such selective inhibition of the late responses to electrical stimulation of afferent fibers by CP-96,345 in vivo has been confirmed subsequently by other workers in extracellular experiments (Toda and Hayashi, 1993). In contrast, the response to C-fiber activation by a single pulse is not affected by CP-96,345 or by CP-

99,994, indicating that a brief C-fiber input may not be releasing sufficient substance P to generate a significant physiological response (De Koninck and Henry 1991; Radhakrishnan and Henry, 1995).

Similar phenomena have been seen in nociceptive spinal reflex studies, wherein the baseline responses to application of brief noxious heat stimuli to the tail of the rat are not affected by NK-1 receptor antagonists (Yashpal and Henry, 1984; Cridland and Henry, 1988a; Garces et al.,

1993), but the facilitation induced in these responses by intense noxious stimulation (Cridland and Henry, 1988a; Yashpal et al., 1993), or by intrathecal administration of substance P (Yashpal and Henry, 1984; Yashpal et al., 1993), is blocked by NK-1 receptor antagonists.

Non-noxious stimulation of the skin by movement of hairs usually elicits fast, brisk responses from dorsal horn neurons. CP-96,345 and CP-99,994 do not affect these fast responses. It is quite likely that these fast responses are not mediated by a slow acting transmitter, such as substance P (Radhakrishnan and Henry, 1995), but may be mediated via activation of excitatory amino acid receptors (Radhakrishnan and Henry, 1993a). This confirms the observation that iontophoretic application of substance P fails to excite non-nociceptive neurons in the dorsal horn (Henry, 1976; Radhakrishnan and Henry, 1991; Salter and Henry, 1991).

Cellular effects of substance P

At the cellular level, substance P may be operating via more than a single mechanism to account for the slow, prolonged effects seen (Krnjević, 1977; Otsuka and Yoshioka, 1993). It is to be noted that, although most of the studies elucidating the mechanism of action of substance P have been done on brain neurons, it is quite likely that a similar mechanism operates at the spinal neuronal level.

A number of cellular mechanisms by which substance P has been reported to elicit its effects are as follows.

Inhibition of an inwardly rectifying potassium channel current

Whole-cell patch-clamp studies have shown that substance P inhibits an inwardly rectifying K$^+$ current in cultured neuronal cells from rat basal forebrain nuclei and locus coeruleus (Stanfield et al., 1985; Yamaguchi et al., 1990; Nakajima et al., 1991). Nakajima et al. (1988, 1993) have shown that this inhibition is mediated through a pertussis toxin-insensitive G protein mechanism.

Inhibition of muscarine-sensitive potassium current (M-current)

A voltage- and time-dependent K$^+$ current inhibited by muscarine is known as the M-current (Brown and Adams, 1980). Substance P has been shown to inhibit this M-current, in mammalian spinal neurons (Hösli et al., 1981; Nowak and Macdonald, 1982; Murase et al., 1986) and in bullfrog sympathetic neurons (Adams et al., 1983; Jones, 1985).

Inhibition of calcium-activated potassium current

An inhibition of calcium-activated potassium current by substance P has been shown in guinea-pig submucosal neurons (Akasu and Tokimasa, 1989; Shen and Surprenant, 1993).

Activation of calcium-sensitive current

In rat dorsal horn neurons in the spinal slice, substance P enhances a slow, persistent, calcium-sensitive current (Murase et al., 1986). An enhancement of low- and high-voltage activated calcium currents by substance P has also been demonstrated in these neurons (Ryu and Randić, 1990). However, in mammalian and non-mammalian sympathetic neurons, a suppression of voltage-gated calcium currents by substance P has also been reported (Bley and Tsien, 1990; Elmslie, 1992; Shapiro and Hille, 1993).

Elevation of intracellular calcium

Womack et al. (1988) reported an elevation of intracellular calcium concentration by substance P in single isolated postnatal rat dorsal horn neurons monitored with the calcium indicator fura-2. Substance P-induced elevation of intracellular calcium has also been demonstrated in non-neuronal tissues (Arkle et al., 1989; Matthews et al., 1989), possibly by a release of calcium from intracellular stores via an inositol 1,4,5-trisphosphate mechanism (Merritt and Rink, 1987; Mochizuki-Oda et al., 1993; Seabrook and Fong, 1993) and by an increase in the influx of calcium (Matthews et al., 1989; Mochizuki-Oda et al., 1993). Inositol trisphosphate has also been shown to activate calcium influx (Mochizuki-Oda et al., 1993).

Activation of intra- / intercellular messenger systems

Inositol phospholipid hydrolysis. NK-1 receptors are G protein-coupled (Boyd et al., 1991), and activation of these receptors by substance P has been shown to activate the enzyme phospholipase C via a G protein mechanism (Taylor et al., 1986).

This results in the hydrolysis of membrane-bound inositol phospholipids, leading to the formation of two second messengers, inositol trisphosphate and diacylglycerol (Hanley et al., 1980; Watson and Downes, 1983; Mantyh et al., 1984). Inositol trisphosphate activates the release of calcium from intracellular stores (Merritt and Rink, 1987; Mochizuki-Oda et al., 1993; Seabrook and Fong, 1993), and diacylglycerol activates protein kinase C and facilitates the opening of voltage-sensitive

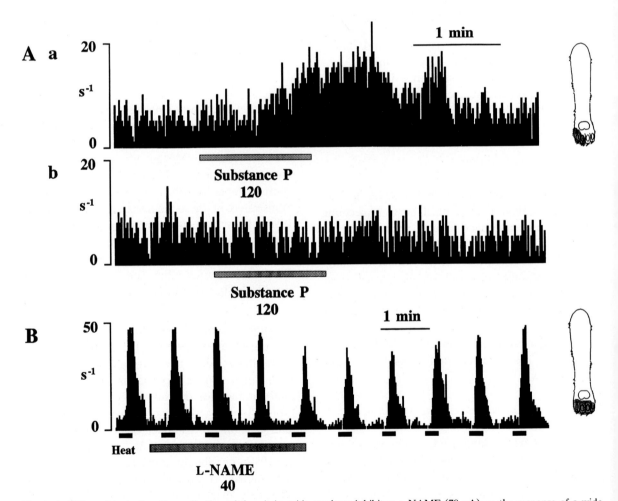

Fig. 4. A. Effect of iontophoretic application of the nitric oxide synthase inhibitor, L-NAME (70 nA) on the response of a wide dynamic range neuron to iontophoretic application of substance P (120 nA). a. The response of the neuron to substance P before the application of L-NAME. L-NAME was applied for 2 min at the end of the record shown. b. The response of the same neuron to substance P applied one min after L-NAME was given. B. Effect of iontophoretic application of L-NAME (40 nA) on the response of a wide dynamic range neuron to noxious thermal stimulation of the receptive field.

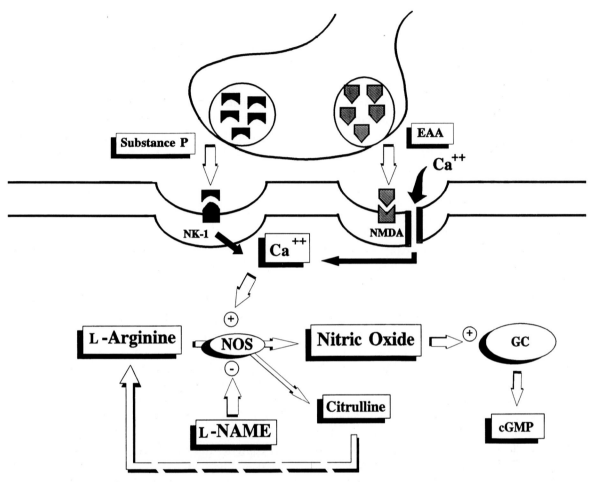

Fig. 5. Schematic representation of the steps involved in the activation of L-arginine-nitric oxide pathway following the release of substance P and excitatory amino acids (EAA) from the primary afferent terminals. NMDA, *N*-methyl-D-aspartate receptor; NOS, nitric oxide synthase; GC, soluble guanylate cyclase; cGMP, cyclic guanosine monophosphate; +, activation; −, inhibition. Evidence suggests that nitric oxide formed in the stimulated neuron may not be activating the formation of cGMP in the same neuron because the elevated intracellular calcium in the neuron may be inhibiting the activation of guanylate cyclase. Nitric oxide, being an easily diffusible gas, may diffuse into the neighboring neurons and activate guanylate cyclase in those target neurons to form cGMP from guanosine triphosphate.

calcium channels and, thereby, influx of calcium into the cells (Gallacher et al., 1990).

Cyclic adenosine monophosphate (cAMP). In rat and human brain neurons (Duffy and Powell, 1975; Mistry and Vijayan, 1987; Moser, 1990; Krause et al., 1993), and in transfected Chinese hamster ovary cells (Nakajima et al., 1992; Takeda et al., 1992) and rat KNRK kidney cells (Mitsu-

hashi et al., 1992), substance P has been shown to elevate intracellular cAMP levels.

Nitric oxide and cyclic guanosine monophosphate (cGMP). There is also indication that substance P may activate cGMP formation in non-neuronal cells (Sjödin et al., 1980; Schini et al., 1990). cGMP in endothelial and neuronal cells can be formed by the activation of the L-arginine-nitric oxide pathway. Nitric oxide, formed from L-arginine by the action of the enzyme nitric oxide synthase, activates the soluble guanylate cyclase in the cells to generate cGMP from guanosine triphosphate (Garthwaite et al., 1988; Knowles et al., 1989; Bredt et al., 1990; Knowles et al., 1990). The formation of nitric oxide is a calcium-dependent process (Garthwaite et al., 1988) and, therefore, this mechanism may be tied in with others mentioned above. Substance P-induced relaxation of rabbit aortic rings and vasodilation in dogs are antagonized by an endothelial nitric oxide synthase inhibitor (Lewis and Henderson, 1987; Moncada et al., 1991; Persson et al., 1991), indicating the involvement of nitric oxide in the mediation of substance P effects in these peripheral tissues as well.

Our recent studies have indicated that the nitric oxide synthase inhibitor, N^G-nitro-L-arginine methyl ester (L-NAME) attenuates the responses of dorsal horn neurons to iontophoretic application of substance P (Radhakrishnan and Henry, 1993b). Also, L-NAME effectively inhibits the responses of the neurons to noxious thermal (Fig. 4) and mechanical stimulation of the cutaneous receptive field, suggesting the mediation of these responses via a nitric oxide pathway (Radhakrishnan and Henry, 1993b). We have shown earlier that these nociceptive responses are mediated by activation of NK-1 receptors (Radhakrishnan and Henry, 1991). Taken together, these data suggest that NK-1 receptor activation triggers the formation of nitric oxide and, subsequently, an elevation of cGMP in dorsal horn nociceptive cells. A schematic representation of the steps involved in such a mechanism is illustrated in Fig. 5.

Physalaemin

The non-mammalian tachykinin, physalaemin shows preferential affinity for the NK-1 type of neurokinin receptor (Mohini et al., 1985) and is sometimes used as a natural substance P analog. Iontophoretic application of physalaemin to dorsal horn neurons preferentially excites nocicep-

tive neurons, although a proportion of non-nociceptive neurons is also excited (Salter and Henry, 1991). Intrathecal administration of physalaemin facilitates the tail-flick reflex and the effects are indistinguishable from those of substance P (Cridland and Henry, 1986). Physalaemin, like substance P and neurokinin A, has also been shown to potentiate adenosine receptor-mediated inhibition of nociceptive neurons in cat spinal cord (Salter and Henry, 1988).

Neurokinin A

Neurokinin A, another member of the tachykinin family along with substance P, has also been localized in the dorsal horn (Hua et al., 1985; Duggan et al., 1990). It acts preferentially on the NK-2 type of neurokinin receptor (Quirion, 1985; Buck and Shatzer, 1988; Maggi et al., 1993). An earlier study from our laboratory has shown that iontophoretic application of neurokinin A to dorsal horn neurons, evokes a slow, prolonged response, similar to that of substance P (Salter and Henry, 1991). However, in contrast to substance P, which excites only nociceptive neurons, neurokinin A was found to excite both nociceptive and non-nociceptive neurons (Salter and Henry, 1991). Neurokinin A has also been found to potentiate the response of dorsal horn neurons to excitatory amino acids such as NMDA, quisqualate and AMPA without affecting responses to kainate (Rusin et al., 1993a,b). There is some evidence to suggest that spinal NK-2 receptors mediate the responses to brief cutaneous thermal stimulation, high-threshold afferent fiber stimulation or capsaicin in rats (Fleetwood-Walker et al., 1993; Nagy et al., 1993; Thompson et al., 1993; Urban et al., 1993). Intrathecal administration of neurokinin A has been shown to facilitate a nociceptive spinal reflex in tail-flick studies, though to a lesser degree than does substance P (Cridland and Henry, 1986). Potentiation of adenosine receptor-mediated inhibition of nociceptive neurons by neurokinin A has also been reported (Salter and Henry, 1988).

Calcitonin gene-related peptide (CGRP)

The presence of CGRP-like immunoreactivity in the superficial dorsal horn (Gibson et al., 1984; Carlton et al., 1987; Ju et al., 1987; Yashpal et al., 1992), co-localization of this peptide with substance P (Wiesenfeld-Hallin et al., 1984), and release of CGRP in the spinal cord by various noxious stimuli (Morton and Hutchison, 1989), are indications that this peptide may play a significant role in nociceptive transmission. Iontophoretic application of CGRP has been shown to activate some dorsal horn neurons (Miletić and Tan, 1988). A synergistic interaction between substance P and CGRP has also been suggested based on the potentiation of substance P-induced responses by CGRP (Wiesenfeld-Hallin et al., 1984; Biella et al., 1991). Iontophoretic application of CGRP potentiates the responses of dorsal horn neurons to noxious cutaneous stimulation as well as to application of substance P (Biella et al., 1991). A facilitation of bombesin-mediated nociceptive responses by CGRP has also been reported (Mao et al., 1992). These in vivo electrophysiological results have been substantiated by other lines of evidence. For example, intrathecal administration of CGRP facilitates the tail-flick reflex in rats (Cridland and Henry, 1988b), and dorsal horn neuronal responses to NMDA are also potentiated by CGRP (Murase et al., 1989). CGRP has been shown to induce a slow depolarization of dorsal horn neurons (Ryu et al., 1988).

Opioid peptides

Opioid peptides constitute another class of peptides implicated in dorsal horn synaptic function. The presence of opioid peptides, such as methionine-enkephalin, leucine-enkephalin and dynorphin (Hökfelt et al., 1977; Aronin et al., 1981; Medina et al., 1993; Sharma et al., 1993), and their receptors (μ, δ and κ) (Besse et al., 1992; Besse et al., 1990; Hunter et al., 1989) has also been demonstrated in the dorsal horn of spinal cord. Noxious stimulation of the skin (Cesselin et al., 1989), stimulation of afferent fibers (Hutchi-

son et al., 1990; Lucas and Yaksh, 1990), acupuncture-like stimulation (Bing et al., 1991) and perfusion with substance P or potassium (Yaksh and Elde, 1980, 1981; Cesselin et al., 1985) evoke release of opioid peptides in the spinal cord.

Duggan and colleagues (1976, 1977) have shown that iontophoretic application of Met-enkephalin selectively inhibits the responses of nociceptive neurons in the dorsal horn. Similar observations have been reported by others (Randić and Miletić 1978; Zieglgänsberger and Tulloch, 1979; Sastry and Goh, 1983). The selectivity for nociceptive neurons appears to be restricted to superficial layers since an inhibition of both nociceptive and non-nociceptive neurons is observed in deeper laminae (Duggan et al., 1977). Intracellular studies in vitro revealed a hyperpolarization induced by enkephalin in dorsal horn neurons in rats (Murase et al., 1982; Yoshimura and North, 1983) and a blockade of depolarizing responses induced by electrical or chemical stimulation of afferents (Jeftinija et al., 1993). The inhibitory effects of enkephalin on dorsal horn neurons may be via its action on δ or μ receptors (Dickenson et al., 1986; Jeftinija, 1988; Sullivan et al., 1989; Jeftinija et al., 1993). An inhibition of the responses of nociceptive neurons by application of morphine has also been demonstrated (Piercey et al., 1980; Henry, 1983; Homma et al., 1983; Dickenson and Sullivan, 1986). Morphine selectively inhibits the responses to C-fiber-, but not A-fiber-evoked responses (Dickenson and Sullivan, 1986; Kellstein et al., 1990) and does not antagonise the facilitatory responses to substance P (Piercey et al., 1980; Henry, 1983). In addition to the direct postsynaptic effects of opioid peptides (Duggan et al., 1976; Murase et al., 1982; Yoshimura and North, 1983), a presynaptic mechanism, probably by inhibiting the release of substance P (Jessell and Iversen, 1977; Hirota et al., 1985; Aimone and Yaksh, 1989) is also likely. Co-localization of substance P and enkephalin immunoreactivities in the superficial dorsal horn has been recently reported (Ribeiro-da-Silva et al., 1991).

Somatostatin

Somatostatin, another peptide present in the dorsal horn (Hannan and Ho, 1992; Lu and Ho, 1992; El-Bohy and LaMotte, 1993; Proudlock et al., 1993) and released following noxious stimuli (Kuraishi et al., 1985, 1991; Morton et al., 1989), has been shown to depress the activity of nociceptive (Randić and Miletić, 1978) but not non-nociceptive (Sandkühler et al., 1990) dorsal horn neurons. An inhibition of the responses to noxious thermal stimulation in cats (Sandkühler et al., 1990) and to subcutaneous injection of formalin in rats (Chapman and Dickenson, 1992) has been observed. Intracellular studies have indicated that somatostatin hyperpolarizes the membrane of the dorsal horn cells in lamprey spinal cord (Christenson et al., 1991) in a manner similar to the effects of enkephalin (Murase et al., 1982).

Bombesin, neuromedin B and neuromedin C

The presence of bombesin-like immunoreactivity in the superficial laminae of mammalian dorsal horn, and a reduction in this immunoreactivity after dorsal rhizotomy, suggest a strong correlation of an analogous peptide to primary afferents and sensory transmission (Fuxe et al., 1983; Massari et al., 1983; O'Donohue et al., 1984). Furthermore, the binding of [^{125}I]bombesin is restricted to the superficial laminae and this binding decreases after dorsal rhizotomy (Massari et al., 1983; O'Donohue et al., 1984), suggesting a predominantly presynaptic localization of the receptors. Iontophoretic application of bombesin and its related mammalian peptides, neuromedin B and neuromedin C, has been shown to preferentially depress the activity of nociceptive neurons of the superficial dorsal horn in cats (De Koninck and Henry, 1989). This inhibition is unaffected by naloxone, bicuculline and caffeine, suggesting that it is a pharmacologically distinct effect and not mediated via opioid, $GABA_A$ or purinergic inhibitory systems (De Koninck and Henry, 1989). Other reports indicate that, in rats, bombesin and the related peptides may induce an excitation of

spinal reflexes. In an isolated rat spinal cord preparation, bath application of bombesin or its related peptides has been shown to induce a depolarizing response as recorded from the ventral roots (Guo et al., 1993a,b). A facilitation of the tail-flick reflex has been observed following administration of bombesin, neuromedin B or neuromedin C in rats (Cridland and Henry, 1992). Bombesin also has been shown to induce nociceptive behavioral responses in rats (Mao et al., 1992).

Other peptides

A number of other peptides has also been implicated. For example, peptides such as vasoactive intestinal polypeptide (Knyihár-Csillik et al., 1991, 1993; Klein et al., 1992; Yamamoto and Yaksh, 1992), galanin (Klein et al., 1992; Zhang et al., 1993), neurotensin (Todd et al., 1992; Proudlock et al., 1993; Zhang et al., 1993), cholecystokinin (Jacquin et al., 1992; El-Bohy and LaMotte, 1993; Verge et al., 1993; Zhang et al., 1993), thyrotropin-releasing hormone (Coffield et al., 1986; Ulfhake et al., 1987) and neuropeptide Y (Kar and Quirion, 1992; Doyle and Maxwell, 1993; Rowan et al., 1993) have also been demonstrated in primary afferents and in nerve terminals of the dorsal horn.

Iontophoretic application of vasoactive intestinal polypeptide (Jeftinija et al., 1982), neurotensin (Miletić and Randić, 1979; Stanzione and Zieglgänsberger, 1983) and cholecystokinin (Jeftinija et al., 1981) has been shown to excite both nociceptive and non-nociceptive neurons of the dorsal horn, implying that these peptides may participate non-selectively in the transmission of both nociceptive and non-nociceptive signals. The inhibition of nociceptive neuronal responses brought about by morphine is attenuated by cholecystokinin and enhanced by cholecystokinin antagonists, suggesting a role of the peptide in nociception (Kellstein et al., 1991; Stanfa and Dickenson, 1993). Jackson and White (1988) have demonstrated that application of thyrotropin-releasing hormone increases the excitability of dorsal horn neurons to the actions of glutamate. Nistri and colleagues have demonstrated that the increase in excitability seen after thyrotropin-releasing hormone administration in spinal motoneurons is due to the blockade of a potassium current (Nistri et al., 1990; Fisher and Nistri, 1993). Intrathecal administration of vasoactive intestinal polypeptide has been shown to facilitate tail flick reflex in rats (Cridland and Henry, 1988b), while that of galanin increases the reaction time in tail flick paradigms (Cridland and Henry, 1988b), potentiates the spinal analgesic effect of morphine (Wiesenfeld-Hallin et al., 1990) and antagonizes the facilitatory effect of substance P in the spinal nociceptive reflex (Xu et al., 1989).

Conclusions

The evidence cited thus indicates that the dorsal horn, being the first relay station of primary afferent signals, plays a pivotal role in the integration of sensory information. The multitude of neurotransmitters and neuromodulators, including the neuropeptides, amino acids and other chemicals distributed in the dorsal horn, subserve this integratory role. Noxious stimulation of the periphery induces the release of both excitatory and inhibitory neuropeptides along with other neurotransmitters in the spinal cord. The differential actions of these peptides on the dorsal horn neurons, thus may bring in a myriad of complex changes to regulate the overall excitability of the neurons and, thereby, regulate the flow of information from the spinal cord to the higher areas.

However, at the end of this survey, a number of questions remain unanswered. For example, electrophysiologists have not yet addressed fully the functional significance of the co-localization of several neuropeptides in one terminal or even the co-localization of neuropeptides with other classes of chemical. While evidence is emerging on the links between expression of NK-1 receptor activation and expression of NMDA receptor activation, little is known about other possible interactions. Nor is there a complete understanding of how so many different neuropeptides are found in the dorsal horn, particularly in the substantia gelatinosa. Given the notably longer time course of the actions of neuropeptides compared to that for most of the other classes of chemical, this may mean that closer scrutiny needs to be paid to longer term changes induced at synapses. This would, of course include plastic changes, which have been tied particularly with nociceptive function. Finally, it is clear that more electrophysiological studies need to focus on the peptides for which relatively little is known; these would include not only the obvious, such as vasoactive intestinal polypeptide, neuropeptide Y, neurotensin, somatostatin, galanin and dynorphin, but also proctolin, peptide YY, atrial natriuretic peptide and brain natriuretic peptide (Fone et al., 1991; Hösli et al., 1992), which have also been found in the spinal cord, but for which little if any physiological information is available.

References

Aanonsen, L.M., Kajander, K.C., Bennett, G.J. and Seybold, V.S. (1992) Autoradiographic analysis of ^{125}I-substance P binding in rat spinal cord following chronic constriction injury of the sciatic nerve. Brain Res., 596: 259–268.

Adams, P.R., Brown, D.A. and Jones, S.W. (1983) Substance P inhibits the M-current in bullfrog sympathetic neurones. Br. J. Pharmacol., 79: 330–333.

Aimone, L.D. and Yaksh, T.L. (1989) Opioid modulation of capsaicin-evoked release of substance P from rat spinal cord in vivo. Peptides, 10: 1127–1131.

Akasu, T. and Tokimasa, T. (1989) Potassium currents in submucous neurons of guinea-pig caecum and their synaptic modification. J. Physiol. (London), 416: 571–588.

Arkle, S., Michalek, R. and Templeton, D. (1989) The relationship of intracellular free calcium activity to amylase secretion in substance P- and isoprenaline-stimulated rat parotid acini. Biochem. Pharmacol., 38: 1257–1261.

Aronin, N., DiFiglia, M., Liotta, A.S. and Martin, J.B. (1981) Ultrastructural localization and biochemical features of immunoreactive leu-enkephalin in monkey dorsal horn. J. Neurosci., 1: 561–577.

Barber, R.P., Vaughn, J.E., Slemmon, J.R., Salvaterra, P.M., Roberts, E. and Leeman, S.E. (1979) The origin, distribution and synaptic relationships of substance P axons in rat spinal cord. J. Comp. Neurol., 184: 331–352.

188

Battaglia, G. and Rustioni, A. (1988) Coexistence of glutamate and substance P in dorsal root ganglion neurons of the rat and monkey. *J. Comp. Neurol.*, 277: 302–312.

Bernau, N.A., Dawson, S.D., Kane, L.A. and Pubols, L.M. (1993) Changes in substance P and 5-HT binding in the spinal cord dorsal horn and lamina 10 after dorsolateral funiculus lesions. *Brain Res.*, 613: 106–114.

Besse, D., Lombard, M.C., Zajac, J.M., Roques, B.P. and Besson, J.M. (1990) Pre- and postsynaptic distribution of μ, δ and kappa opioid receptors in the superficial layers of the cervical dorsal horn of the rat spinal cord. *Brain Res.*, 521: 15–22.

Besse, D., Lombard, M.C. and Besson, J.M. (1992) Time-related decreases in μ and δ opioid receptors in the superficial dorsal horn of the rat spinal cord following a large unilateral dorsal rhizotomy. *Brain Res.*, 578: 115–121.

Biella, G., Panara, C., Pecile, A. and Sotgiu, M.L. (1991) Facilitatory role of calcitonin gene-related peptide (CGRP) on excitation induced by substance P (SP) and noxious stimuli in rat spinal dorsal horn neurons. An iontophoretic study in vivo. *Brain Res.*, 559: 352–356.

Bing, Z., Cesselin, F., Bourgoin, S., Clot, A.M., Hamon, M. and Le Bars, D. (1991) Acupuncture-like stimulation induces a heterosegmental release of Met-enkephalin-like material in the rat spinal cord. *Pain*, 47: 71–77.

Bley, K.R. and Tsien, R.W. (1990) Inhibition of Ca^{2+} and K^+ channels in sympathetic neurons by neuropeptides and other ganglionic transmitters. *Neuron*, 4: 379–391.

Boyd, N.D., MacDonald, S.G., Kage, R., Luber-Narod, J. and Leeman, S.E. (1991) Substance P receptor: biochemical characterization and interactions with G proteins. *Ann. NY Acad. Sci.*, 632: 79–93.

Bredt, D.S., Hwang, P.M. and Snyder, S.H. (1990) Localization of nitric oxide synthase indicating a neural role for nitric oxide. *Nature*, 347: 768–770.

Brodin, E., Linderoth, B., Cazelius, B. and Ungerstedt, V. (1987) In vivo release of substance P in cat dorsal horn studied with microdialysis. *Neurosci. Lett.*, 76: 357–362.

Brown, D.A. and Adams, P.R. (1980) Muscarinic suppression of a novel voltage-sensitive K^+ current in a vertebrate neurone. *Nature*, 283: 673–676.

Buck, S.H. and Shatzer, S.A. (1988) Agonist and antagonist binding to tachykinin peptide NK-2 receptors. *Life Sci.*, 42: 2701–2708.

Carlton, S.M., McNeill, D.L., Chung, K. and Coggeshall, R.E. (1987) A light and electron microscopic level analysis of calcitonin gene-related peptide (CGRP) in the spinal cord of the primate: An immunohistochemical study. *Neurosci. Lett.*, 82: 145–150.

Cesselin, F., Le Bars, D., Bourgoin, S., Artaud, F., Gozlan, H., Clot, A.M., Besson, J.M. and Hamon, M. (1985) Spontaneous and evoked release of methionine-enkephalin-like material from the rat spinal cord in vivo. *Brain Res.*, 339: 305–313.

Cesselin, F., Bourgoin, S., Clot, A.M., Hamon, M. and Le Bars, D. (1989) Segmental release of met-enkephalin-like material from the spinal cord of rats, elicited by noxious thermal stimuli. *Brain Res.*, 484: 71–77.

Chapman, V. and Dickenson, A.H. (1992) The effects of sandostatin and somatostatin on nociceptive transmission in the dorsal horn of the rat spinal cord. *Neuropeptides*, 23: 147–152.

Christenson, J., Alford, S., Grillner, S. and Hökfelt, T. (1991) Co-localized GABA and somatostatin use different ionic mechanisms to hyperpolarize target neurons in the lamprey spinal cord. *Neurosci. Lett.*, 134: 93–97.

Coffield, J.A., Miletić, V., Zimmermann, E., Hoffert, M.J. and Brooks, B.R. (1986) Demonstration of thyrotropin-releasing hormone immunoreactivity in neurons of the mouse spinal dorsal horn. *J. Neurosci.*, 6: 1194–1197.

Cridland, R.A. and Henry, J.L. (1986) Comparison of the effects of substance P, neurokinin A, physalaemin and eledoisin in facilitating a nociceptive reflex in the rat. *Brain Res.*, 381: 93–99.

Cridland, R.A. and Henry, J.L. (1988a) Facilitation of the tail-flick reflex by noxious cutaneous stimulation in the rat: antagonism by a substance P analogue. *Brain Res.*, 462: 15–21.

Cridland, R.A. and Henry, J.L. (1988b) Effects of intrathecal administration of neuropeptides on a spinal nociceptive reflex in the rat: VIP, galanin, CGRP, TRH, somatostatin and angiotensin II. *Neuropeptides*, 11: 23–32.

Cridland, R.A. and Henry, J.L. (1992) Bombesin, neuromedin C and neuromedin B given intrathecally facilitate the tail flick reflex in the rat. *Brain Res.*, 584: 163–168.

Cuello, A.C. (1987) Peptides as neuromodulators in primary sensory neurons. *Neuropharmacology*, 7: 971–979.

Cuello, A.C., Jessell, T.M., Kanazawa, I. and Iversen, L.L. (1977) Substance P-localization in synaptic vesicles in rat central nervous system. *J. Neurochem.*, 29: 747–751.

Cuello, A.C. and Kanazawa, I. (1978) The distribution of substance P immunoreactive fibers in the rat central nervous system. *J. Comp. Neurol.*, 178: 129–156.

De Biasi, S. and Rustioni, A. (1988) Glutamate and substance P coexist in primary afferent terminals in the superficial laminae of spinal cord. *Proc. Natl. Acad. Sci. USA*, 85: 7820–7824.

De Koninck, Y. and Henry, J.L. (1989) Bombesin, neuromedin B and neuromedin C selectively depress superficial dorsal horn neurones in the cat spinal cord. *Brain Res.*, 498: 105–117.

De Koninck, Y. and Henry, J.L. (1991) Substance P-mediated slow excitatory postsynaptic potential elicited in dorsal horn neurons in vivo by noxious stimulation. *Proc. Natl. Acad. Sci. USA*, 88: 11344–11348.

Dickenson, A.H. and Sullivan, A.F. (1986) Electrophysiological studies on the effects of intrathecal morphine on nociceptive neurones in the dorsal horn. *Pain*, 24: 211–222.

Dickenson, A.H., Sullivan, A., Feeney, C., Fournie-Zaluski, M.C. and Roques, B.P. (1986) Evidence that endogenous enkephalins produce delta-opiate receptor mediated neuronal inhibitions in rat dorsal horn. *Neurosci. Lett.*, 72: 179–182.

Dougherty, P.M. and Willis, W.D. (1991) Enhancement of spinothalamic neuron responses to chemical and mechanical stimuli following combined micro-iontophoretic application of N-methyl-D-aspartic acid and substance P. *Pain*, 47: 85–93.

Dougherty, P.M., Palecek, J., Zorn, S. and Willis, W.D. (1993) Combined application of excitatory amino acids and substance P produces long-lasting changes in responses of primate spinothalamic tract neurons. *Brain Res. Rev.*, 18: 227–246.

Doyle, C.A. and Maxwell, D.J. (1993) Neuropeptide Y-immunoreactive terminals form axo-axonic synaptic arrangements in the substantia gelatinosa (lamina II) of the cat spinal dorsal horn. *Brain Res.*, 603: 157–161.

Duffy, M.J. and Powell, D. (1975) Stimulation of brain adenylate cyclase activity by the undecapeptide substance P and its modulation by the calcium ion. *Biochim. Biophys. Acta*, 385: 275–280.

Duggan, A.W. (1992) Neuropeptide release in the spinal cord in response to noxious and non-noxious stimulation. *Neuropeptides*, 22: 19.

Duggan, A.W., Hall, J.G. and Headley, P.M. (1976) Morphine, enkephalin and the substantia gelatinosa. *Nature*, 264: 456–458.

Duggan, A.W., Hall, J.G. and Headley, P.M. (1977) Enkephalins and dorsal horn neurons of the cat: effects on responses to noxious and innocuous skin stimuli. *Br. J. Pharmacol.*, 61: 399–408.

Duggan, A.W., Morton, C.R., Zhao, Z.Q. and Hendry, I.A. (1987) Noxious heating of the skin releases immunoreactive substance P in the substantia gelatinosa of the cat: a study with antibody microprobes. *Brain Res.*, 403: 345–349.

Duggan, A.W., Hendry, I.A., Morton, C.R., Hutchison, W.D. and Zhao, Z.Q. (1988) Cutaneous stimuli releasing immunoreactive substance P in the dorsal horn of the cat. *Brain Res.*, 451: 261–273.

Duggan, A.W., Hope, P.J., Jarrott, B., Schaible, H.-G. and Fleetwood-Walker, S.M. (1990) Release, spread and persistence of immunoreactive neurokinin A in the dorsal horn of the cat following noxious cutaneous stimulation. Studies with antibody microprobes. *Neuroscience*, 35: 195–202.

El-Bohy, A. and LaMotte, C.C. (1993) Deafferentation-induced changes in neuropeptides of the adult rat dorsal horn following pronase injection of the sciatic nerve. *J. Comp. Neurol.*, 336: 545–554.

Elmslie, K.S. (1992) Calcium current modulation in frog sympathetic neurons: multiple neurotransmitters and G proteins. *J. Physiol. (London)*, 451: 229–246.

Fisher, N.D. and Nistri, A. (1993) A study of the barium-sensitive and -insensitive components of the action of thyrotropin-releasing hormone on lumbar motoneurons of the rat isolated spinal cord. *Eur. J. Neurosci.*, 5: 1360–1369.

Fleetwood-Walker, S.M., Parker, R.M.C., Munro, F.E., Young, M.R., Hope, P.J. and Mitchell, R. (1993) Evidence for a role of tachykinin NK_2 receptors in mediating brief nociceptive inputs to rat dorsal horn (laminae III–V) neurons. *Eur. J. Pharmacol.*, 242: 173–181.

Fone, K.C.F., Johnson, J.V., Putland, A.P. and Bennett, G.W. (1991) Ventral horn neuropeptides modulate the release of noradrenaline from tissue slices of rat brainstem and ventral thoracic spinal cord. *J. Neurochem.*, 57: 845–851.

Fuxe, K., Agnati, L.F., McDonald, T., Locatelli, V., Hökfelt, T., Dalsgaard, C.-J., Battistini, N., Yanaihara, N., Mutt, V. and Cuello, A.C. (1983) Immunohistochemical indications of gastrin releasing peptide bombesin-like immunoreactivity in the nervous system of the rat. Codistribution with substance P-like immunoreactive terminal systems and coexistence with substance P-like immunoreactivity in dorsal root ganglion cell bodies. *Neurosci. Lett.*, 37: 17–22.

Gallacher, D.V., Hanley, M.R., Petersen, O.H., Roberts, M.L., Squire-Pollard, L.G. and Yule, D.I. (1990) Substance P and bombesin elevate cytosolic Ca^{2+} by different molecular mechanisms in a rat pancreatic acinar cell line. *J. Physiol. (London)*, 426: 193–207.

Garces, Y.I., Rabito, S.F., Minshall, R.D. and Sagen, J. (1993) Lack of potent antinociceptive activity by substance P antagonist CP-96,345 in the rat spinal cord. *Life Sci.*, 52: 353–360.

Garthwaite, J., Charles, S.L. and Chess-Williams, R. (1988) Endothelium-derived relaxing factor release on activation of NMDA receptors suggests role as intracellular messenger in the brain. *Nature*, 336: 385–388.

Gibson, S.J., Polak, J.M., Bloom, S.R., Sabate, I.M., Mulderry, P.M., Ghatei, M.A., McGregor, G.P., Morrison, J.F., Kelly, J.S., Evans, R.M. and Rosenfeld, M.G. (1984) Calcitonin gene-related peptide immunoreactivity in the spinal cord of man and eight other species. *J. Neurosci.*, 4: 3101–3111.

Go, V.L.W. and Yaksh, T.L. (1987) Release of substance P from the cat spinal cord. *J. Physiol. (London)*, 391: 141–167.

Gouarderes, C., Jhamandas, K., Cridland, R., Cros, J., Quirion, R. and Zajac, J.M. (1993) Opioid and substance P receptor adaptations in the rat spinal cord following sub-chronic intrathecal treatment with morphine and naloxone. *Neuroscience*, 54: 799–807.

Guard, S., Boyle, S.J., Tang, K.-W., Watling, K.J., McKnight, A.T. and Woodruff, G.N. (1993) The interaction of the NK_1 receptor antagonist CP-96,345 with L-type calcium channels and its functional consequences. *Br. J. Pharmacol.*, 110: 385–391.

Guo, J.-Z., Yoshioka, K., Yanagisawa, M., Hagan, R.M. and Otsuka, M. (1993a) Blockade of cutaneous nerve-evoked responses by GR71251 in the isolated spinal cord preparation of newborn rat. *Regul. Peptides*, 46: 309–310.

Guo, J.-Z., Yoshioka, K., Yanagisawa, M., Hosoki, R., Hagan, R.M. and Otsuka, M. (1993b) Depression of primary afferent-evoked responses by GR71251 in the isolated spinal cord of the neonatal rat. *Br. J. Pharmacol.*, 110: 1142–1148.

Hanley, M.R., Lee, C.M., Jones, L.M. and Mitchell, R.H. (1980) Similar effects of substance P and related peptides on salivation and on phosphatidylinositol turnover in rat salivary glands. *Mol. Pharmacol.*, 18: 78–83.

Hannan, L.J. and Ho, R.H. (1992) Anatomical evidence for interactions between somatostatin neurites in lamina II of the rat spinal cord. *Peptides*, 13: 329–337.

Henry, J.L. (1976) Effects of substance P on functionally identified units in cat spinal cord. *Brain Res.*, 114: 439–451.

Henry, J.L. (1983) Naloxone fails to block substance P-induced excitation of spinal nociceptive units. *Brain Res. Bull.*, 10: 727–730.

Henry, J.L. (1993) Participation of substance P in spinal physiological responses to peripheral aversive stimulation. *Regul. Peptides*, 46: 138–143.

Henry, J.L. and Ben Ari, Y. (1976) Actions of p-chlorophenyl derivative of GABA, Lioresal, on nociceptive and non-nociceptive units in the spinal cord of the cat. *Brain Res.*, 117: 540–544.

Henry, J.L., Krnjević, K. and Morris, M.E. (1975) Substance P and spinal neurons. *Can. J. Physiol. Pharmacol.*, 53: 423–432.

Hirota, N., Kuraishi, Y., Hino, Y., Sato, Y., Satoh, M. and Takagi, H. (1985) Met-enkephalin and morphine but not dynorphin inhibit noxious stimuli-induced release of substance P from rabbit dorsal horn in situ. *Neuropharmacology*, 24: 567–570.

Homma, E., Collins, J.G. and Kitahata, L.M. (1983) Effects of intrathecal morphine on activity of dorsal horn neurons activated by noxious heat. In: JJ. Bonica, U. Lindblom and A. Iggo (Eds.), *Advances in Pain Research and Therapy, Vol. 5.* Raven Press, New York, pp. 481–485.

Hökfelt, T., Kellerth, J.-O., Nilsson, G. and Pernow, B. (1975a) Experimental immunohistochemical studies on the localization and distribution of substance P in cat primary sensory neurons. *Brain Res.*, 100: 235–252.

Hökfelt, T., Kellerth, J.-O., Nilsson, G. and Pernow, B. (1975b) Substance P: localization in the central nervous system and in some primary sensory neurons. *Science*, 190: 889–891.

Hökfelt, T., Ljungdahl, A., Terenius, L., Elde, R. and Nilsson, G. (1977) Immunohistochemical analysis of peptide pathways possibly related to pain and analgesia: enkephalin and substance P. *Proc. Natl. Acad. Sci. USA*, 74: 3081–3085.

Hösli, L., Hösli, E., Zehntner, C. and Landolt, H. (1981) Effects of substance P on neurones and glial cells in cultured rat spinal cord. *Neurosci. Lett.*, 24: 165–168.

Hösli, L., Hösli, E., Kaeser, H. and Lefkovits, M. (1992) Colocalization of receptors for vasoactive peptides on astrocytes of cultured rat spinal cord and brain stem: electrophysiological effects of atrial and brain natriuretic peptide,

neuropeptide Y and bradykinin. *Neurosci. Lett.*, 148: 114–116.

Hua, X.-Y., Theodorsson-Norheim, E., Brodin, E., Lundberg, J.M. and Hökfelt, T. (1985) Multiple tachykinins (neurokinin A, neuropeptide K and substance P) in capsaicin-sensitive neurons in the guinea-pig. *Regul. Peptides*, 13: 1–19.

Hunter, J.C., Birchmore, B., Woodruff, R. and Hughes, J. (1989) Kappa opioid binding sites in the dog cerebral cortex and spinal cord. *Neuroscience*, 31: 735–743.

Hutchison, W.D., Morton, C.R. and Terenius, L. (1990) Dynorphin A: in vivo release in the spinal cord of the cat. *Brain Res.*, 532: 299–306.

Jackson, D.A. and White, S.R. (1988) Thyrotropin releasing hormone (TRH) modifies excitability of spinal cord dorsal horn cells. *Neurosci. Lett.*, 92: 171–176.

Jacquin, M.F., Beinfeld, M.C., Chiaia, N.L. and Zahm, D.S. (1992) Cholecystokinin concentrations and peptide immunoreactivity in the intact and deafferented medullary dorsal horn of the rat. *J. Comp. Neurol.*, 326: 22–43.

Jeftinija, S. (1988) Enkephalins modulate excitatory synaptic transmission in the superficial dorsal horn by acting at mu-opioid receptor sites. *Brain Res.*, 460: 260–268.

Jeftinija, S., Miletić, V. and Randić, M. (1981) Cholecystokinin octapeptide excites dorsal horn neurons both in vivo and in vitro. *Brain Res.*, 213: 231–236.

Jeftinija, S., Murase, K., Nedeljkov, V. and Randić, M. (1982) Vasoactive intestinal polypeptide excites mammalian dorsal horn neurons both in vivo and in vitro. *Brain Res.*, 243: 158–164.

Jeftinija, S., Urban, L. and Kojić, L. (1993) The selective activation of dorsal horn neurons by potassium stimulation of high threshold primary afferent neurons *in vitro*. *Neuroscience*, 56: 473–484.

Jessell, T.M. and Iversen, L.L. (1977) Opiate analgesics inhibit substance P release from rat trigeminal nucleus. *Nature*, 268: 549–551.

Jones, S.W. (1985) Muscarinic and peptidergic excitation of bull-frog sympathetic neurones. *J. Physiol. (London)*, 366: 63–87.

Ju, G., Hökfelt, T., Brodin, E., Fahrenkrug, J., Fischer, J.A., Frey, P., Elde, R.P. and Brown, J.C. (1987) Primary sensory neurons of the rat showing calcitonin gene-related peptide immunoreactivity and their relation to substance P-, somatostatin-, galanin-, vasoactive intestinal polypeptide-and cholecystokinin-immunoreactive ganglion cells. *Cell Tissue Res.*, 247: 417–431.

Kangrga, I. and Randić, M. (1990) Tachykinins and calcitonin gene-related peptide enhance release of endogenous glutamate and aspartate from the rat spinal dorsal horn slice. *J. Neurosci.*, 10: 2026–2038.

Kar, S. and Quirion, R. (1992) Quantitative autoradiographic localization of [^{125}I]neuropeptide Y receptor binding sites in rat spinal cord and the effects of neonatal capsaicin, dorsal rhizotomy and peripheral axotomy. *Brain Res.*, 574: 333–337.

Kawagoe, R., Onodera, K. and Takeuchi, A. (1986) The release of endogenous glutamate from the newborn rat spinal cord induced by dorsal root stimulation and substance P. *Biomed. Res.*, 7: 253–259.

Kellstein, D.E., Price, D.D., Hayes, R.L. and Mayer, D.J. (1990) Evidence that substance P selectively modulates C-fiber-evoked discharges of dorsal horn nociceptive neurons. *Brain Res.*, 526: 291–298.

Kellstein, D.E., Price, D.D. and Mayer, D.J. (1991) Cholecystokinin and its antagonist lorglumide respectively attenuate and facilitate morphine-induced inhibition of C-fiber evoked discharges of dorsal horn nociceptive neurons. *Brain Res.*, 540: 302–306.

Klein, C.M., Coggeshall, R.E., Carlton, S.M. and Sorkin, L.S. (1992) The effects of A- and C-fiber stimulation on patterns of neuropeptide immunostaining in the rat superficial dorsal horn. *Brain Res.*, 580: 121–128.

Knowles, R.G., Palacios, M., Palmer, R.M.J. and Moncada, S. (1989) Formation of nitric oxide from L-arginine in the central nervous system: a transduction mechanism for stimulation of the soluble guanylate cyclase. *Proc. Natl. Acad. Sci. USA*, 86: 5159–5162.

Knowles, R.G., Palacios, M., Palmer, R.M.J. and Moncada, S. (1990) Kinetic characteristics of nitric oxide synthase from rat brain. *Biochem. J.*, 269: 207–210.

Knyihár-Csillik, E., Kreutzberg, G.W., Raivich, G. and Csillik, B. (1991) A case for transmitter plasticity at the molecular level: axotomy-induced VIP increase in the upper spinal dorsal horn is related to blockade of retrograde axoplasmic transport of nerve growth factor in the peripheral nerve. *Acta Histochem. (Jena)*, 91: 77–83.

Knyihár-Csillik, E., Kreutzberg, G.W. and Csillik, B. (1993) Fine structural correlates of VIP-like immunoreactivity in the upper spinal dorsal horn after peripheral axotomy: possibilities of a neuro-glial translocation of a neuropeptide. *Acta Histochem.*, 94: 1–12.

Krause, J.E., Bu, J.-Y., Takeda, Y., Blount, P., Raddatz, R., Sachais, B.S., Chou, K.B., Takeda, J., McCarson, K. and DiMaggio, D. (1993) Structure, expression and second messenger-mediated regulation of the human and rat substance P receptors and their genes. *Regul. Peptides*, 46: 59–66.

Krnjević, K. (1977) Effects of substance P on central neurons in cats. In: U.S. von Euler and B. Pernow (Eds.), *Substance P*. Raven Press, New York, pp. 217–230.

Kuraishi, Y., Hirota, N., Sato, Y., Hino, Y., Satoh, M. and Takagi, H. (1985) Evidence that substance P and somatostatin transmit separate information related to pain in the spinal dorsal horn. *Brain Res.*, 325: 294–298.

Kuraishi, Y., Minami, M. and Satoh, M. (1991) Serotonin, but neither noradrenaline nor GABA, inhibits capsaicin-evoked

release of immunoreactive somatostatin from slices of rat spinal cord. *Neurosci. Res.*, 9: 238–245.

Laird, J.M.A., Hargreaves, R.J. and Hill, R.G. (1993) Effect of RP 67580, a non-peptide neurokinin$_1$ receptor antagonist, on facilitation of a nociceptive spinal flexion reflex in the rat. *Br. J. Pharmacol.*, 109: 713–718.

Lembeck, F. (1953) Zur Frage der zentralen Übertragung afferenter Impulse. III. Mitteilung. Das Vorkommen und die Bedeutung der Substanz P in den dorsalen Wurzeln des Rückenmarks. *Arch. Exp. Pathol. Pharmakol.*, 219: 197–213.

Lewis, M.J. and Henderson, A.H. (1987) A phorbol ester inhibits the release of endothelium-derived relaxing factor. *Eur. J. Pharmacol.*, 137: 167–171.

Light, A.R. and Perl, E.R. (1979) Spinal termination of functionally identified primary afferent neurons with slowly conducting myelinated fibers. *J. Comp. Neurol.*, 186: 133–150.

Lu, J. and Ho, R.H. (1992) Evidence for dorsal root projection to somatostatin-immunoreactive structures in laminae I–II of the spinal dorsal horn. *Brain Res. Bull.*, 28: 17–26.

Lucas, D. and Yaksh, T.L. (1990) Release in vivo of met-enkephalin and encrypted forms of met-enkephalin from brain and spinal cord of the anesthetized cat. *Peptides*, 11: 1119–1125.

Maehara, T., Suzuki, H., Yoshioka, K. and Otsuka, M. (1993) Substance P-evoked release of amino acid transmitters from the newborn rat spinal cord. *Regul. Peptides*, 46: 354–356.

Maggi, C.A., Patacchini, R., Rovero, P. and Giachetti, A. (1993) Tachykinin receptors and tachykinin receptor antagonists. *J. Auton. Pharmacol.*, 13: 23–93.

Mantyh, P.W., Pinnock, R.D., Downes, C.P., Goedert, M. and Hunt, S.P. (1984) Correlation between inositol phospholipid hydrolysis and substance P receptors in rat CNS. *Nature*, 309: 795–797.

Mao, J., Coghill, R.C., Kellstein, D.E., Frenk, H. and Mayer, D.J. (1992) Calcitonin gene-related peptide enhances substance P-induced behaviors via metabolic inhibition: in vivo evidence for a new mechanism of neuromodulation. *Brain Res.*, 574: 157–163.

Massari, V.J., Tizabi, Y., Park, C.H., Moody, T.W., Helke, C.J. and O'Donohue, T.L. (1983) Distribution and origin of bombesin, substance P and somatostatin in rat spinal cord. *Peptides*, 4: 673–681.

Matthews, G., Neher, E. and Penner, R. (1989) Second messenger-activated calcium influx in rat peritoneal mast cells. *J. Physiol. (London)*, 418: 105–130.

McLean, S., Ganong, A.H., Seeger, T., Bryce, D.K., Pratt, K.G., Reynolds, L.S., Siok, C.J., Lowe, J.A., III and Heym, J. (1991) Activity and distribution of binding sites in brain of a nonpeptide substance P (NK$_1$) receptor antagonist. *Science*, 251: 437–439.

McLean, S., Ganong, A., Seymour, P.A., Snider, R.M., Desai, M.C., Rosen, T., Bryce, D.K., Longo, K.P., Reynolds, L.S.,

192

Robinson, G., Schmidt, A.W., Siok, C. and Heym, J. (1993) Pharmacology of CP-99,994; a nonpeptide antagonist of the tachykinin neurokinin-1 receptor. *J. Pharmacol. Exp. Ther.*, 267: 472–479.

Medina, V.M., Wang, L. and Gintzler, A.R. (1993) Spinal cord dynorphin: positive region-specific modulation during pregnancy and parturition. *Brain Res.*, 623: 41–46.

Merighi, A., Polak, J.M. and Theodosis, D.T. (1991) Ultra-structural visualization of glutamate and aspartate immunoreactivities in the rat dorsal horn, with special reference to the co-localization of glutamate, substance P and calcitonin-gene related peptide. *Neuroscience*, 40: 67–80.

Merritt, J.E. and Rink, T.J. (1987) The effects of substance P and carbachol on inositol tri- and tetrakisphosphate formation and cytosolic free calcium in rat parotid acinar cells. A correlation between inositol phosphate levels and calcium entry. *J. Biol. Chem.*, 262: 14912–14916.

Miletić, V. and Randić, M. (1979) Neurotensin excites cat spinal neurons located in laminae I–III. *Brain Res.*, 169: 600–604.

Miletić, V. and Tan, H. (1988) Iontophoretic application of calcitonin gene-related peptide produces a slow and prolonged excitation of neurons in the cat lumbar dorsal horn. *Brain Res.*, 446: 169–172.

Mistry, A. and Vijayan, E. (1987) Differential responses of hypothalamic cAMP and cGMP to substance P and neurotensin in ovariectomized rats. *Brain Res. Bull.*, 18: 169–173.

Mitsuhashi, M., Ohashi, Y., Shichijo, S., Christian, C., Sudduth-Klinger, J., Harrowe, G. and Payan, D.G. (1992) Multiple intracellular signaling pathways of the neuropeptide substance P receptor. *J. Neurosci. Res.*, 32: 437–443.

Mochizuki-Oda, N., Nakajima, Y., Nakanishi, S. and Ito, S. (1993) Substance P-induced elevation of intracellular calcium in transfected Chinese hamster ovary cells: Role of inositol trisphosphate. *Regul. Peptides*, 46: 450–452.

Mohini, P., Bahouth, S.W., Brundish, D.E. and Musaccaio, J.M. (1985) Specific labelling of rat brain substance P receptors with physalaemin. *J. Neurosci.*, 5: 2078–2085.

Moncada, S., Palmer, R.M.J. and Higgs, E.A. (1991) Nitric oxide: Physiology, pathophysiology, and pharmacology. *Pharmacol. Rev.*, 43: 109–142.

Morton, C.R. and Hutchison, W.D. (1989) Release of sensory neuropeptides in the spinal cord: studies with calcitonin gene-related peptide and galanin. *Neuroscience*, 31: 807–815.

Morton, C.R., Hutchison, W.D., Hendry, I.A. and Duggan, A.W. (1989) Somatostatin: evidence for a role in thermal nociception. *Brain Res.*, 488: 89–96.

Moser, A. (1990) Guanine nucleotides regulate the effect of substance P on striatal adenylate cyclase of the rat. *Biochem. Biophys. Res. Commun.*, 167: 211–215.

Murase, K., Nedeljkov, V. and Randić, M. (1982) The actions of neuropeptides on dorsal horn neurons in the rat spinal cord slice preparation: an intracellular study. *Brain Res.*, 234: 170–176.

Murase, K., Ryu, P.D. and Randić, M. (1986) Substance P augments a persistent slow inward calcium-sensitive current in voltage-clamped spinal dorsal horn neurons of the rat. *Brain Res.*, 365: 369–376.

Murase, K., Ryu, P.D. and Randić, M. (1989) Excitatory and inhibitory amino acids and peptide-induced responses in acutely isolated rat spinal dorsal horn neurons. *Neurosci. Lett.*, 103: 56–63.

Nagy, I., Maggi, C.A., Dray, A., Woolf, C.J. and Urban, L. (1993) The role of neurokinin and *N*-methyl-D-aspartate receptors in synaptic transmission from capsaicin-sensitive primary afferents in the rat spinal cord in vitro. *Neuroscience*, 52: 1029–1037.

Nakajima, Y., Nakajima, S. and Inoue, M. (1988) Pertussis toxin-insensitive G protein mediates substance P-induced inhibition of potassium channels in brain neurons. *Proc. Natl. Acad. Sci. USA*, 85: 3643–3647.

Nakajima, Y., Stanfield, P.R., Yamaguchi, K. and Nakajima, S. (1991) Substance P excites cultured cholinergic neurons in the basal forebrain. *Adv. Exp. Med. Biol.*, 295: 157–167.

Nakajima, Y., Tsuchida, K., Negishi, M., Ito, S. and Nakanishi, S. (1992) Direct linkage of three tachykinin receptors to stimulation of both phosphatydylinositol hydrolysis and cyclic AMP cascades in transfected Chinese hamster ovary cells. *J. Biol. Chem.*, 267: 2437–2442.

Nakajima, Y., Koyano, K., Velimirovic, B.M., Grigg, J.J. and Nakajima, S. (1993) Signal transduction mechanisms of substance P effects on ion channels. *Regul. Peptides*, 46: 110–113.

Nicoll, R.A., Schenker, C. and Leeman, S.E. (1980) Substance P as a transmitter candidate. *Ann. Rev. Neurosci.*, 3: 227–268.

Ninkovic, M., Beaujouan, J.C., Torrens, Y., Saffroy, M., Hall, M.D. and Glowinski, J. (1984) Differential localization of tachykinin receptors in rat spinal cord. *Eur. J. Pharmacol.*, 106: 463–464.

Nistri, A., Fisher, N.D. and Gurnell, M. (1990) Block by the neuropeptide TRH of an apparently novel K^+ conductance of rat motoneurones. *Neurosci. Lett.*, 120: 25–30.

Nowak, L.M. and Macdonald, R.L. (1982) Substance P: ionic basis for depolarizing responses of mouse spinal cord neurons in cell culture. *J. Neurosci.*, 2: 1119–1128.

O'Donohue, T.L., Massari, J.V., Christopher, P.J., Chronwall, B.M., Shults, C.W., Quirion, R., Chase, T.N. and Moody, T.W. (1984) A role for bombesin in sensory processing in the spinal cord. *J. Neurosci.*, 4: 2956–2962.

Otsuka, M. and Yanagisawa, M. (1990) Pain and neurotransmitters. *Cell. Mol. Neurobiol.*, 10: 293–302.

Otsuka, M. and Yoshioka, K. (1993) Neurotransmitter functions of mammalian tachykinins. *Physiol. Rev.*, 73: 229–308.

Pernow, B. (1953) Studies on substance P. Purification, occurrence and biological actions. *Acta Physiol. Scand.*, 29(Suppl. 105): 1–90.

Persson, M.G., Hedqvist, P. and Gustafsson, L.E. (1991) Nerve-induced tachykinin-mediated vasodilatation in skeletal muscle is dependent on nitric oxide formation. *Eur. J. Pharmacol.*, 205: 295–301.

Pickel, V.M., Reis, D.J. and Leeman, S.E. (1977) Ultrastructural localization of substance P in neurons of rat spinal cord. *Brain Res.*, 122: 534–540.

Piercey, M.F., Einsphar, F.J., Dorbry, P.J.K., Schroeder, L.A. and Hollister, R.P. (1980) Morphine does not antagonize the substance P mediated excitation of dorsal horn neurons. *Brain Res.*, 186: 421–434.

Proudlock, F., Spike, R.C. and Todd, A.J. (1993) Immunocytochemical study of somatostatin, neurotensin, GABA, and glycine in rat spinal dorsal horn. *J. Comp. Neurol.*, 327: 289–297.

Quirion, R. (1985) Multiple tachykinin receptors. *Trends Neurosci.*, 8: 183–185.

Radhakrishnan, V. and Henry, J.L. (1991) Novel substance P antagonist, CP-96,345, blocks responses of cat spinal dorsal horn neurones to noxious cutaneous stimulation and to substance P. *Neurosci. Lett.*, 132: 39–43.

Radhakrishnan, V. and Henry, J.L. (1993a) Excitatory amino acid receptor mediation of sensory inputs to functionally identified dorsal horn neurons in cat spinal cord. *Neuroscience*, 55: 531–544.

Radhakrishnan, V. and Henry, J.L. (1993b) L-NAME blocks responses to NMDA, substance P and noxious cutaneous stimuli in cat dorsal horn. *NeuroReport*, 4: 323–326.

Radhakrishnan, V. and Henry, J.L. (1995) Antagonism of nociceptive responses of cat spinal dorsal horn neurons *in vivo* by the NK-1 receptor antagonists CP-96,345 and CP-99,994, but not by CP-96,344. *Neuroscience*, 64: 943–958.

Randić, M. and Miletić, V. (1977) Effect of substance P in cat dorsal horn neurones activated by noxious stimuli. *Brain Res.*, 128: 164–169.

Randić, M. and Miletić, V. (1978) Depressant actions of methionine-enkephalin and somatostatin in cat dorsal horn neurones activated by noxious stimuli. *Brain Res.*, 152: 196–202.

Randić, M., Hecimovic, H. and Ryu, P.D. (1990) Substance P modulates glutamate-induced currents in acutely isolated rat spinal dorsal horn neurones. *Neurosci. Lett.*, 117: 74–80.

Randić, M., Jiang, M.C., Rusin, K.I., Cerne, R. and Kolaj, M. (1993) Interactions between excitatory amino acids and tachykinins and long-term changes of synaptic responses in the rat spinal dorsal horn. *Regul. Peptides*, 46: 418–420.

Ribeiro-da-Silva, A., Pioro, E.P. and Cuello, A.C. (1991) Substance P- and enkephalin-like immunoreactivities are colocalized in certain neurons of the substantia gelatinosa of the rat spinal cord: an ultrastructural double-labeling study. *J. Neurosci.*, 11: 1068–1080.

Rowan, S., Todd, A.J. and Spike, R.C. (1993) Evidence that neuropeptide Y is present in GABAergic neurons in the superficial dorsal horn of the rat spinal cord. *Neuroscience*, 53: 537–545.

Rusin, K.I., Ryu, P.D. and Randić, M. (1992) Modulation of excitatory amino acid responses in rat dorsal horn neurons by tachykinins. *J. Neurophysiol.*, 68: 265–286.

Rusin, K.I., Bleakman, D., Chard, P.S., Randić, M. and Miller, R.J. (1993a) Tachykinins potentiate N-methyl-D-aspartate responses in acutely isolated neurons from the dorsal horn. *J. Neurochem.*, 60: 952–960.

Rusin, K.I., Jiang, M.C., Cerne, R. and Randić, M. (1993b) Interactions between excitatory amino acids and tachykinins in the rat spinal dorsal horn. *Brain Res. Bull.*, 30: 329–338.

Ryu, P.D. and Randić, M. (1990) Low- and high-voltage-activated calcium currents in rat spinal dorsal horn neurons. *J. Neurophysiol.*, 63: 273–285.

Ryu, P.D., Gerber, G., Murase, K. and Randić, M. (1988) Actions of calcitonin gene-related peptide on rat spinal dorsal horn neurons. *Brain Res.*, 441: 357–361.

Salter, M.W. and Henry, J.L. (1985) Effects of adenosine 5'-monophosphate and adenosine 5'-triphosphate on functionally identified units in the cat spinal dorsal horn. Evidence for a differential effect of adenosine 5'-triphosphate on nociceptive vs non-nociceptive units. *Neuroscience*, 15: 815–825.

Salter, M.W. and Henry, J.L. (1987a) Evidence that adenosine mediates the depression of spinal dorsal horn neurons induced by peripheral vibration in the cat. *Neuroscience*, 22: 631–650.

Salter, M.W. and Henry, J.L. (1987b) Purine-induced depression of dorsal horn neurons in the cat spinal cord: enhancement by tachykinins. *Neuroscience*, 23: 903–915.

Salter, M.W. and Henry, J.L. (1988) Tachykinins enhance the depression of spinal nociceptive neurons caused by cutaneously applied vibration in the cat. *Neuroscience*, 27: 243–249.

Salter, M.W. and Henry, J.L. (1991) Responses of functionally identified neurons in the dorsal horn of the cat spinal cord to substance P, neurokinin A and physalaemin. *Neuroscience*, 43: 601–610.

Sandkühler, J., Fu, Q.-G. and Helmchen, C. (1990) Spinal somatostatin superfusion *in vivo* affects activity of cat nociceptive dorsal horn neurons: comparison with spinal morphine. *Neuroscience*, 34: 565–576.

Sastry, B.R. and Goh, J.W. (1983) Actions of morphine and met-enkephaline-amide on nociceptor driven neurones in substantia gelatinosa and deeper dorsal horn. *Neuropharmacology*, 22: 119–122.

Schini, V.B., Katusic, Z.S. and Vanhoutte, P.M. (1990) Neurohypophyseal peptides and tachykinins stimulate the production of cyclic GMP in cultured porcine aortic endothelial cells. *J. Pharmacol. Exp. Ther.*, 255: 994–1000.

Schmidt, A.W., McLean, S. and Heym, J. (1992) The substance P receptor antagonist CP-96,345 interacts with Ca^{2+} channels. Eur. J. Pharmacol., 215: 351–352.

Seabrook, G.R. and Fong, T.M. (1993) Thapsigargin blocks the mobilisation of intracellular calcium caused by activation of human NK1 (long) receptors expressed in chinese hamster ovary cells. Neurosci. Lett., 152: 9–12.

Shapiro, M.S. and Hille, B. (1993) Substance P and somatostatin inhibit calcium channels in rat sympathetic neurons via different G protein pathways. Neuron, 10: 11–20.

Sharma, H.S., Nyberg, F., Thörnwall, M. and Olsson, Y. (1993) Met-enkephalin-Arg[6]-Phe[7] in spinal cord and brain following traumatic injury to the spinal cord: influence of p-chlorophenylalanine. An experimental study in the rat using radioimmunoassay technique. Neuropharmacology, 32: 711–717.

Shen, K.-Z. and Surprenant, A. (1993) Common ionic mechanisms of excitation by substance P and other transmitters in guinea-pig submucosal neurones. J. Physiol. (London), 462: 483–501.

Sjödin, L., Conlon, T.P., Gustavson, C. and Uddholm, K. (1980) Interaction of substance P with dispersed pancreatic acinar cells from the guinea pig. Stimulation of calcium outflux, accumulation of cyclic GMP and amylase release. Acta Physiol. Scand., 109: 107–110.

Skilling, S.R., Harkness, D.H. and Larson, A.A. (1992) Experimental peripheral neuropathy decreases the dose of substance P required to increase excitatory amino acid release in the CSF of the rat spinal cord. Neurosci. Lett., 139: 92–96.

Sluka, K.A. and Westlund, K.N. (1993) Spinal cord amino acid release and content in an arthritis model: the effects of pretreatment with non-NMDA, NMDA, and NK1 receptor antagonists. Brain Res., 627: 89–103.

Snider, R.M., Constantine, J.W., Lowe, J.A., III, Longo, K.P., Lebel, W.S., Woody, H.A., Drozda, S.E., Desai, M.C., Vinick, F.J., Spencer, R.W. and Hess, H.-J. (1991) A potent nonpeptide antagonist of the substance P (NK1) receptor. Science, 251: 435–437.

Stanfa, L.C. and Dickenson, A.H. (1993) Cholecystokinin as a factor in the enhanced potency of spinal morphine following carrageenin inflammation. Br. J. Pharmacol., 108: 967–973.

Stanfield, P.R., Nakajima, Y. and Yamaguchi, K. (1985) Substance P raises neuronal membrane excitability by reducing inward rectification. Nature, 315: 498–501.

Stanzione, P. and Zieglgänsberger, W. (1983) Action of neurotensin on spinal cord neurons in the rat. Brain Res., 268: 111–118.

Sugiura, Y., Lee, C.L. and Perl, E.R. (1986) Central projections of identified, unmyelinated (C) afferent fibers innervating mammalian skin. Science, 234: 358–361.

Sullivan, A.F., Dickenson, A.H. and Roques, B.P. (1989) δ-Opioid mediated inhibitions of acute and prolonged nox-

ious-evoked responses in rat dorsal horn neurones. Br. J. Pharmacol., 98: 1039–1049.

Takahashi, T. and Otsuka, M. (1975) Regional distribution of substance P in the spinal cord and nerve roots of the cat and the effect of dorsal root section. Brain Res., 87: 1–11.

Takano, M., Takano, Y. and Yaksh, T.L. (1993) Release of calcitonin gene-related peptide (CGRP), substance P (SP), and vasoactive intestinal polypeptide (VIP) from rat spinal cord: Modulation by α_2 agonists. Peptides, 14: 371–378.

Takeda, Y., Blount, P., Sachais, B.S., Hershey, A.D., Raddatz, R. and Krause, J.E. (1992) Ligand binding kinetics of substance P and neurokinin A receptors stably expressed in Chinese hamster ovary cells and evidence for differential stimulation of inositol 1,4,5-trisphosphate and cyclic AMP second messenger responses. J. Neurochem., 59: 740–745.

Taylor, C.W., Merritt, J.E., Putney, J.W. and Rubin, R.P. (1986) A guanine nucleotide-dependent regulatory protein couples substance P receptors to phospholipase C in rat parotid gland. Biochem. Biophys. Res. Commun., 136: 362–368.

Tiseo, P.J., Adler, M.W. and Liu-Chen, L.-Y. (1990) Differential release of substance P and somatostatin in the rat spinal cord in response to noxious cold and heat; effect of dynorphin $A_{(1-17)}$. J. Pharmacol. Exp. Ther., 252: 539–545.

Toda, T. and Hayashi, H. (1993) The inhibitory effect of substance P antagonist, CP-96,345, on the late discharges of nociceptive neurons in the rat superficial spinal dorsal horn. Neurosci. Lett., 158: 36–38.

Todd, A.J., Russell, G. and Spike, R.C. (1992) Immunocytochemical evidence that GABA and neurotensin exist in different neurons in laminae II and III of rat spinal dorsal horn. Neuroscience, 47: 685–691.

Thompson, S.W.N., Urban, L. and Dray, A. (1993) Contribution of NK_1 and NK_2 receptor activation to high threshold afferent fibre evoked ventral root responses in the rat spinal cord in vitro. Brain Res., 625: 100–108.

Ulfhake, B., Arvidsson, U., Cullheim, S., Hökfelt, T. and Visser, T.J. (1987) Thyrotropin-releasing hormone (TRH)-immunoreactive boutons and nerve cell bodies in the dorsal horn of the cat L7 spinal cord. Neurosci. Lett., 73: 3–8.

Urban, L. and Randić, M. (1984) Slow excitatory transmission in rat dorsal horn: possible mediation by peptides. Brain Res., 290: 336–341.

Urban, L., Dray, A., Nagy, I. and Maggi, C.A. (1993) The effects of NK-1 and NK-2 receptor antagonists on the capsaicin evoked synaptic response in the rat spinal cord in vitro. Regul. Peptides, 46: 413–414.

Verge, V.M.K., Wiesenfeld-Hallin, Z. and Hökfelt, T. (1993) Cholecystokinin in mammalian primary sensory neurons and spinal cord: in situ hybridization studies in rat and monkey. Eur. J. Neurosci., 5: 240–250.

Vita, G., Haun, C.K., Hawkins, E.F. and Engel, W.K. (1990) Effects of experimental spinal cord transection on substance P receptors: a quantitative autoradiography study. *Neuropeptides*, 17: 147–153.

Warden, M.K. and Young, W.S. (1988) Distribution of cells containing mRNAs encoding substance P and neurokinin B in the rat central nervous system. *J. Comp. Neurol.*, 272: 90–113.

Watling, K.J. (1992) Nonpeptide antagonists herald new era in tachykinin research. *Trends Pharmacol. Sci.*, 13: 266–269.

Watson, S.P. and Downes, C.P. (1983) Substance P induced hydrolysis of inositol phospholipids in guinea-pig ileum and rat hypothalamus. *Eur. J. Pharmacol.*, 93: 245–253.

Wiesenfeld-Hallin, Z., Hökfelt, T., Lundberg, J.M., Forssmann, W.G., Reinecke, M., Tschopp, F.A. and Fischer, J. (1984) Immunoreactive calcitonin gene-related peptide and substance P coexist in sensory neurons to the spinal cord and interact in spinal behavioral responses of the rat. *Neurosci. Lett.*, 52: 199–204.

Wiesenfeld-Hallin, Z., Xu, X.-J., Villar, M.J. and Hökfelt, T. (1990) Intrathecal galanin potentiates the spinal analgesic effect of morphine: behavioural and electrophysiological studies. *Neurosci. Lett.*, 109: 217–221.

Womack, M.D., MacDermott, A.B. and Jessell, T.M. (1988) Sensory transmitters regulate intracellular calcium in dorsal horn neurons. *Nature*, 334: 351–353.

Xu, X.-J., Wiesenfeld-Hallin, Z., Villar, M.J. and Hökfelt, T. (1989) Intrathecal galanin antagonizes the facilitatory effect of substance P on the nociceptive flexor reflex in the rat. *Acta Physiol. Scand.*, 137: 463–464.

Yaksh, T.L. and Elde, R.P. (1980) Release of methionine-enkephalin immunoreactivity from the rat spinal cord in vivo. *Eur. J. Pharmacol.*, 63: 359–362.

Yaksh, T.L. and Elde, R.P. (1981) Factors governing release of methionine-enkephalin-like immunoreactivity from mesencephalon and spinal cord of the cat in vivo. *J. Neurophysiol.*, 46: 1056–1075.

Yamaguchi, K., Nakajima, Y., Nakajima, S. and Stanfield, P.R. (1990) Modulation of inwardly rectifying channels by substance P in cholinergic neurones from rat brain in culture. *J. Physiol. (London)*, 426: 499–520.

Yamamoto, T. and Yaksh, T.L. (1992) Effects of intrathecal capsaicin and an NK-1 antagonist, CP,96–345, on the thermal hyperalgesia observed following unilateral constriction of the sciatic nerve in the rat. *Pain*, 51: 329–334.

Yashpal, K. and Henry, J.L. (1984) Substance P analogue blocks SP-induced facilitation of a spinal nociceptive reflex. *Brain Res. Bull.*, 13: 597–600.

Yashpal, K., Dam, T.V. and Quirion, R. (1990) Quantitative autoradiographic distribution of multiple neurokinin binding sites in rat spinal cord. *Brain Res.*, 506: 259–266.

Yashpal, K., Radhakrishnan, V. and Henry, J.L. (1991) NMDA receptor antagonist blocks the facilitation of the tail flick reflex in the rat induced by intrathecal administration of substance P and by noxious cutaneous stimulation. *Neurosci. Lett.*, 128: 269–272.

Yashpal, K., Kar, S., Dennis, T. and Quirion, R. (1992) Quantitative autoradiographic distribution of calcitonin gene-related peptide (hCGRPα) binding sites in the rat and monkey spinal cord. *J. Comp. Neurol.*, 322: 224–232.

Yashpal, K., Radhakrishnan, V., Coderre, T.J. and Henry, J.L. (1993) CP-96,345, but not its stereoisomer, CP-96,344, blocks the nociceptive responses to intrathecally administered substance P and to noxious thermal and chemical stimuli in the rat. *Neuroscience*, 52: 1039–1047.

Yoshimura, M. and North, R.A. (1983) Substantia gelatinosa neurons in vitro hyperpolarized by enkephalin. *Nature*, 305: 529–530.

Zhang, X., Ju, G., Elde, R. and Hökfelt, T. (1993) Effect of peripheral nerve cut on neuropeptides in dorsal root ganglia and the spinal cord of monkey with special reference to galanin. *J. Neurocytol.*, 22: 342–381.

Zieglgänsberger, W. and Tulloch, I.F. (1979) The effects of methionine- and leucine-enkephalin on spinal neurones of the cat. *Brain Res.*, 167: 53–64.

F. Nyberg, H.S. Sharma and Z. Wiesenfeld-Hallin (Eds.)
Progress in Brain Research, Vol 104

CHAPTER 12

Release of neuropeptides in the spinal cord

A.W. Duggan

Department of Preclinical Veterinary Sciences, University of Edinburgh, Royal (Dick) School of Veterinary Studies, Summerhall, Edinburgh EH9 1QH, UK

Introduction

There are several questions requiring answers in studies of the central release of neuropeptides. These include the cell types containing and releasing a particular compound, the adequate stimuli producing release, the sites of release, the events interposed between the invasion of a terminal by an action potential and the actual process of release, physiological controls of release and the spread and inactivation of released compounds. The present account will deal briefly with all of these processes with the exception of events occurring within releasing terminals.

With the description of a novel compound suspected of being a neurotransmitter, as a first step, it is important to determine whether such a compound is released, in a calcium-dependent manner, from an in vitro preparation following a non-discriminatory electrical or chemical stimulus. Such studies are not considered in detail within this account. Beyond this first stage, many studies of release of neuroactive compounds attempt to produce release by discrete physiological stimuli, with the ultimate aim of contributing to an understanding of the physiology and pharmacology of particular processes or events within the nervous system.

The coexistence of more than one neuroactive compound within nerve terminals has brought about some rethinking of the significance of release studies. Whereas 15 years ago, the demonstration that substance P (SP) was released in the spinal cord by impulses in nociceptive afferents would have been considered compelling evidence that this neuropeptide was the transmitter of information in some of these fibres, that is not the case now. Elsewhere in this volume, considerable attention is given to the coexistence of a number of neuroactive compounds within primary afferent fibres and neurons of the spinal cord. The combinations are multiple and varied and include coexistent neuropeptides (Gibbins et al., 1985; Ju et al., 1987b; Cameron et al., 1988) and peptides coexistent with an excitant-amino acid (Battaglia and Rustioni, 1988). It is the latter combination in particular which makes it less likely that the co-existent neuropeptide is signalling accurately the onset, offset and intensity of a peripheral stimulus. Encoding a rapid onset and offset of a stimulus requires a short latency, rapidly inactivated compound, and what is known of some neuropeptides in the periphery does not favour such an action. Considerable evidence suggests that some neuropeptides released from primary afferent fibres act to alter the efficacy of transmission of impulses by rapidly degraded compounds and such alterations can last for relatively prolonged periods.

When a neuropeptide coexists with another neuroactive compound, such as an amino acid, it does not necessarily follow that the neuropeptide and the amino acid will be released in a similar manner by invading impulses. Thus, a patterning of impulses such as short bursts, may be more efficacious in releasing one class of compound and a regular firing pattern may be better for the other.

Despite these caveats, there is accumulating evidence that within the central nervous system neuropeptides have roles in functionally defined systems. By defining the stimuli producing release, controls of release and the degradation of released compounds, release studies can contribute to an understanding of such systems.

Methodologies

In vitro techniques

At the simplest level, spinal cord slices, incubated in vitro, can be used to study release of neuropeptides in the spinal cord (Clarke et al., 1984; Pang and Vasko, 1986; Linderoth and Brodin, 1988; Donnerer and Amann, 1992). From a physiological view point, the technique has many limitations. Thus when using elevated potassium levels as a stimulus, virtually all neurons and axon terminals in the slice will be depolarised and the source of the released compounds are conjectural. A spinal cord slice contains intrinsic neurons but also severed endings of propriospinal, supraspinally derived and primary afferent fibres.

Defined stimuli to produce release are mainly used under in vivo conditions but there are exceptions. Thus capsaicin has been perfused over dorsal horn slices in an attempt to produce release selectively from the central terminals of nociceptors (Aimone and Yaksh, 1989). By analogy with the action of capsaicin in the periphery (Holzer, 1991), this probably is a selective stimulus, but whether the concentrations used have effects on other structures in a slice preparation is unknown. The hemisected immature spinal cord with attached dorsal roots can be maintained in vitro (Sakuma et al., 1991) and, in this case, electrical stimulation of the dorsal roots can be employed. As with smaller slices, measurements of the relevant compound are made in the perfusate.

Beyond non-discriminatory release, the next obvious question is what discrete physiological stimuli produce release under in vivo conditions? There are two components to this question which require separate consideration: the method of detection and the nature of the stimulus, and the latter has both qualitative and quantitative considerations.

In vivo techniques

Under in vivo conditions, release of neuropeptides in the spinal cord has been studied by perfusing the surface of the spinal cord, by perfusing localised areas within the cord by push-pull cannulae or microdialysis tubes, or by binding released molecules at the site of release with antibody microprobes.

Perfusing the surface of the spinal cord (Yaksh, 1984) clearly cannot localise sites of release, and contributions to what is measured in the perfusate can come from neuropeptide-containing nerves to the dura and pia-arachnoid. If inactivation of released neuropeptides occurs predominantly within the spinal cord, then a surface perfusate will collect very little of what is released, although metabolites may be more readily detected. The push-pull cannula (Philippu, 1984) is a relatively large device (outer diameter typically 500 μm) and flow rates of approximately one μl min^{-1} must result in distortion of tissue at the tip of the cannula, since the perfusate is actively expelled from one channel of the device. The push-pull cannula, however, will collect virtually any class of diffusible molecule in the extracellular space.

Microdialysis tubing employs a membrane window to allow exchange of compounds with the extracellular space (Ungerstedt, 1984). Although excellent for small molecules, recovery rates for most neuropeptides are low, and this probably explains the relative paucity of reports on the release of neuropeptides within the central nervous system using this method. Tubing diameters as small as 300 μm have been used, but this is still relatively large when compared with the thickness of spinal laminae in the cat and particularly the rat.

The antibody microprobe uses antibodies immobilised to the outer surface of glass micropipettes to capture molecules at sites of release (Duggan et al., 1988a; Duggan, 1991). The bound molecules are detected on autogradiograph as deficits in the binding of a radiolabelled ligand in which the microprobes are incubated after withdrawal from the nervous system. Microprobes remain in the spinal cord or brain for periods of 5–30 min depending on the neuropeptide being studied and/or the stimulus being used. It is the least traumatic of currently used devices, but has to operate within the constraint of antibody specificity, and hence cannot give exact chemical identity to what is detected. An important advantage of the antibody microprobe is its spatial resolution. It is estimated (Duggan, 1991) that sites of release of 100-μm diameter can be detected with this device.

Stimuli

To apply all the stimuli which might produce spinal release of a neuropeptide is an enormous task. Any spinal ganglia may supply a host of tissues such as skin, muscle, joints, bones and viscera and, within each of these tissues, specialised receptors exist which respond to defined stimuli. Viewed in this way, many of the studies subsequently discussed in relation to particular neuropeptides may appear to be using relatively gross stimuli. This is correct from the viewpoint of defining types of primary afferent neuron which release a neuropeptide centrally when information is transmitted to the spinal cord. It is rare, however, for a real environmental stimulus to activate one receptor type. Thus the immersion of part of an extremity in water of a defined temperature may not be precise in terms of knowing which receptors are activated, but it is important to know whether this real life stimulus results in the central release of a neuropeptide which can influence how the afferent information is processed within the spinal cord.

The methods employed by sensory physiologists to activate peripheral sensory receptors are applicable to studies of neuropeptide release in the spinal cord but in general stimuli need to be applied for relatively prolonged periods. Thus, for example, whereas noxious heating of the skin for 15–30 sec is adequate to study the firing of a peripheral fibre or a spinal neuron, the same stimulus may need 5–15 min application for central release of a neuropeptide to be detected. Peripheral sensory receptors may adapt, seen as a reduction in firing rate with continued application of a stimulus. The implication for release studies is the need to apply stimuli intermittently for a given total period. The need to use prolonged stimuli creates other problems. The volume of peripheral tissues affected by a prolonged thermal stimulus may exceed that of a brief stimulus, and what may be a cutaneous stimulus with brief application may be a subcutaneous and cutaneous stimulus with prolonged stimulation. Probably more important with noxious stimuli, however, is that prolonged intense stimuli may produce tissue damage. There is now abundant evidence that the endings of many afferent fibres sensitise when exposed to inflammatory exudates (Schaible and Schmidt, 1985a). The effect of this is to lower the threshold for excitation and, for example, both mechanical and thermal stimuli which were previously inadequate under normal conditions can cause sensitised nociceptors to fire. Such work has emphasised the need to cross from the realm of physiology to that of pathology when considering the function of nociceptors, and this has proved to be important with some neuropeptides.

The sensitisation of nerve fibres, moreover, has implications for the effects of peripheral nerve stimulation. Electrical stimulation of nerves is used commonly to evoke release of neuropeptides both peripherally and centrally. Although stimulus strength can be graded, electrical stimulation always simultaneously activates fibres of many functionally different types. Thus stimulus strengths adequate to excite unmyelinated afferents, even when coupled with anodal block to prevent impulses in large myelinated fibres reaching the spinal cord, results in impulses in nociceptors, thermoreceptors and some low-threshold mechanoreceptors reaching the spinal cord. Studies on sensitised fibres have described a group which cannot be fired under normal conditions by any natural stimulus, but will do so when sensitised by adjacent inflammation (Schaible and Schmidt, 1985a; Schaible and Grubb, 1993). These have been termed silent nociceptors but they too will be excited by high intensity electrical stimulation.

The problem of sources of release

Although it may be quite clear that a stimulus produces release of a particular compound, defining the structure or structures producing release within the central nervous system is often partly conjectural. Reference nearly always has to be made to histochemistry, and it is rare that a compound of interest occurs only within one class of neural structure. Calcitonin gene-related peptide (CGRP) however is contained within a proportion of primary afferent fibres of the cat and rat, and also within motoneurons, but virtually no other spinal neural structure (Chung et al., 1988). Thus release of CGRP into the spinal cord following a peripheral stimulus almost certainly results from release only from the central terminals of primary afferents. If release can be localised anatomically with some precision, then the probability of release from a known structure is increased. Although substance P-containing neurons occur in various areas of the spinal cord and within descending fibres (particularly in the ventral horn), the detection, by antibody microprobes, of release in the region of the substantia gelatinosa of spinal cats following a peripheral noxious stimulus almost certainly represents release predominantly from the central terminals of nociceptors (Hokfelt et al., 1977; Difiglia et al., 1982; Lindh et al., 1989).

This difficulty of relating release to a structure is at its worst when examining a likely widely used transmitter such as L-glutamate. If the technology used collects the compound diffusely from the whole spinal cord, such as with surface perfusion in vivo or perfusion of a spinal cord in vitro, then localising sources of release is usually not possible.

Quantification

All of these methods produce numbers of one type or another and the usual use of these numbers is to show a significant change produced by a defined stimulus. Thus release is equated with increased extracellular levels of a compound following a stimulus. This is not the only explanation, since a stimulus could cause the release of a compound protecting a previously present compound from degradation. There is evidence that this may happen through CGRP decreasing degradation of SP.

An important consideration is whether more use can be made of the measurements from various detection methods. With a rapidly degraded transmitter the answer is probably no. Thus concentrations within synaptic clefts almost certainly decline very rapidly, are initially well in excess of the K_d values of the relevant receptors and the amounts escaping from synapses and detected by a collection method are of little physiological significance. This is probably the situation with amino acid transmitters.

Peptides are degraded by enzymes which may be relatively non-selective in their substrates and little is known of the proximity of degrading enzymes to peptide-releasing synapses (McKelvey and Blumberg, 1986). There is increasing evidence that peptides differ in their rates of degradation following release in the central nervous system. Slowly degraded compounds will diffuse away from sites of release and thus have the potential to activate receptors remote from sites of release. The concept of remote action has been termed 'volume transmission' (Fuxe and Agnati, 1991).

The ability of a release detection system to produce meaningful measures of the changes in extracellular level of a given compound relates both to the frequency with which extracellular levels can be sampled and to the rate of degradation of the substance being studied. With a compound having a half-life of the order of twice the collection period, the estimates of the extracellular levels can be meaningful in terms of possible function when related to the K_d of the relevant receptors. Morton et al. (1989) prepared curves for antibody microprobes exposed to differing concentrations of somatostatin in vitro, and related these to the images of microprobes inserted into the spinal cord. This is illustrated in Fig. 5. The peak level of somatostatin in the region of the substantia gelatinosa was equivalent to an in vitro concentration 10^{-6} M. This is sufficient to activate receptors for somatostatin. Irrespective of this interpretation, it is valid to state that microprobes found 100-times more somatostatin in the area of the substantia gelatinosa when compared with the dorsal columns.

Studies of the release of individual neuropeptides

Tachykinins

Release of the tachykinins has been intensively investigated in the spinal cord. Of the tachykinin family of peptides, substance P (SP), neurokinin A (NKA), neurokinin B, neurokinin K and neuropeptide K occur in vertebrates. Although neuropeptide K has been identified in human cerebrospinal fluid (Toresson et al., 1990), release studies in the spinal cord in vivo have only dealt with SP and NKA.

Virtually all studies have been directed at the possible functions of SP contained within primary afferent fibres. From a functional viewpoint, this is best studied by giving adequate stimuli to intact peripheral tissues and hence under in vivo conditions. In vitro methods will be discussed when considering possible controls of SP release.

Within dorsal root ganglion, SP is contained within a proportion of small diameter ganglion cells (Hökfelt et al., 1976). This has directed attention to nociceptors and hence many studies have examined the ability of peripheral noxious stimuli to evoke spinal release of SP.

Substance P release in normal animals

Spinal cord perfusion. Perfusion of the surface of the spinal cord of the anaesthetised cat has shown a release of immunoreactive (ir) SP following electrical stimulation of high-threshold primary afferent fibres (Yaksh et al., 1980). In subsequent experiments (Go and Yaksh, 1987), intense heat (metal plates at 75°C applied to the hind limbs intermittently for 30 min) produced small increases in irSP in the spinal perfusate. In view of the ease with which noxious heating of the skin has produced release of irSP within the spinal cord when studied by other methods, this result with surface perfusion illustrates the limitations of this methodology.

Push-pull cannulae and microdialysis. Using push-pull cannulae inserted into the spinal cords of rabbits to measure irSP, Kuraishi et al. (1985) found that noxious mechanical, but not thermal stimuli, produced a 10-fold increase in levels of irSP in the cannulae perfusates. The thermal stimulus used was a focused light bulb and the temperatures attained were measured with a subcutaneous thermocouple. The maximum temperature attained was 48.5°C, and it was stated that subdermal temperatures of 44°C were exceeded for more than 11 min of the 20-min stimulus period. In a subsequent study (Kuraishi et al., 1989), this group found that severe thermal stimuli did result in a spinal release of irSP, and they suggested an association with peripheral tissue damage, since subcutaneous formalin also increased release. Rather puzzling are the observations of McCarson and Goldstein (1991), who also used the push-pull cannula method and found that noxious mechanical cutaneous stimulation increased release of irSP in the spinal cord of the rat, but that injection of formalin subcutaneously decreased release. Others have found enhanced release of SP in the spinal cord when inflammation develops in the periphery (discussed later).

Brodin et al. (1987) inserted 500-μm microdialysis tubing into the spinal cords of cats and showed release of irSP following ipsilateral sciatic nerve

202

A

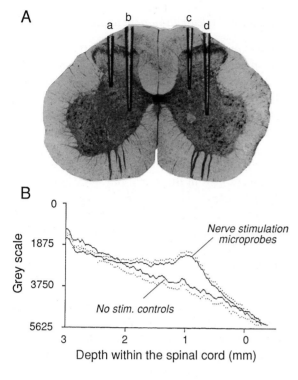

B

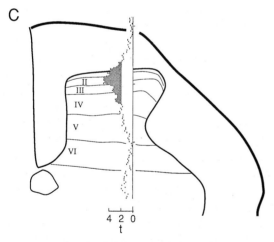

C

Fig. 1. Detection by antibody microprobes of irSP released by peripheral nerve stimulation. A. Photographic enlargement of autoradiographs of microprobes bearing antibodies to SP have been appropriately superimposed on a similar enlargement of an unstained transverse section of the lumbar spinal cord of the cat. The microprobes were either 20 or 30 min in the spinal cord and under differing conditions. Microprobe (a), no added stimulus; microprobe (b), large diameter fibres of the ipsilateral tibial nerve were stimulated; microprobes (c) and (d), both large- and small-diameter fibres of the ipsilateral tibial nerve were stimulated. B. Mean image analyses (in 30-μm intervals) of two groups of microprobes bearing antibodies to SP and inserted 3 mm into the spinal cord of the cat.

stimulation in the lower lumbar segments. Sustained isometric contraction of muscle produces rises in blood pressure and respiratory rate. Wilson et al. (1993) found that this stimulus was associated with increased release of irSP in the dorsal horn of the anaesthetized cat. These experiments employed a microdialysis probe with 3 mm of exposed membrane and, as with the study of Brodin et al. (1987), no fine localisation of sites of release was possible.

Antibody microprobes. The original studies with antibody microprobes found that, in the anaesthetised spinal cat, electrical stimulation of large-diameter primary afferents of the tibial nerve did not produce release of irSP within the spinal cord, but that increasing the stimulus strength to include unmyelinated (C) fibres resulted in release of this peptide in the region of the substantia gelatinosa of the ipsilateral dorsal horn (Duggan and Hendry, 1986). This result is illustrated in Fig. 1A–C. The stimulus frequencies used varied from 2 to 30 Hz and microprobes remained in the spinal cord from 10 to 30 min.

When using noxious peripheral stimuli applied to the skin, a release of irSP was produced both in the region of the substantia gelatinosa of the spinal cat and also at the cord surface by noxious thermal, mechanical and chemical stimuli (Duggan et al., 1988b). With noxious heat, the hind paw was immersed in a water bath and, although temperatures of 45–48°C are generally regarded as painful both in man and cat (Zimmerman, 1976), a bath temperature of 50°C was needed to produce release of irSP in the dorsal horn. The

The 'no stim controls' group comprised 16 microprobes while the 'nerve stimulation microprobes' represents 33 microprobes present in the spinal cord during electrical stimulation of both large- and small-diameter fibres of the ipsilateral tibial nerve. With both groups, a line joins the mean image density at each point but the standard error of each mean is plotted separately. C. The *t*-statistics derived from the differences of the means of the two groups of microprobes plotted in (B) are appropriately superimposed on a diagram of a transverse section of the spinal cord of the cat at the L7 segment.

noxious mechanical stimulus was pinching of the skin of digital pads with small alligator clips. Non-noxious mechanical stimulation did not result in irSP release. The noxious chemical stimulus was painting the skin of digital pads with methylene chloride, and this produced considerable swelling of the hind paws. Although these early experiments required stimulus times of 15–30 min, later microprobe experiments (Duggan et al., 1992; Schaible et al., 1992) have shown release of irSP with 10 min of noxious pinch or 2 min of nerve stimulation (Schaible et al., 1992).

Experiments with antibody microprobes have shown release of irSP centred on the superficial dorsal horn (Laminae I and II) but extending beyond it. Importantly this technique consistently shows a presence of irSP extending into the dorsal columns. Since there is no evidence for SP-releasing terminals in the dorsal columns this must represent diffusion away from sites of release. The significance of this will be discussed subsequently.

What are the sources of SP measured in this variety of ways? Although all of the experiments cited have produced increased activity in fine-diameter primary afferents, SP contained within these afferents and from within intrinsic neurons of the spinal cord and brain stem-derived fibres could all contribute to what was measured. Although not definitive, the results from the microprobe experiments favour release from primary afferents. These experiments were in spinal animals, so release from supraspinally derived fibres can be discounted. In some microprobe experiments, release has been restricted to a 300-μm zone of the superficial dorsal horn (see Fig. 2), and this coincides well with the zone of termination of nociceptive cutaneous afferents. Sectioning the dorsal roots has been found to lower substance P levels in the spinal cord by 50–80% (Ogawa et al., 1983), but the localised loss in Lamina I by sectioning the sciatic nerve is near 100% as shown by immunocytochemistry (Wall et al., 1981). Thus release centred on Lamina II following stimulation of cutaneous nociceptive afferents probably results predominantly from release from the central terminals of nociceptors.

There are many gaps in knowledge concerning the adequate stimuli producing spinal release of SP in normal animals. Nothing is known of the effects of stimulation of viscera and data from deep tissues are scant.

Spinal release of substance P with the development of peripheral inflammation

Because of the need to use relatively severe stimuli to produce release of irSP into the substantia gelatinosa, it was suggested that tissue damage was the more effective stimulus. This has led to studies of spinal release of substance P as arthritis develops. Arthritis is known to produce sensitisation of peripheral nociceptors, and to produce firing in the so-called 'silent nociceptor' group (Schaible and Schmidt, 1985b).

Oku et al. (1987) examined irSP release with push-pull cannulae inserted into the spinal cords of rats made polyarthritic by injection of Freund's adjuvant 2–3 weeks previously. Joint movement of arthritic but not normal joints increased levels of irSP in cannulae perfusates.

Schaible et al. (1988b) examined the effects of acute inflammation by using antibody microprobes to measure spinal release of irSP in the cat, before and after induction of inflammation in a knee joint by injection of kaolin and carrageenan (Schaible et al., 1990). Both before, and from 3 to 8 h after joint injection, joint movement failed to produce a central release of irSP. Beyond that period, joint flexion produced a massive release of SP both in the superficial dorsal horn and deep in spinal Laminae VI and VII. Compression of an inflamed joint resulted in a similarly large release of SP. When compression of an inflamed joint resulted in a widespread presence of irSP in the dorsal horn, noxious pinch to the uninflamed digital pads of these animals resulted in a discrete zone of release restricted to the region of the substantia gelatinosa. The significance of these contrasting patterns, which are illustrated in Fig. 2, will be discussed subsequently when considering degradation of released tachykinins. Prior to that, it is necessary to consider studies of the release of another tachykinin, neurokinin A (NKA).

**Flex inflamed
knee**

**Pinch normal
digits**

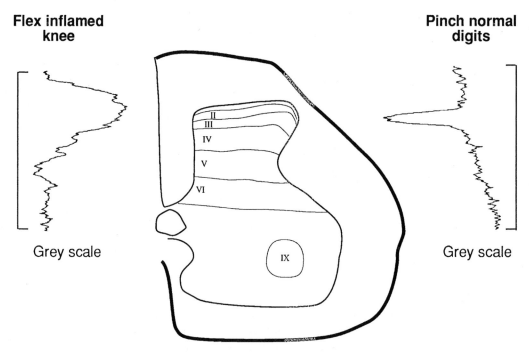

Grey scale

Grey scale

Fig. 2. Comparison of the focal release of irSP from pinching normal digits with the widespread release of irSP from flexing an inflamed knee joint. The traces on either side of the outline of a transverse section of the lumbar spinal cord of the cat are optical scans of the autoradiographs of single microprobes inserted into the spinal cord of the same cat. Whereas flexion of the inflamed knee (prior injection of kaolin and carrageenan) showed a diffuse presence of irSP throughout the superficial dorsal horn and dorsal columns, pinching the normal digits of the foot of the same side resulted in release of irSP predominantly in Lamina II.

Spinal release of neurokinin A. NKA is a tachykinin which extensively coexists with substance P in dorsal root fibres of the rat (Dalsgaard et al., 1985). Virtually all dorsal root ganglion cells containing NKA also contain SP, although the converse is not true.

Linderoth and Brodin (1988) superfused the rat spinal cord in vitro and in vivo, and found equimolar release of both irNKA and irSP following peripheral nerve stimulation or superfusion of the spinal cord with capsaicin (10^{-5} M) or potassium (4×10^{-2} M). No release was detected when noxious thermal, mechanical or chemical stimuli were applied to the skin.

Antibody microprobe experiments have found release of irNKA following noxious thermal or mechanical stimuli but important differences from the release of irSP were observed. In the anaes-thetised cat, peripheral cutaneous thermal and mechanical stimuli produced a spinal release of irNKA (Duggan et al., 1990). Unlike the relatively focal release of irSP in the substantia gelatinosa, irNKA was detected widely in the dorsal horn. Because of the relative resistance of NKA to enzyme degradation (Nyberg et al., 1984) it was suggested that this neuropeptide diffused widely from sites of release and thus could affect neurons within relatively large areas of the spinal cord. Further support for this proposal came from experiments in which irNKA was found to require 60–90 min to return to basal levels following 30 min of peripheral nerve stimulation (Hope et al., 1990).

Spinal release of irNKA was also studied following the induction of peripheral arthritis (Hope et al., 1990). Unlike substance P, spinal release of irNKA occurred immediately after joint injection and widespread presence in the spinal cord was observed. Indeed, for the duration of each experiment, microprobes indicated that irNKA was detectable throughout the whole of the spinal grey matter sampled within 30 min of injecting one knee joint with kaolin and carrageenan. Thus NKA and SP gave very different release patterns in this model of arthritis. IrNKA appeared with joint injection and persisted in the spinal cord irrespective of any peripheral stimulus, whereas irSP release did not occur until some hours after joint injection and required an active stimulus. These results have an interesting peripheral counterpart, where arthroscopy of joints in humans was associated with detectable levels of NKA in synovial fluid but not of SP (Larsson et al., 1991).

An important corollary to these studies on the release of irNKA, is that protecting SP from degradation should result in a release pattern similar to that of NKA. Such an effect was shown by Duggan et al. (1992), following microinjection of the mixed peptidase inhibitor, kelatorphan, into the superficial dorsal horn of the cat. Under these conditions, released irSP not only diffused widely in the spinal cord but also persisted for prolonged periods following release. Whereas the increased amounts in the grey matter could represent protection of previously undetectable amounts at sites of release, this reasoning cannot apply to the widespread presence of irSP in the dorsal columns which must have diffused from distal sites of release.

Additional experiments with microinjection of CGRP suggested that the sites accessed by synaptically released SP may be under physiological control through a mechanism of varied rate of degradation. Le Greves et al. (1985) showed that CGRP is a potent inhibitor of an endopeptidase degrading SP. CGRP is often colocalised with SP in primary afferent neurons (Gibson et al., 1985; Ju et al., 1987a; Villar et al., 1991; Hökfelt et al., 1992) and is likely coreleased. When applied topically to the spinal cord CGRP prolonged facilita-

tion of a flexor reflex by SP (Woolf and Wiesenfeld-Hallin, 1986), a result consistent with an inhibition of SP degradation. Experiments with antibody microprobes have shown that microinjection of CGRP into the superficial dorsal horn gave results similar to those obtained with synthetic peptidase inhibitors: irSP released by noxious stimuli diffused widely in the dorsal horn when compared with release prior to injection (Schaible et al., 1992). This action of CGRP is illustrated in Fig. 3.

It is possible that the relatively massive release of SP observed with the development of peripheral joint inflammation represents protection of SP by co-released CGRP. Both in vitro (Garry and Hargreaves, 1992) and in vivo (Collin et al., 1993) studies have provided evidence for enhanced spinal release of CGRP when inflammation develops in the periphery.

Substance P and neurokinin A as transmitters

These extensive experiments on release of irSP and irNKA do permit some conclusions on the possible roles of these compounds when released from the central terminals of primary afferents. The results with SP indicate that this compound could function as a neurotransmitter released by polymodal nociceptors derived from skin and other tissues. The experiments dealing with degradation of SP and NKA suggest an alternate or additional role for these neuropeptides, particularly if they are co-released with a fast-acting, rapidly degraded compound such as L-glutamate. Release of L-glutamate would be appropriate to an accurate depiction of the hard-wired somatotopic map of the periphery in the spinal cord with accurate signalling of the onset, offset and intensity of a peripheral stimulus. An additional release of SP and/or NKA would result in raised levels of excitability of neurons, both within and without this hard wired map, and such changes would outlast the stimulus producing release. The functional significance of this may be to simply result in the perception of pain outlasting the

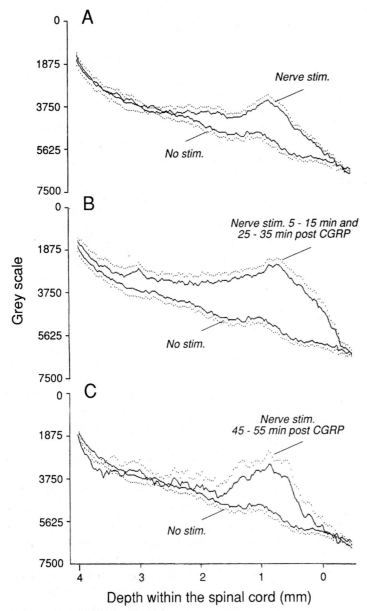

Fig. 3. The effect of microinjection of CGRP on the pattern of nerve stimulus-evoked release of irSP in the spinal cord of the cat. A. The two groups of microprobes are those present in the spinal cord for 10 min in the absence of any stimulus and prior to microinjection of CGRP (no stim, $n = 19$) and those present during ipsilateral tibial nerve stimulation but prior to CGRP injection (nerve stim., $n = 23$). B. The two groups are 'no stim' as in (A) but the 'nerve stim group' comprises 12 microprobes present in the spinal cord during peripheral nerve stimulation, but either 5, 15 or 25, 35 min after microinjection of CGRP 10^{-3} M in volumes of approximately 0.125 μ1 at 1, 1.5, 2.0 and 2.5 mm from the dorsal spinal cord surface. C. The groups are as in (B) but the 'nerve stim' group were present in the spinal cord 45, 55 min following microinjection of CGRP. (Reproduced, with permission, from Schaible *et al.*, (1992.)

stimulus, but it may also produce hyperalgesia in tissues adjacent to an injured focus with the ultimate aim of immobility as an aid to healing.

Two studies (Duggan et al., 1979; Yoshimura et al., 1993) have found SP to have little effect on neurons of the substantia gelatinosa, the area of peak release, and a recent study of the distribution of NK_1 receptors (Liu et al., 1994) has found a paucity of such receptors in the substantia gelatinosa. Collectively this evidence suggests that released tachykinins have roles in transmission of nociceptive information, which is different to that of conventional neurotransmission and which depends on their ability to resist rapid degradation. If the demonstrated action of CGRP in protecting SP is indeed a physiological control, then neurotransmission from nociceptive primary afferents is potentially a very plastic situation.

Inhibitory control of tachykinin release

Presynaptic inhibition acting on the central terminals of nociceptors is an attractive mechanism of analgesia since it is obviously selective in reducing the onward transmission of information transmitted in a particular type of sensory information. When opioid peptides were found to have powerful inhibitory effects in the substantia gelatinosa (Duggan et al., 1976), and to reduce substance P release from a slice preparation including this area (Jessell and Iversen, 1977), a presynaptic mechanism acting on the central terminals of nociceptors was proposed. When evidence has been sought to support such proposals, however, establishing presynaptic inhibition as an effective control acting on release of substances from nociceptors has proved to be controversial.

Presynaptic inhibition of transmitter release from the central terminals of large-diameter muscle afferents is well established (Schmidt, 1971). Such a control has a structural basis in axo-axonic synapses and pharmacological evidence indicates that γ-aminobutyric acid (GABA) is released at such synapses as the mediator of presynaptic inhibition (Curtis et al., 1977). The mechanism is believed to be a terminal depolarization by GABA

with a resultant reduced calcium entry with each invading action potential.

Given the considerable evidence that GABA release occurs at axo-axonic synapses on large-diameter afferents, such structures were sought on the central terminals of small-diameter fibres when it was proposed that enkephalins acted presynaptically on the central terminals of nociceptors. Fine-structure studies failed to find significant numbers of axo-axonic synapses in the superficial dorsal horn with immunoreactive-enkephalin in the presynaptic element (Glazer and Basbaum, 1981; Ruda, 1982; Sumal et al., 1982). Indeed, axo-axonic synapses of any type have been reported as relatively uncommon in the superficial dorsal horn of the species examined, with estimates of 0.8% of all synapses in this area in the rat (Zhu et al., 1981) and 1.7% in the cat (Duncan and Morales, 1978). More recent accounts, however, do refer to such structures in relation to particular compounds and these will be discussed later.

The concept of volume transmission was mentioned earlier in this review, and this hypotheses implies that released compounds could act on receptors not necessarily located at synapses, although the mechanism of the resultant inhibition is unknown. It could involve block of impulse propagation into axon terminals (McLachlan, 1978).

Inhibitory controls of tachykinin release have been examined from two viewpoints: can physiological mechanisms be shown to inhibit such release or does the administration of exogenous compounds result in reduced release?

Kuraishi et al. (1982) found that sectioning the spinal cord of the rabbit did increase irSP release evoked by a noxious mechanical stimulus and measured with a push-pull cannula. Thus a tonic inhibition of SP release and of brain stem origin was proposed. The variance in the data, however, casts some doubts on this conclusion. Thus evoked release was 136 fmol/min ± 37 SEM before, and 265 fmol/min ± 139 SEM after, cord transection. Tonic inhibition of SP release was investigated in the cat using the antibody microprobe technique

(Duggan et al., 1988c). When release of irSP was measured in the superficial dorsal horn of the seventh lumbar segment, in response to either a noxious thermal stimulus or electrical stimulation of the ipsilateral tibial nerve, this was not altered either by cooling a lower thoracic segment of the spinal cord or sectioning the cord at this level.

A segmental control of transmitter release from the central terminals of nociceptors was proposed by Melzack and Wall (1965) in their gate hypothesis. Morton and Hutchison (1989), however, could find no inhibition of evoked release of irSP in the dorsal horn of the cat when A-fibres of the spinal nerve were electrically stimulated continuously while a noxious peripheral stimulus was applied.

Exogenous compounds

Opioids have been extensively investigated for effects on tachykinin release in the spinal cord. Many studies have administered opioids topically and measured release of irSP from slice preparation of the brain or spinal cord. Inhibition of irSP release by opioids was first shown by Jessell and Iversen (1977) in a slice preparation of rat trigeminal nucleus. The stimulus used was 47 mM potassium in the perfusate. This will depolarize virtually all neural elements in the slice and hence the source of SP becomes uncertain. Furthermore, the concentration of morphine used was high (10^{-5} M). Support for the proposal that opiates impair substance P release from the central terminals of nociceptors came from the experiments of Yaksh et al. (1980) and Go and Yaksh (1987), in which morphine (10^{-4} M) added to a superfusate of intact cat spinal cord in vivo reduced the release of substance P into the perfusate following electrical stimulation of unmyelinated primary afferents. Lembeck and Donnerer (1985) measured irSP levels in the perfusate of the isolated rat spinal cord. Field stimulation of the cord or adding capsaicin to the perfusate produced release of irSP which was reduced by lofentanil 10^{-6} M.

This uniform inhibition of release by μ opioid agonists applied topically, either in vitro or in vivo, has not been observed by other laboratories. Thus Mauborgne et al. (1987) found that, whilst the μ agonist [D-Ala^2,M-Me-Phe^4,Gly-ol]-enkephalin (DAGO, 10^{-5} M), increased both high potassium- and capasaicin-induced release of SP from dorsal horn slices, the δ receptor agonist [D-Thr^2-Leu^5]-enkephalin-Thr (DTLET, 3×10^{-6} M) reduced release in the same preparation. The K agonist, U50488H ($0.5–50 \times 10^{-6}$ M), did not affect release of SP (Hamon et al., 1988; Pohl et al., 1989).

More recently, Suarez-Roca et al. (1992) found concentration-dependent effects of morphine on high potassium-evoked release of irSP from a trigeminal nucleus slice. On the basis of the effects of antagonists they proposed: inhibition of release by 10^{-9} M morphine acting at μ_1 receptors, increased release by 10^{-7} M morphine (μ receptors), inhibition of release by 3×10^{-6} M morphine (δ receptors), and increased release by 3×10^{-5} M morphine (κ receptors).

The studies cited have all superfused opioids to a spinal cord preparation. When morphine has been administered intravenously in analgesic or higher doses, no group has found a reduction in stimulus-evoked release of SP. Thus Kuraishi et al. (1983) and Hirota et al. (1985) used the push-pull cannula technique to study irSP release in spinal rabbits. Release of irSP by a noxious mechanical stimulus was not reduced by systemic morphine in analgesic (1 mg/kg) or supra-analgesic (10 mg/kg) doses (Kurashi et al., 1983). Release of SP was reduced, however, in a naloxone-reversible manner by administering morphine or Met^5-enkephalin (10^{-5} M) through the perfusion system. Studies with antibody microprobes have also found no inhibition of SP, NKA or CGRP release following analgesic doses of systemically administered morphine. Morton et al. (1990) found that morphine, administered in either a low (0.3–4.0 mg/kg) or a high (10–20 mg/kg) dose regime, had no effect on noxious stimulus-evoked release of SP measured with antibody microprobes. Superfusing the spinal cord surface with 10^{-5} M morphine did slightly reduce SP release, but this was not reversed by systemic naloxone.

Lang et al. (1991) used antibody microprobes to study noxious stimulus-evoked release of NKA in the superficial dorsal horn. Because of the persistence of NKA in the spinal cord of the cat following its release by a noxious peripheral stimulus, morphine needed to be administered prior to the delivery of such a stimulus. Neither morphine, nor naloxone after morphine, had any influence on the spinal release of NKA.

If there are physiological controls of tachykinin release involving opioids in the dorsal horn then they have not been defined in terms of adequate stimuli. Similarly, concentration-dependent effects (which may relate to activation of differing receptor populations) reported by different laboratories do not permit conclusions on which peptides are likely to underlie such physiological controls. There is near uniform agreement that when opioids are added in some concentration to the perfusate of a spinal cord slice, or to the surface of the spinal cord, that release of SP can be altered. As will be discussed later, when considering release of CGRP, this method of administration can affect receptors along the length of nerve fibres, as well as those at nerve terminals, and cannot necessarily be related to physiological controls. It is still unknown whether microinjecting opioid peptides near the spinal terminals of unmyelinated primary afferents alters release of SP from those terminals.

The differing concentration-dependent effects of opioids added to superfusates does prevent any prediction of the effects of therapeutically relevant doses of systemic morphine or related opiates. No laboratory has found reduced substance P release with these doses, although whether this results from mixed effects at different receptors, the low concentrations relative to those attained in vitro or the insensitivity of currently used measures of release cannot be decided.

Noradrenaline, neuropeptide Y (NPY) and substance P (SP) release

Noradrenaline and NPY extensively coexist in brain stem neurons of the rat and the cat (Everitt et al., 1984; Holets et al., 1988). Such coexistence

has not been demonstrated in supraspinal fibres of the superficial dorsal horn, but the question has not been directly addressed. Ultrastructural studies have failed to find axo-axonic synapses with tyrosine hydroxylase (Doyle and Maxwell, 1991a) or dopamine β-hydroxylase (Doyle and Maxwell, 1991b) in the presynaptic component in the superficial dorsal horn of the cat. A more recent study, however, has observed irNPY boutons making triadic arrangements with dendrites and the central element (axonal) of glomeruli in the superficial dorsal horn of the cat (Doyle and Maxwell, 1993).

Both in the peripheral and central nervous systems there are several instances where NPY has been shown to have effects on nerve terminals consistent with an impairment of transmitter release (Colmers et al., 1991; Haas et al., 1987). Two experimental approaches have provided evidence that NPY does reduce the release of SP from the central terminals of primary afferent fibres. Bleakman et al. (1991) cultured dorsal root ganglion cells and showed that 10^{-7} M NPY reduced the high K^+-evoked release of SP into the perfusate of such neurons. Such experiments cannot necessarily be related to the function of nociceptors since the stimulus was non-specific. Duggan et al. (1991) used antibody microprobes to examine spinal release of irSP in the cat following electrical stimulation of unmyelinated primary afferents of the ipsilateral tibial nerve or to a noxious stimulus. NPY (10^{-7}–10^{-5} M) was microinjected into the superficial dorsal horn and reduced evoked release of SP for up to 40 min after microinjection. Kar and Quirion (1992) have demonstrated a high density of ^{125}I-NPY binding sites in the superficial dorsal horn of the rat and a significant reduction in such binding following dorsal rhizotomy, peripheral nerve section and neonatal capsaicin administration. Such a reduction suggests the presence of binding sites on the intraspinal terminations of primary afferent fibres and, when considered with the ultrastructural observations (Doyle and Maxwell, 1993) the case for a role for NPY in reducing release of SP in the spinal cord is substantial.

Noradrenaline suppresses the nociceptive responses of dorsal horn neurons when administered microiontophoretically in the substantia gelatinosa (Headley et al., 1978) or near the neurons being studied (Fleetwood-Walker et al., 1985). Adrenoceptors of the α_2 variety underlie these antinociceptive actions (Fleetwood-Walker et al., 1985; Zhao and Duggan, 1987). Noradrenaline has been shown to hyperpolarize neurons of the substantia gelatinosa in vitro (North and Yoshimura, 1984) but, nevertheless, presynaptic actions on nociceptor central terminals have been sought.

Noradrenaline added to the perfusate of a push-pull cannula in a concentration of 10^{-5} M was found to reduce noxious stimuli-evoked release of SP in the dorsal horn of the rabbit (Kuraishi et al., 1982). In a slice preparation of the rat spinal cord, 10^{-5} M noradrenaline reduced high K^+-evoked release of SP (Pang and Vasko, 1986) and 10^{-5} M clonidine reduced veratridine-evoked release (Ono et al., 1991). When 10^{-3} M noradrenaline or 10^{-3} M medetomidine were microinjected into the dorsal horn of the anaesthetized cat and nerve stimulus-evoked release of SP measured with antibody microprobes, no significant inhibition of release was observed.

Anatomical studies have failed to find any basis for a control of SP release by noradrenaline (Doyle and Maxwell, 1991a,b). The situation has parallels with that discussed previously in relationship to opiates, and more information is needed on the ultrastructural location of adrenoceptors in relation to primary afferents and other structures of the upper dorsal horn.

5-Hydroxytryptamine (5HT)

The evidence supporting a functional role for 5HT in controlling tachykinin release is not convincing. Anatomical studies have not found axoaxonal contacts in the superficial dorsal horn containing 5-HT in the presynaptic element (Ruda and Gobel, 1980). When examined for effects on SP release, the affects of 5HT have been variable. A reduced release was observed when SP was measured in a superfusate of the trigeminal nu-

cleus caudalis and the tooth pulp stimulated (Yonehara et al., 1991). Two studies (Pang and Vasko, 1986; Saria et al., 1991) have found no effect of 5HT on high potassium-stimulated release of SP from spinal cord slices. In the study of Saria et al. (1991), antagonists of $5HT_3$ receptors reduced release of NKA and CGRP, implying a physiological enhancement of release by 5HT. With the multiplicity of 5HT receptor subtypes now described there is scope for further study of this question.

GABA

It is unknown if GABA-containing terminals establish presynaptic contacts with the central terminals of unmyelinated nociceptors, although recently such contacts have been demonstrated with the terminations of small myelinated high-threshold mechanoceptors (Alvarez et al., 1992). Although one study found no inhibition of potassium-stimulated release of SP by GABA superfused over a spinal cord slice (Pang and Vasko, 1986), in the experiments of Malcangio and Bowery (1993) the GABA-β agonist, baclofen, did release nerve stimulus-evoked release of SP from a spinal cord slice. When given intravenously, however, baclofen did not alter nerve stimulus-evoked released of irSP measured with antibody microprobes (Morton et al., 1992).

Spinal release of calcitonin gene-related peptide (CGRP)

CGRP is contained within many dorsal root ganglion neurons, including both small- and large-diameter cell bodies (Gibson et al., 1984; Ju et al., 1987b; Carlton et al., 1988). Within the rat spinal cord, CGRP is unusual in that it is found in motoneurons but in no other intrinsic neuron (Chung et al., 1988). Hence release of CGRP in the spinal cord following impulses in primary afferents can be reasonably attributed to release only from these fibres. Among peptides in dorsal root ganglion neurons, CGRP is also unusual because of its presence in both large and small cells raising the possibility that it might be released by innocuous cutaneous stimuli.

This was not however observed by Morton and Hutchison (1989). Noxious thermal and mechanical stimulation of the skin did produce a release of irCGRP in the superficial dorsal horn of the cat, but innocuous stimuli and electrical stimulation of large-diameter primary afferent fibres were ineffectual. This study used antibody microprobes, and the area of the superficial dorsal horn over which it CGRP was detected, was similar to that of SP. Unlike SP, however, a significant basal level of CGRP was detected.

Pohl et al. (1992) measured CGRP in a perfusate of the surface of the lower medulla and upper spinal cord of the anaesthetized rat. Levels of CGRP were increased by noxious heating of the muzzle but not by noxious mechanical stimulation of this area. A significant basal presence of CGRP was observed, though the reason for this was obscure since surgery is scarcely a stimulus to thermal nociceptors.

Earlier in this review it was suggested that CGRP protected SP from degradation, and that this may be a factor in the relatively massive release and spread of SP occurring when inflammation develops peripherally. Enhanced release of CGRP and SP has been observed in dorsal horn slice preparations taken from animals with peripheral carageenan-induced inflammation (Garry and Hargreaves, 1992) or with Freund's adjuvant-induced polyarthritis (Nanayana, 1989). Collin et al. (1993b) superfused the spinal cord surface of rats with polyarthritis of 3–4 week's standing and found elevated levels of CGRP compared with normal animals, suggesting enhanced basal release of this neuropeptide.

The evidence is now substantial that when inflammation develops in the periphery the relevant segments of the spinal cord are subject to enhanced release both of the tachykinins and of CGRP. It has not been demonstrated however, that this is a unique situation: it may simply represent what happens with repetitive firing of both normal and peripherally sensitized receptors. Although these neuropeptides might be expected to increase the excitability of neurons bearing the relevant receptors, and hence increase the messages transmitted to the brain which ultimately result in pain perception, the situation is more complicated. Later in this account the enhanced release of dynorphin and galanin with peripheral inflammation is described, and these compounds may be inhibitory to spinal transmission of nociceptive information. There is evidence for increased sensitivity to opioids when inflammation develops. Although this overall picture is complex, it does offer possibilities that disturbances of the release and/or function of one of these neuropeptides could be relevant to aberrant pain states.

Controls of spinal release of CGRP

Because of the anatomical evidence that CGRP within the spinal cord is almost exclusively of primary afferent origin, this is an advantageous situation for studying controls of the release of a neuropeptide from the central terminals of some primary afferents. Thus, even when using a slice preparation and non-specific stimuli such as electrical field stimulation, elevated potassium in the perfusate of the slice or the addition of capsaicin, it is highly probable that release of CGRP can be related to activity in the central terminals of primary afferent fibres. Under these conditions, it has been shown that CGRP release is reduced by adenosine (Santicioli et al., 1992), α2-adrenoceptor agonists (Takano et al., 1993; but see Bourgoin et al., 1993), GABA-A agonists (Bourgoin et al., 1992) and 5HT acting on $5HT_3$ receptors (Barnes, 1991; but see Bourgoin et al., 1993). In all of these experiments, the inhibiting compound was added to the perfusate and hence could act at receptors along the whole length of the primary afferents within the slice, as well as at the terminations. There is evidence for 5HT receptors on the peripheral branches of unmyelinated primary afferents (Neto, 1978) and for GABA-A receptors on undefined peripheral nerve fibres (Sakatani et al., 1991). Importantly, application of GABA (10^{-4} M) to the hemisected spinal cord of the neonatal

212

rat reduced the amplitude of the compound action potential resulting from propagation of impulses along dorsal column fibres (Sakatani et al., 1993). This effect, which was blocked by bicuculline, would reduce transmitter release at the relevant terminals. Thus caution is needed in interpreting effects observed when adding a compound to a perfusate as necessarily revealing physiological controls acting at spinal terminations. Nevertheless, the evidence is substantial that activation of a number of receptor types, located somewhere along primary afferent fibres, can reduce CGRP release in the spinal cord.

Morton and Hutchison (1990) found that intravenous morphine (up to 10 mg/kg) had no effect on noxious stimulus-evoked release of CGRP in the region of the substantia gelatinosa of the anaesthetized cat. This study used antibody microprobes. Collin et al. (1993a) also found no effect by intravenous morphine (20 mg/kg) on the spontaneous release of CGRP into a surface perfusate of the anaesthetized rat. They found evidence, however, that simultaneous activation of μ and κ opiate receptors did reduce spontaneous CGRP release in the rat. In rats with polyarthritism, however, activity at μ receptors alone could reduce CGRP levels measured in a surface perfusate (Collin et al., 1993b).

Probably the more significant results from this group are the findings that intravenous naloxone (Collin et al., 1993a) or low-intensity electrical stimulation of the skin of the muzzle of the rat (Pohl et al., 1992) reduced the spontaneous release of CGRP. This implies a physiological mechanism. Figure 4 illustrates varying effects of skin stimulation on release of CGRP. Many years ago, anatomists searched avidly in the dorsal horn for axo-axonic synapses containing enkephalins in the presynaptic element and failed to find significant numbers (Glazer and Basbaum, 1981; Ruda, 1982; Sumal et al., 1982). If peptides do diffuse significant distances from sites of release, then such a search may have been in vain since opiate receptors on axon terminals may occur independently of axo-axonic synapses. When antibodies to opiate receptors become freely available, one can anticipate that ultrastructural studies on opiate receptor locations in the superficial dorsal horn will help settle this controversy.

Somatostatin

Somatostatin was discovered through its action in inhibiting pituitary secretion of growth hormone, and hence its presence in dorsal root ganglion neurons (considered wholly excitatory neurons) of the rat (Hökfelt et al., 1976) was surprising. In the original report, Hökfelt et al. (1976) described the separateness of rat DRG neurons containing somatostatin from those containing substance P.

It is a consistent finding that immunoreactive-somatostatin is released in the dorsal horn following noxious heating of the skin. This has been observed in the rabbit (Kuraishi et al., 1985; push-pull cannulae), the rat (Tiseo et al., 1990; push-pull cannulae), and cat (Morton et al., 1989; antibody microprobes). In these studies innocuous peripheral stimuli, noxious mechanical stimuli and noxious cold stimuli did not produce release of immunoreactive-somatostatin.

Morton et al. (1989) localized release of immunoreactive-somatostatin to the superficial dorsal horn and observed a large basal presence of this neuropeptide when compared with substance P. Since there was no reason to attribute this to activity in thermal nociceptors, these authors drew attention to the difficulties of determining the sources of release with a compound present in primary afferents, intrinsic neurons and propriospinal and supraspinally derived fibres. When somatostatin has been applied near spinal neurons (Randic and Miletic, 1978; Fleetwood-Walker et al., 1992), or applied topically to the spinal cord (Sandkuhler et al., 1990; Chapman and Dickenson, 1992), the results have been predominantly inhibitory and this action is difficult to reconcile with that of an excitatory transmitter released from the central terminals of thermal

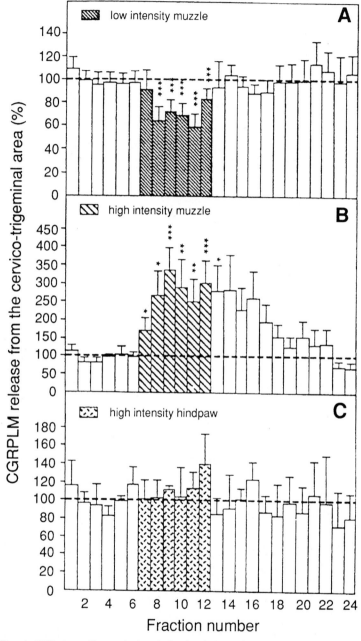

Fig. 4. Differing effects of electrical stimulation of various skin areas on CGRP release into a surface perfusate of the cervico-trigeminal area of the anaesthetised rat. The perfusate collection periods were 5 min and CGRP was measured by radioimmunoassay. Electrical stimulation was by means of percutaneous steel needles and low intensity stimulation (0.2-ms pulses, 0.5 mA) was considered to activate only large myelinated fibres. High intensity stimulation (2.0-ms pulses, 25 mA) probably activated both myelinated and unmyelinated fibres. (Reproduced, with permission, from Pohl *et al.*, (1992.)

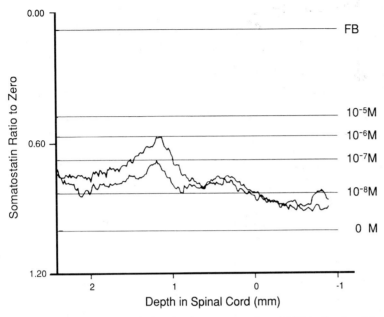

Fig. 5. Estimation of the equivalent in vitro concentration of irSS in the dorsal horn during cutaneous thermal stimulation. The grey scale of image density scans of microprobes exposed to standard concentrations of SS in vitro prior to incubation in ^{125}I-SS have been expressed as a ratio of the mean grey scale of 60 microprobes exposed to ^{125}I-SS (in vitro zero group). The mean scans for each concentration were then calculated and plotted as single line averages. The image density scans of microprobes inserted in the spinal cord for 5 min during 41°C (lower scan, $n = 14$) or 52°C (upper scan, $n = 15$) stimulation of the ipsilateral hind paw have similarly been expressed as ratios to the in vitro zero group. Standard errors have been omitted for clarity. FB, film background. (Reproduced, with permission, from Morton et al., (1989.)

nociceptors. Excitatory action of somatostatin-28 have been described (Fleetwood-Walker et al., 1992), but this neuropeptide is a minor component of the forms of somatostatin present within primary afferents fibres (Tessler et al., 1986).

Given that somatostatin does exist within a small proportion of DRG neurons of the rat (Hokfelt et al., 1976) and cat (Leah et al., 1985) it is probable that at least some of that found to be released in the superficial dorsal horn following noxious thermal stimuli is derived from the central terminals of primary afferents. Whether this represents co-release with (for example) L-glutamate, and somatostatin is acting to inhibit release from other fibres or to inhibit neurons remote from those excited by L-glutamate is unknown. There remains the distinct possibility that a proportion of the somatostatin released by noxious thermal stimuli is derived from intrinsic neurons of the spinal cord.

Galanin

There is dispute among investigators on the abundance of galanin-containing neurons in dorsal root ganglia of the rat with estimates varying from rare ($\ll 5\%$; Villar et al., 1990) to more common than neurons containing CGRP (Klein et al., 1990). Galanin also occurs within intrinsic neurons of the spinal cord and fibres of supraspinal origin (Ch'ng et al., 1985; Melander et al., 1986; Holets et al., 1988). It is predominantly small diameter DRG neurons which contain this peptide, and hence release studies have been directed towards nociception and inflammation.

Morton and Hutchison (1989) used antibody microprobes to detect immunoreactive-galanin in the spinal cord of the cat. A basal presence was detected in the region of Lamina II (substantia gelatinosa) and at the spinal cord surface. Electrical stimulation of both A- and C-fibres of the tibial nerve (10 Hz) failed to produce a spinal release of immunoreactive-galanin. Similarly ineffective were peripheral noxious thermal and mechanical stimuli. These results suggested that the basal presence of galanin in the dorsal horn was not derived from primary afferents. A different approach was used by Klein et al. (1992). They employed immunocytochemistry on spinal cord sections of the rat, comparing levels on the two sides following stimulation of one tibial nerve. Stimulation of A- and C-fibres at 1 Hz for 20 min reduced staining for immunoreactive-galanin on the stimulated side which was interpreted as stimulus-evoked release.

Hope et al. (1994) studied spinal release of immunoreactive-galanin in normal rats and in those in which inflammation of one ankle region had been induced 4–6 days previously. A basal presence of immunoreactive-galanin was observed diffusely in the dorsal horns of normal rats and those with peripheral inflammation. In the normal rat, noxious and non-noxious peripheral stimuli failed to elicit spinal release of galanin. In inflamed animals, repeated flexion of the inflamed ankle eventually produced a spinal release of galanin but subsequent noxious compression of the inflamed ankle caused a near disappearance of galanin from the spinal cord. The authors suggested that this was not the release pattern of a compound released from many primary afferents, and that release from intrinsic neurons was significant. The apparent inhibition of release with severe stimuli was unusual and the mechanism was unknown.

Little is known of the function of galanin in the spinal cord. Following intrathecal administration in relatively low doses, galanin has been variously found to produce hyperalgesia to mechanical but not thermal noxious stimuli (Cridland and Henry,

1988), to result in vocalisation to innocuous mechanical peripheral stimuli (Cridland and Henry, 1988) and to enhance reflexes to peripheral noxious thermal but not mechanical stimuli (Wiesenfeld-Hallin et al., 1991). In contrast to these enhanced responses, a number of depressant actions of intrathecal galanin have also been observed, but following doses generally higher than those producing increased responses. These depressant actions include decreased responses in hot plate and tail flick tests (Post et al., 1988), and decreased flexor reflexes produced by peripheral nerve stimulation (Wiesenfeld-Hallin et al., 1991). Whether these varied effects represent an excitant action of galanin released from primary afferents, and a depressant action of galanin released from intrinsic and/or descending fibres, requires further evidence.

Opioid peptides

The opioids present difficulties in release studies through their sheer number. For example, in the dynorphin series, release of dynorphin, dynorphin(1–13), or dynorphin(1–8) could occur. The products potentially released from processing of preproenkephalin include Met^5-enkephalin, Met^5-enkephalin-Arg^6,Phe^7, Met^5-enkephalin-Arg^6,Gly^7,Leu^8 and peptide E. There is, as yet, no consensus as to whether a major opioid peptide is released by itself, or is always accompanied by release of longer or shorter derivative peptides. The opioids also do not occur to any significant extent within primary afferent fibres, and hence the relatively simple experiment of stimulating these fibres will not necessarily be adequate to produce release of opioids within the spinal cord.

Despite this, release of Met^5-enkephalin has been demonstrated in a perfusate of the spinal cord of the cat (Yaksh and Elde, 1981) and rat (Cesselin et al., 1985) following electrical stimulation of unmyelinated primary afferents of the sciatic nerve. In the experiments of Yaksh and Elde (1981), cold block of the thoracic region of the spinal cord did not alter evoked release from lower spinal segments, indicating lack of brain control under the conditions used.

In both rat and cat, there is evidence that extended forms of Met[5]-enkephalin are released in the spinal cord following high-intensity sciatic nerve stimulation. Iadarola et al. (1986) identified Met[5]-enkephalin [Arg[6],Gly[7],Leu[8]] and a higher molecular weight compound in a perfusate of the rat cord, and Nyberg et al. (1983) obtained evidence for simultaneous release of Met[5]-enkephalin and Met[5]-enkephalin-Lys[6] from the cat spinal cord.

Somewhat different results were obtained by Le Bars et al. (1987). They perfused the surface of the lower spinal cord of the anaesthetised rat and found a basal presence of ir-Met[5]-enkephalin, which was increased by noxious stimuli to the muzzle and by i.p. acetic acid, but prolonged inhibition of basal release followed pinching the tail. Thus a heterosegmental inhibitory process involving opioids was proposed. This has a physiological parallel in the diffuse noxious inhibitory controls of Le Bars et al. (1990). The same laboratory (Bing et al., 1991) found that acupuncture also produced a heterosegmental release of ir-Met[5]-enkephalin from the spinal cord.

Draisci and Iadarola (1989) have shown an increased expression of the preproenkephalin message with the development of peripheral inflammation. Bourgourn et al. (1988) found that the basal levels of ir-Met[5]-enkephalin were reduced in rats with a Freund's adjuvant-induced arthritis of 4 week's duration. Moving the inflamed hind paw produced release of Met[5]-enkephalin.

The likely source of the enkephalins measured in these experiments is intrinsic neurons of the spinal cord. Since all the cited experiments perfused the surface of the spinal cord, none could localize sites of release. This is of some importance since, while there are reports of naloxone electrophysiological sensitive events in the ventral horn (Morton et al., 1982; Clarke et al., 1988), such inhibition is not consistently found when studying neurons of the dorsal horn.

Nyberg et al. (1983) found a complex mixture of opioids in a surface perfusate of the cat spinal cord following high-intensity sciatic nerve stimulation and a major component was dynorphin(1–13). Hutchison et al. (1990) also studied dynorphin release in normal anaes-

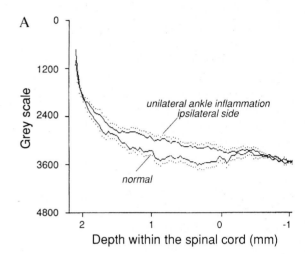

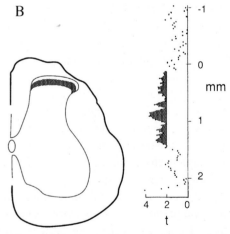

Fig. 6. Enhanced basal release of immunoreactive-dynorphin(1–8) in rats with lateral ankle inflammation. A. The mean image analyses of two groups of microprobes are illustrated: those inserted 2.25 mm into the lumbar spinal cords of normal rate for 20 min (normal, $n = 22$), and those inserted into the side of the spinal cord ipsilateral to an inflamed ankle region ($n = 23$). B. The differences between these groups indicate a significantly enhanced basal release of immunoreactive-dynorphin(1–8) in the nucleus proprius region of the dorsal horn.

thetized cats but used antibody microprobes. The latter bore immobilized antibodies to dynorphin(1–17). They found a basal presence of ir dynorphin in Lamina I of the dorsal horn and this was increased by electrical stimulation of unmyelinated primary afferents of the ipsilateral tibial nerve at frequencies of 50–100 Hz. No release occurred with stimulation at 10 Hz. Evoked release was abolished by spinal transection suggesting that release came from intrinsic spinal neurons activated by supraspinally derived fibres. Possibly relevant to this hypothesis is the finding that adding corticotropin-releasing factor to a perfusate of the isolated mouse spinal cord produced a release of immunoreactive-dynorphin (Song and Takemori, 1992).

Iadarola et al. (1988) showed that when inflammation developed peripherally there followed a marked and prolonged increase in the levels of dynorphin(1–8). Similar observations have been reported for dynorphin(1–17) (Millan et al., 1986; Weihe et al., 1989). Riley et al. (1994) investigated this by inserting microprobes bearing immobilized antibodies to dynorphin(1–8) into the spinal cords of rats with unilateral arthritis of 4 day's duration. Immunoreactive-dynorphin levels were elevated diffusely throughout the spinal cord on the side ipsilateral to the inflammation when compared with the contralateral side and normal animals. This action is illustrated in Fig. 5.

Concluding remarks

Apart from the detailed aspects of the release of particular peptides, there are some general principles concerning the release of neuropeptides and studies in the spinal cord to date which require some comment.

Although coexistence of a peptide with another peptide or a small neuroactive compound appears to be common, co-release from defined fibre types has yet to be demonstrated experimentally in the spinal cord. The heterogeneity of the spinal cord, together with the need to stimulate many nerve terminals to detect release, has prevented such experiments. The situation in the periphery is much more favourable. It is similarly unknown whether differing impulse patterns favour release of one class of compound when compared with another.

Measurements of the spatial spread of neuropeptides after release has given unexpected results and has given support to proposals that some neuroactive compounds diffuse away from sites of release, and thus can activate receptors relatively distant from such sites. The neuropeptides studied to date appear to differ in such behaviour and much work remains to clarify these distinctions. The diffusion of neuropeptides highlights the need to define receptor locations at the ultrastructural level, and with antibodies to defined sequences of receptors becoming increasingly available, such information can be obtained.

Controls of neuropeptides released from primary afferent fibres remain a controversial subject with convincing evidence being obtained for their presence mainly from in vitro experiments, but less so from in vivo experiments and a distinct lack of support from structural studies. Information on receptor location may help resolve these differences and, if extrasynaptic receptors are shown in large numbers on the intraspinal terminations of defined primary afferents, transmitter release from these fibres is clearly a pharmacological target without necessarily being of physiological significance.

There is considerable scope for improvement in the technology of release of neuropeptides. On-line detection has not been achieved but, given the minute amounts to be detected and the close structural similarities between members of a neuropeptide family, this is a formidable task.

References

Aimone, L.D. and Yaksh, T.L. (1989) Opioid modulation of capsaicin-evoked release of substance P from rat spinal cord in vivo. *Peptides*, 10: 1127–1131.

Alvarez, F.J., Kavookjian, A.M. and Light, A.R. (1992) Synaptic connections between GABA-immunoreactive profiles and the terminals of functionally defined myelinated nociceptors in the monkey and cat spinal cord. *J. Neurosci.*, 12: 2901–2917.

218

Barnes, P.J. (1991) Neurogenic inflammation in airways. *Int. Arch. Allergy Appl. Immunol.*, 94: 303–309.

Battaglia, G. and Rustioni, A. (1988) Co-existence of glutamate and substance P in dorsal root ganglia neurons of the rat and monkey. *J. Comp. Neurol.*, 277: 302–312.

Bing, Z., Cesselin, F., Bourgoin, S., Clot, A.M., Hamon, M. and Le Bars, D. (1991) Acupuncture-like stimulation induces a heterosegmental release of Met-enkephalin-like material in the rat spinal cord. *Pain*, 47: 71–77.

Bleakman, D., Colmers, W.F., Fournier, A. and Miller, R.J. (1991) Neuropeptide Y inhibits Ca^{2+} influx into cultured dorsal root ganglion neurons of the rat via a Y2 receptor. *Br. J. Pharmacol.*, 103: 1781–1789.

Bouhassira, D., Bing, Z. and Le Bars, D. (1990) Studies of the brain structures involved in diffuse noxious inhibitory controls: the mesencephalon. *J. Neurophysiol.*, 64: 1712–1723.

Bourgoin, S., Le Bars, D., Clot, A.M., Hamon, M. and Cesselin, F. (1988) Spontaneous and evoked release of met-enkephalin-like material from the spinal cord of arthritic rats in vivo. *Pain* 32: 107–114.

Bourgoin, S., Pohl, M., Benoliel, J.J., Mauborgne, A., Collin, E., Hamon, M. and Cesselin, F. (1992) Gamma-aminobutyric acid, through $GABA_A$ receptors, inhibits the potassium-stimulated release of calcitonin gene-related peptide- but not that of substance P-like material from rat spinal cord slices. *Brain Res.*, 583: 344–348.

Bourgoin, S., Pohl, M., Mauborgne, A., Benoliel, J.J., Collin, E., Hamon, M. and Cesselin, F. (1993) Monoaminergic control of the release of calcitonin gene-related peptide- and substance P-like materials from rat spinal cord slices. *Neuropharmacology*, 32: 633–640.

Brodin, E., Linderoth, B., Gazelius, B. and Ungerstedt, U. (1987) In vivo release of substance P in cat dorsal horn studied with microdialysis. *Neurosci. Lett.*, 76: 357–362.

Cameron, A.A., Leah, J.D. and Snow, P.J. (1988) The coexistence of neuropeptides in feline sensory neurons. *Neuroscience*, 27: 969–979.

Carlton, S.M., McNeill, D.L., Chung, K. and Coggeshall, R.E. (1988) Organization of calcitonin gene-related peptide immunoreactive terminals in the primate dorsal horn. *J. Comp. Neurol.*, 276: 527–536.

Cesslin, F., Le Bars, D., Bougoin, S., Artaud, F., Gozlan, H., Clot, A.M., Besson, J.M. and Hamon. M. (1985) Spontaneous and evoked release of methionine-enkephalin-like materials from the rat spinal cord in vivo. *Brain Res.*, 339: 305–338.

Ch'ng, J.L.C., Christofides, P., Anand, S.J., Gibson, S., Allen, H.C., Su, K., Tatemoto, J.F.B., Morrison, J.M., Polak, J.M. and Blomm, S.R. (1985) Distribution of galanin immunoreactivity in the central nervous system and responses of galanin-containing neuronal pathways to injury. *Neuroscience*, 16: 343–354.

Chapman, V. and Dickenson, A.H. (1992) The effects of sandostatin and somatostatin on nociceptive transmission in the dorsal horn of the rat spinal cord. *Neuropeptides*, 23: 147–152.

Chung, K., Lee, W.T. and Carlton, S.M. (1988) The effects of dorsal rhizotomy and spinal cord isolation on calcitonin gene-related peptide-labeled terminals in the rat lumbar dorsal horn. *Neurosci. Lett.*, 90: 17–32.

Clarke, P.B.S., Pert, C.B. and Pert, A. (1984) Autoradiographic distribution of nicotine receptors in rat brain. *Brain Res.* 323: 390.

Clarke, R.W., Ford, T.W. and Taylor, J.S. (1988) Adrenergic and opioidergic modulation of a spinal reflex in the decerebrated rabbit. *J. Physiol.*, 404: 407: 417.

Collin, E., Frechilla, D., Pohl, M., Bourgoin, S., LeBars, D., Hamon, M. and Cesselin, F. (1993a) Opioid control of the release of calcitonin gene-related peptide-like material from the rat spinal cord in vivo. *Brain Res.*, 609: 211–222.

Collin, E., Mantelet, S., Frechilla, D., Pohl, M., Bourgoin, S., Hamon, M. and Cesselin, F. (1993b) Increased in vivo release of calcitonin gene-related peptide-like material from the spinal cord in arthritic rats. *Pain*, 54: 203–211.

Colmers, W.F., Klapstein, G.J., Fournier, A., St-Pierre, S. and Treherne, K.A. (1991) Presynaptic inhibition by neuropeptide Y in rat hippocampal slice in vitro is mediated by a Y2 receptor. *Br. J. Pharmacol.*, 102: 41–44.

Cridland, R.A. and Henry, J.L. (1988) Effects of intrathecal administration of neuropeptides on a spinal nociceptive reflex in the rat: VIP, galanin, CGRP, TRH, somatostatin and angiotensin II. Neuropeptides, 11: 23–32.

Curtis, D.R., Lodge, D. and Brand, S.J. (1977) GABA and spinal afferent terminal excitability in the cat. *Brain Res.* 130: 360–363.

Dalsgaard, C-J., Haegerstrand, A., Theodorsson-Norheim, E., Brodin, E. and Hökfelt, T. (1985) Neurokinin-A like immunoreactivity in rat primary sensory neurons: coexistence with substance P. *Histochemistry*, 83: 37–40.

Difiglia, M., Aronin, N. and Leeman, S.E. (1982) Light microscopic and ultrastructural localization of immunoreactive substance P in the dorsal horn of monkey spinal cord. *Neuroscience* 7: 1127–1140.

Donnerer, J. and Amann, R. (1992) Time course of capsaicin-evoked release of CGRP from rat spinal cord in vitro. Effect of concentration and modulations by ruthenium red. *Ann. NY Acad. Sci.*, 657: 491–492.

Doyle, C.A. and Maxwell, D.J. (1991a) Ultrastructural analysis of noradrenergic nerve terminals in the cat lumbosacral spinal dorsal horn: A dopamine-β-hydroxylase immunocytochemical study. *Brain Res.*, 563: 329–333.

Doyle, C.A. and Maxwell, D.J. (1993) Neuropeptide Y immunoreactive terminals form axo-axonic synaptic arrangements in the substantia gelatinosa (lamina II) of the cat spinal cord. *Brain Res.*, 603: 157–161.

Draisci, G. and Iadarola, M.J. (1989) Temporal analysis of increase in c-*fos*, preprodynorphin and preproenkephalin mRNAs in rat spinal cord. *Mol. Brain Res.*, 6: 31–37.

Duggan, A.W. (1991) Antibody Microprobes. In: *Monitoring Neuronal Activity: A Practical Approach*, J. Stamford, Ed., Oxford University Press, Oxford.

Duggan, A.W. and Hendry, I.A. (1986) Laminar localization of the sites of release of immunoreactive substance P in the dorsal horn with antibody coated microelectrodes. *Neurosci. Lett.*, 68: 134–140.

Duncan, D. and Morales, R. (1978) Relative numbers of several types of synaptic connections in the substantia gelatinosa of the cat spinal cord. *J. Comp. Neurol.*, 182: 601–610.

Duggan, A.W., Hall, J.G. and Headley, P.M. (1976) Morphine, enkephalin and the substantia gelatinosa. *Nature*, 264: 456–458.

Duggan, A.W., Greirsmith, B.T., Headley, P.M. and Hall, J.G. (1979) Lack of effect of substance P at sites in the substantia gelatinosa where met-enkephalin reduces the transmission of nociceptive information. *Neurosci. Lett.*, 12: 313–317.

Duggan, A.W., Hendry, I.A., Green, J.L., Morton, C.R. and Hutchison, W.D. (1988a) The preparation and use of antibody microprobes. *J. Neurosci. Methods*, 23: 241–247.

Duggan, A.W., Hendry, I.A., Green, J.L., Morton, C.R. and Zhao, Z.Q. (1988b) Cutaneous stimuli releasing immunoreactive substance P in the dorsal horn of the cat. *Brain Res.*, 451: 261–273.

Duggan, A.W., Morton, C.R., Hutchison, W.D. and Hendry, I.A. (1988c) Absence of tonic supraspinal control of substance P release in the substantia gelatinosa of the anaesthetized cat. *Exp. Brain Res.*, 71: 597–602.

Duggan, A.W., Hope, P.J., Jarrott, B., Schaible, H.-G. and Fleetwood-Walker, S.M. (1990) Release, spread and persistence of immunoreactive neurokinin A in the dorsal horn of the cat following noxious cutaneous stimulation. Studies with antibody microprobes. *Neuroscience*, 35: 195–202.

Duggan, A.W., Hope, P.J. and Lang, C.W. (1991) Microinjection of neuropeptide Y into the superficial dorsal horn reduces stimulus evoked release of immunoreactive substance P in the anaesthetized cat. *Neuroscience*.

Duggan, A.W., Schaible, H.-G., Hope, P.J. and Lang, C.W. (1992) Effect of peptidase inhibition on the pattern of intraspinally released immunoreactive substance P detected with antibody microprobes. *Brain Res.*, 579: 261–269.

Everitt, B.J., Hokfelt, T., Terenius, L., Tatemoto, K., Mutt, V. and Goldstein, M. (1984) Differential co-existence of neuropeptide Y (NPY)-like immunoreactivity with catecholamine in the central nervous system of the rat. *Neuroscience*, 11: 443–462.

Fleetwood-Walker, S.M., Mitchell, R., Hope, P.J., Molony, V. and Iggo, A. (1985) An alpha 2 receptor mediates the selective inhibition by noradrenaline of nociceptive responses of identified dorsal horn neurons. *Brain Res.*, 334: 243–254.

Fleetwood-Walker, S.M., Hope, P.J., Molony, V., Parker, R.M.C., Munro, F.E. and Mitchell, R. (1992) Distinct ef-

fects of somatostatin-14 and somatostatin-28 on nociceptive responses of spinal dorsal horn neurons. *Br. J. Pharmacol.*, 105: 132.

Fuxe, K. and Agnati, L.F. (1991) Two principal modes of electrochemical communication in the brain: volume versus wiring transmission. In: K. Fuxe (Ed.) *Volume Transmission in the Brain*, Raven Press, New York, pp. 1–9.

Garry, M.G. and Hargreaves, K.M. (1992) Enhanced release of immunoreactive CGRP and substance P from spinal dorsal horn slices occurs during carrageenan inflammation. *Brain Res.*, 582: 139–142.

Gibbins, I.L., Furness, J.B., Costa, M., MacIntyre, I., Hillyard, C.J. and Girgis, S. (1985) Colocalization of calcitonin gene-related peptide-like immunoreactivity with substance P in cutaneous, vascular and visceral sensory neurons of guinea pigs. *Neurosci. Lett.*, 57: 125–130.

Gibson, S.J., Polak, J.M., Bloom, S.R., Sabate, I.M., Mulderry, P.M., Ghatei, M.A., McGregor, G.P., Morrison, J.F., Kelly, J.S., Evans, R.M. and Rosenfeld, M.G. (1984) Calcitonin gene-related peptide immunoreactivity in the spinal cord of man and eight other species. *Neuroscience*, 4: 3101–3111.

Gibson, S.J., McCrossan, M.V. and Polak, J.M. (1985) A sub-population of calcitonin gene-related peptide (CGRP)-immunoreactive neurons in the dorsal root ganglia also display substance P, somatostatin or gelanin immunoreactivity. *Proc. XII Int. Anatomy Congress*, 232.

Glazer, E.J. and Basbaum, A.I. (1981) Immunohistochemical localization of leucine-enkephalin in the spinal cord of the cat: enkephalin-containing marginal neurons and pain modulation. *J. Comp. Neurol.*, 196: 377–390.

Go, V.L.W. and Yaksh, T.L. (1987) Release of substance P from the cat spinal cord. *J. Physiol.*, 391: 141–167.

Haas, H.L., Hermann, A., Greene, R.W. and Chan-Palay, V. (1987) Action and location of neuropeptide tyrosine (Y) on hippocampal neurons of the rat in slice preparations. *Comp. Neurol.*, 257: 208–215.

Hamon, M., Bourgoin, S., Le Bars, D. and Cesselin, F. (1988) In vivo and in vitro release of central neurotransmitters in relation to pain and analgesia. In: H.L. Fields and J.-M. Besson, (Eds.) *Pain Modulation. Progress in Brain Research*, Elsevier Science Publishers, Amsterdam, pp. 431–444.

Headley, P.M., Duggan, A.W. and Griersmith, B.T. (1978) Selective reduction by noradrenaline and 5-hydroxytryptamine of nociceptive responses of cat dorsal horn neurons. *Brain Res.*, 145: 185–189.

Hirota, N., Kuraishi, Y., Hino, U., Sato, Y., Satoh, M. and Takagi, H. (1985) Met-enkephalin and morphine but not dynorphin inhibit noxious stimulus-induced release of substance P from rabbit dorsal horn in situ. *Neuropharmacology*, 24: 567–570.

Hökfelt, T., Elde, R., Johansson, O., Luft, R., Nilsson, G. and Arimura, A. (1976) Immunohistochemical evidence for separate populations of somatostatin-containing and substance

P-containing primary afferent neurons in the rat. *Neuroscience*, 1: 131–136.

Hökfelt, T., Ljungdahl, A., Terenius, L., Elde, R. and Nilsson, G. (1977) Immunohistochemical analysis of peptide pathways possibly related to pain and analgesia: enkephalin and substance P. *Proc. Natl. Acad. Sci. USA*, 74: 3081–3085.

Hökfelt, T., Arvidsson, U., Ceccatelli, S., Cort,s, R., Cullheim, S., Dagerlind, Å., Johnson, H., Orazzo, C., Piehl, F., Pieribone, V., Schalling, M., Terenius, L., Ulfhake, B., Verge, V.M., Villar, M., Wiesenfeld-Hallin, Z., Xu, X.-J. and Xu, Z. (1992) Calcitonin gene-related peptide in the brain, spinal cord and some peripheral systems. *Ann. NY Acad. Sci.*, 657: 119–134.

Holets, V.R., Hökfelt, T., Rokaeus, A., Terenius, L. and Goldstein, M. (1988) Locus coeruleus neurons in the rat containing neuropeptide Y, tyrosine hydroxylase or galanin and their efferent projections to the spinal cord, cerebral cortex and hypothalamus. *Neuroscience*, 24: 893–906.

Holzer, P. (1991) Capsaicin: cellular targets, mechanisms of action and selectively for thin sensory neurons. *Pharm. Rev.*, 43: 143–202.

Hope, P.J., Jarrott, B., Schaible, H.-G., Clarke, W. and Duggan, A.W. (1990a) Release and spread of immunoreactive neurokinin A in the cat spinal cord in a model of acute arthritis. *Brain Res.*, 533: 292–299.

Hope, P.J., Lang, C.W. and Duggan, A.W. (1990b) Persistence of immunoreactive neurokinins in the dorsal horn of barbiturate anaesthetised and spinal cats, following release by tibial nerve stimulation. *Neurosci. Lett.*, 118: 25–28.

Hope, P.J., Lang, C.W., Grubb, B.D. and Duggan, A.W. (1994) Release of immunoreactive galanin in the spinal cord of rats with ankle inflammation: studies with antibody microprobes. *Neuroscience*, 60: 801–807.

Hutchison, W.D. and Morton, C.R. (1989) Electrical stimulation of primary afferent A fibres does not reduce substance P release in the dorsal horn of the cat. *Pain*, 37: 357–363.

Hutchison, W.D., Morton, C.R. and Terenius, L. (1990) Dynorphin A: in vivo release in the spinal cord of the cat. *Brain Res.*, 532: 299–306.

Iadarola, M.J., Brady, L.S., Draisci, G. and Dubner, R. (1988) Enhancement of dynorphin gene expression in spinal cord following experimental inflammation: stimulus specificity, behavioural parameters and opioid receptor binding. *Pain*, 35: 313–326.

Jessell, T.M. and Iversen, L.L. (1977) Opiate analgesics inhibit substance P release from rat trigeminal nucleus. *Nature*, 268: 549–551.

Ju, G., Hokfelt, T., Brodin, E., Fahrenkrug, J. and Fischer, J.A. (1987a) Primary sensory neurons of the rat showing calcitonin gene-related peptide immunoreactivity and their relation to substance P-, somatostatin-, galanin-, vasoactive intestinal polypetide- and cholecystolcinin-immunoreactive ganglion cells. *Cell Tissue Res.*, 247: 417–431.

Ju, G., Hokfelt, T., Brodin, E., Fahrenkrug, J., Fischer, J.A., Frey, P., Elde, R.P. and Brown, J.C. (1987b) Primary sensory neurons of the rat showing calcitonin gene-related peptide immunoreactivity and their relation to substance P, somatostatin-, galanin-, vasoactive intestinal polypeptide- and cholecystokinin-immunoreactive ganglion cells. *Cell Tissue Res.*, 247: 417–431.

Kar, S. and Quirion, R. (1992) Quantitative autoradiographic localization of [125I]neuropeptide Y receptor binding sites in rat spinal cord and the effects of neonatal capsaicin, dorsal rhizotomy and peripheral axotomy. *Brain Res.*, 574: 333–337.

Klein, C.M., Westlund, K.N. and Coggeshall, R.E. (1990) Percentages of dorsal root axons immunoreactive for galanin are higher than those immunoreactive for calcitonin gene-related peptide. *Brain Res.*, 519: 97–101.

Klein, C.M., Coggeshall, R.E., Carlton, S.M. and Sorkin, L.S. (1992) The effects of A- and C-fiber stimulation on patterns of neuropeptide immunostaining in the rat superficial dorsal horn. *Brain Res.*, 580: 121–128.

Kuraishi, Y., Hirota, N., Sato, Y., Kaneto, S., Satoh, M. and Takagi, H. (1982) Noradrenergic inhibition of the release of substance P from the primary afferents in the rabbit spinal dorsal horn. *Brain Res.*, 359: 177–182.

Kuraishi, Y., Hirota, N., Sugimoto, M., Sato, M. and Tagaki, H. (1983) Effects of morphine on noxious stimuli induced release of substance P from the rabbit dorsal horn. *Life Sci.*, 33: 693–696.

Kuraishi, Y., Hirota, N., Sato, Y., Hino, Y., Satoh, M. and Takagi, H. (1985) Evidence that substance P and somatostatin transmit separate information related to pain in the spinal dorsal horn. *Brain Res.*, 325: 294–298.

Kuraishi, Y., Hirota, N., Sato, Y. and Hanashima, N. (1989) Stimulus specificity of peripherally evoked substance P release from rabbit dorsal horn in situ. *Neuroscience*, 30: 241–250.

Lang, C.W., Duggan, A.W. and Hope, P.J. (1991) Analgesic doses of morphine do not reduce noxious stimulus-evoked release of immunoreactive neurokinins in the dorsal horn of the spinal cat. *Br. J. Pharmacol.*, 103: 1871–1876.

Larsson, J., Ekblom, A., Henriksson, K., Lundeberg, T. and Theodorsson, E. (1991) Concentration of substance P, neurokinin A, calcitonin gene-related peptide, neuropeptide Y and vasoactive intestinal polypeptide in synovial fluid from knee joints in patients suffering from rheumatoid arthritis. *Scand. J. Rheumatol.*, 20: 326–335.

Le Greves, P., Nyberg, F., Terenius, L. and Hokfelt, T. (1985) Calcitonin gene-related peptide is a potent inhibitor of substance P degradation. *Eur. J. Pharmacol.*, 115: 309–311.

Leah, J.D., Cameron, A.A., Kelly, W.L. and Snow, P.J. (1985) Coexistence of peptide immunoreactivity in sensory neurons of the cat. *Neuroscience*, 16: 683–690.

Lembeck, F. and Donnerer, J. (1985) Opioid control of the function of primary afferent substance P fibres. *Eur. J. Pharmacol.*, 114: 241–246.

Linderoth, B. and Brodin, E. (1988) Tachykinin release from rat spinal cord in vitro and in vivo in response to various stimuli. *Regul. Peptides*, 21: 129–140.

Lindh, B., Lundberg, J.M. and Hokfelt, T. (1989) NPY-, galanin-, VIP/PHI-, CGRP- and substance P-immunoreactive neuronal subpopulations in cat autonomic and sensory ganglia and their projections. *Cell Tissue Res.*, 256: 259–273.

Liu, H., Brown, J.L., Jasmin, L., Maggio, J.E., Vigna, S.R., Mantyh, P.W. and Basbaum, A.I. (1994) Synaptic relationship between substance P and the substance P receptor: light and electron microscopic characterization of the mismatch between neuropeptides and their receptors. *Proc. Natl. Acad. Sci. USA*, 91: 1009–1013.

Malcangio, M. and Bowery, N.G. (1993) gamma-Aminobutyric acidB, but not gamma-aminobutyric acidA receptor activation, inhibits electrically evoked substance P-like immunoreactivity release from the rat spinal cord in vitro. *J. Pharmacol. Exp. Ther.*, 266: 1490–1496.

Mauborgne, A., Lutz, O., Legrand, J.C., Hamon, M. and Cesselin, F. (1987) Opposite effects of delta and mu opioid receptor agonists on the in vitro release of substance P-like mateial from the rat spinal cord. *J. Neurochem.*, 48: 529–537.

McCarson, K.E. and Goldstein, B.D. (1991) Release of substance P into the superficial dorsal horn following nociceptive activation of the hindpaw of the rat. *Brain Res.*, 568: 109–115.

McKelvey, J.F. and Blumberg, S. (1986) Inactivation and metabolism of neuropeptides. *Annu. Rev. Neurosci.*, 9: 415–434.

McLachlan, E.M. (1978) The statistics of transmitter release at chemical synapses. In: R. Porter (Ed.) *Neurophysiology III*, University Park Press, Baltimore, pp. 49–117.

Melander, T.T., Hokfelt, T. and Rokaeus, A. (1986) Distribution of galanin-like immunoreactivity in the rat central nevous system. *J. Comp. Neurol.*, 248: 475–517.

Melzack, R. and Wall, P.D. (1965) Pain mechanisms: a new theory. *Science*, 150: 973–979.

Morton, C.R. and Hutchison, W.D. (1989) Release of sensory neuropeptides in the spinal cord: studies with calcitonin gene-related peptide and galanin. *Neuroscience*, 31: 807–815.

Morton, C.R. and Hutchison, W.D. (1990) Morphine does not reduce the intraspinal release of calcitonin gene-related peptide in the cat. *Neurosci. Lett.*, 117: 319–324.

Morton, C.R., Hutchison, W.D., Hendry, I.A. and Duggan, A.W. (1989) Somatostatin:evidence for a role in thermal nociception. *Brain Res.*, 488: 89–96.

Morton, C.R., Hutchison, W.D., Duggan, A.W. and Hendry, I.A. (1990) Morphine and substance P release in the spinal cord. *Exp. Brain Res.*, 82: 89–96.

Morton, C.R., Hutchison, W.D. and Lacey, G. (1992) Baclofen and the release of neuropeptides in the cat spinal cord. *Eur. J. Neurosci.*, 4: 243–250.

Morton, C.R., Zhao, Z.Q. and Duggan, A.W. (1982) A function of opioid peptides in the spinal cord of the cat: intracellular studies of motoneurones during naloxone administration. *Neuropeptides*, 3: 83–90.

Neto, F.R. (1978) The depolarizing action of 5-HT on mammalian non-myelinated nerve fibres. *Eur. J. Pharmacol.*, 49: 351–352.

North, R.A. and Yoshimura, M. (1984) The actions of noradrenaline on neurons of the rat substantia gelatinosa in vitro. *J. Physiol.*, 349: 43–56.

Nyberg, F., Le Greves, P., Sundqvist, C. and Terenius, L. (1984) Characterization of substance P(1–7) and (1–8) generating enzyme in human cerebrospinal fluid. *Biochem. Biophys. Res. Commun.*, 125: 244–250.

Ogawa, I., Kanazawa, I. and Kimura, S. (1983) Regional distribution of substance P, neurokinin A and neurokinin B in the rat spinal cord, nerve roots and dorsal root ganglia and the effects of dorsal root or spinal transection. *Brain Res.*, 359: 132–157.

Oku, R., Satoh, M. and Tagaki, H. (1987) Release of substance P from the dorsal horn is enhanced in polyarthritic rats. *Neurosci. Lett.*, 74: 315–319.

Ono, H., Mishima, A., Ono, S., Fukuda, H. and Vasko, M.R. (1991) Inhibitory effects of clonidine and tizanidine on release of substance P from slices of rat spinal cord and antagonism by α-adrenergic receptor antagonists. *Neuropharmacology*, 30: 585–589.

Pang, I.H. and Vasko, M.R. (1986) Morphine and norepinephrine but not 5-hydroxytryptamine and γ-aminobutyric acid inhibit the potassium-simulated release of substance P from rat spinal cord slices. *Brain Res.*, 376: 268–279.

Philippu, A. (1984) Use of push-pull cannulae to determine the release of endogenous neurotransmitters in distinct brain areas of anaesthetized and freely moving animals. In: C.A. Marsden (Ed.) *Measurement of Neurotransmitter Release In Vivo*, John Wiley, New York, pp. 3–38.

Pohl, M., Mauborgne, A., Bourgoin, S., Benoliel, J.J., Hamon, M. and Cesselin, F. (1989) Neonatal capsaicin treatment abolishes the modulations by opioids of substance P release from rat spinal cord slices. *Neurosci. Lett.*, 96: 102–107.

Pohl, M., Collin, E., Bourgoin, S., Clot, A.M., Hamon, M., Cesselin, F. and LeBars, D. (1992) In vivo release of calcitonin gene-related peptide-like material from the cervicotrigeminal area in the rat. Effects of electrical and noxious stimulations of the muzzle. *Neuroscience*, 50: 697–706.

Post, C., Alari, L. and Hokfelt, T. (1988) Intrathecal galanin increases the latency in the tail flick and hot plate tests in the mouse. *Acta Physiol. Scand.*, 132: 583–584.

Randic, M. and Miletic, V. (1978) Depressent actions of methionine-enkephalin and somatostatin in cat dorsal horn neurons activated by noxious stimuli. *Brain Res.*, 152: 196–202.

Ruda, M.A. (1982) Opiates and pain pathways: demonstration of enkephalin synapses on dorsal horn projection neurons. *Science*, 215: 1523–1525.

Ruda, M.A. and Gobel, S. (1980) Ultrastructural characterization of axonal endings in the substantia gelatinosa which take up ^{3}H-serotonin. *Brain Res.*, 184: 57–84.

Sakatani, K., Chesler, M. and Hassan, A.Z. (1991) GABAA receptors modulate axonal conduction in dorsal columns of neonatal rat spinal cord. *Brain Res.*, 542: 273–279.

Sakatani, K., Chesler, M., Hassan, A.Z., Lee, M. and Young, W. (1993) Non-synaptic modulation of dorsal column conduction by endogenous GABA in neonatal rat spinal cord. *Brain Res.*, 622: 43–50.

Sakuma, M., Yoshioka, K., Suzuki, H., Yanagisawa, M., Onishi, Y., Kobayashi, N. and Otsuka, M. (1991) Substance P-evoked release of GABA from isolated spinal cord of the newborn rat. *Neuroscience*, 45: 323–330.

Sandkuhler, J., Fu, Q.G. and Helmchen, C. (1990) Spinal somatostatin superfusion 'in vivo' affects activity of cat nociceptive dorsal horn neuron: comparison with spinal morphine. *Neuroscience*, 34: 565–576.

Santicioli, P., Del Bianco, E., Tramontana, M. and Maggi, C.A. (1992) Adenosine inhibits action potential-dependent release of calcitonin gene-related peptide- and substance P-like immunoreactivities from primary afferents in rat spinal cord. *Neurosci. Lett.*, 144: 211–214.

Saria, A., Javorsky, F., Humpel, C. and Gamse, R. (1991) Endogenous 5-hydroxytryptamine modulates the release of tachykinins and calcitonin gene-related peptide from the rat spinal cord via 5-HT3 receptors. *Ann. NY Acad. Sci.*, 632: 464–465.

Schaible, H.-G. and Grubb, B.D. (1993) Afferent and spinal mechanisms of joint pain. *Pain*, 55: 5–54.

Schaible, H.-G. and Schmidt, R.F. (1985a) Effects of an experimental arthritis on the sensory properties of fine articular afferent units. *J. Neurophysiol.*, 54: 1109–1122.

Schaible, H.-G. and Schmidt, R.F. (1985b) Effects of an experimental arthritis on the sensory properties of fine articular afferents. *Neurophysiology*, 54: 1109–1122.

Schaible, H-G., Jarrott, B., Hope, P.J. and Duggan, A.W. (1990) Release of immunoreactive substance P in the spinal cord during development of acute arthritis in the knee joint of the cat: a study with antibody microprobes. *Brain Res.*, 529: 214–223.

Schaible, H-G., Hope, P.J., Lang, C.W. and Duggan, A.W. (1992) Calcitonin gene-related peptide causes intraspinal spreading of substance P released by peripheral stimulation. *Eur. J. Neurosci.*, 4: 750–757.

Schmidt, R.F. (1971) Presynaptic inhibition in the vertebrate nervous system. *Rev. Physiol.*, 63: 20–101.

Suarez-Roca, H., Abdullah, L., Zuniga, J., Madison, S. and Maixner, W. (1992) Multiphasic effect of morphine on the release of substance P from rat trigeminal nucleus slices. *Brain Res.*, 579: 187–194.

Sumal, K.K., Pickel, V.M., Miller, R.J. and Reis, D.J. (1982) Enkephalin containing neurons in substantia gelatinosa of spinal trigeminal complex: ultra structure and synaptic interaction with primary sensory afferents. *Brain Res.*, 248: 223–236.

Takano, M., Takano, Y. and Yaksh, T.L. (1993) Release of calcitonin gene-related peptide (CGRP), substance P (SP) and vasoactive intestinal polypeptide (VIP) from rat spinal cord: Modulation by $\alpha 2$ agonists. *Peptides*, 14: 371–378.

Tessler, A., Himes, B.T., Gruber-Bollinger, J. and Reichin, S. (1986) Characterization of forms of immunoreactive somatostatin in sensory neurons in normal and deafferented spinal cord. *Brain Res.*, 370: 232–240.

Tiseo, P.J., Adler, M.W. and Liu-Chen, L. (1990) Differential release of substance P and somatostatin in the rat spinal cord in response to noxious heat and cold; effect of dynorphin A(1–17). *J. Pharmacol. Exp. Ther.*, 252: 539–545.

Toresson, G., Carreras, C. de las, Brodin, E. and Bertilsson, L. (1990) Neuropeptide K is present in human cerebrospinal fluid. *Life Sci.*, 46, 23.: 1707–1714.

Ungerstedt, U. (1984) Measurement of neurotransmitter release by intracranial dialysis. In: Marsden. C.A. (Ed.) *Measurement of Neurotransmitter Release In Vivo*, John Wiley, New York, pp. 81–106.

Villar, M.J., Cortes, R., Theodorsson, E., Wiesenfeld-Hallin, Z., Schalling, M., Fahrenkrug, J., Emson, P.C. and Hokfelt, T. (1990) Neuropeptide expression in rat dorsal root ganglion cells and spinal cord after peripheral nerve injury with special reference to galanin. *Neuroscience*, 33: 587–604.

Villar, M.J., Wiesenfeld-Hallin, Z., Xu, X.-J., Theodorsson, E., Emson, P.C. and Hökfelt, T. (1991) Further studies on galanin-, substance P- and CGRP-like immunoreactivities in primary sensory neurons and spinal cord: Effects of dorsal rhizotomies and sciatic nerve lesions. *Exp. Neurol.*, 112: 29–39.

Wall, P.D., Fitzgerald, M. and Gibson, S.J. (1981) The response of rat spinal cord cells to ummyelinated afferents after peripheral nerve section and changes in substance P levels. *Neuroscience*, 6: 2205–2216.

Weihe, E., Millan, M.J., Hollt, V., Nohr, D. and Herz, A. (1989) Induction of the gene encoding pro-dnyorphin by experimentally induced arthritis enhances staining for dynorphin in the spinal cord of rats. *Neuroscience*, 31: 77–95.

Wiesenfeld-Hallin, Z., Xu, X.-J., Håkanson, R., Feng, D.M., Folkers, K., Kristensson, K., Villar, M.J., Fahrenkrug, J. and Hökfelt, T. (1991) On the role of substance P, galanin, vasoactive intestinal peptide and calcitonin gene-related peptide in mediation of spinal reflex excitability in rats with intact and sectioned peripheral nerves. *Ann. NY Acad. Sci.*, 632: 198–211.

Wilson, L.B., Fuchs, I.E. and Mitchell, J.H. (1993) Effects of graded muscle contractions on spinal cord substance P release, arterial blood pressure and heart rate. *Circ. Res.*, 73: 1024–1031.

Woolf, C.J. and Wiesenfeld-Hallin, Z. (1986) Substance P and calcitonin gene-related peptide synergistically modulate the gain of the nociceptive flexor withdrawal reflex in the rat. *Neurosci. Lett.*, 66: 226–230.

Yaksh, T. (1984) Spinal perfusion in the rat and cat. In: C.A. Marsden (Ed.) *Measurement of Neurotransmitter Release In Vivo*. John Wiley, New York, pp. 107–126.

Yaksh, T.L. and Elde, R.P. (1981) Factors governing release of methionine enkephalin-like immune reactivity from mesencephalin and spinal cord of the cat in vivo. *J. Neurophysiol.*, 46: 1056–1075.

Yaksh, T.L., Jessell, T.M., Gamse, R., Mudge, A.W. and Leeman, S.E. (1980) Intrathecal morphine inhibits substance P release from mammalian spinal cord in vivo. *Nature*, 286: 155–157.

Yonehara, N., Shibutani, T., Imai, Y., Ooi, Y., Sawada, T. and Inoki, R. (1991) Serotonin inhibits release of substance P evoked by tooth pulp stimulation in trigeminal nucleus caudalis in rabbits. *Neuropharmacology*, 30: 5–14.

Yoshimura, M., Shimizu, T., Yajiri, Y., Inokuchi, H. and Nishi, S. (1993) Primary afferent-evoked slow EPSPs and responses to substance P of dorsal horn neurons in the adult rat spinal cord slices. *Regul. Peptides*, 46: 407–409.

Zhao, Z.-Q. and Duggan, A.W. (1987) Clonidine and the hyper-responsiveness of dorsal horn neurons following morphine withdrawal in the spinal cat. *Neuropharmacology*, 26, No.10: 1499–1502.

Zhu, C.G., Sandri, C. and Akert, K. (1981) Morphological identification of axo-axonic and dendro-dendrtic synapses in the rat substantia gelatinosa. *Brain Res.*, 230: 25–40.

Zimmerman, M. (1976) *International Review of Physiology: Neurophysiology II*, University Park Press, Baltimore.

F. Nyberg, H.S. Sharma and Z. Wiesenfeld-Hallin (Eds.)
Progress in Brain Research, Vol 104

CHAPTER 13

Interaction of neuropeptides and excitatory amino acids in the rat superficial spinal dorsal horn

M. Randić, M. Kolaj, Lj. Kojić, R. Cerne, G. Cheng and R.A. Wang

Department of Veterinary Physiology and Pharmacology, Iowa State University, Ames, IA 50011, USA

Introduction

The superficial spinal dorsal horn (SDH), including substantia gelatinosa (SG), is an area where primary afferent fibers arising predominantly from skin, but also the viscera and muscles terminate and form the first synaptic relay with dendrites of dorsal horn (DH) neurons. For this reason, the SDH has been regarded as an important site for the initial processing of afferent signals directly related to the transmission and modulation of cutaneous information, including pain. Most nociceptive primary afferent fibers terminate in this region (Christensen and Perl, 1970; Sugiura et al., 1986).

It is now established that the primary afferent fibers use glutamate, or a related amino acid, as a principal excitatory transmitter (Zieglgänsberger and Puil, 1973; Watkins and Evans, 1981; Jahr and Jessell, 1985; Mayer and Westbrook, 1987; Sillar and Roberts, 1988; Gerber and Randić, 1989a; Kangrga and Randić, 1990, 1991; Yoshimura and Jessell, 1990; Dougherty et al., 1992; King and Lopez-Garcia, 1993; Yoshimura and Nishi, 1993). Neuronal excitatory amino acids (EAAs), including glutamate, produce their effects through two broad categories of receptors called ionotropic and metabotropic (Watkins et al., 1990; Schoepp et al., 1991). Three EAA ionotropic receptor subtypes are classified on the basis of their selectivity to such synthetic agonists as *N*-methyl-D-aspartate (NMDA), α-amino-3-hydroxy-5-methyl-4-isoxazolepropionic acid (AMPA), and kainate (KA) receptors (Watkins et al., 1990). Molecular studies have demonstrated that these EAA receptor subtypes are hetero-oligomeric assemblies of subunits (Gasic and Hollmann, 1992; Sommer and Seeburg, 1992; Wisden and Seeburg, 1993). The presence of all three binding sites in the mammalian spinal cord has been reported (Monaghan et al., 1989; Jansen et al., 1990; Tölle et al., 1993). The activation of EAA receptors in the spinal cord is important for both physiological and pathophysiological functions. Non-NMDA receptor activation is essential for fast excitatory transmission in the CNS, including spinal cord. At a pathological level, regulation of the voltage-dependent Mg^{2+} ion block of NMDA receptors is, at least in part, responsible for the central sensitization of pain perception (Davies and Lodge, 1987; Chen and Huang, 1992; Woolf and Thompson, 1991). The metabotropic glutamate receptors appear to be coupled to phospholipase C through G-proteins. Their activation causes an increase in turnover of polyphosphoinositides and release of Ca^{2+} from intracellular stores (Schoepp et al., 1991). The increase in $[Ca^{2+}]_i$, in turn, may lead to activation of second messenger systems with consequent changes in the properties of EAA receptor channel complexes that contribute to slow excitatory synaptic transmission (Charpak and Gähwiler, 1991) and to long-term influences on the fast excitatory synaptic transmission (Cerne et al., 1992; Kojic and Randić, 1993), neuronal excitability (Collingridge and Singer, 1990; Siegelbaum and Kandel, 1991; Johnston et al., 1992; Malenka and Nicoll, 1993) and gene expression (Szekely et al., 1989).

The role of neuropeptides, such as tachykinins and opioid peptides in long-term modulation of synaptic transmission related to pain is now well established (Rustioni and Weinberg, 1989; Coderre et al., 1993; Duggan and Fleetwood-Walker, 1993; McMahon et al., 1993). Tachykinins produce their effects in nervous tissue through at least three molecularly distinct subtypes of receptors (Masu et al., 1987; Yokota et al., 1989; Shigemoto et al., 1990). The neurokinin (NK) receptors, NK_1, NK_2 and NK_3 are preferentially activated by the endogenous peptides, substance P (SP), neurokinin A (NKA) and neurokinin B. SP, the most extensively characterized member of tachykinin peptide family, is released in the spinal DH by impulses in peripheral nociceptors (Yaksh et al., 1980; Duggan et al., 1987). It has been shown to depolarize DH neurons (Murase and Randić, 1984), to stimulate low- and high-voltage activated Ca^{2+} channels (Ryu and Randić, 1990), to increase $[Ca^{2+}]_i$ in these neurons (Womack et al., 1988), to modify a number of voltage-dependent potassium currents (Murase et al., 1989; Yamaguchi et al., 1990), to stimulate phosphoinositide turnover (Mantyh et al., 1984) and cyclic AMP formation (Nakajima et al., 1992). Tachykinins appear to be functionally involved in the slow excitatory synaptic transmission (Urbán and Randić, 1984; Randić et al., 1986, 1987; De Koninck and Henry, 1991). Immunocytochemical studies have demonstrated that glutamate coexists with SP in many small dorsal root ganglia neurons and their terminals in the superficial laminae of the rat spinal DH (DeBiasi and Rustioni, 1988). However, the physiological significance of this phenomenon for primary afferent neurotransmission is not understood.

The DH of the spinal cord contains both endogenous opioid peptides derived from proopiomelanocortin, preproenkephalin and preprodynorphin (Simon, 1991) and at least three subtypes (μ, δ and κ) (Martin et al., 1964; Lord et al., 1977) of the opioid receptors, which are present both on the primary sensory and DH neurons (Atweh and Kuhar, 1977; Fields et al., 1980; Slater and Patel, 1983; Morris and Herz, 1987; Sharif et al., 1988; Allerton et al., 1989). Recently, direct evidence for the presence of molecularly distinct μ, δ and κ opioid receptor subtypes in central neurons has been obtained (Reisine and Bell, 1993). Endogenous opioid peptides methionine- and leucine-enkephalin, regarded as likely endogenous ligands for δ and μ receptors, and dynorphin A for κ receptors, are also present within the spinal DH, where they occur in local neurons (Hunt et al., 1980; Botticelli et al., 1981; Glazer and Basbaum, 1981; Miller and Seybold, 1987, 1989; Fallon and Ciofi, 1990), in descending neurons (Hökfelt et al., 1983) and in afferent fibers (Jessell and Dodd, 1989). Functional studies made in adult spinal cord support the involvement of μ and δ opioid receptors in spinal nociception. Evidence for the involvement of κ receptors is less clear (Coderre et al., 1993; Duggan and Fleetwood-Walker, 1993). However, the cellular mechanism(s) and the role of different subtypes of opioid receptors and opioid peptides in the regulation of sensory information, including pain, at the spinal level remains controversial. Previous studies have shown that the activation of opioid receptors produces inhibitory (Calvillo et al., 1974; Zieglgänsberger and Bayerl, 1976; Duggan et al., 1976a,b, 1977a,b; Randic and Miletic, 1978; Sastry and Goh, 1983; Willcockson et al., 1986; Fleetwood-Walker et al., 1988; Dong et al., 1991) and excitatory (Belcher and Ryall, 1978; Willcockson et al., 1986; Knox and Dickenson, 1987; Hylden et al., 1991) effects in DH neurons studied in vivo. In the CNS, the suppression of synaptic responses by opioids has been reported (McFadzean et al., 1987; Allerton et al., 1989; Hori et al., 1992; Pinnock, 1992; Wagner et al.,

1992; Rhim et al., 1993; Weisskopf et al., 1993; Glaum et al., 1994). Both, presynaptic and postsynaptic sites of action have been suggested (Millan, 1990; Duggan and Fleetwood-Walker, 1993). Presynaptically, μ and δ opioids suppress the release of neurotransmitters (North, 1993), including glutamate (Kangrga and Randić, 1991; Hori et al., 1992) and SP (Jessell and Iversen, 1977), from primary sensory neurons in slice. Postsynaptically, opioids produce a hyperpolarization in DH neurons (Murase et al., 1982; Yoshimura and North, 1983; Grudt and Williams, 1993); they increase K^+ conductance or decrease Ca^{2+} conductance (Grudt and Williams, 1993; North, 1993). At the molecular level, activation of opioid receptors leads to inhibition of adenylate cyclase through the action of G-proteins (Childers, 1993). Opioid peptides also modulate the responses to glutamate and its analogs. Thus the δ receptor-preferring ligand enkephalin inhibits the glutamate-evoked activity of spinal neurons (Barker et al., 1978a,b; Zieglgänsberger and Tulloch, 1979; Willcockson et al., 1986), whereas μ and κ receptor agonists such as morphine and dynorphin, either depress or enhance the glutamate activity of spinal neurons (Zieglgänsberger and Bayerl, 1976; Zieglgänsberger and Tulloch, 1979; Willcockson et al., 1986; Aanonsen and Wilcox, 1987). However, the specific subtypes of opioid and glutamate receptors involved, and the cellular mechanisms underlying the modulation of glutamate receptor-activated conductance by μ and κ opioids, have only recently been investigated (Chen and Huang, 1991; Rusin and Randić, 1991; Kolaj et al., 1992, 1993a,b; 1995; Cerne et al., 1993a).

This review focuses on recent information derived from neurophysiological work done in vitro, using spinal slice preparation and acutely isolated spinal DH neurons of young rats. The emphasis of this review is placed on interaction of sensory neuropeptides (tachykinins and μ and κ opioid receptor-preferring peptide ligands) and excitatory amino acids and their potential role in long-term changes in synaptic transmission related to pain.

Interaction of tachykinins and EAAs

The functional role of tachykinins in the rat spinal DH could be related, at least in part, to an interaction with glutamate receptor at the postsynaptic site. It has been reported that glutamate-activated conductance in rat spinal DH neurons is enhanced by SP (Randić et al., 1990), but the specific subtypes of glutamate and tachykinin receptors involved and the cellular mechanisms underlying the SP enhancement have not been studied until recently (Rusin et al., 1992, 1993a,b). The use of acutely isolated DH neurons under whole-cell voltage clamp conditions, permitted analysis of direct postsynaptic interactions between tachykinin and EAA receptors. A simultaneous application of NMDA and SP for several seconds reversibly enhanced (Fig. 1B) the peak amplitude of the NMDA-induced current in 60% of the examined cells and reduced it in 27% of the cells. In addition, pretreatment of DH cells with SP for several minutes produced an initial decrease followed by an increase (Fig. 1A) in the AMPA-induced currents. For a given tachykinin concentration, SP was more effective in producing an increased NMDA receptor-mediated current response, both in the amplitude of the peak currents generated and in the percentage of cells that responded to this peptide. As opposed to SP, a simultaneous application of NMDA and NKA reversibly suppressed the peak amplitude of the NMDA-induced current in more than half of the examined cells. Similar to SP, however, the NMDA-induced currents were enhanced (Fig. 1B) by NKA up to 20 min after removal of the peptide. These effects were observed at tachykinin concentrations as low as 10^{-11} M. Exposure of DH cells to SP or NKA for several minutes had two distinct effects on the peak amplitude of the NMDA-induced current, consisting of an initial depression followed by a marked potentiation. The enhancing effect in some cells lasted up to 1 hour. The SP potentiation of NMDA-induced current was blocked by a nonselective antagonist of neurokinin receptors, spantide II (Folkers et al., 1990), suggesting that the SP effect is likely to be a true tachykinin receptor-mediated event. Moreover, the interaction between tachykinins and NMDA receptors appears to be mediated by both NK_1 and NK_2 receptors.

The exact molecular mechanisms underlying the enhancement of NMDA receptor-activated conductance by tachykinins have yet to be elucidated. The possibility that SP directly modifies kinetic properties of single NMDA channels, or

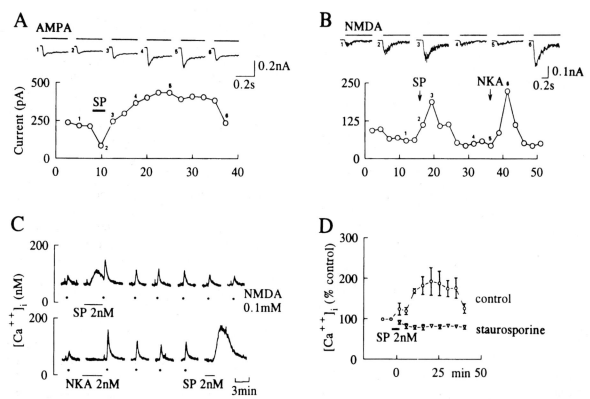

Fig. 1. NMDA- and AMPA-induced current responses in DH neurons are potentiated by substance P (SP) and neurokinin A (NKA). A. The traces show inward current responses evoked by 10 μM AMPA recorded at 2.5-min intervals from a DH neuron held at -60 mV before (trace 1), during (trace 2) and after (traces 3,4,5,6) superfusion of the cell with SP (1 nM for 2.5 min). Time course of changes in the AMPA-induced current responses recorded before, during and after the superfusion with SP in the same DH neuron is shown in the graph. B. The traces show inward current responses evoked by 0.1 mM NMDA recorded at 2.5-min intervals at high-speed on a digital oscilloscope diskette from a DH neuron held at -60 mV before (trace 1) and during 10 sec application of 0.1 mM NMDA plus 2 nM SP (trace 2) or 0.1 mM NMDA plus 2 nM NKA (trace 5). Time course of changes in the peak amplitude of the NMDA-induced current responses recorded before, during and after SP + NMDA or NKA + NMDA co-administration in the same neuron is shown in the graph. TTX (5×10^{-7} M) was present throughout. A,B. Thirteen-day-old rats. C,D. Tachykinin effects on NMDA (100 μM)-dependent increases in $[Ca^{2+}]_i$ in single DH neurons and blockade by staurosporine. C. The potentiation of NMDA responses by SP (2 nM) in a single cell. The traces were taken at 10, 18, 26, 37 and 45 min after the application of SP (upper row); and at 11, 20 and 28 min for NKA (lower row). This experiment also shows that the cell still responds to SP with an increase in the $[Ca^{2+}]_i$ after the NKA failed to produce such a response. D. The effect of 2 nM SP (open circles) for eight of the 17 cells in which a potentiation of the NMDA response was observed. Staurosporine (200 nM) prevented the potentiating effects of SP on NMDA (100 μM) responses in DH neurons (open triangles, $n = 7$ cells). The time course of the response in pooled data from 5-min bins of data is shown. (Reproduced with permission, from Rusin et al., 1993a, and Randic et al., 1993b.)

unmasks silent NMDA receptor-channel complexes, seems unlikely because the NMDA-activated single channel currents recorded in cultured cerebral cortical neurons in the presence of high external glycine, were not significantly modified by SP (Randić et al., 1990). Alternatively, SP may act at one or more of regulatory sites known to be associated with the NMDA receptor-ion channel complex. The best characterized modulation of the NMDA receptor activity is by glycine (Johnson and Ascher, 1987). Glycine is known to enhance the activity of NMDA channels and the strychnine-resistant, high-affinity glycine binding site is located at the NMDA receptor-ion channel complex. Glycine is presently thought to act either as a co-agonist (Kleckner and Dingledine, 1988) or a regulator of the rate of desensitization at NMDA receptors (Mayer et al., 1989; Benveniste et al., 1990; Vyklicky et al., 1990). Glycine (50 nM–1 μM) reduced or abolished the SP-induced potentiation of the NMDA response observed when using nominally glycine-free solutions. Moreover, 7-chlorokynurenic acid, a competitive antagonist at the glycine regulatory site of the NMDA receptor-channel complex (Watkins et al., 1990), led to a re-establishment of the SP effect. Although molecular mechanism(s) underlying the dependence of the SP-induced enhancement of the NMDA receptor-activated conductance on external glycine concentration is presently unknown. Modulation of glycine affinity for NMDA receptors by extracellular calcium has been reported (Gu and Huang, 1994).

Another, even more likely way in which the activation of SP receptors may modify glutamate and NMDA receptor-activated conductances of DH neurons is indirectly through the regulation of intracellular mechanisms (Mantyh et al., 1984). Evidence indicates that NMDA, non-NMDA, and tachykinin (SP, NKA) receptors are coexpressed on single DH neurons (Rusin et al., 1992). Furthermore, it is known that there is a convergent regulation of $[Ca^{2+}]_i$ in rat DH neurons by SP (Womack et al., 1988) and glutamate receptor agonists (MacDermott et al., 1986). SP and glutamate both can increase intracellular Ca^{2+} concentration, $[Ca^{2+}]_i$, by activating the IP_3 system to release Ca^{2+} from intracellular stores and by triggering Ca^{2+} influx either through NMDA receptor-operated channels or through voltage-gated Ca^{2+} channels following activation of non-NMDA and NK_1 receptors (Womack et al., 1988; Ryu and Randić, 1990; Rusin et al., 1993a). The hypothesis that the SP-induced enhancement of the responses of acutely isolated rat spinal DH neurons to NMDA might be causally related to the changes in $[Ca^{2+}]_i$ was suggested by the observation that the potentiation of NMDA currents was depressed by loading the cells with BAPTA (Rusin et al., 1992). Indeed, potentiation of NMDA currents by Ca^{2+} ionophores has been reported (Markram and Segal, 1991). However, the results of a recent study clearly dissociate the ability of tachykinins to increase $[Ca^{2+}]_i$ from their ability to enhance NMDA effects (Rusin et al., 1993a). Thus, both SP and NKA enhanced NMDA effects, whereas only SP increased basal $[Ca^{2+}]_i$ (Fig. 1C). Moreover, SP enhanced NMDA effects both in cells where it did and did not increase $[Ca^{2+}]_i$ by itself. Therefore, it is possible that the inhibitory effects caused by BAPTA are not indicative of a role for Ca^{2+} as a second messenger in this case, but of the necessity of having a basal $[Ca^{2+}]_i$ high enough to allow effective G-protein function and operation of signal transduction pathways in general (Beech et al., 1991).

The enhancing effects of tachykinins in freshly dissociated DH neurons are relatively slow to appear and decay, which is suggestive of a second messenger/phosphorylation-mediated mechanism. The intracellular pathway linking SP receptor activation to changes in NMDA responsiveness may involve protein kinase C (PKC) (Nishizuka, 1984, 1988) since perfusion of rat spinal cord slices with phorbol esters enhanced the depolarizing responses to NMDA and glutamate in DH neurons (Gerber et al., 1989). Experiments using *Xenopus* oocytes have also shown that phorbol esters markedly increase NMDA-induced currents (Kelso et al., 1992). Consistent with these results, it has been reported that active phorbol esters potentiate the NMDA-induced current responses (Rusin et al., 1992), and also the NMDA-dependent increases in $[Ca^{2+}]_i$ (Rusin et al., 1993a) in DH neurons. Furthermore, the PKC (and protein kinase A, PKA) inhibitor staurosporine prevented (Fig. 1D) the SP-induced potentiation of the NMDA response (Rusin et al., 1992). It has been demonstrated that heteromeric NMDA receptors reconstructed in vitro from cloned subunits can be directly potentiated by PKC, and this effect can be blocked by staurosporine (Kutsuwada et al., 1992). Previous studies in non-neuronal preparations have demonstrated that SP can activate PKC (Gallacher et al., 1990). The possibility that the tachykinin-mediated enhancement of the effects of NMDA is due to PKC-mediated phosphorylation is consistent with the structure of the recently cloned rat brain NMDA receptor that possesses consensus phosphorylation sites for Ca^{2+}-calmodulin-dependent protein kinase type II and protein kinase C (Moriyoshi et al., 1991; Kutsuwada et al., 1992). Exactly how the function of the NMDA receptor is altered is not clear.

Recent results suggest the possibility that the tachykinin-caused alteration in $[Ca^{2+}]_i$ and consequential changes in at least three second messenger systems may be involved in the regulation of the activity of neuronal NMDA receptors. It has been reported (Rusin et al., 1992, 1993a) that NMDA currents of isolated spinal DH neurons, and NMDA-induced increases in $[Ca^{2+}]_i$, are also modulated by the activity of PKA. The finding that NMDA-evoked current was potentiated (Rusin et al., 1992; Cerne et al., 1993b) by treatment of these neurons with an activator of adenylate cyclase, forskolin or 8-Br cAMP, as well as by intracellular application of cAMP or catalytic subunit of PKA, is consistent with the results obtained in DH neurons using the spinal slice preparation (Gerber et al., 1989; Cerne et al., 1992), and the observations made in *Xenopus* oocytes injected with rat brain mRNA (McVaugh and Waxham, 1992). However, the finding of the enhancement of macroscopic NMDA currents by PKA in the spinal DH differs from the results

obtained in the hippocampus, where whole-cell and single channel analysis in cultured rat hippocampal neurons revealed no obvious alterations of the NMDA channel properties (Greengard et al., 1991; Wang et al., 1991). This difference in the results may arise from different experimental protocols used, or from differential expression of NMDA receptor subtypes in the two preparations studied. The mechanism underlying the potentiation of NMDA current by PKA remains to be determined. Several possibilities could be considered. Thus NMDA receptor-channel complexes might be directly phosphorylated by PKA or, alternatively, regulation of the receptor channels could be indirect by means of regulatory proteins associated with channels. The latter possibility appears to be more likely, since the various subunits of the cloned rat NMDA receptor contain no consensus sequence for PKA (Moriyoshi et al., 1991; Kutsuwada et al., 1992). In addition Ca^{2+}/calmodulin-dependent protein kinase II enhances DH neuronal responses to NMDA (Kolaj et al., 1994). However, in view of the multiplicity of NMDA receptor subtypes (Tölle et al., 1993), further study is needed to determine whether NMDA receptor is directly phosphorylated by known protein kinases.

Modulation of synaptic and EAA responses in the superficial DH of rat spinal cord by dynorphin A

The opioid peptide dynorphin A(1–17) (dynorphin) is thought to be the endogenous ligand for κ opioid receptors (Chavkin et al., 1982; Stevens and Yaksh, 1986). Two forms of dynorphin have been isolated from mammalian brain, dynorphin A and dynorphin B (Vincent et al., 1982; Cruz and Basbaum, 1985). The precise functions of the dynorphin peptides in the spinal cord are not known, although several lines of evidence strongly suggest involvement in spinal nociceptive mechanism (Millan, 1990; Herrero and Headley, 1991; Coderre et al., 1993; Duggan and Fleetwood-Walker, 1993). Immunohistochemical studies have revealed prodynorphin-derived peptides in both superficial and deeper laminae of the rat spinal DH (Miller and Seybold, 1987, 1989; Cho and Basbaum, 1989). Electrical stimulation of unmyelinated primary afferent fibers has been shown to cause a spinal release of dynorphin (Nyberg et al., 1983; Hutchison et al., 1990).

Kappa receptors are present in deep as well as SDH, where they appear to be concentrated in the SG (Gouarderes et al., 1982, 1985; Slater and Patel, 1983; Morris and Herz, 1987; Sharif et al., 1988). In ligand binding studies, the highly selective arylacetamide ligand [^{3}H]U 69,593 has revealed, in both rat (Allerton et al., 1989; James et al., 1990) and dog (Hunter et al., 1989) spinal cords, a small population of well-characterized κ receptors in adult animals, with a significantly higher density being observed in young rats. It is possible that these sites represent only a subpopulation of κ_1 receptors, since other distinct κ subtypes (κ_2, κ_3) have been proposed (Attali et al., 1982; Zukin et al., 1988; Clark et al., 1989; Rothman et al., 1990; Nock et al., 1993). A substantial proportion of the κ receptors are postsynaptic since about half remain after dorsal rhizotomy (Besse et al., 1990).

Both the presynaptic and postsynaptic κ opioid actions have been reported at a level of a single neuron (Duggan and Fleetwood Walker, 1993; North, 1993). Presynaptically, dynorphin inhibits voltage-dependent calcium current in cultured dorsal root ganglion cells (Macdonald and Werz, 1986; Gross and Macdonald, 1987; Bean, 1989; Gross et al., 1990); postsynaptically, κ opioids increase K^+-conductance of DH neurons (Grudt and Williams, 1993) and decrease Ca^{2+} conductance in DH cells (Bean, 1989) and in nucleus tractus solitarii (Rhim and Miller, 1993). It has been a widely held view that a reduction in voltage-dependent calcium current at the nerve terminal could underlie the presynaptic inhibition of transmitter release (North, 1993). However, only an increase (Bakshi et al., 1990; Skilling et al., 1992) in the release of glutamate and aspartate in the spinal cord with nanomolar concentrations of dynorphin has been reported. Moreover, the modulation of the release of SP from peripheral and central sensory structures by stimulation of κ opioid receptors is controversial. In vivo experiments have failed to demonstrate any modulatory action of high micromolar concentrations of the κ opioid receptor selective agonist U 50,488H, on SP release (Yaksh, 1988). In vitro studies have also reported conflicting results (Chang et al., 1989; Pohl et al., 1989). Recently, a dual modulation of K^+-evoked SP release from rat trigeminal nucleus caudalis has been reported (Suarez-Roca and Maixner, 1993). Thus, nanomolar concentrations of U 50,488H increased SP release, whereas higher concentrations produced an inhibitory effect. Previous in vivo studies have shown that the activation of κ opioid receptors produces generally inhibitory effects on spinal DH neurons (Willcockson et al., 1986; Knox and Dickenson, 1987; Fleetwood-Walker et al., 1988; Hope et al., 1990; Hylden et al., 1991), although excitatory effects were also observed (Willcockson et al., 1986; Knox and Dickenson, 1987; Hylden et al., 1991). Topical application of dynorphin and U 50,488H has resulted in both a facilitation and inhibition of the C-fiber-evoked nociceptive responses, but the effects were relatively insensitive to naloxone antagonism (Knox and Dickenson, 1987). It is known that, besides opioid, κ agonists can display strong non-opioid effects on motor functions (Przewlocki et al., 1983; Faden and Jacobs, 1984), neurotoxicity (Stewart and Isaac, 1989) and can cause apparent attenuation of μ agonist-caused antinociception (Dickenson and Knox, 1987; Schmauss and Herz, 1987).

Dual modulation of excitatory transmission by dynorphin in the superficial DH

It is known that the transmission of cutaneous sensory information from the periphery to the CNS is mediated by primary sensory neurons that terminate predominantly on neurons in Laminae I and II of the dorsal horn (Réthelyi, 1977; Light and Perl, 1979; Rustioni and Weinberg, 1989). Although the mechanisms underlying chemical transmission at Aδ- and C-fiber synapses in the

DH are still not resolved, the use of in vitro spinal cord slice preparation enabled a more detailed analysis of primary afferent neurotransmission. Thus, intracellular recordings from spinal cord slices isolated from rats or hamsters has demonstrated that stimulation of primary afferent fibers evokes both fast and slow EPSPs in DH neurons (Urban and Randić, 1984; Randić et al., 1986, 1987; King et al., 1988; Schneider and Perl, 1988; Gerber and Randić, 1989a,b; Yoshimura and Jessell, 1989a; Gerber et al., 1991). Some fast EPSPs were sensitive to excitatory amino acid antagonists, supporting the concept that L-glutamate, or a related compound, is a fast-acting primary afferent transmitter. However, the monosynaptic nature of the afferent input to DH neurons and the class of afferent fibers responsible for the postsynaptic excitation was studied more recently. The experiments provided results that are consistent with the conclusion that primary afferent fibers release glutamate and that the synaptic activation of the non-NMDA receptors of SG neurons predominantly mediates the DR-evoked, presumably monosynaptic, EPSP (Fig. 2) (Yoshimura and Jessell, 1990; Jiang and Randić, 1991; Randić et al., 1993a; Yoshimura and Nishi, 1993). These findings are consistent with other published reports for spinal neurons examined in

vitro (Dale and Roberts, 1985; Forsythe and Westbrook, 1988; King and Lopez-Garcia, 1993) and in vivo (Dougherty et al., 1992).

The role of dynorphin in regulation of EPSPs at primary afferent synapses with SG neurons was examined recently by intracellular recording in a transverse slice preparation of young rat spinal cord (Randić et al., 1994). The results indicate that the role of endogenous dynorphin in the excitatory synaptic transmission is extremely complex. Dynorphin causes a dual modulation of primary afferent stimulation-evoked EPSPs: it decreased (Fig. 3A,B) and increased (Fig. 3D,E) synaptic responses at nanomolar concentrations and increased EPSPs at micromolar concentrations. Both responses to dynorphin were slow in onset and long-lasting, frequently requiring 30–60 min for recovery (Fig. 3B,E). Similar changes in synaptic responses were observed in a proportion of SG cells when dynorphin had no effect on membrane potential or input resistance. Although the dynorphin-induced depression and enhancement of EPSPs remained under conditions in which NMDA-, GABA- and glycine-mediated synaptic responses were blocked by selective antagonists, D-2-amino-5-phosphonovaleric acid, bicuculline and strychnine, respectively. The proportion of cells with enhanced EPSPs was reduced. The unequivocal interpretation of results obtained in pharmacological experiments is difficult unless the opioid compound has selectivity for one type of receptor. Dynorphin A(1–17) has relatively high affinity for κ sites, but it also has affinity for the μ and somewhat less for δ sites (Corbett et al., 1993). In addition, DH neurons are known to contain a heterogenous population of opioid receptors. Under these conditions use of selective agonists and antagonists are essential for defining the type of receptor which mediates the inhibitory and excitatory actions of dynorphin on synaptic responses. To characterize the spinal opioid receptor type(s) responsible for the depression and potentiation of synaptic responses by dynorphin, two κ_1 receptor-preferring ligands U 50,488H and U 69,593 (VonVoigtlander et al., 1983; Lahti et al., 1985; Nock et al., 1990), as well

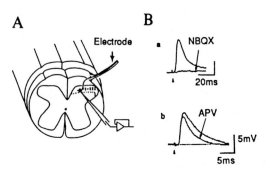

Fig. 2. Schematic arrangement for intracellular recording and dorsal root stimulation. A. Dorsal root was stimulated by a coaxial stainless steel stimulating electrode (arrow). B. Presumed monosynaptic EPSPs evoked by single electrical shocks (a and b) are shown before and during bath application of 5 μM NBQX (a) and 100 μM APV (b). (Reproduced with permission, from Randic et al., 1993a.)

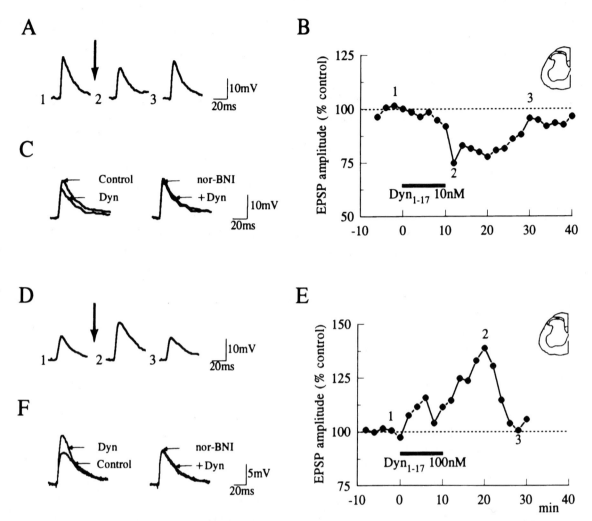

Fig. 3. Dual modulation of primary afferent fiber-evoked EPSPs by dynorphin A(1–17). The graphs (B,E) show the time course of depression (B) and potentiation (E) in the peak amplitude of EPSPs caused by 10 nM (B) and 100 nM (E) dynorphin. The EPSPs were recorded intracellularly at 2-min intervals from SG neurons (inset) in response to single electrical stimuli applied to a lumbar dorsal root. Exposure of slices to nor-binaltorphimine (nor-BNI, 100 nM in C, 10 μm in F) prevented both the depression (C) and potentiation (F) of EPSPs. The individual, apparently monosynaptic EPSPs, are displayed in A and D. A,B. V_m = -81 mV, 21-day-old rat. C. V_m = -76 mV, 24-day-old rat. D,E. V_m = -72 mV, 25-day-old rat. F. V_m = -73 mV, 26-day-old rat.

as a non-selective opioid receptor antagonist, naloxone, and a claimed selective κ_1 opioid receptor antagonist, norbinaltorphimine (nor-BNI) (Portoghese et al., 1987; Takemori et al., 1988), were used. Whereas dual modulation of EPSPs was observed with U 50,488H in control solution, a depression was exclusively seen with nanomolar concentrations of U 69,593 when GABA$_A$-,

glycine-, NMDA-, and μ- and δ-opioid receptors were blocked. Although pretreatment of slices with naloxone or nor-BNI antagonized the depressant effect (Fig. 3C), the enhancing effect of dynorphin was infrequently blocked (Fig. 3F). These results suggest that depression of primary afferent neurotransmission by dynorphin, U 50,488H and U 69,593 is likely to be mediated by

κ_1 receptors. This conclusion is consistent with the report (Allerton et al., 1989; James et al., 1990) that κ_1 receptors predominate in spinal cord of young rats. Studies of the guinea-pig dentate gyrus (Wagner et al., 1992, 1993) support a role for the κ_1 receptor in reducing AMPA-mediated excitatory synaptic transmission. An interesting recent finding (Caudle et al., 1994), is that a receptor that bears similar pharmacology to that reported for the κ_2/ϵ binding site (Nock et al., 1988, 1990, 1993; Zukin et al., 1988; Rothman et al., 1992) inhibits NMDA receptor-mediated synaptic responses in the hippocampus. However, the pharmacological properties and anatomical distribution of the κ_2 receptors remains controversial, due to the fact that there are no selective κ_2 receptor ligands.

At present we do not know the mechanism of the κ_1 opioid receptor-mediated modulation of synaptic responses. In principle, dynorphin could regulate excitatory synaptic transmission in the spinal DH by modulating the presynaptic release of glutamate or the postsynaptic actions of glutamate. The inability of κ opioids to affect passive membrane properties of neurons in several brain regions (McFadzean et al., 1987; Pinnock, 1992; Wagner et al., 1992; Rhim et al., 1993; Weisskopf et al., 1993), including the deep DH (Allerton et al., 1989), as well as postsynaptic glutamate responses, and the finding that, in dorsal root ganglion neurons, κ agonists depress a voltage-sensitive calcium-conductance of the N-type (Gross and Macdonald, 1987), led to the concept that κ agonists act presynaptically to reduce transmitter release, and that this action may account for their depressant effect on the synaptic responses. However, as noted above, dynorphin A(1–13) and U 50,488H enhance glutamate/aspartate release in the spinal DH in vivo (Bakshi et al., 1990; Skilling et al., 1992), and alter K^+-evoked SP release in a bimodal fashion from rat trigeminal neurons in vitro (Suarez-Roca and Maixner, 1993). Thus, in the absence of significant changes in resting membrane potential and neuronal input resistance, the increased synaptic efficacy, as manifested by the increase in the amplitude of the evoked EPSP in a subset of the SG neurons, could be due, at least in part, to increased probability of release of transmitter(s) presynaptically. However, findings indicate additional postsynaptic site of action of κ opioids (Kolaj et al., 1992, 1993a; Cerne et al., 1993a; Grudt and Williams, 1993).

Dynorphin, and non-peptide κ agonists, could affect the excitability of a DH neuron postsynaptically by several mechanisms including: (1) hyperpolarization or depolarization of the neuronal membrane either by directly opening or closing ion channels or through intracellular second messengers; (2) acting as neuromodulators, namely having little effect on ionic conductances per se but altering the actions of other neuroactive compounds, including glutamate; and (3) acting as receptor antagonists. In contrast to the well-known direct hyperpolarizing action of μ receptor agonists (Murase et al., 1982; Yoshimura and North, 1983; Duggan and North, 1984; North, 1993), the actions of κ opioid receptor agonists at the single cell level in the spinal cord remained unknown until recently. Using an in vitro slice preparation from guinea pig spinal trigeminal nucleus, Grudt and Williams (1993) showed that a subset of SG neurons was hyperpolarized by U 69,593 via an increase of potassium conductance, and that nor-BNI blocked the hyperpolarization. Although, dynorphin also caused hyperpolarization, the effect was only reduced by naloxone and a higher concentration of nor-BNI. The data suggested that dynorphin was acting at μ opioid receptors, but it was not possible to rule out an additional action at κ_2 receptors. However, about equal proportions of SG cells exhibited depolarization in the presence of the κ agonists. Although nor-BNI reduced or prevented the dynorphin hyperpolarization, depolarization was not antagonized in a few cells. Whereas in a smaller proportion of the SG neurons tested with dynorphin there was no apparent change in input resistance, a small increase or a decrease was observed in a majority of the cells. Dual modulation of the membrane potential and input resistance (Randić et al., 1994) by κ opioids may involve alteration of multiple voltage-dependent ionic conductances of postsynaptic membrane. Besides K^+ conductance (Grudt and Williams, 1993), κ opioids may modify the inward rectifier current in DH neurons (Yoshimura and Jessell, 1989b). The hyperpolarization of presynaptic nerve terminals in the ciliary ganglion by κ opioids appears to result from inhibition of the Na^+-K^+ inward rectifier current, whereas the depolarization may result from a decrease in membrane potassium conductance (Fletcher and Chiapinelli, 1993). Ca^{2+} conductance in DH neurons and $[Ca^{2+}]_i$ might also be altered by κ opioids (Rhim and Miller, 1993). In most CA3 hippocampal neurons, the voltage-dependent K^+ current, known as the M-current, was uniquely sensitive to the κ opioids with the direction of response dependent upon the κ opiate receptor type and concentration (Moore et al., 1994). However, under conditions of blockade of synaptic transmission with tetrodotoxin, and μ- and δ- opioid receptors, we recently found that dynorphin and U-69,593 hyperpolarize most of rat substantia gelatinosa neurons and decrease their input resistance (Randić et al., 1995). There is no convincing evidence that opioids act as antagonists at receptors for other neuroactive compounds.

Several heuristic models have been proposed to account for the variable effects of dynorphin in other brain regions and may also apply to the SDH. One possible explanation for the bimodal pattern of the modulation of excitatory transmission by κ opioids is that individual SG neurons have different κ opioid receptor subtypes that are selectively activated by different dynorphin concentrations or dynorphin fragments that produce qualitatively different responses. Indeed, it is known that dynorphin is a preferential κ agonist at low concentrations (Chavkin et al., 1982), whereas at high concentrations it displays also affinity for μ and δ receptors (Corbett et al., 1993). Moreover, there is evidence for multiple κ binding sites (κ_1, κ_2, κ_3) in the rat spinal DH (Zukin et al., 1988; Allerton et al., 1989; Traynor, 1989; James et al., 1990; Nock et al., 1990, 1993). A range of endogenous opioids resulting from the

processing of pre-prodynorphin precursors with differing profiles of receptor selectivity are found in the DH, particularly in the marginal zone and substantia gelatinosa. It is further possible that the enzymatic cleavage patterns occurring in particular cells may differ so as to provide releasable opioids with different profiles of activity. In addition, the specificity of dynorphin and κ agonists for opioid receptors has been brought into question because of the often reported inability to block these effects by naloxone (Walker et al., 1982; Faden and Jacobs, 1984; Moises and Walker, 1985; Knox and Dickenson, 1987; Caudle and Isaac, 1988; Hylden et al., 1991).

Although it is an attractive idea that the excitatory actions of opioids on DH cells (Willcockson et al., 1986; Knox and Dickenson, 1987) might be due to activation of a particular κ opiate receptor subtype, the possibility that the κ opioids cause inhibition of a neighboring inhibitory interneuron resulting in a disinhibition cannot be excluded. Thus, the excitatory effects may represent a κ opioid-mediated depression of the activity of local GABA-ergic interneurons. GABA is present in cell bodies and axons in Laminae I–III of the spinal DH (Ribeiro-da-Silva and Coimbra, 1980; Hunt et al., 1981; Barber et al., 1982). Modulation of postsynaptic $GABA_A$ receptors by μ opioids in freshly isolated spinal DH neurons has been recently observed (Kolaj et al., 1993b; Wang and Randić, 1994). Excitations due to μ, δ and κ opioids have been reported in hippocampus (Nicoll et al., 1980; Vidal et al., 1984; Zieglgänsberger, 1986), where a disinhibitory mechanism involving GABA-ergic interneurons has been postulated. Whether a similar disinhibitory mechanism due to κ opioids operates in the SG neurons is presently unknown. Another possibility is that dynorphin, and other κ opioids, may act as μ opiate receptor antagonists (Dickenson and Knox, 1987; Corbett et al., 1993; Rothman et al., 1993). This opens the possibility that dynorphin might reduce tonic opiate action and produce disinhibition in this manner. In addition, there is evidence that κ opioids may increase K^+-evoked SP release from rat trigeminal nucleus caudalis slice

(Suarez-Roca and Maixner, 1993), which would be expected to produce depolarization and raise the excitability of neurons (Murase and Randić, 1984). This type of mechanism may in part contribute to the spinal excitatory effects of κ opioids. Finally, κ opioids can display very pronounced excitatory non-opioid effects (Crain and Shen, 1990; Faden, 1990; Millan, 1990; Dubner and Ruda, 1992).

Effects of κ and μ agonists on EAA-evoked responses in acutely isolated neurons from the SDH

The neuromodulatory hypothesis about mechanism of postsynaptic action of opioids (morphine, enkephalins) was originally suggested by Zieglgänsberger and his colleagues (Zieglgänsberger, 1986). These investigators could detect no consistent effects of opioids on the membrane potential, input resistance or action potential waveform of cat spinal neurons, including DH neurons, studied in vivo, but the opioids did depress the depolarization and associated decrease in membrane resistance following iontophoretic administration of L-glutamate. Since glutamate increases the membrane permeability, predominantly to sodium ions, they concluded that opioids block the same sodium conductance that is physiologically activated by glutamate. Such a modulatory effect of enkephalins was also observed in cultured mouse spinal neurons (Barker et al., 1978a,b), where enkephalin depressed glutamate-evoked responses in a noncompetitive manner. However, the neuromodulatory role of κ opioids in the SDH has not been studied until more recently (Kolaj et al., 1992, 1993a, 1995; Cerne et al., 1993a).

To examine whether the activation of κ and μ opioid receptors affects the sensitivity of postsynaptic glutamate receptors, the actions of the κ receptor-preferring ligands dynorphin, U 50,488H and U 69,593, and the μ opioid receptor agonist Tyr-D-Ala^2-Gly-N-Me-Phe^4-Gly-ol^5-enkephalin (DAGO) on the responses of DH neurons to selective ionotropic glutamate receptor agonists AMPA, KA and NMDA were examined.

Under whole-cell voltage-clamp conditions, dynorphin caused a dose-dependent and reversible decrease in the peak amplitude of the initial transient component of the AMPA-activated current in more than a half of the examined cells (Fig. 4A,B). However, an increase in the magnitude of AMPA current was seen with lower (< 1 nM) concentrations of the peptide. The depression of AMPA response was associated with slowing of the response kinetics, including both rise time and the time constant of decay. The depressant effect of dynorphin appears to be independent of any direct effect of the peptide on membrane input resistance, the result indicating a direct modulatory effect on the AMPA-induced current. The AMPA activated currents were modified by dynorphin, not only during the co-administration, but up to an hour after removal of the peptide. In about 40% of the examined cells the peak AMPA current was increased by dynorphin. Both, the initial depression and the late potentiation of the peak AMPA response remained when intracellular dialysis solution-containing K^+ instead of Cs^+ ions was used, and in the presence of APV. It should be noted, however, that the depressant effect was more prominent when intracellular cesium was used to reduce outward potassium currents. There was no apparent correlation between the incidence of cells showing the dynorphin-induced depression of the AMPA responses and the cell types isolated. KA-induced inward currents were also affected by dynorphin. Dynorphin decreased the magnitude of the KA-induced current in about half of the examined cells (Fig. 4C,D). Similar to dynorphin, pretreatment of cells with U 50,488H had two distinct effects on the peak amplitude of the AMPA-induced current consisting of an initial depression followed by a potentiation. In contrast to the bimodal effects of dynorphin and U 50,488H, U 69,593 caused only a sustained depression of the AMPA response. Naloxone and nor-BNI (5 or 100 nM) reduced or prevented the development of the depression of the AMPA-induced current by κ opioids, whereas the antagonists by themselves did not show any appreciable effect on the AMPA response. This antagonistic effect of

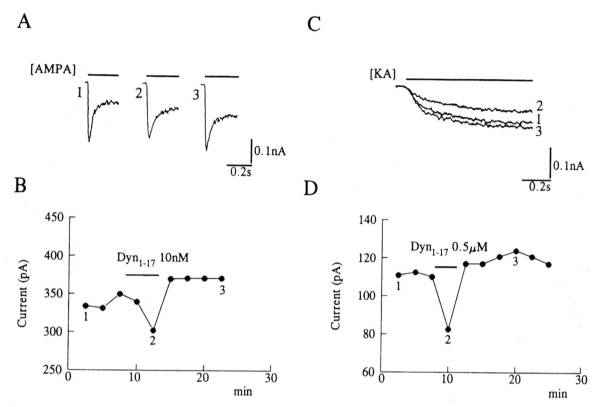

Fig. 4. A. The traces show inward current responses evoked by 10 μM AMPA recorded at 2.5-min intervals from a DH neuron held at −60 mV before (trace 1), during (trace 2) and after (trace 3) dynorphin (10 nM for 5 min) application. Whereas the transient component of AMPA-induced current was slightly depressed during co-administration with dynorphin the steady-state component was enhanced both during and after the removal of peptide. B. The time course of the peak AMPA current responses recorded before, during and after dynorphin administration is shown in the graph. Internal solution contained (mM) 3 Mg^{2+}-ATP, 0.1 GTP (12-day-old rat). C. The superimposed traces of inward current responses evoked by 5 sec pressure application of 50 μM KA to a DH neuron held at −60 mV recorded before (trace 1), during (trace 2) and after (trace 3) 0.5 μM dynorphin application. D. The time course of the changes in the peak amplitude of KA-induced current responses recorded before, during and after dynorphin co-administration is shown in the graph (12-day-old rat).

naloxone or nor-BNI suggests that the depressant effect of dynorphin, U 50,488H and U 69,593 on the AMPA-activated conductance is a true opioid, probably κ_1 opioid receptor-mediated event.

The effects of dynorphin, U 50,488H and U 69,593 on the NMDA-induced current responses of single DH neurons were also examined. Both initial-peak and steady-state components of the NMDA-induced current demonstrated typical properties of NMDA channels; they were potentiated by glycine (Johnson and Ascher, 1987) and reduced by Mg^{2+} (Mayer et al., 1984; Nowak et al., 1984). Pressure application of 1 nM dynorphin

enhanced the peak amplitude of the NMDA-induced current, as shown in Fig. 5A. In contrast, higher concentration of dynorphin (1 μM) in the same cell (Fig. 5A,B), produced two distinct effects on the NMDA response consisting of an initial reversible depression followed by a small potentiation. Similar to the AMPA response, U 69,593 caused only a sustained depression of the NMDA-induced current. The depressant and enhancing effects of dynorphin were present under conditions of superfusion with glycine-enriched solution. Inhibitory (Fig. 5) action of dynorphin was sensitive to nor-BNI indicating that the effect

238

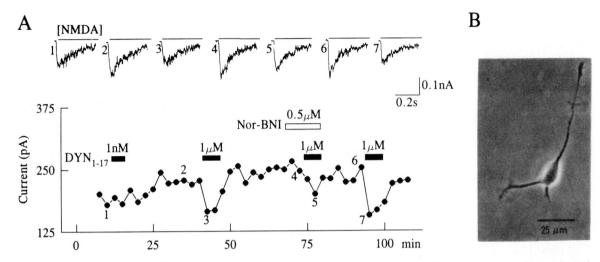

Fig. 5. Dynorphin modulated NMDA-induced current responses of cultured DH neurons. A. The time course of changes in peak amplitude of the initial transient component of NMDA (0.1 mM, 5–8 sec)-induced current responses recorded at 2.5-min intervals before, during and after superfusion with dynorphin from a DH neuron (B) held at −60 mV. Dynorphin at low concentration (1 nM for 5 min) produced a prolonged enhancement of NMDA-induced current responses. At high concentrations (1 μM for 5 min), dynorphin transiently depressed NMDA-induced current responses. nor-BNI (0.5 μM for 10 min) prevented the depressant effect of 1 μM dynorphin. The numbers denote individual NMDA-induced current responses illustrated above the graph. B. The neuron was obtained from a 7-day-old rat and maintained in culture medium for 3 days.

is likely to be mediated by κ receptors. Overall, these findings indicate that dynorphin A(1–17) is an endogenous ligand for κ_1 receptors in the superficial spinal DH of young rats and that these receptors regulate AMPA, KA and NMDA receptor function. In addition, the results support previous findings (Besse et al., 1990) that a substantial number of κ receptors are present on somas and proximal dendrites of DH neurons and, when activated, they modulate the sensitivity of postsynaptic AMPA and KA subtypes of glutamate receptor. Although exact molecular mechanisms underlying the modulation of the ionotropic glutamate receptor-activated conductances have not been studied in detail, an increase in the basal $[Ca^{2+}]_i$ was observed after micromolar dynorphin and U 69,593 application in the cultured DH neurons (Cerne et al., 1995). Moreover, intracellular application of a protein inhibitor of cyclic AMP-dependent protein kinase or staurosporine prevented the dynorphin-induced depression of the AMPA and NMDA responses.

The exact molecular mechanism(s) underlying the modulation of the EAA receptor-activated conductances by κ opioids have yet to be elucidated. Kappa opioids could directly modify kinetic properties of single AMPA, KA and NMDA channels. Whereas the effects of activation of κ receptors on AMPA/KA-activated single channel currents have not been as yet reported, dynorphin caused a significant reduction in the probability of NMDA channel openings in rat trigeminal neurons, but had no effect on single channel conductance or the mean open time of the channel (Chen and Huang, 1993).

Another way in which the activation of κ receptors may modify glutamate receptor-activated conductances of DH neurons is indirectly through the regulation of intracellular mechanisms. Kappa opioid receptors are thought to belong to a family of membrane receptors that transduce their intracellular signals via G protein-coupled pathways (Childers, 1993; Cox, 1993; North, 1993). Kappa agonists, including dynorphin, inhibit adenylate cyclase activity in rat spinal cord-dorsal root ganglion cultures in an Na-dependent manner (Attali et al., 1989a) and reduce dorsal root ganglion calcium currents (Macdonald and Werz, 1986; Gross and Macdonald, 1987; Attali et al., 1989b; Gross et al., 1990; Rhim and Miller, 1993). Most of the electrophysiological evidence suggests that the adenylate cyclase/cAMP system does not play a direct role in the effects of κ opioids on the calcium channels; the κ opioid receptors couple to ion channels directly through G-proteins (Attali et al., 1989b; Gross et al., 1990; North, 1993). However, one possible exception to this general finding may be the spinal cord. Crain and colleagues (Chen et al., 1988) showed that opioid effects on Ca^{2+}-conductance in cultured sensory ganglion neurons may be mediated by cyclic AMP-dependent protein kinase. They reported that selective μ, δ and κ agonists can elicit excitatory modulation of the calcium-dependent action potential of dorsal root ganglion neurons when applied at low concentrations, and inhibitory modulation at high micromolar concentrations. They provided additional evidence that excitatory effects of opioids on these neurons are mediated by opioid receptors that are positively coupled via a G_s-like protein to adenylyl cyclase and cAMP-dependent voltage-sensitive Ca^{2+}-conductance. By contrast, inhibitory effects are mediated by opioid receptors linked to pertussis-sensitive G proteins, G_i and G_o.

The intracellular pathway linking κ opioid receptor activation to changes in EAA responses in rat DH neurons, may involve the adenylate cyclase/cAMP-dependent protein kinase system for several reasons. The spinal DH contains a high density of binding sites for forskolin (Worley et al., 1986), and exposure of spinal slices to forskolin, or a membrane permeant analog of cAMP, 8Br-cAMP, or a phosphodiesterase inhibitor IBMX, enhanced the depolarizing responses to AMPA, KA and NMDA in DH neurons (Cerne et al., 1992). Evidence has also been provided that glutamate receptor gated by kainate in white perch horizontal cells, mammalian hippocampal neurons, and GluR6, glutamate receptor tran-

siently expressed in mammalian cells can be regulated by cAMP-dependent protein phosphorylation (Liman et al., 1989; Greengard et al., 1991; Raymond et al., 1993). We have shown that inhibition of PKA blocked the depressant effect of dymorphin (Kolaj et al., 1995). The possibility that the dynorphin-mediated depression of the AMPA and KA responses related due to PKA-mediated phosphorylation is consistent with the structure of the recently cloned rat brain AMPA and KA receptors that possess a number of consensus phosphorylation sites, including for those for PKA (Sommer and Seeburg, 1992; Wisden and Seeburg, 1993). On the other hand, regulation of the NMDA receptor channels by dynorphin could be indirect by means of regulatory proteins associated with channels (Moriyoshi et al., 1991; Kutsuwada et al., 1992). Exactly how the function of AMPA and NMDA receptors is altered by dynorphin is at present not clear.

Receptor-mediated stimulation of phosphatidylinositol (PI) turnover is another second messenger system linked to some neuropeptides. Since changes in Ca^{2+} flux have been associated with κ opioid receptor function (Attali et al., 1989b), and since κ opioids are coupled to G-proteins, one potential opioid-coupled second messenger system is PI turnover. Although, recent data have suggested that κ agonists at high doses stimulate PI turnover (Periyasamy and Hoss, 1990), the pharmacological experiments have not yet confirmed the κ opioid selectivity of this response. However, staurosporine reduced the dynorphin depressant effect on the AMPA-induced currents in DH neurons (Kolaj et al., 1995). These results suggest the possibility that at least two second messenger systems may be involved in the regulation of the activity of neuronal AMPA and NMDA receptors.

The interaction between κ opioids and EAA receptors may have important implications for the functioning of synapses in the DH of the spinal cord, where both dynorphin and glutamate are present in the primary afferent terminals and intrinsic neurons. It is likely that the stimulation parameters required for the release of these two compounds are different and that release of dynorphin would have a higher threshold (Verhage et al., 1991). Thus, at high rates of stimulation, the release of dynorphin could modify the postsynaptic actions of glutamate and synaptic transmission.

Effects of DAGO on AMPA- and NMDA-induced current responses in acutely isolated DH neurons

In acutely dissociated DH neurons, DAGO, an opioid agonist with a preference for the μ receptor, causes a long-lasting potentiation of both AMPA- and NMDA-induced current responses, after an initial period of depression (Fig. 6) (Rusin and Randić, 1991; Kolaj et al., 1993b; Randic and Kolaj, 1993). Both effects were reduced or prevented by the μ opioid receptor antagonists, naloxone (Fig. 6C) and β-funaltrexamine (Corbett et al., 1993). The magnitude and the duration of the depressant effect of DAGO was increased when the intracellular dialysis solution contained MgATP and GTP. These findings indicate that DAGO has dual effects in the rat spinal DH. Postsynaptically, DAGO enhances AMPA and NMDA receptor-mediated glutamate responses of acutely isolated rat DH neurons (Rusin and Randić, 1991; Kolaj et al., 1993b; Randic and Kolaj, 1993), and NMDA responses of trigeminal neurons (Chen and Huang, 1991). Presynaptically, DAGO inhibits glutamate and aspartate release (Kangrga and Randić, 1991). Thus the net effect of DAGO on excitatory transmission in the DH will depend on balance between its presynaptic and postsynaptic actions.

The exact molecular mechanisms underlying the modulation of AMPA and NMDA receptor-activated conductances by DAGO have yet to be elucidated. DAGO might directly modify the kinetic properties of single AMPA or NMDA channels, or alternatively in the case of the NMDA receptor, act at a glycine binding site closely associated with the NMDA receptor-ion channel complex. It has been reported that, in the presence of glycine, the enhancement of the NMDA response was significantly reduced (Rusin and Randić, 1991). In addition, it is known that AMPA receptors are subject to modulation through the adenylate cyclase cascade (Greengard et al., 1991; Wang et al., 1991) and NMDA receptor through protein kinase C (Chen and Huang, 1991). Consistent with these results, recent findings that the AMPA and NMDA responses of DH cells were potentiated by phorbol esters, 8Br-cAMP, and by intracellularly applied PKC or the catalytic subunit of PKA (Cerne et al., 1993b; Cerne and Randić, 1993). The relation between AMPA or NMDA receptor-mediated Ca^{2+} fluxes, voltage-gated Ca^{2+} channels and the release of intracellular Ca^{2+} following activation of opioid receptors remains to be elucidated. Evidence indicates that protein phosphorylation of glutamate-gated ionotropic channels by PKC and PKA can modulate the channels and produce long-term changes in synaptic strength.

Possible functional implications of the neuropeptide-induced modulation of EAA responses

The efficiency of synaptic transmission in the CNS, including spinal cord, is not constant and can be modulated by the rate of activity in presynaptic pathways. In a variety of brain structures, repetitive activation of synaptic connections can lead to long-term potentiation (LTP) or long-term depression (LTD) of excitatory synaptic transmission (Madison et al., 1991; Siegelbaum and Kandel, 1991; Johnston et al., 1992). However, the presence of the similar phenomena in the spinal cord has not until recently been demonstrated (Randić et al., 1993a). Brief repetitive activation of primary afferent synapses with neurons in the superficial laminae (Laminae I–III) of DH of the rat spinal cord results in a substantial increase or decrease in synaptic strength that can last more than an hour. Both the AMPA and the NMDA receptor-mediated components of synaptic transmission can exhibit LTP and LTD of synaptic responses. These results are in agreement with other data showing that the AMPA receptor plays a key role in mediating expression of both forms

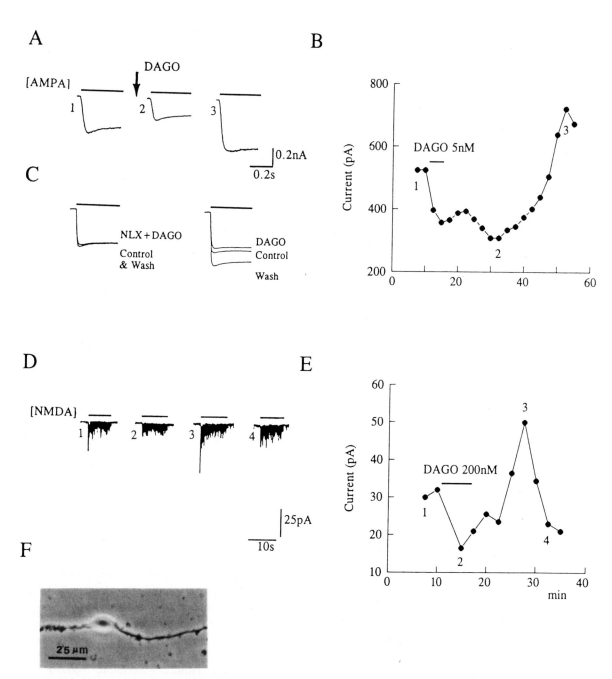

Fig. 6. The traces shown in A are inward current responses induced by 15 μM AMPA applied for 5 sec before (trace 1), during (trace 2) and after (trace 3) 5 nM DAGO application. B. The time course of the peak AMPA current responses is shown in the graph (12-day-old rat). C. The left superimposed traces are inward current responses induced by 25 μM AMPA recorded from a DH neuron (F) before, during, and after the combined application of naloxone (NLX, 100 nM for 7 min) plus DAGO (10 nM for 3 min). Thirty-five minutes after the removal of naloxone the same concentration of DAGO produced two distinct effects on the AMPA response, consisting of an initial depression followed by a late potentiation. This is shown in the right superimposed traces recorded before, during and after the application of DAGO alone (10-day-old rat). D. The traces show inward current responses elicited by 0.1 mM NMDA recorded from a DH neuron held at -60 mV prior to and after DAGO (200 nM for 5 min) application. First trace shows a control response to NMDA, whereas other traces show responses recorded after the removal of DAGO at the times indicated in the graph (E). E. Time course of the peak NMDA current responses is shown in the graph (12-day-old rat).

of plasticity in the CNS, and that LTP can also be expressed by the pharmacologically isolated NMDA receptor-mediated EPSP (Bashir et al., 1991; Xie and Lewis, 1991). The induction of LTP or LTD was not abolished in the presence of a GABA$_A$ receptor antagonist, bicuculline.

By analogy with other examples of synaptic plasticity in the mammalian brain, LTP in the DH has distinct induction and maintenance phases, although the molecular mechanisms underlying these phenomena in the spinal DH have yet to be elucidated. A role for NMDA receptors in the induction phase of LTP has been suggested (Randić et al., 1993a). Recent studies in the hippocampus show that NMDA receptor activation does not exclusively lead to generation of LTP. Instead, activation of NMDA receptors may cause multiple forms of synaptic plasticity including short-term potentiation and long-term depression. Mechanistic relationships between these different phenomena are presently poorly understood (Malenka and Nicoll, 1993). The role of PKC in LTP has been reviewed, and PKC modulation of NMDA currents has been suggested as an important link for LTP induction (Ben-Ari et al., 1992). PKC modulates synaptic transmission of NMDA receptor-mediated responses and mimics features of LTP in the rat spinal DH (Gerber et al., 1989). A number of diverse inputs, including tachykinins and activation of glutamate metabotropic receptors, could lead to PKC activation in the spinal DH, and there are cellular mechanisms other than phosphorylation of NMDA ion channels that might result in prolonged excitability increases seen during LTP. Multiple cellular mechanisms could participate in synaptic plasticity in the DH including: the activation of metabotropic glutamate receptor (Bortollotto and Collingridge, 1992; Kojic and Randić, 1993), activation of voltage-sensitive Ca^{2+} channels (Kullman et al., 1992), nitric oxide (Schuman and Madison, 1991), inhibition of voltage- or calcium-dependent K$^+$ channels (Aniksztejn and Ben-Ari, 1991; Charpak and Gähwiler, 1991), and arachidonic acid generation. Potentiation of NMDA receptor-activated conductance by a metabotropic glutamate receptor agonist, trans-ACPD (Cerne and Randić, 1992), and arachidonic acid (Miller et al., 1992) has been demonstrated. Presynaptic increases in the release of glutamate could be potentially produced by PKC (Gerber et al., 1989), PKA (Greengard et al., 1991) and calcium/calmodulin-dependent protein kinase.

Although anatomical and neurochemical studies suggest that endogenous opioids and tachykinins act as neurotransmitters, their roles in normal and pathophysiological regulation of synaptic transmission are not defined. Recent evidence indicates that opioids (Martinez et al., 1990) can enhance synaptic transmission and LTP in the rat mossy fiber-CA3 system, whereas naloxone is reported to prevent LTP induction (Derrick et al., 1991). In addition, two recent reports suggest that dynorphin may reduce LTP in the hippocampus in a naloxone-reversible manner, at least in part by a presynaptic action (Wagner et al., 1993; Weisskopf et al., 1993). Whether it exerts a similar action on spinal neurons is not known.

Contribution of neuropeptides and EAAs to central hyperexcitability triggered by noxious inputs

Repetitive activity in unmyelinated sensory afferent neurons arising from electrical stimulation, tissue injury or nerve damage, can induce long-lasting sensitization in DH neurons (Woolf and Wall, 1986; Woolf, 1991). This sensitization is manifested by an increase in activity of DH neurons, an expansion of receptive fields and a lowering of a threshold to afferent inputs. Although the precise cellular mechanisms responsible have not yet been elucidated (Schaible et al., 1991; Wilcox, 1991; Dubner and Ruda, 1992; Coderre et al., 1993), the NMDA receptor has been shown to have a major role (Duggan et al., 1988, 1990; Haley et al., 1990; Dougherty and Willis, 1991a; Woolf and Thompson, 1991; Coderre et al., 1993; Dougherty et al., 1993), as have tachykinins acting on NK$_1$ and NK$_2$ receptors (Xu et al., 1992a,b;

Nagy et al., 1993). In addition, recent evidence suggests that nitric oxide may have a mediator role in the phenomenon of central sensitization (McMahon et al., 1993).

The results of electrophysiological and behavioral experiments indicate a functional interaction between SP and glutamate in the mammalian spinal DH, compatible with the hypothesis that co-release of SP and glutamate from primary afferent neurons may enhance nociception. Neuropeptides and EAAs coexist in the central terminals of primary afferent neurons (De Biasi and Rustioni, 1988). Dougherty and Willis (1991b) demonstrated increased responsiveness of primate spinothalamic tract (STT) neurons after the combined administration of EAA (AMPA, QA, KA and NMDA) and SP. The effects of SP on the responses of DH neurons to NMDA were prevented by NK_1 receptor antagonist, CP-96,345 (Snider et al., 1991), while the changes in the responses to AMPA were not. The potentiating effect of SP lasted for hours and was accompanied by an increase in the responses of the STT cells to mechanical stimulation of skin. Participation of EAAs and SP in the generation of a long-lasting potentiation of various nociceptive reflexes (Mjellem-Joly et al., 1991), and in the development of prolonged increase of spinal cord excitability after repetitive stimulation of C-afferents, has also been demonstrated (Wiesenfeld-Hallin et al., 1991). It is likely that neuropeptides produce their effects via presynaptic and postsynaptic mechanisms. Tachykinins (SP, NKA) and CGRP have been shown to increase release of endogenous glutamate and aspartate (Kangrga and Randić, 1990) and tachykinins, as discussed above, enhance the responses of freshly dissociated DH neurons to EAAs (Randić et al., 1990; Rusin et al., 1992, 1993a,b). Thus, besides contributing via voltage-dependent regulation of NMDA receptors, tachykinins may participate in central sensitization by directly modulating the NMDA receptor-ion channel complex, as it has been suggested both by in vivo and in vitro experiments.

Although the above data suggest that glutamate acting at NMDA receptors and tachykinins are essential mediators of the central hyperexcitability, the molecular mechanisms underlying hyperalgesia and neuroplasticity in nociceptive systems are not well understood. Recent evidence suggests that changes in $[Ca^{2+}]_i$, second messenger systems and protein kinases can cause a prolonged change in membrane excitability.

Activation of NK_1 receptors by SP (Mantyh et al., 1984) or metabotropic glutamate receptors (Sugiyama et al., 1987) stimulates the hydrolysis of inositol phospholipids with resulting formation of two intracellular messengers, inositol trisphosphate (IP_3) and diacylglycerol (DAG). IP_3 stimulates the release of Ca^{2+} from internal stores, whereas DAG activates PKC. When activated by DAG, the C kinase phosphorylates specific substrate proteins that contribute to various cellular processes including neurotransmitter release and receptor-transducing mechanisms (Nishizuka, 1984, 1988). Gerber et al., (1989) have demonstrated that phorbol esters increase the basal and the dorsal root stimulation-evoked release of endogenous glutamate and aspartate in the spinal slice, synaptic responses, and also the depolarizing responses of DH neurons to exogenous glutamate and NMDA. The activation of metabotropic glutamate receptors also enhances NMDA currents in hippocampal neurons (Aniksztejn et al., 1991) and EPSPs, and AMPA and NMDA current responses in DH neurons (Cerne and Randić, 1992). This effect may be mediated by PKC since the effects of metabotropic receptor activation were blocked by inhibitors of PKC (Ben-Ari et al., 1992). Recent behavioral experiments suggest a contribution of PKC to persistent nociception following tissue injury in rats (Coderre, 1992). A possible mechanism of the modulation of excitatory synaptic transmission by PKC is indicated by the finding that PKC increases NMDA-activated currents in acutely dissociated trigeminal neurons by increasing the probability of channel openings and by reducing the voltage-dependent Mg^{2+} block of NMDA receptor-ion channels (Chen and Huang, 1992). This would result in a greater NMDA receptor response at resting membrane potential, increase in $[Ca^{2+}]_i$, PKC activity and the excitability of the neuron. This positive feedback loop may be important for the induction or maintenance of the central sensitization. The model is compatible with the in vivo findings that NMDA receptor antagonists can prevent central sensitization, or reduce it once it has been established (Woolf and Thompson, 1991).

Increase in $[Ca^{2+}]_i$ as a result of Ca^{2+} influx, either through NMDA receptor-operated channels or through voltage-gated Ca^{2+} channels following activation of non-NMDA and NK_1 receptors (Womack et al., 1988; Rusin et al., 1993a), may be involved in triggering the production of immediate early gene (IEG) transcription factors such as c-*fos*. Transcriptional factors encoded by IEGs are rapidly induced in DH neurons by noxious stimulation (Hunt et al., 1987), glutamate, NMDA and quisqualate (Szekely et al., 1987), kainate (Lerea et al., 1992), and SP in spinal cord neurons (Bigot et al., 1989). There is evidence indicating that a c-*fos* protein is involved in the transcriptional control of genes encoding various neuropeptides, including tachykinins and opioid peptides, in the rat spinal cord. Thus peripheral inflammation, nerve lesions and activation of PKC induce c-*fos* and the genes encoding pro-dynorphin (Höllt et al., 1987; Ruda et al., 1988), pro-enkephalin (Iadarola et al., 1988) and prepro-tachykinin A (Noguchi et al., 1988). Analgesic doses of morphine and the κ-selective agonist U 50,488H suppress c-*fos* induction in the spinal cord following noxious stimulation (Hammond et al., 1992). These results indicate that both enkephalin and dynorphin may be involved in the modulation of the development of central plasticity and hyperalgesia following noxious stimulation.

A multitude of different possible mechanisms could produce central sensitization. Presently, it is not known if a single mechanism is involved, or if the increased excitability can be produced by nociceptive afferents through a number of different processes. Understanding of the cellular mechanisms has implications both for the understanding of somatosensory processing in the spinal dorsal horn, as well as for the development of novel analgesic strategies to prevent post-injury pain hypersensitivity.

Acknowledgements

Our work has been supported by grants from the National Institute for Neurological Disorders and Stroke, the National Science Foundation and the United States Department of Agriculture.

References

Aanonsen, L.M. and Wilcox, G.L. (1987) Nociceptive action of excitatory amino acids in the mouse: effects of spinally administered opioids, phencyclidine and sigma agonists. *J. Pharm. Exp. Ther.*, 243: 9–19.

Allerton, C.A., Smith, J.A.M., Hunter, J.C., Hill, R.G. and Hughes, J. (1989) Correlation of ontogeny with function of $[^3H]U$-69,593 labelled κ opioid binding sites in the rat spinal cord. *Brain Res.*, 502: 149–157.

Aniksztejn, L. and Ben-Ari, Y. (1991) Novel form of long-term potentiation produced by a K^+ channel blocker in the hippocampus. *Nature (London)*, 349: 67–69.

Aniksztejn, L., Bregestovski, P. and Ben-Ari, Y. (1991) Selective activation of quisqualate metabotropic receptor potentiates NMDA but not AMPA responses. *Eur. J. Pharmacol.* 205: 327–328.

Attali, B., Gouarderes, C., Mazarguil, H., Audigier, Y. and Cros, J. (1982) Evidence for multiple 'Kappa' binding sites by use of opioid peptides in the guinea-pig lumbo-sacral spinal cord. *Neuropeptides*, 3: 53–64.

Attali, B., Saya, D. and Vogel, Z. (1989a) κ-Opiate agonists inhibit adenylate cyclase and produce heterologous desensitization in rat spinal cord. *J. Neurochem.*, 52: 360–369.

Attali, B., Saya, D., Nah, S-Y. and Vogel, Z. (1989b) κ-Opiate agonists inhibit Ca^{2+} influx in rat spinal cord-dorsal root ganglion cocultures: involvement of a GTP-binding protein. *J. Biol. Chem.*, 264: 347–353.

Atweh, S.F. and Kuhar, M.J. (1977) Autoradiographic localization of opiate receptors in rat brain. I. Spinal cord and lower medulla. *Brain Res.*, 124: 53–67.

Bakshi, R., Newman, A.H. and Faden, A.I. (1990) Dynorphin A (1–17) induces alterations in free fatty acids, excitatory amino acids, and motor function through an opiate receptor-mediated mechanism. *J. Neurosci.*, 10: 3793–3800.

Barber, R.P., Vaughn, J.E. and Roberts, E. (1982) The cytoarchitecture of GABAergic neurons in rat spinal cord. *Brain Res.*, 238: 305–328.

Barker, J.L., Neale, J.H., Smith, T.G. Jr. and Macdonald R.C.

(1978a) Opiate peptide modulation of amino acid responses suggests novel form of neuronal communication. *Science*, 199: 1451–1453.

Barker, J.L., Smith, T.G. Jr. and Neale, J.H. (1978b) Multiple membrane actions of enkephalin revealed using cultured spinal neurons. *Brain Res.*, 154: 153–158.

Bashir, Z.I., Alford, S., Davies, S.N., Randall, A.D. and Collingridge, G.L. (1991) Long-term potentiation of NMDA receptor-mediated synaptic transmission in the hippocampus. *Nature (London)*, 349: 156–158.

Bean, B.P. (1989) Neurotransmitter inhibition of neuronal calcium currents by changes in channel voltage dependence. *Nature (London)*, 340: 153–156.

Beech, D.J., Bernheim, L., Mathie, A. and Hille, B. (1991) Intracellular Ca^{2+} buffers disrupt muscarinic suppression of Ca^{2+} current and M current in rat sympathetic neurons. *Proc. Natl. Acad. Sci. USA*, 88: 652–656.

Belcher, G. and Ryall, R.W. (1978) Differential excitatory and inhibitory effects of opiates on non-nociceptive and nociceptive neurones in the spinal cord of the cat. *Brain Res.*, 145: 303–314.

Ben-Ari, Y., Aniksztejn, L. and Bregestovski, P. (1992) Protein kinase C modulation of NMDA currents: an important link for LTP induction. *Trends Neurosci.*, 15: 333–339.

Benveniste, M., Clements, J., Vyklicky, L. Jr. and Mayer, M.L. (1990) A kinetic analysis of the modulation of *N*-methyl-D-aspartate acid receptors by glycine in mouse cultured hippocampal neurones. *J. Physiol. (London)*, 428: 333–357.

Besse, D., Lombard, M.C., Zajac, J.M., Roques, B.P. and Besson, J.M. (1990) Pre- and postsynaptic distribution of mu, delta and kappa opioid receptors in the superficial layers of the cervical dorsal horn of the rat spinal cord. *Brain Res.*, 521: 15–22.

Bigot, D., Evan, G. and Hunt, S.P. (1989) Rapid induction of c-*fos* protein in glial and neuronal cells studied in vitro. *Neurosci. Lett.*, Suppl. 36: S75.

Bortolotto, Z.A. and Collingridge, G.L. (1992) Activation of glutamate metabotropic receptors induces long-term potentiation. *Eur. J. Pharmacol.*, 214: 297–298.

Botticelli, L.J., Cox, B.M. and Goldstein, A. (1981) Immunoreactive dynorphin in mammalian spinal cord and dorsal root ganglia. *Proc. Natl. Acad. Sci. USA*, 78: 7783–7786.

Calvillo, O., Henry, J.L. and Neuman, R.S. (1974) Effects of morphine and naloxone on dorsal horn neurones in the cat. *Can. J. Physiol. Pharmacol.*, 52: 1207–1211.

Caudle, R.M. and Isaac, L. (1988) Influence of dynorphin (1–13) on spinal reflexes in the rat. *J. Pharmacol. Exp. Ther.*, 246: 508–513.

Caudle, R.M., Chavkin, C. and Dubner, R. (1994) κ_2 opioid receptors inhibit NMDA receptor-mediated synaptic currents in guinea pig CA3 pyramidal cells. *J. Neurosci.*, 14: 5580–5589.

Cerne, R. and Randić, M. (1992) Modulation of AMPA and NMDA responses in rat spinal dorsal horn neurons by trans-1-aminocyclopentane-1,3-dicarboxylic acid. *Neurosci. Lett.*, 144: 180–184.

Cerne, R. and Randić, M. (1993) Modulation of NMDA and AMPA responses by cAMP-dependent protein kinase and protein kinase C in spinal dorsal horn neurons. *Neurosci. Abstr.*, 19: 1531.

Cerne, R., Jiang, M.C. and Randić, M. (1992) Cyclic adenosine 3',5'-monophosphate potentiates excitatory amino acid and synaptic responses of rat spinal dorsal horn neurons. *Brain Res.*, 596: 111–123.

Cerne, R., Kolaj, M., Jiang, M.C. and Randić, M. (1993a) Dynorphin reduces synaptic and excitatory amino acid responses of rat spinal dorsal horn neurons. In: *Proc. 32nd Int. Congr. Physiol. Sci.*, 299. 7/0.

Cerne, R., Kolaj, M., Parpura, V. and Randić, M. (1995). Dynorphin modulates N-Methyl-D-aspartate responses in acutely isolated neurons from the dorsal horn. *J. Neurosci.*, in press.

Cerne, R., Rusin, K.I. and Randić, M. (1993b) Enhancement of the *N*-methyl-D-aspartate response in spinal dorsal horn neurons by cAMP-dependent protein kinase. *Neurosci. Lett.*, 161: 124–128.

Chang, H.M., Berde, C.B., Holz, G.G. VI, Steward, G.F. and Kream, R.M. (1989) Sufentanil, morphine, Met-enkephalin, and kappa-agonist (U 50,488H) inhibit substance P release from primary sensory neurons: A model for presynaptic spinal opioid actions. *Anesthesiology*, 70: 672–677.

Charpak, S. and Gähwiler, B.H. (1991) Glutamate mediates a slow synaptic response in hippocampal slice cultures. *Proc. Roy. Soc. London Ser. B*, 243: 221–226.

Chavkin, C., James, I.F. and Goldstein, A. (1982) Dynorphin is a specific endogenous ligand of the κ opioid receptor. *Science*, 215: 413–415.

Chen, L. and Huang, L.-Y.M. (1991) Sustained potentiation of NMDA receptor-mediated glutamate responses through activation of protein kinase C by a μ opioid. *Neuron*, 7: 319–326.

Chen, L. and Huang, L.-Y.M. (1992) Protein kinase C reduces Mg^{2+} block of NMDA-receptor channels as a mechanism of modulation. *Nature (London)*, 356: 521–523.

Chen, L. and Huang, L.-Y.M. (1993) Dynorphin actions on NMDA-activated currents in trigeminal neurons: a single channel analysis. *Neurosci. Abstr.*, 19: 1157.

Chen, G-G., Chalazonitis, A., Shen, K-F. and Crain, S.M. (1988) Inhibitor of cyclic AMP-dependent protein kinase blocks opioid-induced prolongation of the action potential of mouse sensory ganglion neurons in dissociated cell cultures. *Brain Res.*, 462: 372–377.

Childers, S.R. (1993) Opioid receptor-coupled second messenger systems. Opioids I. In: A. Herz (Ed.), *Handbook of Experimental Pharmacology, Vol. 104/I*, Springer-Verlag, Berlin, Heidelberg, pp. 189–216.

Christensen, B.N. and Perl, E.R. (1970) Spinal neurons specifically excited by noxious or thermal stimuli: marginal zone of the dorsal horn. *J. Neurophysiol.*, 33: 293–307.

Cho, H.J. and Basbaum, A.I. (1989) Ultrastructural analysis of dynorphin B-immunoreactive cells and terminals in the superficial dorsal horn of the deafferented spinal cord of the rat. *J. Comp. Neurol.*, 281: 193–205.

Clark, J.A., Liu, L., Price, M., Hersh, B., Edelson, M. and Pasternak, G.W. (1989) Kappa opiate receptor multiplicity: evidence for two U 50,488-sensitive κ_1 subtypes and a novel κ_3 subtype. *J. Pharmacol. Exp. Ther.*, 251: 461–468.

Coderre, T.J. (1992) Contribution of protein kinase C to central sensitization and persistent nociception following tissue injury. *Neurosci. Lett.*, 140: 181–184

Coderre, T.J., Katz, J., Vaccarino, A.L. and Melzack, R. (1993) Contribution of central neuroplasticity to pathological pain: review of clinical and experimental evidence. *Pain*, 52: 259–285.

Collingridge, G.L. and Singer, W. (1990) Excitatory amino acid receptors and synaptic plasticity. *Trends Pharmacol. Sci.*, 11: 290–296.

Corbett, A.D., Paterson, S.J. and Kosterlitz, H.W. (1993) Selectivity of ligands for opioid receptors. Opioids I. In: A. Herz (Ed.) *Handbook of Experimental Pharmacology, Vol. 104/I*, Springer-Verlag, Berlin, Heidelberg, pp. 645–679.

Cox, B.M. (1993) Opioid receptor-G protein interactions: acute and chronic effects of opioids. Opioids I. In: A. Herz (Ed.) *Handbook of Experimental Pharmacology, Vol. 104/I*, Springer-Verlag, Berlin, Heidelberg, pp. 145–188.

Crain, S.M. and Shen, K.-F. (1990) Opioids can evoke direct receptor-mediated excitatory effects on sensory neurons. *Trends Pharmacol. Sci.*, 11: 77–81.

Cruz, L. and Basbaum, A.I. (1985) Multiple opioid peptides and the modulation of pain: immunohistochemical analysis of dynorphin and enkephalin in the trigeminal nucleus caudalis and spinal cord of the cat. *J. Comp. Neurol.*, 240: 331–348.

Dale, N. and Roberts, A. (1985) Dual-component amino-acid-mediated synaptic potentials: excitatory drive for swimming in *Xenopus* embryos. *J. Physiol. (London)*, 363: 35–59.

Davies, S.N. and Lodge, D. (1987) Evidence for involvement of N-methylaspartate receptors in 'wind-up' of class 2 neurones in the dorsal horn of the rat. *Brain Res.*, 424: 402–406.

De Biasi, S. and Rustioni, A. (1988) Glutamate and substance P coexist in primary afferent terminals in the superficial laminae of spinal cord. *Proc. Natl. Acad. Sci. USA*, 85: 7820–7824.

DeKoninck, Y. and Henry, J.L. (1991) Substance P-mediated slow excitatory postsynaptic potential elicited in dorsal horn neurones in vivo by noxious stimulation. *Proc. Natl. Acad. Sci. USA*, 88: 11344–11348.

Derrick, B.E., Weinberger, S.B. and Martinez, J.L. (1991) Opioid receptors are involved in an NMDA receptor-independent mechanism of LTP induction at hippocampal mossy fiber-CA3 synapses. *Brain Res. Bull.*, 27: 219–223.

Dickenson, A.H. and Knox, R.J. (1987) Antagonism of mu-opioid receptor-mediated inhibitions of nociceptive neurones by U50488H and dynorphin A_{1-13} in the rat dorsal horn. *Neurosci. Lett.*, 75: 229–234.

Dong, X.W., Parsons, C.G. and Headley, P.M. (1991) Effects of intravenous μ and κ opioid receptor agonists on sensory responses of convergent neurones in the dorsal horn of spinalized rats. *Br. J. Pharmacol.*, 103: 1230–1236.

Dougherty, P.M. and Willis, W.D. (1991a) Modification of the responses of primate spinothalamic neurons to mechanical stimulation by excitatory amino acids and N-methyl-D-aspartate antagonist. *Brain Res.*, 542: 15–22.

Dougherty, P.M. and Willis, W.D. (1991b) Enhancement of spinothalamic neuron responses to chemical and mechanical stimuli following combined micro-iontophoretic application of N-methyl-D-aspartic acid and substance P. *Pain*, 47: 85–93.

Dougherty, P.M., Palecek, J., Paleckova, V., Sorkin, L.S. and Willis, W.D. (1992) The role of NMDA and non-NMDA excitatory amino acid receptors in the excitation of primate spinothalamic tract neurones by mechanical, chemical, thermal and electrical stimuli. *J. Neurosci.*, 12: 3025–3041.

Dougherty, P.M., Palecek, J., Zorn, S. and Willis, W.D. (1993) Combined application of excitatory amino acids and substance P produces long-lasting changes in responses of primate spinothalamic tract neurons. *Brain Res. Rev.*, 18: 227–246.

Dubner, R. and Ruda, M.A. (1992) Activity-dependent neuronal plasticity following tissue injury and inflammation. *Trends Neurosci.*, 15: 96–103.

Duggan, A.W. and Fleetwood-Walker, S.M. (1993) Opioids and sensory processing in the central nervous system. Opioids I. In A. Herz (Ed.) *Handbook of Experimental Pharmacology, Vol. 104/I*, Springer-Verlag, Berlin, Heidelberg, p. 731–771.

Duggan, A.W. and North, R.A. (1984) Electrophysiology of opioids. *Pharmacol. Rev.*, 35: 219–281.

Duggan, A.W., Davies, J. and Hall, J.G. (1976a) Effects of opiate agonists and antagonists on central neurons of the cat. *J. Pharm. Exp. Ther.*, 196: 107–120.

Duggan, A.W., Hall, J.G. and Headley, P.M. (1976b) Morphine, enkephalin and the substantia gelatinosa. *Nature (London)*, 264: 456–458.

Duggan, A.W., Hall, J.G. and Headley, P.M. (1977a) Suppression of transmission of nociceptive impulses by morphine: selective effects of morphine administered in the region of the substantia gelatinosa. *Br. J. Pharmacol.*, 61: 65–76.

Duggan, A.W., Hall, J.G. and Headley, P.M. (1977b) Enkephalins and dorsal horn neurones of the cat: effects on responses to noxious and innocuous skin stimuli. *Br. J. Pharmacol.*, 61: 399–408.

Duggan, A.W., Morton, C.R., Zhao, Z.Q. and Hendry I.A. (1987) Noxious heating of the skin releases immunoreactive substance P in the substantia gelatinosa of the cat: a study with antibody microprobes. *Brain Res.*, 403: 345–349.

Duggan, A.W., Hendry, I.A., Morton, C.R., Hutchison, W.D. and Zhao, Z.Q. (1988) Cutaneous stimuli releasing immunoreactive substance P in the dorsal horn of the cat. *Brain Res.*, 451: 261–273.

Duggan, A.W., Hope, P.J., Jarrott, B., Schaible, H.G. and Fleetwood-Walker, S.M. (1990) Release, spread and persistence of immunoreactive neurokinin A in the dorsal horn of the cat following noxious cutaneous stimulation. Studies with antibody microprobes. *Neuroscience*, 35: 195–202.

Faden, A.I. (1990) Opioid and nonopioid mechanisms may contribute to dynorphin's pathophysiological actions in spinal cord injury. *Ann. Neurol.*, 27: 67–74.

Faden, A.I. and Jacobs, T.P. (1984) Dynorphin-related peptides cause motor dysfunction in the rat through a non-opiate action. *Br. J. Pharmacol.*, 81: 271–276.

Fallon, J.H. and Ciofi, P. (1990) Dynorphin containing neurons. In: A. Björklund, T. Hökfelt and Kuhar M. (Eds.) *Neuropeptides in the CNS, Part II, Handbook of Chemical Neuroanatomy, Vol. 9*, Elsevier, Amsterdam, pp. 1–130.

Fleetwood-Walker, S.M., Hope, P.J., Mitchell, R., El-Yassir, N. and Molony, V. (1988) The influence of opioid receptor subtypes on the processing of nociceptive inputs in the spinal dorsal horn of the cat. *Brain Res.*, 451: 213–226.

Fletcher, G.H. and Chiappinelli, V.A. (1993) The actions of the κ_1 opioid agonist U 50,488 on presynaptic nerve terminals of the chick ciliary ganglion. *Neuroscience*, 53: 239–250.

Fields, H.L., Emson, P.C., Leigh, B.K., Gilbert, R.F.T. and Iversen, L.L. (1980) Multiple opiate receptor sites on primary afferent fibres. *Nature (London)*, 284: 351–353.

Folkers, K., Feng, D.-M., Asano, N., Håkanson, R., Wiesenfeld-Hallin, Z. and Leander, S. (1990) Spantide II, an effective tachykinin antagonist having high potency and negligible neurotoxicity. *Proc. Natl. Acad. Sci. USA*, 87: 4833–4835.

Forsythe, I.D. and Westbrook, G.L. (1988) Slow excitatory postsynaptic currents mediated by *N*-methyl-D-aspartate receptors on cultured mouse central neurones. *J. Physiol. (London)*, 396: 515–533.

Gallacher, D.V., Hanley, M.R., Peterson, O.H., Roberts, M.L., Squire-Pollard, L.G. and Yule, D.I. (1990) Substance P and bombesin elevate cytosolic Ca^{2+} by different molecular mechanisms in a rat pancreatic acinar cell line. *J. Physiol. (London)*, 426: 193–207.

Gasic, G.P. and Hollmann, M. (1992) Molecular neurobiology of glutamate receptors. *Annu. Rev. Physiol.*, 54: 507–536.

Gerber, G. and Randić, M. (1989a) Excitatory amino acid-mediated components of synaptically evoked input from dorsal roots to deep dorsal horn neurons in the rat spinal cord slice. *Neurosci. Lett.*, 106: 211–219.

Gerber, G. and Randić, M. (1989b) Participation of excitatory amino acid receptors in the slow excitatory synaptic transmission in the rat spinal dorsal horn in vitro. *Neurosci. Lett.*, 106: 220–228.

Gerber, G., Kangrga, I., Ryu, P.D., Larew, J.S. and Randić, M. (1989) Multiple effects of phorbol esters in the rat spinal dorsal horn. *J. Neurosci.*, 9: 3606–3617.

Gerber, G., Cerne, R. and Randić, M. (1991) Participation of excitatory amino acid receptors in the slow excitatory synaptic transmission in rat spinal dorsal horn. *Brain Res.*, 561: 236–251.

Glaum, S.R., Miller, R.J. and Hammond, D.L. (1994) Inhibitory actions of δ_1-, δ_2-, and μ-opioid receptor agonists on excitatory transmission in lamina II neurons of adult rat spinal cord. *J. Neurosci.* 14: 4965–4971.

Glazer, E.J. and Basbaum, A.I. (1981) Immunohistochemical localization of leucine-enkephalin in the spinal cord of the cat: enkephalin-containing marginal neurons and pain modulation. *J. Comp. Neurol.*, 196: 377–389.

Gouardères, C., Audigier, Y. and Cros, J. (1982) Benzomorphan binding sites in rat lumbo-sacral spinal cord. *Eur. J. Pharmacol.*, 78: 483–486.

Gouardères, C., Cros, J. and Quirion, R. (1985) Autoradiographic localization of mu, delta and kappa opioid receptor binding sites in rat and guinea pig spinal cord. *Neuropeptides*, 6: 331–342.

Greengard, P., Jen, J., Nairn, A.C. and Stevens, C.F. (1991) Enhancement of the glutamate response by cAMP-dependent protein kinase in hippocampal neurons. *Science*, 253: 1135–1138.

Gross, R.A. and Macdonald, R.L. (1987) Dynorphin A selectively reduces a large transient (N-type) calcium current of mouse dorsal root ganglion neurons in cell culture. *Proc. Natl. Acad. Sci. USA*, 84: 5469–5473.

Gross, R.A., Moises, H.C., Uhler, M.D. and Macdonald, R.L. (1990) Dynorphin A and cAMP- dependent protein kinase independently regulate neuronal calcium currents. *Proc. Natl. Acad. Sci. USA*, 87: 7025–7029.

Grudt, T.J. and Williams, J.T. (1993) κ-Opioid receptors also increase potassium conductance. *Proc. Natl. Acad. Sci. USA*, 90: 11429–11432.

Gu, Y. and Huang, L.-Y.M. (1994) Modulation of glycine affinity for NMDA receptors by extracellular Ca^{2+} in triqeminal neurons. *J. Neurosci.*, 14: 4561–4570.

Haley, J.E., Sullivan, A.F. and Dickenson, A.H. (1990) Evidence for spinal *N*-methyl-D-aspartate receptor involvement in prolonged chemical nociception in the rat. *Brain Res.*, 518: 218–226.

Hammond, D.L., Presley, R., Gogas, K.R. and Basbaum, A.I. (1992) Morphine or U 50,488 suppresses Fos protein-like immunoreactivity in the spinal cord and nucleus tractus solitarii evoked by a noxious visceral stimulus in the rat. *J. Comp. Neurol.*, 315: 244–253.

Herrero, J.F. and Headley, P.M. (1991) The effects of sham and full spinalization on the systemic potency of μ- and κ-opioids on spinal nociceptive reflexes in rats. *Br. J. Pharmacol.*, 104: 166–170.

Hope, P.J., Fleetwood-Walker, S.M. and Mitchell, R. (1990) Distinct antinociceptive actions mediated by different opioid receptors in the region of lamina I and laminae III–V of the dorsal horn of the rat. *Br. J. Pharmacol.*, 101: 477–483.

Hori, Y., Endo, K. and Takahashi, T. (1992) Presynaptic

inhibitory action of enkephalin on excitatory transmission in superficial dorsal horn of rat spinal cord. *J. Physiol. (London)*, 450: 673–685.

Hökfelt, T., Skirboll, L., Lundberg, J.M., Dalsgaard, C.-J., Johansson, O., Pernow, B. and Jancsó, G. (1983) Neuropeptides and pain pathways. In: J.J. Bonica, U. Lindblom and A. Iggo (Eds.) *Advances in Pain Research and Therapy, Vol. 5*, Raven Press, New York, pp. 227–246.

Höllt, V., Haarmann, I., Millan, M.J. and Herz, A. (1987) Prodynorphin gene expression is enhanced in the spinal cord of chronic arthritic rats. *Neurosci. Lett.*, 73: 90–94.

Hunt, S.P., Kelly, J.S. and Emson, P.C. (1980) The electron microscopic localization of methionine-enkephalin within the superficial layers (I and II) of the spinal cord. *Neuroscience*, 5: 1871–1890.

Hunt, S.P., Kelly, J.S., Emson, P.C., Kimmel, J.R., Miller, R.J and Wu J.-Y. (1981) An immunohistochemical study of neuronal populations containing neuropeptides or γ-aminobutyrate within the superficial layers of the rat dorsal horn. *Neuroscience*, 6: 1883–1898.

Hunt, S.P., Pini, A. and Evan, G. (1987) Induction of c-*fos*-like protein in spinal cord neurones following sensory stimulation. *Nature (London)*, 328: 632–634.

Hunter, J.C., Birchmore, B., Woodruff, R. and Hughes, J. (1989) Kappa opioid binding sites in the dog cerebral cortex and spinal cord. *Neuroscience*, 31: 735–743.

Hutchison, W.D., Morton, C.R. and Terenius, L. (1990) Dynorphin A: in vivo release in the spinal cord of the cat. *Brain Res.*, 532: 299–306.

Hylden, J.L.K., Nahin, R.L., Traub, R.J. and Dubner, R. (1991) Effects of spinal kappa-opioid receptor agonists on the responsiveness of nociceptive superficial dorsal horn neurons. *Pain*, 44: 187–193.

Iadarola, M.J., Douglass, J., Civelli, O. and Naranjo, J.R. (1988) Differential activation of spinal cord dynorphin and enkephalin neurons during hyperalgesia: evidence using cDNA hybridization. *Brain Res.*, 455: 205–212.

Jahr, C.E. and Jessell, T.M. (1985) Synaptic transmission between dorsal root ganglion and dorsal horn neurons in culture: antagonism of monosynaptic excitatory postsynaptic potentials and glutamate excitation by kynurenate. *J. Neurosci.*, 5: 2281–2289.

James, I.F., Bettaney, J., Perkins, M.N., Ketchum, S.B. and Dray, A. (1990) Opioid receptor ligands in the neonatal rat spinal cord: binding and in vitro depression of the nociceptive responses. *Br. J. Pharmacol.*, 99: 503–508.

Jansen, K.L., Faull, R.L., Dragunow, M. and Waldvogel, H. (1990) Autoradiographic localization of NMDA, quisqualate and kainic acid receptors in human spinal cord. *Neurosci. Lett.*, 108: 53–57.

Jessell, T.M. and Dodd, J. (1989) Functional chemistry of primary afferent neurons. In: P.D. Wall and R. Melzack (Eds.) *Textbook of Pain*, 2nd Edn., Churchill Livingstone, Edinburgh, pp. 82–99.

Jessell, T.M. and Iversen, L.L. (1977) Opiate analgesics inhibit substance P release from rat trigeminal nucleus. *Nature (London)*, 268: 549–551.

Jiang, M.C. and Randić, M. (1991) Long-lasting modification in synaptic efficacy at primary afferent synapses with neurons in rat superficial spinal dorsal horn. *Third IBRO World Congr. Neurosci. Abstr.*, p. 307.

Johnson, J.W. and Ascher, P. (1987) Glycine potentiates the NMDA response in cultured mouse brain neurons. *Nature (London)*, 325: 529–531.

Johnston, D., Williams, S., Jaffe, D. and Gray, R. (1992) NMDA-receptor independent long-term potentiation. *Annu. Rev. Physiol.*, 54: 489–505.

Kangrga, I. and Randić, M. (1990) Tachykinins and calcitonin gene-related peptide enhance release of endogenous glutamate and aspartate from the rat spinal dorsal horn slice. *J. Neurosci.*, 10: 2026–2038.

Kangrga, I. and Randić, M. (1991) Outflow of endogenous aspartate and glutamate from the rat spinal dorsal horn in vitro by activation of low- and high-threshold primary afferent fibers. Modulation by μ-opioids. *Brain Res.*, 553: 347–352.

Kelso, S.R., Nelson, T.E. and Leonard, J.P. (1992) Protein kinase C-mediated enhancement of NMDA currents by metabotropic glutamate receptors in *Xenopus* oocytes. *J. Physiol. (London)*, 449: 705–718.

King, A.E. and Lopez-Garcia, J.A. (1993) Excitatory amino acid receptor-mediated neurotransmission from cutaneous afferents in rat dorsal horn in vitro. *J. Physiol. (London)*, 472: 443–457.

King, A.E., Thompson, S.W., Urban, L. and Woolf, C.J. (1988) The responses recorded in vitro of deep dorsal horn neurons to direct and orthodromic stimulation in the young rat spinal cord. *Neuroscience*, 27: 231–242.

Kleckner, N.W. and Dingledine, R. (1988) Requirement for glycine in activation of NMDA receptors expressed in *Xenopus* oocytes. *Science*, 241: 835–837.

Knox, R.J. and Dickenson, A.H. (1987) Effects of selective and non-selective κ-opioid receptor agonists on cutaneous C-fiber-evoked responses of rat dorsal horn neurones. *Brain Res.*, 415: 21–29.

Kojić, Lj. and Randić, M. (1993) Modulation of excitatory synaptic responses in rat spinal dorsal horn neurons by (1*S*,3*R*-1-aminocyclopentane-1,3-dicarboxylic acid. *Neurosci. Abstr.*, 19: 1526.

Kolaj, M., Cerne, R., Jiang, M.C., Lanthorn, T.H. and Randić, M. (1992) The effects of dynorphin A (1–13) on glutamate and synaptic responses of rat spinal dorsal horn neurons. *Neurosci. Abstr.*, 18: 281.

Kolaj, M., Cerne, R. and Randić, M. (1993a) Kappa opioid receptor activation modulates excitatory amino acid responses in acutely isolated neurons from the dorsal horn. *Neurosci. Abstr.*, 19: 1382.

Kolaj, M., Wang, R.A. and Randić, M. (1993b) DAGO modulates AMPA and GABA$_A$ receptor sensitivity in acutely isolated neurons from the spinal dorsal horn. *Abstract of the 7th World Congress on Pain*, Paris, France, p. 470.

Kolaj, M., Cerne, R., Cheng, G., Brickey, D.A. and Randić M. (1994) Alpha subunit of calcium/calmodulin-dependent protein kinase enhances excitatory amino acid and synaptic responses of rat spinal dorsal horn neurons. *J. Neurophysiol.*, 72: 2525–2531.

Kolaj, M., Cerne, R. and Randić, M. (1995) Modulation of excitatory amino acid responses in rat dorsal horn neurons by κ-opioids. *Brain Res.*, 671: 227–244.

Kullmann, D.M., Perkel, D.J., Manabe, T. and Nicoll, R.A. (1992) Ca^{2+} entry via postsynaptic voltage-sensitive Ca^{2+} channels can transiently potentiate excitatory synaptic transmission in the hippocampus. *Neuron*, 9: 1175–1183.

Kutsuwada, T., Kashiwabuchi, N., Mori, H., Sakimura, K., Kushiya, E., Araki, K., Meguro, H., Masaki, H., Kumanishi, T., Arakawa, M. and Mishina, M. (1992) Molecular diversity of the NMDA receptor channel. *Nature (London)*, 358: 36–41.

Lahti, R.A., Mickelson, M.M., McCall, J.M. and Von-Voigtlander, P.F. (1985) [^{3}H]U 69,593, a highly selective ligand for the opioid κ-receptor. *Eur. J. Pharmacol.*, 109: 281–284.

Lerea, L.S., Butler, L.S. and McNamara, J.O. (1992) NMDA and non-NMDA receptor-mediated increase of c-*fos* mRNA in dentate gyrus neurons involves calcium influx via different routes. *J. Neurosci.*, 12: 2973–2981.

Light A.R. and Perl, E.R. (1979) Spinal termination of functionally identified primary afferent neurons with slowly conducting myelinated fibers. *J. Comp. Neurol.*, 186: 133–150.

Liman, E.R., Knapp, A.G. and Dowling, J.E. (1989) Enhancement of kainate-gated currents in retinal horizontal cells by cyclic AMP-dependent protein kinase. *Brain Res.*, 481: 399–402.

Lord, J.A.H., Waterfield, A.A., Hughes, J. and Kosterlitz, H.W. (1977) Endogenous opioid peptides: multiple agonists and receptors. *Nature (London)*, 267: 495–499.

MacDermott, A.B., Mayer, M.L., Westbrook, G.L., Smith, S.J. and Barker, J.L. (1986) NMDA-receptor activation increases cytoplasmatic calcium concentration in cultured spinal cord neurones. *Nature (London)*, 321: 519–522.

Macdonald, R.L. and Werz, M.A. (1986) Dynorphin A decreases voltage-dependent calcium conductance of mouse dorsal root ganglion neurones. *J. Physiol. (London)*, 377: 237–249.

Madison, D.V., Malenka, R.C. and Nicoll, R.A. (1991) Mechanisms underlying long-term potentiation of synaptic transmission. *Annu. Rev. Neurosci.*, 14: 379–397.

Malenka, R.C. and Nicoll, R.A. (1993) NMDA-receptor-dependent synaptic plasticity: multiple forms and mechanisms. *Trends Neurosci.*, 16: 521–527.

Mantyh, P.W., Pinnock, R.D., Downes, C.P., Goedert, M. and Hunt, S.P. (1984) Correlation between inositol phospholipid hydrolysis and substance P receptors in rat CNS. *Nature (London)*, 309: 795–797.

Markram, H. and Segal, M. (1991) Calcimycin potentiates responses of rat hippocampal neurons to *N*-methyl-D-aspartate. *Brain Res.*, 540: 322–324.

Martin, W.R., Eades, C.G., Fraser, H.F. and Wikler, A. (1964) Use of hindlimb reflexes of the chronic spinal dog for comparing analgesics. *J. Pharmacol. Exp. Ther.*, 144: 8–11.

Martinez, J.L., Janak, P.H., Weinberger, S.B., Schulteis, G., Derrick, B.E. (1990) Enkephalin influences on behavioral and neural plasticity: mechanisms of action. In: L. Erinoff (Ed.) *Neurobiology of Drug Abuse: Learning and Memory, Natl. Inst. Drug Abuse Res. Monogr.*, Natl. Inst. Drug Abuse, Washington, DC, pp. 48–78.

Masu, Y., Nakayama, K., Tamaki, H., Harada, Y., Kuno, M. and Nakanishi, S. (1987) cDNA cloning of bovine substance-K receptor through oocyte expression system. *Nature (London)*, 329: 836–838.

Mayer, M.L. and Westbrook, G.L. (1987) The physiology of excitatory amino acids in the vertebrate central nervous system. *Prog. Neurobiol.*, 28: 197–276.

Mayer, M.L., Westbrook, G.L. and Guthrie, P.B. (1984) Voltage-dependent block by Mg^{2+} of NMDA responses in spinal cord neurones. *Nature (London)*, 309: 261–263.

Mayer, M.L., Vyklicky, L. Jr. and Clements, J. (1989) Regulation of NMDA receptor desensitization in mouse hippocampal neurons by glycine. *Nature (London)*, 338: 425–427.

McFadzean, I., Lacey, M.G., Hill, R.G. and Henderson, G. (1987) Kappa opioid receptor activation depresses excitatory synaptic input to rat locus coeruleus neurons in vitro. *Neuroscience*, 20: 231–239.

McMahon, S.B., Lewin, G.R. and Wall, P.D. (1993) Central hyperexcitability triggered by noxious inputs. *Curr. Opin. Neurobiol.*, 3: 602–610.

McVaugh, W.B. and Waxham, M.N. (1992) Augmentation of NMDA currents by cyclic AMP and forskolin. *Neurosci. Abstr.*, 18: 651.

Meller, S.T., Pechman, P.S., Gebhart, G.F. and Maves, T.J. (1992) Nitric oxide mediates the thermal hyperalgesia produced in a model of neuropathic pain in the rat. *Neuroscience*, 50: 7–10.

Millan, M.J. (1990) κ-Opioid receptors and analgesia. *Trends Pharmacol. Sci.*, 11: 70–76.

Miller, K.E. and Seybold, V.S. (1987) Comparison of met-enkephalin-, dynorphin A-, and neurotensin-immunoreactive neurons in the cat and rat spinal cords. I. Lumbar cord. *J. Comp. Neurol.*, 255: 293–304.

Miller, K.F. and Seybold, V.S. (1989) Comparison of met-enkephalin, dynorphin A, and neurotensin-immunoreactive neurons in the cat and rat spinal cords. II. Segmental differences in the marginal zone. *J. Comp. Neurol.*, 279: 619–628.

Miller, B., Sarantis, M., Traynelis, S.F. and Attwell, D. (1992) Potentiation of NMDA receptor currents by arachidonic acid. *Nature (London)*, 355: 722–725.

Mjellem-Joly, N., Lund, A., Berge, O.-G. and Hole, K. (1991) Potentiation of a behavioural response in mice by spinal coadministration of substance P and excitatory amino acid agonists. *Neurosci. Lett.*, 133: 121–124.

Moises, H.C. and Walker, J.M. (1985) Electrophysiological

250

effects of dynorphin peptides on hippocampal pyramidal cells in rat. *Eur. J. Pharmacol.*, 108: 85–98.

Monaghan, D.T., Bridges, R.J. and Cotman, C.W. (1989) The excitatory amino acid receptors: their classes, pharmacology, and distinct properties in the function of the central nervous system. *Ann. Rev. Pharmacol. Toxicol.*, 29: 365–402.

Moore, S.D., Madamba, S.G., Schweitzer, P. and Siggins, G.R. (1994) Voltage-dependent effects of opioid peptides on hippocampal CA3 pyramidal neurons in vitro. *J. Neurosci.*, 14: 809–820.

Moriyoshi, K., Masu, M., Ishii, T., Shigemoto, R., Mizuno, N. and Nakanishi, S. (1991) Molecular cloning and characterization of the rat NMDA receptor. *Nature (London)*, 354: 31–37.

Morris, B.J. and Herz, A. (1987) Distinct distribution of opioid receptor types in rat lumbar spinal cord. *Naunyn-Schmiedeberg's Arch. Pharmacol.*, 336: 240–243.

Murase, K. and Randić, M. (1984) Actions of substance P on rat spinal dorsal horn neurones. *J. Physiol. (London)*, 346: 203–217.

Murase, K., Nedeljkov, V. and Randić, M. (1982) The actions of neuropeptides on dorsal horn neurons in the rat spinal cord slice preparation: an intracellular study. *Brain Res.*, 234: 170–176.

Murase, K., Ryu, P.D. and Randić, M. (1989) Tachykinins modulate multiple ionic conductances in voltage-clamped rat spinal dorsal horn neurons. *J. Neurophysiol.*, 61: 854–865.

Nagy, J.I., Maggi, C.A., Dray, A., Woolf, C.J. and Urban, L. (1993) The role of neurokinin and *N*-methyl-D-aspartate receptors in synaptic transmission from capsaicin-sensitive primary afferents in the rat spinal cord in vitro. *Neuroscience*, 52: 1029–1037.

Nakajima, Y., Tsuchida, K., Negishi, M., Ito, S. and Nakanishi, S. (1992) Direct linkage of three tachykinin receptors to stimulation of both phosphatidylinositol hydrolysis and cyclic AMP cascades in transfected chinese hamster ovary cells. *J. Biol. Chem.*, 267: 2437–2442.

Nicoll, R.A., Alger, B.E. and Jahr, C.E. (1980) Enkephalin blocks inhibitory pathways in the vertebrate CNS. *Nature (London)*, 287: 22–25.

Nishizuka, Y. (1984) The role of protein kinase C in cell surface signal transduction and tumour promotion. *Nature (London)*, 308: 693–698.

Nishizuka, Y. (1988) The molecular heterogeneity of protein kinase C and its implications for cellular regulation. *Nature (London)*, 334: 661–665.

Nock, B., Rajpara, A., O'Connor, L.H. and Cicero, T.J. (1988) Autoradiography of [^{3}H]U 69,593 binding sites in rat brain: evidence for κ opioid receptor subtypes. *Eur. J. Pharmacol.*, 154: 27–34.

Nock, B., Giordano, A.L., Cicero, T.J. and O'Connor, L.H. (1990) Affinity of drugs and peptides for U 69,593-sensitive and -insensitive kappa opiate binding sites: the U 69,593-insensitive site appears to be the beta endorphin-specific epsilon receptor. *J. Pharm. Exp. Ther.*, 254: 412–419.

Nock, B., Giordano, A.L., Moore, B.W. and Cicero, T.J. (1993) Properties of the putative epsilon opioid receptor: identification in rat, guinea pig, cow, pig and chicken brain. *J. Pharmacol. Exp. Ther.*, 264: 349–359.

Noguchi, K., Morita, Y., Kiyama, H., Ono, K. and Tohyama, M. (1988) A noxious stimulus induces the preprotachykinin-A gene expression in the rat dorsal root ganglion: A quantitative study using in situ hybridization histochemistry. *Brain Res.*, 464: 31–35.

North, R.A. (1993) Opioid actions on membrane ion channels. Opioids I. In: A. Herz (Ed.) *Handbook of Experimental Pharmacology, Vol. 104 / I*, Springer-Verlag, Berlin, Heidelberg, pp. 773–797.

Nowak, L., Bregestovski, P., Ascher, P., Herbet, A. and Prochiantz, A. (1984) Magnesium gates glutamate-activated channels in mouse central neurones. *Nature (London)*, 307: 462–465.

Nyberg, F., Yaksh, T.L. and Terenius, L. (1983) Opioid activity released from cat spinal cord by sciatic nerve stimulation. *Life Sci.*, 33(Suppl. 1): 17–20.

Periyasamy, S. and Hoss, W. (1990) Kappa opioid receptors stimulate phosphoinositide turnover in rat brain. *Life Sci.*, 47: 219–225.

Pinnock, R.D. (1992) A highly selective κ-opioid receptor agonist, CI-977, reduces excitatory synaptic potentials in the rat locus coeruleus in vitro. *Neuroscience*, 47: 87–94.

Pohl, M., Mauborgne, A., Bourgoin, S., Benoliel, J.J., Hamon, M. and Cesselin, F. (1989) Neonatal capsaicin treatment abolishes the modulations by opioids of substance P release from rat spinal cord slices. *Neurosci. Lett.*, 96: 102–107.

Portoghese, P.S., Lipkowski, A.W. and Takemori, A.E. (1987) Binaltorphimine and nor-binaltorphimine, potent and selective κ-opioid receptor antagonists. *Life Sci.*, 40: 1287–1292.

Przewlocki, R., Shearman, G.T. and Herz, A. (1983) Mixed opioid/non-opioid effects of dynorphin and dynorphin-related peptides after their intrathecal injection in rats. *Neuropeptides*, 3: 233–240.

Randić, M. and Kolaj, M. (1993) Modulation of AMPA response by μ-opioid receptor agonist DAGO in acutely isolated neurons from the dorsal horn. *Neurosci. Abstr.*, 19: 302.

Randić, M. and Miletic, V. (1978) Depressant actions of methionine-enkephalin and somatostatin in cat dorsal horn neurones activated by noxious stimuli. *Brain Res.*, 152: 196–202.

Randić, M., Ryu, P.D. and Urban, L. (1986) Effects of polyclonal and monoclonal antibodies to substance P on slow excitatory transmission in rat spinal dorsal horn. *Brain Res.*, 383: 15–27.

Randić, M., Murase, K., Ryu, P.D. and Gerber, G. (1987) Slow excitatory transmission in the rat spinal dorsal horn: possible mediation by tachykinins. *Biomed Res.*, 8(Suppl.): 71–82.

Randić, M., Hecimovic, H. and Ryu, P.D. (1990) Substance P modulates glutamate-induced currents in acutely isolated rat spinal dorsal horn neurons. *Neurosci. Lett.*, 117: 74–80.

Randić, M., Jiang, M.C. and Cerne, R. (1993a) Long-term potentiation and long-term depression of primary afferent neurotransmission in the rat spinal cord. *J. Neurosci.*, 13: 5228–5241.

Randić, M., Jiang, M.C., Rusin, K.I., Cerne, R. and Kolaj, M. (1993b) Interactions between excitatory amino acids and tachykinins and long-term changes of synaptic responses in the rat spinal dorsal horn. *Regul. Peptides*, 46: 418–420.

Randić, M., Cheng, G. and Kojić, Lj. (1994) Kappa opioid receptor activation modulates excitatory synaptic responses of the rat spinal dorsal horn neurons. *Can. J. Physiol. Pharmacol.*, 72 (suppl. 1): 348.

Raymond, L.A., Blackstone, C.D. and Huganir, R.L. (1993) Phosphorylation and modulation of recombinant GluR6 glutamate receptors by cAMP-dependent protein kinase. *Nature (London)*, 361: 637–641.

Reisine, T. and Bell, G.I. (1993) Molecular biology of opioid receptors. *Trends Neurosci.*, 16: 506–510.

Réthelyi, M. (1977) Preterminal and terminal axon arborizations in the substantia gelatinosa of cat's spinal cord. *J. Comp. Neurol.*, 172: 511–521.

Rhim, H. and Miller, R.J. (1993) Opioid modulation of evoked calcium signals in acutely dissociated neurons from the rat nucleus tractus solitarius (NTS). *Neurosci. Abstr.* 19: 420.

Rhim, H., Glaum, S.R. and Miller, R.J. (1993) Selective opioid agonists modulate afferent transmission in the rat nucleus tractus solitarius. *J. Pharmacol. Exp. Ther.*, 264: 795–800.

Ribeiro-da-Silva, A. and Coimbra, A. (1980) Neuronal uptake of [^{3}H]GABA and [^{3}H]glycine in laminae I–III (substantia gelatinosa Rolandi) of the rat spinal cord. An autoradiographic study. *Brain Res.*, 188: 449–464.

Rothman, R.B., Bykov, V., de Costa, B.R., Jacobson, A.E., Rice, K.C. and Brady, L.S. (1990) Interaction of endogenous opioid peptides and other drugs with four kappa opioid binding sites in guinea pig brain. *Peptides*, 11: 311–331.

Rothman, R.B., Bykov, V., Xue, B.G., Xu, H., De Costa, B.R., Jacobson, A.E., Rice, K.C., Kleinman, J.E. and Brady, L.S. (1992) Interaction of opioid peptides and other drugs with multiple kappa receptors in rat and human brain. Evidence for species differences. *Peptides*, 13: 977–987.

Rothman, R.B., Holaday J.W. and Porreca, F. (1993) Allosteric coupling among opioid receptors: evidence for an opioid receptor complex. Opioids I. In: A. Herz (Ed.) *Handbook of Experimental Pharmacology, Vol. 104 / I*, Springer-Verlag, Berlin, Heidelberg, pp. 217–237.

Ruda, M.A., Iadarola, M.J., Cohen, L.V. and Young, W.S. III (1988) In situ hybridization histochemistry and immunocytochemistry reveal an increase in spinal dynorphin biosynthesis in a rat model of peripheral inflammation and hyperalgesia. *Proc. Natl. Acad. Sci. USA*, 85: 622–626.

Rusin, K.I. and Randić, M. (1991) Modulation of NMDA-induced currents by μ-opioid receptor agonist DAGO in acutely isolated rat spinal dorsal horn neurons. *Neurosci. Lett.*, 124: 208–212.

Rusin, K.I., Ryu, P.D. and Randić, M. (1992) Modulation of excitatory amino acid responses in rat dorsal horn neurons by tachykinins. *J. Neurophysiol.*, 68: 265–286.

Rusin, K.I., Bleakman, D, Chard, P.S., Randić, M. and Miller, R.J. (1993a) Tachykinins potentiate N-methyl-D-aspartate responses in acutely isolated neurons from the dorsal horn. *J. Neurochem.*, 60: 952–960.

Rusin, K.I., Jiang, M.C., Cerne, R. and Randić, M. (1993b) Interactions between excitatory amino acids and tachykinins in the rat spinal dorsal horn. *Brain Res. Bull.*, 30: 329–338.

Rustioni, A. and Weinberg, R.J. (1989) The somatosensory system. In: A. Björklund, T. Hökfelt and L.W. Swanson (Eds.), *Handbook of Chemical Neuroanatomy, Vol. 7, Integrated Systems of the CNS, Part II*, Elsevier, Amsterdam, pp. 219–321.

Ryu, P.D. and Randić, M. (1990) Low- and high-voltage-activated calcium currents in rat spinal dorsal horn neurons. *J. Neurophysiol.*, 63: 273–285.

Sastry, B.R. and Goh, J.W. (1983) Actions of morphine and met-enkephalin-amide on nociceptor driven neurones in substantia gelatinosa and deeper dorsal horn. *Neuropharmacology*, 22: 119–122.

Schaible, H.-G., Grubb, B.D., Neugebauer, V. and Dubner, R. (1991) The effects of NMDA antagonists on neuronal activity in cat spinal cord evoked by acute inflammation in the knee joint. *Eur. J. Neurosci.*, 3: 981–991.

Schmauss, C. and Herz, A. (1987) Intrathecally administered dynorphin-(1–17) modulates morphine-induced antinociception differently in morphine-naive and morphine-tolerant rats. *Eur. J. Pharmacol.*, 135: 429–431.

Schneider, S.P. and Perl, E.R. (1988) Comparison of primary afferent and glutamate excitation of neurons in the mammalian spinal dorsal horn. *J. Neurosci.*, 8: 2062–2073.

Schoepp, D., Bockaert, J. and Sladeczek, F. (1991) Pharmacological and functional characteristics of metabotropic excitatory amino acid receptors. In: D. Lodge and G. Collingridge (Eds.) *The Pharmacology of Excitatory Amino Acids. A Special Report*, Elsevier, Cambridge, pp. 74–81.

Sharif, N.A., Hunter, J.C., Hill, R.G. and Hughes, J. (1988) [^{125}I]Dynorphin (1–8) produces a similar pattern of κ-opioid receptor labelling to [^{3}H]dynorphin (1–8) and [^{3}H]etorphine in guinea pig brain: a quantitative autoradiographic study. *Neurosci. Lett.*, 86: 272–278.

Shigemoto, R., Yokota, Y., Tsuchida, K. and Nakanishi, S. (1990) Cloning and expression of a rat neuromedin K receptor cDNA. *J. Biol. Chem.*, 265: 623–628.

Schuman, E.M. and Madison, D.V. (1991) A requirement for the intercellular messenger nitric oxide in long-term potentiation. *Science*, 254: 1503–1506.

Siegelbaum, S.A. and Kandel, E.R. (1991) Learning-related synaptic plasticity: LTP and LTD. *Curr. Opin. Neurobiol.*, 1: 113–120.

Sillar, K.T. and Roberts, A. (1988) Unmyelenated cutaneous afferent neurons activate two types of excitatory amino acid receptor in the spinal cord of *Xenopus laevis* embryos. *J. Neurosci.*, 8: 1350–1360.

Simon, E.J., (1991) Opioid receptors and endogenous opioid peptides. *Med. Res. Rev.*, 11: 357–374.

Skilling, S.R., Sun, X-F., Kurtz, H.J. and Larson, A.A. (1992) Selective potentiation of NMDA-induced activity and release of excitatory amino acids by dynorphin: possible roles in paralysis and neurotoxicity. *Brain Res.*, 575: 272–278.

Slater, P. and Patel, S. (1983) Autoradiographic localization of opiate κ-receptors in the rat spinal cord. *Eur. J. Pharmacol.*, 92: 159–160.

Snider, M.R., Constantine, J.W., Lowe, J.A. III, Longo, K.P., Lebel, W.S., Woody, H.A., Drozda, S.E., Desai, M.C., Vinick, F.J., Spencer, R.W. and Hess, H.-J. (1991) A potent nonpeptide antagonist of the substance P (NK-1) receptor. *Science*, 251: 435–437.

Sommer, B. and Seeburg, P.H. (1992) Glutamate receptor channels: novel properties and new clones. *Trends Pharmacol. Sci.*, 13: 291–296.

Stevens, C.W. and Yaksh, T.L. (1986) Dynorphin A and related peptides administered intrathecally in the rat: a search for putative kappa opiate receptor activity. *J. Pharmacol. Exp. Ther.*, 238: 833–838.

Stewart, P. and Isaac, L. (1989) Localization of dynorphin-induced neurotoxicity in rat spinal cord. *Life Sci.*, 44: 1505–1514.

Suarez-Roca, H. and Maixner, W. (1993) Activation of kappa opioid receptors by U 50,488H and morphine enhances the release of substance P from rat trigeminal nucleus slices. *J. Pharmacol. Exp. Ther.*, 264: 648–653.

Sugiura, Y., Lee, C.L. and Perl, E.R. (1986) Central projections of identified, unmyelinated (C) afferent fibers innervating mammalian skin. *Science*, 234: 358–361.

Sugiyama, H., Ito, I. and Hirono, C. (1987) A new type of glutamate receptor linked to inositol phospholipid metabolism. *Nature (London)*, 325: 531–533.

Szekely, A.M., Barbaccia, M.L. and Costa, E. (1987) Activation of specific glutamate receptor subtypes increases c-*fos* proto-oncogene expression in primary cultures of neonatal rat cerebellar granule cells. *Neuropharmacology*, 26: 1779–1782.

Szekely, A.M., Barbaccia, M.L., Alho, H. and Costa, E. (1989) In primary cultures of cerebellar granule cells the activation of N-methyl-D-aspartate-sensitive glutamate receptors induces c-*fos* mRNA expression. *Mol. Pharmacol.*, 35: 401–408.

Takemori, A.E., Ho, B.Y., Naeseth, J.S. and Portoghese, P.S. (1988) Nor-binaltorphimine, a highly selective kappa-opioid antagonist in analgesic and receptor binding assays. *J. Pharmacol. Exp. Ther.*, 246: 255–258.

Tölle, T.R., Berthele, A., Zieglgänsberger, W., Seeburg, P.H. and Wisden, W. (1993) The differential expression of 16 NMDA and non-NMDA receptor subunits in the rat spinal cord and in periaqueductal gray. *J. Neurosci.*, 13: 5009–5028.

Traynor, J. (1989) Subtypes of the κ-opioid receptor: fact or fiction? *Trends Pharmacol. Sci.*, 10: 52–53.

Urbán, L. and Randić, M. (1984) Slow excitatory transmission in rat dorsal horn: possible mediation by peptides. *Brain Res.*, 290: 336–341.

Verhage, M., McMahon, H.T., Ghijsen, W.E., Boomsma, F., Scholten, G., Wiegant, V.M. and Nicholls, D.G. (1991) Differential release of amino acids, neuropeptides, and catecholamines from isolated nerve terminals. *Neuron*, 6: 517–524.

Vidal, C., Maier, R. and Zieglgänsberber, W. (1984) Effects of dynorphin A_{1-17}, dynorphin A_{1-13} and D-ala^2-D-leu^5-enkepha lin on the excitability of pyramidal cells in CA1 and CA2 of the rat hippocampus in vitro. *Neuropeptides*, 5: 237–240.

Vincent, S.R., Hökfelt, T., Christensson, I. and Terenius, L. (1982) Dynorphin-immunoreactive neurons in the central nervous system of the rat. *Neurosci. Lett.*, 33: 185–190.

VonVoigtlander, P.F., Lahti, R.A. and Ludens, J.H. (1983) U 50,488: a selective and structurally novel non-mu (kappa) opioid agonist. *J. Pharmacol. Exp. Ther.*, 224: 7–12.

Vyklicky, L. Jr., Benveniste, M. and Mayer, M.L. (1990) Modulation of N-methyl-D-aspartate receptor desensitization by glycine in mouse cultured hippocampal neurones. *J. Physiol. (London)*, 428: 313–331.

Wagner, J.J., Caudle, R.M. and Chavkin, C. (1992) κ-Opioids decrease excitatory transmission in the dentate gyrus of the guinea pig hippocampus. *J. Neurosci.*, 12: 132–141.

Wagner, J.J., Terman, G.W. and Chavkin, C. (1993) Endogenous dynorphins inhibit excitatory neurotransmission and block LTP induction in the hippocampus. *Nature (London)*, 363: 451–454.

Walker, J.M., Moises, H.C., Coy, D.H. Baldrighi, G. and Akil, H. (1982) Nonopiate effects of dynorphin and des-Tyr-dynorphin. *Science*, 218: 1136–1138.

Wang, R.A. and Randić, M. (1994) Activation of μ-opioid receptor modulates $GABA_A$ receptor-mediated currents in isolated spinal dorsal horn neurons. *Neurosci. Lett.*, 180 (1994) 109–113.

Wang, L.Y., Salter, M.W. and MacDonald, J.F. (1991) Regulation of kainate receptors by cAMP-dependent protein kinase and phosphatases. *Science*, 253: 1132–1135.

Watkins, J.C. and Evans, R.H. (1981) Excitatory amino acid transmitters. *Ann. Rev. Pharmacol. Toxicol.*, 21: 165–204.

Watkins, J.C., Krogsgaard-Larsen, P. and Honoré, T. (1990) Structure-activity relationships in the development of excitatory amino acid receptor agonists and competitive antagonists. *Trends Pharmacol. Sci.*, 11: 25–33.

Weisskopf, M.G., Zalutsky, R.A. and Nicoll, R.A. (1993) The opioid peptide dynorphin mediates heterosynaptic depression of hippocampal mossy fibre synapses and modulates long-term potentiation. *Nature (London)*, 362: 423–427.

Wiesenfeld-Hallin, Z., Xu, X.-J. and Dalsgaard, C.J. (1991) Central sensitization after C-fiber activation is mediated by NMDA and substance P receptors. *Neurosci. Abstr.*, 17: 728.

Wilcox, G.L. (1991) Excitatory neurotransmitters and pain. In: M.R. Bond, J.E. Charlton and C.J. Woolf (Eds.) *Proceedings of the VIth World Congress on Pain*, Elsevier, Amsterdam, pp. 97–117.

Willcockson, Wm.S., Kim, J., Shin, H.K., Chung, J.M. and Willis, W.D. (1986) Actions of opioids on primate spinothalamic tract neurons. *J. Neurosci.*, 6: 2509–2520.

Wisden, W. and Seeburg, P.H. (1993) Mammalian ionotropic glutamate receptors. *Curr. Opin. Neurobiol.*, 3: 291–298.

Womack, M.D., MacDermott, A.B. and Jessell, T.M. (1988) Sensory transmitters regulate intracellular calcium in dorsal horn neurons. *Nature (London)*, 334: 351–353.

Woolf, C.J. (1991) Central mechanisms of acute pain. In: M.R. Bond, J.E. Charlton and C.J. Woolf (Eds.), *Pain Research and Clinical Menagment, Vol. 4, Proceedings of the VIth World Congress on Pain*, Elsevier, Amsterdam, pp. 25–34.

Woolf, C.J. and Thompson, S.W. (1991) The induction and maintenance of central sensitization is dependent on *N*-methyl-D-aspartic acid receptor activation: implications for the treatment of post-injury pain hypersensitivity states. *Pain*, 44: 293–299.

Woolf, C.J. and Wall, P.D. (1986) Relative effectiveness of C primary afferent fibers of different origins in evoking a prolonged facilitation of the flexor reflex in the rat. *J. Neurosci.*, 6: 1433–1442.

Worley, P.F., Baraban, J.M., De Souza, E.B. and Snyder, S.H. (1986) Mapping second messenger systems in the brain: differential localizations of adenylate cyclase and protein kinase C. *Proc. Natl. Acad. Sci. USA*, 83: 4053–4057.

Xie, C.W. and Lewis, D.V. (1991) Opioid-mediated facilitation of long-term potentiation at the lateral perforant path-dentate granule cell synapse. *J. Pharmacol. Exp. Ther.*, 256: 289–296.

Xu, X.-J., Dalsgaard, C.J. and Wiesenfeld-Hallin, Z. (1992a) Spinal substance P and *N*-methyl-D-aspartate receptors are coactivated in the induction of central sensitization of the nociceptive flexor reflex. *Neuroscience*, 51: 641–648.

Xu, X.-J., Dalsgaard, C.J. and Wiesenfeld-Hallin, Z. (1992b) Intrathecal CP-96,345 blocks reflex facilitation induced in rats by substance P and C-fiber-conditioning stimulation. *Eur. J. Pharmacol.*, 216: 337–344.

Yaksh, T.L. (1988) Substance P release from knee joint afferent terminals: modulation by opioids. *Brain Res.*, 458: 319–324.

Yaksh, T.L., Jessell, T.M., Gamse, R., Mudge, A.W. and Leeman, S.E. (1980) Intrathecal morphine inhibits substance P release from mammalian spinal cord in vivo. *Nature (London)*, 286: 155–157.

Yamaguchi, K., Nakajima, Y., Nakajima, S. and Stanfield, P.R. (1990) Modulation of inwardly rectifying channels by substance P in cholinergic neurones from rat brain in culture. *J. Physiol. (London)*, 426: 499–520.

Yokota, Y., Sasai, Y., Tanaka, K., Fujiwara, T., Tsuchida, K., Shigemoto, R., Kakizuka, A., Ohkubo, H. and Nakanishi, S. (1989) Molecular characterization of a functional cDNA for rat substance P receptor. *J. Biol. Chem.*, 264: 17649–17652.

Yoshimura, M. and Jessell, T.M. (1989a) Primary afferent-evoked synaptic responses and slow potential generation in rat substantia gelatinosa neurons in vitro. *J. Neurophysiol.*, 62: 96–108.

Yoshimura, M. and Jessell, T.M. (1989b) Membrane properties of rat substantia gelatinosa neurons in vitro. *J. Neurophysiol.*, 62: 109–118.

Yoshimura, M. and Jessell, T.M. (1990) Amino acid-mediated EPSPs at primary afferent synapses with substantia gelatinosa neurones in the rat spinal cord. *J. Physiol. (London)*, 430: 315–335.

Yoshimura, M. and Nishi, S. (1993) Blind patch-clamp recordings from substantia gelatinosa neurons in adult rat spinal cord slices: pharmacological properties of synaptic currents. *Neuroscience*, 53: 519–526.

Yoshimura, M. and North, R.A. (1983) Substantia gelatinosa neurones hyperpolarized in vitro by enkephalin. *Nature (London)*, 305: 529–530.

Zieglgänsberger, W. (1986) Central control of nociception. In: V.B. Mountcastle, F.E. Bloom and S.R. Geiger (Eds.) *Handbook of Physiology: The Nervous System, Vol. IV*, Williams and Wilkins, Baltimore, pp. 581–645.

Zieglgänsberger, W. and Bayerl, H. (1976) The mechanism of inhibition of neuronal activity by opiates in the spinal cord of cat. *Brain Res.* 115: 111–128.

Zieglgänsberger, W. and Puil, E.A. (1973) Actions of glutamic acid on spinal neurones. *Exp. Brain Res.*, 17: 35–49.

Zieglgänsberger, W. and Tulloch, I.F. (1979) The effects of methionine- and leucine-enkephalin on spinal neurones of the cat. *Brain Res.*, 167: 53–64.

Zukin, R.S., Eghbali, M., Olive, D., Unterwald, E.M. and Tempel, A. (1988) Characterization and visualization of rat and guinea pig brain κ-opioid receptors: evidence for κ_1 and κ_2 opioid receptors. *Proc. Natl. Acad. Sci. USA*, 85: 4061–4065.

F. Nyberg, H.S. Sharma and Z. Wiesenfeld-Hallin (Eds.)
Progress in Brain Research, Vol 104
© 1995 Elsevier Science BV. All rights reserved.

CHAPTER 14

Peptidergic afferents: physiological aspects

L. Urban[1], S.W.N. Thompson[1], A.J. Fox[2], S. Jeftinija[3] and A. Dray[1]

[1]*Department of Pharmacology, Sandoz Institute for Medical Research, 5 Gower Place, London WC1E 6BN, UK,*
[2]*Department of Thoracic Medicine, National Heart and Lung Institute, Dovehouse Street, London, UK and*
[3]*Department of Anatomy, Iowa State University, Ames, IA 50010, USA*

Introduction

Many primary afferent neurons express a wide array of neuropeptides in varying proportions, which may differ also according to their target tissues (Levin et al., 1993; Lawson et al., 1994) and response to nerve injury (Hökfelt et al., 1994). At first sight, therefore, it is not easy to relate peptide content to a functional modality of the primary afferent. For example, CGRP is present in some small calibre, unmyelinated C-fibres, as well as in a group of large myelinated fibres (Ju et al., 1987). Also, many of the peptidergic fibres contain a variety of neuropeptides. However, there are some physiological characteristics and certain modalities which predict the peptide content of the primary afferent. Thus, small-diameter myelinated and unmyelinated afferent fibres with small-diameter cell bodies are excited by noxious thermal and mechanical stimuli. A particular characteristic of these fibres is that they are also excited by known algogenic and irritant substances such as capsaicin or bradykinin (Nagy et al., 1993; Fig. 1). Considerable evidence indicates that some of these nociceptive fibres contain the neurokinins, substance P (SP) and neurokinin A (NKA) (Gamse et al., 1979; Jancso et al., 1981; Lawson et al., 1984). Furthermore, numerous studies have shown that these peptides are released from primary afferent nerve terminals in

the dorsal horn of the spinal cord (Duggan et al., 1988, 1990) and in peripheral target tissues (Holzer, 1991) in response to high-intensity electrical or noxious thermal, mechanical and chemical stimuli. The nature of all of these stimuli implies that these fibres are involved in nociception.

The exact peptide content of these fibres is discussed elsewhere. Here we will examine the behavioural and physiological characteristics of fine primary afferent fibres which conduct at low velocity, and have a high threshold for electrical stimulation, are activated by algogenic substances, express tetrodotoxin (TTX)-resistant Na-channels, and are the most likely ones, as we will demonstrate, to release substance P (SP) and neurokinin A (NKA) from their terminals in the periphery (neuro-effector functions) and in the spinal cord (central transmission). We will focus primarily on the pharmacological role of neuropeptides in primary afferent nociceptive function.

Characterization of capsaicin-sensitive cutaneous C-primary afferents

Application of capsaicin to peripheral nerves in human subjects evokes intense burning pain (LaMotte et al., 1992). In animal models, the release of neurokinins in the periphery and in the

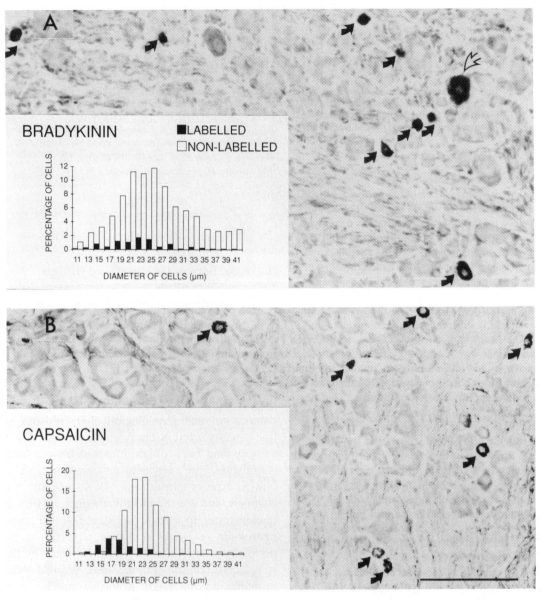

Fig. 1. Dorsal root ganglion cells stained with cobalt after exposure to (A) bradykinin and (B) capsaicin. Dark, labelled cells represent dorsal root ganglion neurons sensitive to bradykinin or capsaicin (arrows). Insert shows the frequency distribution of the longest diameter of cobalt-labelled (filled bars) and non-labelled (open bars) DRG cells for a sample ganglion after capsaicin, and an other ganglion after bradykinin perfusion. Note that the two cell populations did not completely overlap, as bradykinin marks some cells with large diameter (see open arrow in A), while capsaicin staining is restricted to cells with small soma size. (With permission, modified from Nagy et al., 1993b).

spinal cord underlies the pain (see Bevan and Szolcsanyi, 1990; Holzer, 1991). Also, neonatal treatment of rats with capsaicin depletes most of the SP content of the dorsal horn (Nagy et al.,

1983), suggesting that (1) SP is present in the chemosensitive primary afferents and (2) it is released by noxious chemical stimuli.

The technique of recording from single units of

a peripheral nerve has enabled the characterization of primary afferent fibres in terms of their responses to different stimuli. With the in vitro hindpaw skin-saphenous nerve preparation from the rat (Reeh, 1986; Lang et al., 1990), stimuli may be applied directly to identified receptive fields, and we have used this preparation to examine the characteristics of capsaicin-sensitive afferents.

Those fibres responding to capsaicin were also sensitive to mechanical and thermal stimuli and were, therefore, classified as polymodal nociceptor units (Seno and Dray, 1993). Their mechanical threshold was usually high (> 4 g) and they were excited only by a noxious thermal stimulation of a 52°C salt solution applied onto their receptive fields. All mechano-heat sensitive units (MH) were excited by relatively low concentrations of capsaicin (100 nM−1.0 μM superfused to the receptive field for 30 sec, and whilst the majority had conduction velocities between 0.5 and 1 m/sec, characteristic of unmyelinated C-fibres, a small proportion were in the Aδ range (1−5 m/sec). Although these findings were consistent with others obtained from the hairy skin of the rat (Lang et al., 1990) the use of other in vitro preparations suggest that the characteristics of primary afferents vary considerably between different sites (Jänig and McLachlan, 1992).

A distinguishing feature of the small-diameter primary afferents is their sensitivity to a number of chemical stimuli in addition to capsaicin. Thus, a proportion are excited also by bradykinin, histamine, 5-HT and protons (Reeh, 1994). It is apparent, however, that the mechanical and chemical properties of these cutaneous afferents may differ from those of other sites. For example, examination of the afferent fibres innervating the guinea-pig airways showed a number of differences from cutaneous fibres (Fox et al., 1993). Thus airway C- and Aδ-fibres have considerably lower mechanical thresholds than their counterparts in the skin, perhaps reflecting their protective nature. Moreover, in the airways, chemosensitivity appears to be expressed solely by C-fibres, all of which are excited by capsaicin, bradykinin and protons, and at much lower threshold concentrations than seen in the skin. In addition, it appears that these airway C-fibres may be driven to a higher degree by stimuli, such as capsaicin and bradykinin from cutaneous nociceptors, again illustrating their apparently greater sensitivity. Airway C-fibres are, however, insensitive to 5-HT and histamine, again in contrast to those in the skin. The properties of C-fibres innervating the rat skin and guinea-pig airways are summarised in Table I, which illustrates the differences that appear to occur with primary afferent fibres depending on their target.

Despite numerous variations in the modalities of cutaneous and airway fibres, there seems to be one important common feature, namely that C-fibres did not generally fire spontaneously.

Polymodal nociceptors and hyperalgesia

The behaviour of polymodal nociceptors may change dramatically under pathological conditions. When heat hyperalgesia was produced in the hindpaw by ultraviolet (UV-A) irradiation of the glabrous skin (Perkins et al., 1993; Urban et al., 1993), polymodal units became spontaneously active (77% of the polymodal C-fibre population) with a sporadic firing (0.1−2 Hz) of action potentials (Andreev et al., 1994). In addition, responses to capsaicin were enhanced, although the threshold concentration in comparison to control was unchanged. The capsaicin-sensitive population of the cutaneous C-afferents remained basically the same. Although their mechanical threshold was not systematically tested, data from other studies indicate that, during inflammation, the mechanical sensitivity of joint C-fibres increases dramatically (Schmidt, this volume). These findings provide evidence that, during inflammation, cutaneous polymodal C-units became more sensitive to mechanical and chemical irritation.

It is likely that this apparent sensitization occurs as a result of the combined activity of a variety of mediators released during inflammation (Rang, 1991; Reeh, 1994). Using the neonatal rat tail-cord preparation, we have found that 5-HT and bradykinin cause a direct activation of the peripheral terminals of primary afferent fibres as

TABLE 1

Characterization of chemosensitive C-fibres innervating the guinea-pig airways and the rat skin

Modality	Primary afferents	
	Airways	Cutaneous
Conduction velocity (m/sec)	0.9	0.55
Mechanical threshold (g)	0.22	5.6
BK sensitivity	> 30 nM (100%)	10 μM (56%)
Capsaicin sensitivity	> 30 nM (100%)	> 1.0 μM (100%)
Low pH	100% excited (pH 5.0)	38% excited (pH 5.2)
5-HT	no effect	33% excited
Histamine	no effect	37% excited
Heat sensitivity	?	+

Note that the mechanical threshold for capsaicin-sensitive fibres in the trachea is significantly lower than that for cutaneous polymodal units. Their threshold sensitivity to capsaicin and bradykinin is also lower. 5-HT excites only a fraction of cutaneous polymodal units, while airway C-fibres are not sensitive at all. (Data taken from Fox et al., 1993; and from Seno and Dray, 1993; Lang et al., 1992; Fox, Barnes and Dray, unpublished data.)

well as enhancing responses to a noxious heat stimulus (Rueff and Dray, 1993). Similarly, PGE_2 and PGI_2, whilst having no direct excitatory effect, caused increased responses to bradykinin (Rueff and Dray, 1993). This phenomenon of sensitization has been observed with these and other mediators in numerous studies of cutaneous, joint and testicular polymodal nociceptors (see Levine et al., 1993). However we do not know precisely, whether sensitization could also affect larger fibres. For example, in contrast to capsaicin, which excites afferents with small soma size, bradykinin also excites primary afferents with large soma diameter (Nagy et al., 1993b; see Fig. 1).

The increased excitability and enhanced responsiveness of C-polymodals, and perhaps other nociceptor units, and of other fibres imply that the spinal cord will receive an increased primary afferent input during inflammatory conditions. As we have described above, most of these fibres belong to fine unmyelinated C-afferents (at least in the skin nerve model) which terminate in the superficial laminae of the spinal cord. It will therefore predominantly enhance the activity of dorsal horn neurons.

The effects of C-fibre stimulation on spinal cord transmission

The spinal dorsal horn, particularly in the superficial Laminae I and II, receives a large input from fine unmyelinated primary afferents. After immuno-histochemical examinations revealed the presence of SP in these fibres, it was suggested that SP may serve as a pain transmitter in the spinal cord. However subsequent discoveries, that SP and excitatory amino acids (EAAs: glutamate and aspartate) coexist in fine afferents (DeBiasi et al., 1988), and that other peptides may be present as co-transmitters in the same terminals, have led to a re-evaluation of this concept. In addition, some C-fibres contain only EAAs, and experiments suggest that EAA receptor antagonists are powerful blockers of spinal synaptic activity evoked by acute mechanical and thermal nociceptive stimulation (King and Lopez-Garcia, 1993; Yoshimura et al., 1993). In spite of these findings there is still hope for neurokinins to reclaim at least some of their prominence in pain transmission. Firstly, we have to make distinctions between activation and modulation of synaptic events in the dorsal horn, and evidence suggests that SP has well-defined modulatory functions (Coderre and Melzack, 1992; Dougherty and Willis, 1992; Rusin et al., 1992; Xu et al., 1992; Urban et al., 1994). Secondly, during sustained activation of C-fibres in inflammatory hyperalgesia, large quantities of SP are released (Duggan et al., 1988) and, indeed, neurokinin receptor antagonists seem to have analgesic effects in animal models of inflammatory pain (Yamamoto and Yaksh, 1992; Henry et al., 1993).

To study the pharmacological properties of the synaptic mechanisms underlying nociception in the spinal dorsal horn, we have established in vitro hemisected spinal cord models (Urban and Randić, 1984; Urban and Dray, 1992; Jeftinija et al., 1993; Thompson et al., 1993) from both mice and rats (10–30-day-old). Experiments on the isolated spinal cord allow us to study the effects of receptor antagonists against excitatory amino acid (EAA) and neurokinin (NK) receptors present in the spinal cord without their unwanted in vivo side effects on microcirculation and ventilation. To excite primary afferents we have used capsaicin and 50 mM KCl, administered to the dorsal root, or electrical stimulation of the dorsal roots and peripheral nerves (Fig. 2). To achieve stimulation of C-fibres, high-intensity electrical stimuli were required, which activate both large- and small-diameter fibres. Postsynaptic activity was measured either by intracellular recording from single dorsal horn neurons, or from ventral roots via suction electrodes.

Capsaicin (100–500 nM; 30 sec) excited only fibres with slow conduction velocity in the dorsal root (Urban and Dray, 1992) and consequently evoked a long-lasting synaptic activation in about 60–70% of deep dorsal horn neurons in Laminae III–V (see Fig. 2; Nagy et al., 1993). Subsequent experiments showed that this excitation was transmitted predominantly through C-fibres (Fig. 3). High-intensity electrical stimulation of the dorsal root evoked a long-lasting compound postsynaptic potential in dorsal horn neurons. This postsynaptic potential can be separated by using TTX in two distinct groups of postsynaptic potentials in the isolated spinal cord preparation. In the pres-

ence of TTX (1.0–10.0 μM) on the DRG, the early component of the EPSP is blocked, indicating its origin from large, fast conducting fibres, which possess TTX-sensitive sodium channels (Jeftinija et al., 1993). On the other hand, application of a high concentration of capsaicin (1.0–10.0 μM) to the dorsal roots, which blocks C-fibre excitability (Urban and Dray, 1992), selectively inhibits the long latency, prolonged phase of the EPSP (see Fig. 3). Therefore capsaicin was used to selectively excite the C-fibre input to dorsal horn neurons in further experiments on the study of the pharmacology of the synaptic connection.

The contribution of NK_1 and NK_2 receptors to the spinal excitability

We have used selective agonists and antagonists to assess the relative importance of NK_1, NK_2 and N-methyl-D-aspartate (NMDA) receptors in central processing of the primary afferent input. The postsynaptic activity of deep dorsal horn cells evoked by capsaicin-activated C-fibre input was reduced by 76% following superfusion of the spinal cord with the selective NMDA receptor blocker D-2-amino-5-phosphonovaleric acid (D-APV), emphasising a strong involvement of NMDA receptor activation in the processing of the chemosensitive primary afferent input. The selective NK_2 receptor antagonist MEN 10,376 (Maggi et al., 1992) was also effective, as it reduced the amplitude of the synaptic response by 63%. The findings that the same neurons which responded to capsaicin application to the dorsal roots and DRGs were activated by exogenous neurokinin A (NKA), and that the NKA-evoked depolarization was blocked by MEN 10,376, further supports a role for NK_2 receptors.

In contrast, in the presence of the selective NK_1 receptor antagonist, CP 96,345 (Snider et al., 1991), postsynaptic responses to capsaicin were unaltered, despite the fact that superfusion of the exogenous NK_1 receptor agonist, GR 73,632, depolarised all dorsal horn cells with capsaicin-sensitive primary afferent input and that this de-

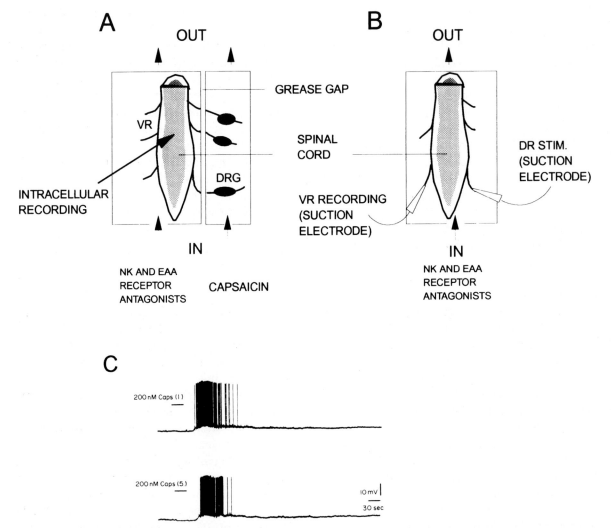

Fig. 2. Experimental arrangements used in our studies. A. Arrangement of the rat hemisected spinal cord dorsal root ganglion preparation. The two compartments are isolated and capsaicin and TTX were perfused to the DRGs, while other drugs were applied to the spinal cord. In separate experiments (B) dorsal roots were stimulated, and ventral root potentials were recorded with suction electrodes. C. Capsaicin activation of a single dorsal horn neuron, recorded intracellularly. Capsaicin was superfused for 30 sec to the dorsal roots, and synaptic activation of a dorsal horn cells was recorded. This figure shows that addition of 1.0 μM Concanavalin A to the superfusate prevents desensitization of the capsaicin response (first and fifth consequent trace, with 30-min perfusion intervals). Recordings from the ventral root are represented in Figs. 4, 5 and 7. (With permission, modified from Nagy et al., 1993.)

polarization was significantly attenuated by CP 96,345 (Nagy et al., 1993a).

On the basis of these results we concluded that, although primary afferent C-fibres release both excitatory amino acids and the neurokinins, SP and NKA (Duggan et al., 1990; Jeftinija et al., 1991), only postsynaptic excitatory amino acid and

NK$_2$ receptors are activated in the dorsal horn neurons following synaptic release of these substances. These data are in good agreement with some other observations that single cell activity in the dorsal horn of the spinal cord, evoked by noxious heat or chemical stimuli, could be attenuated by NK$_2$ but not NK$_1$ receptor antagonists

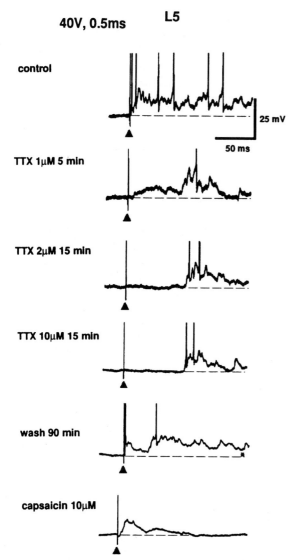

40V, 0.5ms   **L5**

control

25 mV

50 ms

TTX 1µM 5 min

TTX 2µM 15 min

TTX 10µM 15 min

wash 90 min

capsaicin 10µM

Fig. 3. Intracellular recordings from a dorsal horn neuron after the high-intensity electrical stimulation of the L_5 dorsal root (DRG removed) and the effects of the application of TTX and capsaicin on the primary afferent-evoked EPSPs. (Action potentials are truncated.) Application of TTX abolished, in a dose-dependent manner, the activation of the fast primary afferent input and was without effect on the EPSPs evoked by slow conducting fibres. The effect of TTX was reversible (wash). Following the full recovery of synaptic transmission, capsaicin selectively removed the late phase of the synaptic potentials (bottom trace). $V_m = -68$ mV. (With permission, modified from Jeftinija et al., 1993.)

(Fleetwood-Walker et al., 1990, Munro et al., 1993; although see DeKoninck et al., 1991). As

both SP and NKA are produced in primary afferents by the same ppt1 gene (Noguchi et al., 1988), and they are co-released in the dorsal horn following noxious stimulation (Duggan et al., 1988, 1990), a contribution from both NK_1 and NK_2 receptors on dorsal horn neurons would be expected. (Although both ligands excite NK_1 and NK_2 receptors, SP has higher affinity for the NK_1, while NKA has higher affinity for the NK_2 receptors.) In the light of these unexpected results, and particularly because of some unsettled debate on the presence of NK_2 receptor sites in the rat spinal cord (Hagan et al., 1993), we have continued our experiments with a slightly different protocol (Thompson et al., 1993). In these experiments the hemisected spinal cord was also used, but primary afferent fibres were activated by high-intensity electrical stimulation and recordings were made from the ventral roots to monitor the spinal nociceptive reflex (Thompson et al., 1992). In addition to single pulses, we also studied the effects of repetitive dorsal root stimulation, considered to represent spinal 'wind-up'. This is relevant to the spinal reflex activity monitored during several tests of hyperalgesia and pain in vivo (e.g., tail flick, hot plate, paw pressure).

The results are summarised in Fig. 4. Briefly, APV partially blocked the C-fibre-evoked ventral root potential (VRP). Its effect was restricted to a particular segment of the response, which was earlier described as the 'NMDA-component' of the VRP (Thompson et al., 1992). In contrast the NK_2 receptor antagonist, MEN 10,376, attenuated the late phase of the VRP (predicted as peptidergic component). As with the intracellular results, the NK_1 receptor antagonists, CP 96,345 and RP 67,580 did not attenuate the C-fibre evoked VRP. Following repetitive stimulation of dorsal roots, to evoke 'wind-up', this response was only significantly attenuated by APV, but not by NK_1 or NK_2 antagonists (see later in Fig. 6.). These data suggested that blockade of the NK_1 or NK_2 receptors alone was insufficient to prevent central summation of C-fibre-evoked spinal activity. The situation becomes more complex if we look at the results from experiments where the effects of the NMDA receptor antagonist, APV, and one of the NK receptor antagonists, were tested in combination. Co-application of APV with MEN 10,376 caused similar attenuation to that of APV alone. On the other hand, APV and CP 96,345 together inhibited the amplitude of the 'wind-up' significantly more than APV alone, suggesting a possible synergism between the two receptor sites during high-intensity, repetitive stimulation. Indeed, it has been shown that behavioral responses in mice were potentiated by spinal co-application of EAAs and substance P (Mjellem-Joly et al., 1991). In more recent experiments in single dissociated dorsal horn cells (Rusin et al., 1992), and in isolated neonatal spinal cord (Urban et al., 1994), the interaction between EAAs and neurokinins was further confirmed.

The lack of effect of NK_1 receptor antagonists on other dorsal horn responses to capsaicin-stimulation or the high-threshold afferent-evoked VRP, can be explained by the possible rapid degradation of the natural ligand, SP, for mainly

NK_1 receptors by endopeptidases (Duggan et al., 1990; Maggi et al., 1992; Urban et al., 1994). In keeping with this possibility, it has been reported that NKA is more resistant to these enzymes (Nyberg et al., 1991). Following brief stimuli, this mechanism may be responsible for the selective NK_2 receptor activation.

Changes induced by pathological conditions

Although we have shown that, under normal conditions, C-fibre stimulation activates primarily NK_2 receptors in the dorsal horn, it was also apparent in our studies that, under certain conditions, NK_1 receptors may also be activated. This latter observation is in good agreement with in vivo data showing that NK_1 receptor antagonists are potent analgesics (Yamamoto and Yaksh, 1992; Yashpal et al., 1993) following intense nociceptor activation.

Prior to the preparation of the hemisected spinal cord, the left hindpaw of 12-day-old rats

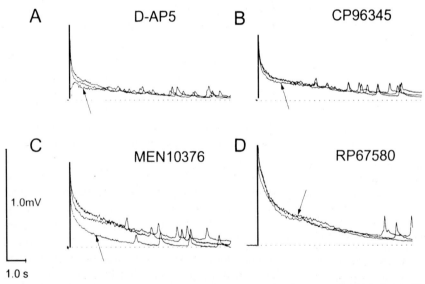

Fig. 4. The effects of NMDA and neurokinin receptor antagonists upon the high-threshold afferent fiber-evoked VRP. A. The effect of 20 μM D-APV applied alone for 20 min. B. The effect of 20 min application of the NK_1 receptor antagonist CP 96,345 (500 nM). C. The effect of a 40-min application of the NK_2 receptor antagonist, MEN 10,376 (100 nM), upon the single shock-evoked VRP. D. The VRP response in the presence of 100 nM RP 67,580. Each panel represents control and wash responses; arrowed traces in each panel are following drug application. In the presence of D-APV and MEN 10,376, the area of the prolonged C-fibre-evoked VRP is significantly reduced from control values. All traces are the average of four responses.

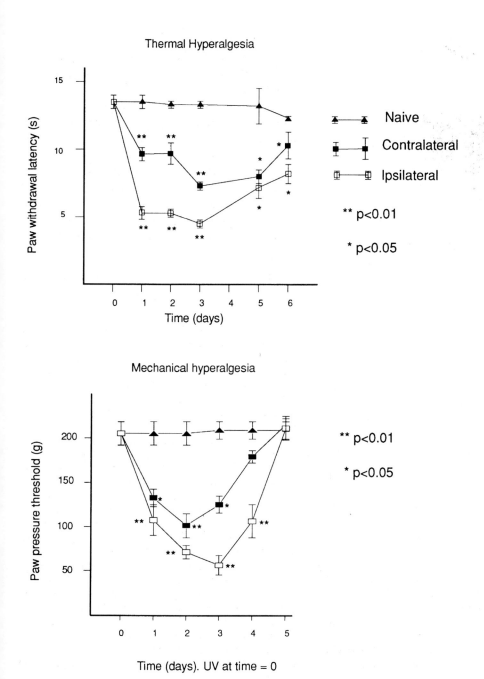

Fig. 5. Time course of thermal and mechanical hyperalgesia observed in the treated (ipsilateral) and untreated (contralateral) hindlimb in the neonatal rat following two successive UV exposures. All animals were between postnatal days 12 and 15 of age at time of behavioural testing. *, $P < 0.05$; **, $P < 0.01$; unpaired t-test. (With permission from Thompson et al., 1993.)

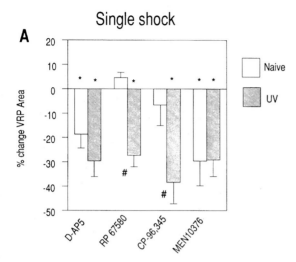

Single shock

A

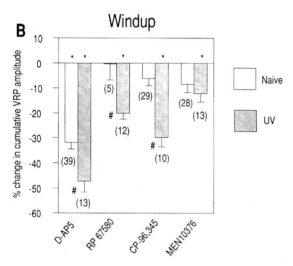

Windup

B

was irradiated with UV-A light (Thompson et al., 1994). Within one day, a hypersensitivity to thermal and mechanical stimuli developed which was maintained for several days (Fig. 5). At the peak of the hypersensitivity (day 2 post-irradiation), animals were anaesthetised, decapitated and the hemisected spinal cord prepared for in vitro examination. The experimental arrangement was identical with that described previously.

In these preparations the spontaneous ventral root activity was higher than in the almost silent control preparation. However, major differences were apparent in the synaptic activation of dorsal horn cells.

(1) The proportion of the C-fibre-evoked VRP

Fig. 6. Pharmacological characterization of C-fibre-evoked ventral root responses. A. The effects of NMDA and neurokinin receptor antagonists upon the high-threshold afferent fibre-evoked VRP. The area under the curve was measured, expressed as a percentage of control and illustrated as deviation from control (baseline) in the presence of the NMDA receptor antagonist, D-APV (20 μM), the NK$_1$ receptor antag-

onists, RP 67,580 (100 nM) and CP 96,345 (500 nM), and the NK$_2$ receptor antagonist, MEN 10,376 (100 nM). Open bars represent data obtained from naive animals, hatched bars from UV-treated animals. In naive animals, D-APV and MEN 10,376 produced a significant inhibition of the response, while neither of the NK$_1$ antagonists worked. In UV-treated animals, all NMDA, NK$_1$ and NK$_2$ receptor antagonists inhibited the VRP. *, $P < 0.05$, ANOVA, in comparison to control responses in the same group without treatment; #, $P < 0.05$, ANOVA, in comparison to similarly treated naive and UV-treated animals. B. The effect of NMDA and neurokinin receptor antagonists upon the C-fibre-evoked summated VRP in naive and UV-treated animals. The percentage change in summated VRP amplitude is shown measured relative to control. D-APV (20 μM) produced a significant reduction from control amplitude in both UV-treated and untreated animals, with a significantly greater effect in UV-treated animals. Neither NK$_1$ antagonist produced any significant effect from control in untreated animals. However, in UV-treated animals, both antagonists produced a significant reduction in summated VRP amplitude from control. The NK$_2$ antagonist, MEN 10,376 (100 nM), did not produce any significant effect in untreated animals, but did produce a small significant depression in UV-treated animals. Symbols are same as in (A). (With permission, modified from Thompson et al., 1994.)

Fig. 7. The effect of NMDA and neurokinin receptor antagonists upon the A-fibre-evoked summated VRP in UV-treated animals. A. The effect of D-APV (20 μM), RP 67,580 (100 nM) and MEN 10,376 (100 nM) upon the amplitude of the summated VRP evoked following 5.0 Hz repetitive stimulation at low intensity (5 V, 20 μsec) for 20 sec, at the time indicated by the horizontal bars in UV-treated animals is shown. Summated VRP amplitudes were measured between the arrows. B. The graph shows the percentage change in VRP amplitude following drug application compared to control value in the absence of drug (100%). All compounds produced a significant reduction in VRP amplitude (*, < 0.05, ANOVA); numbers of observations are in parentheses. (With permission from Thompson et al., 1994.)

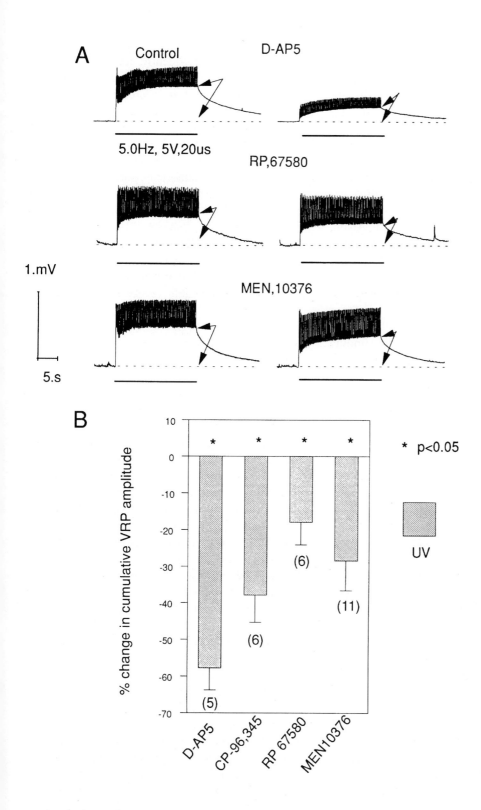

266

sensitive to APV was significantly greater in UV-treated animals. Furthermore, NK_1 receptor antagonists (CP 96,345; RP 67,580) showed potent inhibitory effects on the late phase of the response which was never observed in naive animals. The inhibitory effect of the NK_2 antagonist, MEN 10,376, was unchanged in comparison to that described in the naive spinal cord (Fig. 6.).

(2) The increased importance of NK_1 receptor activation during the course of inflammatory hyperalgesia was further emphasised when the pharmacology of 'wind-up' was analysed. Again, the NMDA receptor antagonist, APV, was the most potent agent reducing the amplitude of the cumulative VRP. It was also significantly more potent than in control spinal cords. However, now in addition to NK_2 antagonists, NK_1 receptor antagonists also significantly reduced the amplitude of the cumulative VRP (Fig. 6). This finding indicates that during inflammatory hyperalgesia the spinal cord undergoes profound dynamic changes, which results in a qualitatively different synaptic connection between primary afferents and dorsal horn neurons. In our preparation the spinal cord was completely separated from the inflamed tissue and dorsal root ganglia, indicating that the hypersensitivity was not due to sustained primary afferent input from the skin, or from the DRG cells (Kajander et al., 1991; Devor et al., 1992), but rather it was now an intrinsic feature of the spinal cord. This phenomenon earlier described as central sensitization (Woolf, 1984), can be induced by an initial sustained (primarily pathological) C-fibre input to dorsal horn cells and, once changes are in place, no futher peripheral input is required for its maintenance.

Possible interaction between NK and NMDA receptors during activity-dependent excitability increase in the dorsal horn

The enhancement of NMDA receptor activity in the dorsal horn by neurokinins following C-fibre acitvation has been discussed elsewhere (Randić, this volume; Urban et al., 1994). Briefly, activation of NK receptors in dorsal horn neurons may induce changes in the phospholipase C-depen-

dent pathway, leading to diacylglycerol (DAG) formation and, consequently, activation of protein kinase C (PKC). Protein kinase C phosphorylates the NMDA receptor and changes its Mg^{2+} binding kinetics (Chen and Huang, 1991; Urban et al., 1994; see also Randić, this volume). Under these conditions NMDA receptors may be activated, even in the presence of normal Mg^{2+} concentration at resting membrane potential level. The involvement of NMDA receptor activation during spinal hyperexcitability has been widely studied (Dickenson and Sullivan, 1987; Woolf and Thompson, 1991; Yashpal et al., 1991), and is believed to be the major component of the increased synaptic activity during hyperalgesia in inflammatory (Schaible et al., 1994) and neuropathic conditions.

Plasticity of peptidergic neurons and spinal dorsal horn cells

The development of the state of central excitability implies that certain dorsal horn cells, which receive input from both C- and A-fibres (WDR neurons), must respond to noxious and innocuous peripheral input in different manners. As we have described in the previous paragraphs, following UV-induced hyperalgesia, C-fibre-evoked responses of dorsal horn neurons develop a significant NK_1 receptor component and an increased NMDA receptor-mediated contribution. We then addressed the question of possible changes in response to innocuous, A-fibre input. Theoretically, as a consequence of the increase in central excitability, the increased number of NMDA receptors would be in a receptive state (see previous paragraph), regardless of the source of excitatory amino acids. Under these conditions, excitatory amino acid release occurring in the absence of peptide release, for example from large-diameter A-fibres, would be able to excite NMDA receptors. This has been recently demonstrated under experimental conditions using the hemisected spinal cord obtained from animals with skin inflammation. In comparison to control animals, where repetitive A-fibre stimulation did not induce cumulative responses (wind-up), in the spinal cords of animals with cutaneous inflammatory hyperalgesia, repetitive stimulation of only myelinated fibres produced enhanced synaptic activity and 'wind-up' (Thompson et al., 1994; Fig. 7). This new phenomenon was seen only in spinal cords which were 'conditioned' during hyperalgesia.

The A-fibre evoked 'wind-up' has some interesting pharmacological characteristics. It was sensitive to NMDA receptor blockers as expected. However, it was clearly also sensitive to both NK_1 and NK_2 receptor antagonists. This latter feature could arise for two reasons: Firstly, an increased leakage of neurokinins from primary afferent terminals (Valtschanoff et al., 1992) could give a sustained peptidergic input to the dorsal horn; and, secondly, some A-fibres under pathological conditions may produce and release some neurokinins (Noguchi et al., 1993).

In summary, these data, together with a wide array of other observations, provide evidence for mechanisms which underlie C-fibre-evoked central sensitization. The inflammation-induced sporadic activity and increased sensitivity of C-nociceptors provide a permanent excitatory amino acid and, more importantly, neurokinin release in the spinal dorsal horn. Activation of neurokinin receptors in dorsal horn neurons 'unmask' NMDA receptors and induce hyperexcitability. Under these conditions, A-fibre activation evokes unusual NMDA-mediated long-lasting responses, different from those in naive animals, and is able to evoke short-term increases in spinal excitability (wind-up). This may be an underlying mechanism of allodynia, tenderness and perhaps some of the clinically observed paraesthesia. It is very likely that the plastic changes observed in the dorsal horn, during hyperalgesia following inflammation, lead to a state whereby the spinal sensory system can be characterised as turning from discriminative to protective.

References

Andreev, N., Urban, L. and Dray, A. (1994) Opioids suppress activity in polymodal nociceptors in rat paw skin induced by ultraviolet irradiation. *Neuroscience*, 58: 793–798.

Bevan, S. and Szolcsanyi, J. (1990) Sensory neuron-specific actions of capsaicin: mechanisms and applications. *Trends Pharmacol. Sci.*, 11: 330–333.

Chen, L. and Huang, L.-Y. (1992) Protein kinase C reduces Mg^{2+} block of NMDA-receptor channels as a mechanism of modulation. *Nature*, 356, 521–523.

Coderre, T.J. and Melzack, R. (1992) The contribution of excitatory amino acids to central sensitisation and persistent nociception after formalin-induced tissue injury. *J. Neurosci.*, 12, 3665–3670.

DeKoninck, Y. and Henry, J.L. (1991) Substance P mediated slow excitatory potential elicited in dorsal horn neurons in vivo by noxious stimulation. *Proc. Natl. Acad. Sci. USA*, 88: 11344–11348.

DeBiasi, S. and Rustioni, A. (1988) Glutamate and substance P coexist in primary afferent terminals in the superficial laminae of the spinal cord. *Proc. Natl. Acad. Sci. USA*, 85: 7820–7824.

Devor, M., Wall, P.D. and Catalan, N. (1992) Systemic lidocaine silences ectopic neuroma and DRG discharge without blocking nerve conduction. *Pain*, 48:261–268.

Dickenson, A.H. and Sullivan, A.F. (1987) Evidence for a role of the NMDA receptor in the frequency dependent potentiation of deep rat dorsal horn nociceptive neurones following C-fibre stimulation. *Neuropharmacology*, 26: 1235–1238.

Dougherty, P.M. and Willis, W.D. (1992) Enhancement of spinothalamic neuron responses to chemical and mechanical stimuli following combined micro-iontophoretic application of NMDA and substance P. *Pain*, 47: 85–93.

Duggan, A.W., Hendry, I.A., Morton, C.R., Hutchinson, W.D. and Zhao, Z.Q. (1988) Cutaneous stimuli releasing immunoreactive substance P in the dorsal horn of cat. *Brain Res.*, 451: 261–273.

Duggan, A.W., Hope, P.J., Jarrott, B., Schaible, H.-G. and Fleetwood-Walker, S.M. (1990) Release, spread and persistence of immunoreactive neurokinin A in the dorsal horn of the cat following noxious cutaneous stimulation. Studies with antibody microprobes. *Neuroscience*, 35: 195–202.

Fleetwood-Walker, S.M., Mitchell, R., Hope, P.J., El-Yassir, N., Molony, V. and Bladon, C.M. (1990) The involvement of neurokinin receptor subtypes in somatosensory processing in the superficial dorsal horn of the cat. *Brain Res.*, 519: 169–182.

Fox, A.J., Barnes, P.J., Urban, L. and Dray, A. (1993) An in vitro study of the properties of single vagal afferents innervating guinea-pig airways. *J. Physiol. (London)*, 469: 21–35.

Gamse, R., Molnar, A. and Lembeck, F. (1979) Substance P release from spinal cord slices by capsaicin. *Life Sci.*, 25: 629–636;

Hagan, R.M., Beresford, I.J.M., Stables, J., Dupere, J., Stubbs, C.M., Elliott, P.J., Sheldrick, R.L.G., Chollet, A., Kawashima, E., McElroy, A.B. and Ward, P. (1993) Characterization, CNS distribution and function of NK2 receptor studied using potent NK2 receptor antagonists. *Regul. Peptides*, 46: 9–19.

Hall, J.M. (1992) Bradykinin receptors: pharmacological properties and biological roles. *Pharmacol. Ther.*, 56: 131–190.

Henry, J.L. (1993) Participation of substance P in spinal physiological responses to peripheral aversive stimulation. *Regul. Peptides*, 46: 138–143.

Holzer, P. (1991) Capsaicin: cellular targets, mechanisms of action, and sensitivity for thin sensory neurons. *Pharm. Rev.*, 43: 143–201.

Hökfelt, T., Zhang, X. and Wiesenfeld-Hallin, Z. (1994) Messenger plasticity in primary sensory neurons following axotomy and its functional implications. *Trends Neurosci.*, 17: 22–30.

Jancso, G., Hökfelt, T., Lundberg, J.M., Kiraly, E., Halasz, N., Nilsson, G., Terenius, L., Rehfeld, J., Steinbusch, H., Verhofstad, A., Elde, R., Said, S. and Brown, M. (1981) Immunohistochemical studies on the effect of capsaicin on spinal medullary peptide and monoamine neurons using antisera to substance P, gastrin/CCK, somatostatin, VIP, enkephalin, neurotensin and 5-hydroxytryptamine. *J. Neurocytol.*, 10: 963–980.

Jänig W. and McLachlan, M. (1992) Characterization of function-specific pathways in the sympathetic nervous system. *Trends Neurosci.*, 15: 475–481.

Jeftinija, S., Jeftinija, K., Korade, Z., Skilling, R.S., Smullin, D.H. and Larson, A.A. (1991) Excitatory amino acids are released from rat primary afferent neurons in vitro. *Neurosci. Lett.*, 135: 191–194.

Jeftinija, S., Urban, L. and Kojić, L. (1993) The selective activation of dorsal horn neurons by potassium stimulation of high threshold primary afferent neurons in vitro. *Neurosciencce*, 56: 473–484.

Ju, G., Hökfelt, T., Brodin, E., Fahrenkrug, J., Fisher, J.A., Frey, P., Elde, R.P. and Brown, J.C. (1987) Primary sensory neurons of the rat showing calcitonin gene-related peptide immunoreactivity and their relation to substance P-, somatostatin-, galanin-, vasoactive intestinal polypeptide- and cholecystokinin-immunoreactive ganglion cells. *Cell Tissue Res.*, 247: 417–431.

Kajander, K., Wakisaka, S. and Bennett, G. (1992) Spontaneous discharge originates in the dorsal root ganglion at the onset of painful peripheral neuropathy in the rat. *Neurosci. Lett.*, 136: 145–150.

King, A.E. and Lopez-Garcia, J.A. (1993) Excitatory amino acid receptor-mediated neurotransmission from cutaneous afferents in rat dorsal horn in vitro. *J. Physiol. (London)*, 472: 443–457.

LaMotte, R.H., Lundberg, L.E.R. and Torebjork, H.E. (1992) Pain, hyperalgesia and activity in nociceptive C units in humans after intradermal injecton of capsaicin. *J. Physiol. (London)*, 448: 749–764.

Lang, E., Novak, A., Reeh, P.W. and Handwerker, H.-O. (1990) Chemosensitivity of fine afferents in vitro. *J. Neurophysiol.*, 63: 887–901.

Lawson, S.N. Crepps, B.A., Bao, J., Brighton, B.W. and Perl, E.R. (1994) Substance P-like immunoreactivity (SP-LI) in guinea-pig dorsal root ganglia (DRGs) is related to sensory receptor type in A- and C-fibre neurons. *J. Physiol. (London)*, 476: 39P.

Levin, J.D., Field, H.L., Basbaum, A.I. (1993) Peptides and the primary afferent nociceptor. *J. Neuroscience*, 13: 2273–2286.

Maggi, C.A., Patacchini, R., Rovero, P. and Giachetti, A. (1992) Tachykinin receptors and tachykinin receptor antagonists. *J. Autonom. Pharmacol.*, 13: 23–93.

Mjellem-Joly, N., Lund, A., Berge, O.G. and Hole, K. (1991) Potentiation of a behavioural response in mice by spinal co-administration of substance P and excitatory amino acid agonists. *Neurosci. Lett.*, 133, 121–124.

Munro, F.E., Fleetwood-Walker, S.M., Parker, R.M.C. and Mitchell, R. (1993) The effects of neurokinin antagonists on mustard oil-evoked activation of rat dorsal horn neurons. *Neuropeptides*, 25: 299–305.

Nagy, I., Maggi, C.A., Woolf, C.J., Dray, A. and Urban, L. (1993a) The role of neurokinin and *N*-methyl-D-apartate receptors in synaptic transmission from capsaicin-sensitive primary afferents in the rat spinal cord in vitro. *Neuroscience*, 52: 1029–1037.

Nagy, I., Pabla, R., Matesz, C., Dray, A., Woolf, C.J. and Urban, L. (1993b) Cobalt uptake enables identification of capsaicin- and bradykinin-sensitive subpopulations of rat dorsal root ganglion cells in vitro. *Neuroscience*, 56: 241–246.

Nagy, J., Iversen, L.L., Goedert, Chapman, D. and Hunt, S.P. (1983) Dose dependent effects of capsaicin on primary sensory neurons in the neonatal rat. *J. Neurosci.*, 3: 399–406.

Noguchi, K., Morita, Y., Kiyama, Y., Ono, K. and Tohyama, M. (1988) A noxious stimulus induces the prepro-tachykinin-A gene expression in the rat dorsal root ganglion: a quantitative study using in situ hybridization histochemistry. *Mol. Brain Res.*, 4: 31–35.

Noguchi, K., Kawai, Y. and Senba, E. (1993) DRG neurons projecting dorsal column nucleus express preprotachykinin mRNA after peripheral axotomy. *IASP Abstr. (Paris)*, 517.13.

Perkins, M.N., Campbell, E. and Dray, A. (1993) Antinociceptive activity of the B1 and B2 receptor antagonists, des-Arg[9], [Leu[8]]-BK and HOE 140, in two models of persistent hyperalgesia in the rat. *Pain*, 53: 191–197.

Nyberg, F., Le Greves, P., Sundquist, C. and Terenius, L. (1991) Characterization of substance P (1–7) and (1–8) generating enzyme in human CSF. *Biochem. Biophys. Res. Commun.*, 125: 244–250.

Rang. H.P. (1991) The nociceptive afferent neurone as a target for new types of analgesic drug. In: M.R. Bond, J.E. Charlton and C.J. Woolf (Eds.) *Proceedings of the VIth Congress on Pain*, Elsevier, Amsterdam, pp. 119–127.

Reeh, P.W. (1986) Sensory receptors in mammalian skin in an in vitro preparation. *Neurosci. Lett.*, 66: 141–146.

Reeh, P.W. (1994) Chemical excitation and sensitization of nociceptors. In L. Urban, (Ed.) *The Cellular Mechanisms of Sensory Processing*, Springer, Amsterdam, pp. 119–131.

Rusin, K.I., Ryu, P.D. and Randić, M. (1992) Modulation of excitatory amino acid responses in rat dorsl horn neurons by tachykinins. *J. Neurophysiol.*, 68: 265–286.

Rueff, A. and Dray, A. (1993) 5-Hydroxytriptamine-induced sensitization and activation of peripheral fibres in the neonatal rat are mediated via different 5-hydroxytriptamine-receptors. *Neuroscience*, 50: 899–905.

Schaible, H.-G., Neugebauer, V. and. Lucke, T. (1994) The involvement of excitatory amino acids and their receptors in the spinal processing of nociceptive input from the normal and inflamed knee joint in the rat. In: L. Urban (Ed.) *The Cellular Mechanisms of Sensory Processing*, Springer, Amsterdam, pp., 195–215.

Schmidt, R.F. (1994) Silent primary afferents. In: L. Urban (Ed.) *The Cellular Mechanisms of Sensory Processing*, Springer, Amsterdam, pp. 289–296.

Seno, N. and Dray, A. (1993) Capsaicin-induced activation of fine afferent fibres from rat skin in vitro. *Neuroscience*, 55: 563–569.

Snider, R.M., Constantine, J.W., Lowe, I.J.A., Longo, K.P., Lebel, W.S., Woody, H.A., Drozda, S.E., Desai, M.C., Vinick, F.J., Spencer, R.W. and Hess, H.J. (1991) A potent nonpeptide antagonist of the substance P (NK1) receptor. *Science*, 251: 435–439.

Szolcsanyi, J. (1977) A Pharmacological approach to elucidation of the role of different nerve fibres and receptor endings in mediation of pain. *J. Physiol. (Paris)*, 73: 251–259.

Thompson, S.W.N., Gerber, G., Sivilotti, L.G. and Woolf, C.J. (1992) Long duration ventral root potentials in the neonatal rat spinal cord in vitro; the effects of ionotropic and metabotropic excitatory amino acid receptor antagonists. *Brain Res.*, 595: 87–97.

Thompson, S.W.N., Urban, L. and Dray, A. (1993) Contribution of NK1 and NK2 receptor activation to high threshold afferent fibre evoked ventral root responses in the rat spinal cord in vitro. *Brain Res.*, 625: 100–108.

Thompson, S.W.N., Dray, A. and Urban, L. (1994) Injury-induced plasticity of spinal reflex activity: NK1 neurokinin

receptor activation and enhanced A- and C-fiber mediated responses in the rat spinal cord in vitro. *J. Neurosci.*, 14: 3672–3687.

Urban, L. and Dray, A. (1992) Synaptic activation of dorsal horn neurons by selective C-fibre excitation with capsaicin in the mouse spinal cord in vitro. *Neuroscience*, 47: 693–702.

Urban L. and Randić, M. (1984) Slow excitsatory transmission in rat dorsal horn.: Possible mediation by peptides. *Brain Res.*, 290: 336–341.

Urban, L., Naeem, S., Patel, I.A. and Dray, A. (1994) Effects of neurokinin antagonists on excitatory amino acid receptor activation in the rat spinal cord in vitro preparation. *Neurosci. Lett.*, 168: 185–188.

Valtschanoff J.G., Weinberg, R.J. and Rustioni, A. (1992) Peripheral injury and anterograde transport of wheat germ agglutitnin-horse radish peroxidase to the spinal cord. *Neuroscience*, 50: 685–696.

Woolf, C.J. (1983) Evidence for a central component of postinjury pain hypersensitivity. *Nature*, 308: 686–688.

Woolf, C.J. and Thompson, S.W.N. (1991) The induction and maintenance of central sensitization is dependent upon N-methyl-D-aspartatic acid receptor activation; implications for the treatment of post-injury hyperactivity states. *Pain*, 44: 293–299.

Xu, X.-J., Dalsgaard, C.-J. and Wiesenfeld-Hallin, Z. (1992) Spinal substance P and N-methyl-D-aspartate receptors are coactivated in the induction of central sensitization of the nociceptive flexor reflex. *Neuroscience*, 51: 641–648.

Yamamoto, T. and Yaksh, T.L. (1991) Stereospecific effects of a nonpeptidic NK1 selective antagonist, CP-96,345: antinociception in the absence of motor dysfunction. *Life Sci.*, 49:1955–1963.

Yashpal, K., Radhakrishnan, V., Coderre, T.J. and J.L. Henry (1993) CP-96,345 but not its stereoisomer, CP-96,344, blocks the nociceptive responses to intrathecally administered substance P and to noxious thermal and chemical stimuli in the rat. *Neuroscience*, 52: 1039–1047.

Yoshimura, M. and Nishi, S. (1993) Blind patch-clamp recordings from substantia gelatinosa neurons in adult rat spinal cord slices: pharmacological properties of synaptic currents. *Neuroscience*, 53: 519–526.

F. Nyberg, H.S. Sharma and Z. Wiesenfeld-Hallin (Eds.)
Progress in Brain Research, Vol 104

CHAPTER 15

Neuropeptides and spinal cord reflexes

Z. Wiesenfeld-Hallin

*Karolinska Institute, Department of Medical Laboratory Sciences and Technology, Division of Clinical Neurophysiology,
Huddinge University Hospital, S-141 86 Huddinge, Sweden*

Introduction

*The use of spinal reflexes in studies of spinal
nociceptive mechanisms*

Spinal reflexes have been extensively used in studies of pain mechanisms in animals and man. The
tail flick test (D'Amour and Smith, 1941), which
can be applied in fully awake or lightly anaesthetized rodents, is a spinal reflex which has been
applied to study both intrinsic pain mechanisms,
as well as many drugs. This response, which involves the removal of the rodent's tail from a
radiant heat stimulus, has the advantage of being
easy to perform and allowing a large number of
animals to be routinely tested, which is clearly
useful in drug screening procedures. But the tail
flick response has a number of serious disadvan-
tages. For example, it has an all-or-none charac-
ter, making it quite insensitive to minor changes
in responsiveness. The same skin area cannot be
tested too often because of the possibility of
damage from the intense heat stimulus needed to
evoke the response. Furthermore, the interpretation of data obtained with the tail flick assay is
complicated by the role of basal skin temperature
on the latency of the response. Basal skin temperature is influenced by a number of drugs which
may have a role in nociceptive transmission, but
also influence the level of vasomotor activity.
Results obtained with this assay are thus confounded by the observation that skin temperature

is negatively correlated with response latency (e.g.,
Berge et al., 1988).

The magnitude of the nocifensive hindpaw
flexor reflex is positively correlated with the activity of dorsal horn neurons that are activated by
both innocuous and noxious stimuli, the so-called
wide dynamic range cells (Schouenborg and
Sjölund, 1983; Carstens et al., 1990). Furthermore, the magnitude of the flexor reflex evoked
by noxious stimulation on the foot and recorded
from the biceps femoris muscle is well correlated
to painful sensations in adult humans (Willer,
1977; Chang and Dallaier, 1989). The cutaneous
flexor reflex in human infants has been useful to
study the postnatal maturation of spinal reflex
mechanisms (Fitzgerald et al., 1988), as well as
nociception (Fitzgerald et al., 1989). The flexor
reflex is a graded, not an all-or-none, response
and is very suitable for both physiological and
pharmacological studies. We have used the
hindlimb flexor reflex as a tool for studying the
role of neuropeptides in spinal nociceptive mechanisms. The preparation used is the decerebrate,
spinalized rat as described by Wall and Woolf
(1984). Since the animals are decerebrated under
the influence of a short-lasting barbiturate, the
responses recorded during the course of the experiment, which starts at least one hour after the
preparation is finished, are not influenced by the
presence of a general anaesthetic. The spinalization procedure removes the tonic descending control exerted by inhibitory pathways originating in

the brainstem (Liebeskind et al., 1973; Willis et al., 1977; Basbaum et. al., 1978). Thus, a very brisk flexor reflex can be evoked by electrical or natural (mechanical or thermal) stimulation of the skin and electrical stimulation of muscle nerves or nerves in the hindlimb. The flexor reflex can be recorded directly from the axons of motorneurons innervating the biceps femoris/semitendinosus muscle or indirectly as electromyographic (EMG) signals from the muscle.

The relationship of the flexor reflex to behavior in intact, conscious animals

The magnitude of the RIII reflex evoked by noxious stimuli in man, which is analogous to the nociceptive hindlimb withdrawal reflex recorded in animals, is highly correlated to perceived pain intensity in man (Willer, 1977). Similarly, the magnitude of the flexor reflex in animals is well correlated with behaviors that reflect nociception or analgesia (see below). It is necessary to establish this correlation, especially in experiments where drugs are used that may have a direct effect on motorneurons. In order to eliminate the possibility that changes in flexor reflex magnitude are due to to direct effects on motorneuron excitability rather than in the dorsal horn, the effect of neuropeptides at concentrations that evoke changes in the flexor reflex are monitored on the amplitude of the monosynaptic reflex (Wiesenfeld-Hallin, 1989; Wiesenfeld-Hallin et al., 1989a).

The effect of conditioning stimulation of unmyelinated afferents on the flexor reflex and its relationship to the release of neuropeptides in the spinal cord

Activation of dorsal horn interneurons and the flexor reflex are under modulatory control, involving both excitation and inhibition (Melzack and Wall, 1966; Besson and Chaouch, 1987). Repetitive activation of C-afferents leads to a gradual increase in the response of dorsal horn interneurons, which has been termed 'wind-up' (Mendell, 1966). In their pioneering study, Wall and Woolf

(1984) demonstrated that a brief conditioning stimulus (CS) train which activates unmyelinated (C) cutaneous afferents leads to wind-up and facilitation of the flexor reflex that considerably exceeds the duration of stimulation. Thus, 20 electric shocks at 1 Hz applied to the cutaneous sural nerve facilitated the flexor reflex for 5–10 min, whereas the same CS applied to muscle afferents in the gastrocnemius nerve facilitated the flexor reflex for about one hour. Such changes in reflex excitability occurred independently of changes in the excitability of afferent terminals or motorneurons (Cook et al., 1986). Thus, prolonged changes in spinal cord excitability may be due to sensitization of dorsal horn interneurons. Corresponding changes in spinal cord excitability may be responsible for some painful conditions in humans, such as hyperalgesia, allodynia and tenderness (Woolf, 1983; Woolf and Chong, 1993). The flexor reflex does not become facilitated if the intensity of the CS is weaker and only activates rapidly conducting ($A\beta$) or slowly conducting ($A\delta$) myelinated afferents (Wall and Woolf, 1984). This difference between the consequences of activation of myelinated and unmyelinated afferents has lead us to consider whether sensory neuropeptides may be involved in the sensitization of the flexor reflex following C-fiber activation.

Assessment of the role of neuropeptides on spinal nociceptive mechanisms with the flexor reflex

The mechanisms of action of a large number of peptides, peptide agonists and antagonists have been examined with the rat flexor reflex model. The results are described below and summarized in Table I.

The role of the tachykinins, substance P and neurokinin A, in flexor reflex hyperexcitability

Substance P-like immunoreactivity (SP-LI) and neurokinin A-LI (NKA-LI) have been found to be colocalized in small dorsal root ganglion cells (Dalsgaard et al., 1985). SP and NKA applied on

TABLE I

Summary of the effects of i.t. neuropeptides, morphine and the cholecystokinin antagonist, CI 988, on the flexor reflex in rats with intact and sectioned sciatic nerves

Peptide	Normal	Axotomy
SP	+	+
NKA	+	nt
SP + NKA	+ +	nt
CGRP	+	+
SP + CGRP	+ +	0
SOM	+	+
SOM + CGRP	+ +	nt
VIP	+	+
VIP + CGRP	+	+ +
GAL	+,−	−−
MO	−−	−
GAL + MO	−−−	nt
GAL + SP	−−	0
GAL + CGRP	−−	−
GAL + VIP	0	−−
GAL + SOM	0	0
CCK	+	+
CI 988	−	−−
CI 988 + MO	−−−	−−−
CCK + MO	−	nt
OXY	+	nt
GAL + OXY	0	nt

SP, substance P; NKA, neurokinin A; CGRP, calcitonin gene-related peptide; SOM, somatostatin; VIP, vasoactive intestinal peptide; GAL, galanin; MO, morphine; CCK, cholecystokinin; OXY, oxytocin; +, reflex facilitation; + +, synergistic reflex facilitaion; −, reflex depression; −− or −−−, synergistic reflex depression; 0, no interaction; nt, not tested.

the spinal cord excite dorsal horn interneurons and may function in nociceptive neurotransmission (Henry, 1976; Fleetwood-Walker et al., 1990). Picomolar quantities of SP or NKA injected intrathecally (i.t.) onto the lumbar spinal cord facilitate the flexor reflex (Wiesenfeld-Hallin, 1986b; Woolf and Wiesenfeld-Hallin, 1986; Xu and Wiesenfeld-Hallin, 1992). Interestingly, the duration of the facilitatory effect of i.t. SP is similar to that evoked by a CS applied to the sural nerve (Woolf and Wiesenfeld-Hallin, 1986). Intrathecal SP facilitates the flexor reflex similarly to both

mechanical and thermal stimuli and thus may be released by polymodal nociceptors (Wiesenfeld-Hallin, 1986b). If NKA and SP are coadministered, the facilitation of the flexor reflex is synergistically increased, exceeding the additive effect of the two peptides (Xu and Wiesenfeld-Hallin., 1992; Wiesenfeld-Hallin and Xu, 1993). The synergistic interaction of SP and NKA may indicate that neuropeptides that are colocalized may interact functionally (also see below).

The role of endogenous SP and NKA in the CNS were difficult to assess before suitable antagonists became available. A number of peptide tachykinin antagonists that have been synthesized (e.g., Folkers et al., 1981) exhibited neurotoxic properties when applied into the CNS (Post and Paulsson, 1985; Wiesenfeld-Hallin and Duranti, 1987a). Spantide II, a non-specific antagonist of both SP and NKA (Folkers et al., 1990), proved to be the first non-toxic tachykinin antagonist with a clear effect in the CNS (Wiesenfeld-Hallin et al., 1990a,b). Spantide II applied i.t. antagonized the scratching/biting behaviour evoked by i.t. SP (Wiesenfeld-Hallin et al., 1990b) and blocked the sensitization of the flexor reflex by SP, as well as following CS of both cutaneous (Wiesenfeld-Hallin et al., 1990a) and muscle (Wiesenfeld-Hallin et al., 1991a) afferents. These results indicated that tachykinins may mediate spinal cord hyperexcitability when released into the spinal cord following activation of both cutaneous and muscle afferents.

More recently, specific antagonists of both SP and NKA have become available. With the use of specific antagonists, it has been possible to demonstrate the differential functions of SP and NKA in the spinal cord (Wiesenfeld-Hallin and Xu, 1993). CP 96,345, a non-peptide antagonist of the NK$_1$ receptor (Snider et al., 1991), effectively blocked facilitation of the flexor reflex following activation of both cutaneous (Xu et al., 1992a) and muscle (Xu and Wiesenfeld-Hallin, unpublished observations) afferents. In contrast, Menarini 10207, a specific antagonist of the NK$_2$ receptor (Maggi et al., 1990), blocked spinal hyperexcitability following CS of muscle, but not cutaneous, afferents (Xu et al., 1991a; Wiesenfeld-Hallin and Xu, 1993). These results indicate that SP released after activation of cutaneous afferents may be responsible for the brief facilitation of the flexor reflex, and co-release of SP and NKA may underly the prolonged facilitation of the flexor reflex following activation of muscle afferents. This differential effect of the activation of NK_1 and NK_2 receptors on spinal reflex hyperexcitability has been recently confirmed with the use of other specific antagonists (Ma et al., 1993).

Based on in vitro studies, it has been suggested that NK_2 receptors may be heterogeneous (Maggi et al., 1990). We have tested selective antagonists for the putative NK_{2A} and NK_{2B} receptors and observed that Menarini 10207 and Menarini 10376, selective NK_{2A} receptor antagonists, blocked the effect of i.t. NKA more potently than R396, a selective NK_{2B} receptor antagonist (Wiesenfeld-Hallin et al., 1994). These results suggest that the NK_2 receptor in rat spinal cord, which mediates the excitatory effect of NKA may belong to the NK_{2A} subpopulation of receptors.

The interaction of SP with other neuroactive substances present in primary afferents

Peptidergic primary afferents exhibit a complex pattern of coexistence where a number of peptides derived from different precursors can be localized in the same afferent (for review, see Hökfelt et al., 1980, 1994). The tachykinins, SP and NKA, are colocalized in primary afferents and synergistically potentiate each other (see above). Tachykinins have been found to be colocalized with other peptides derived from very different precursors. In rats with intact peripheral nerves, SP is colocalized with calcitonin gene-related peptide (CGRP) (Wiesenfeld-Hallin et al., 1984). CGRP-LI, which is very abundant in primary afferents and is found in both small and large dorsal root ganglion cells, may be localized in all cells exhibiting SP-LI. The possible functional consequence of the coexistence of these two peptides was examined in behavioural and physio-

logical studies (Wiesenfeld-Hallin et al., 1984). SP injected onto the lumbar spinal cord in rats with implanted i.t. catheters evoked a brief caudally directed biting/scratching response lasting less than 5 min. CGRP by itself evoked no response, even at high doses. CGRP co-administered with SP potentiated the effect of SP, evoking a much more prolonged and intense biting/scratching behavior. Parallel results were obtained in flexor reflex studies (Woolf and Wiesenfeld-Hallin, 1986). By itself, i.t. CGRP only weakly facilitated the flexor reflex, but synergistically increased the excitatory effect of i.t. SP. The mechanism of action of the interaction between CGRP and SP has been investigated, and CGRP has been found to inhibit the degradation of SP (Le Grevés et al., 1985). The synergistic interaction of SP and CGRP is a further example of functional interaction between coexisting neuropeptides.

SP is also colocalized with the neuropeptide galanin in rat dorsal root ganglion cells and the three peptides, SP, CGRP and galanin, have been identified in the same cell (Ch'ng et al., 1985; Ju et al., 1987). Normally, few DRG cells exhibit galanin-LI in rat, but the expression of this peptide increases remarkably after peripheral nerve injury (Hökfelt et al., 1987; Villar et al., 1989). We have examined the effect of galanin on the flexor reflex both in rats with intact and sectioned sciatic nerves (see below). Galanin has a complex effect on the reflex and has primarily an inhibitory function (Wiesenfeld-Hallin et al., 1989a). Galanin functions as an SP antagonist when the two peptides are coadministered i.t. (Xu et al., 1989, 1990a).

SP is also colocalized with the excitatory amino acid glutamate in dorsal root ganglion cells and their terminals in the spinal cord (Battaglia and Rustioni, 1988; De Biasi and Rustioni, 1988, 1990). Glutamate appears to have an important role in wind-up (Davies and Lodge, 1987) and sensitization of the flexor reflex. The prolonged facilitation of the flexor reflex following C-afferent CS was reduced by blockade of the *N*-methyl-D-aspartate (NMDA) receptor (Woolf and Thompson, 1991). We examined the interaction of the

NK$_1$receptor antagonist, CP 96,345, and the NMDA antagonist, MK-801, on wind-up and on the facilitation of the reflex by CS of cutaneous afferents (Xu et al., 1992b). MK-801 depressed the baseline reflex and reduced wind-up and post-stimulus facilitation. CP 96,345 was less effective in reducing wind-up, but blocked the post-CS facilitation as effectively as MK 801. When the NK$_1$ and NMDA antagonists were coadministered, both wind-up and reflex facilitation were synergistically reduced. Thus, both glutamate and SP may be co-released upon C-fiber stimulation and interact synergistically to induce central sensitization.

The effect of somatostatin on spinal excitability

SOM-LI has been localized in a small population of DRG cells, which is separate from those expressing SP-LI (Hökfelt et al., 1976). Although there is considerable evidence for SOM having a strong inhibitory function (Randić and Miletić, 1978), i.t. SOM evoked an intense scratching behavior and facilitated the flexor reflex (Wiesenfeld-Hallin, 1985). At high doses SOM produced flaccid paralysis and total blocklade of the reflex. In contrast to SP, which facilitated the reflex evoked by both mechanical and thermal stimuli, SOM appeared to have a more selective effect since it evoked reflex facilitation to thermal, but not mechanical, stimuli, suggesting that SOM may be released by thermosensitive C-afferents (Wiesenfeld-Hallin, 1986b). SOM has beeen found to coexist with CGRP-LI in rat DRG (Ju et al., 1987). In behavioral studies i.t. CGRP was found to potentiate SOM-evoked scratching and, in physiological studies, CGRP potentiated SOM-induced facilitation of the flexor reflex (Wiesenfeld-Hallin, 1986a).

The function of galanin and vasoactive intestinal polypeptide on flexor reflex hyperexcitability in rats with intact peripheral nerves

SP, NKA, SOM and CGRP are the major peptides normally identified in rat primary afferents, whereas galanin-LI and vasoactive intestinal polypeptide (VIP)-LI are much less prominent in normal dorsal root ganglia (Hökfelt et al., 1994). Although i.t. VIP facilitates spinal cord reflex excitability in rats with intact peripheral nerves (Wiesenfeld-Hallin, 1987, 1989; Xu and Wiesenfeld-Hallin, 1991), endogenous VIP does not seem to have a role in C-fiber activity-induced spinal sensitization under normal conditions since a VIP antagonist had no effect on CS-induced reflex facilitation in rats with intact sciatic nerves (Wiesenfeld-Hallin et al., 1990c; Xu and Wiesenfeld-Hallin, 1991).

In rats with intact nerves, the entire galanin peptide sequence (1–29) has a complex effect on the flexor reflex with a brief facilitatory effect at low doses, facilitation followed by inhibition at higher doses, and a purely inhibitory effect at the highest dose (Wiesenfeld-Hallin et al., 1988, 1989a). The N-terminal fragment 1–16 had a similar biphasic effect to the full sequence, whereas the C-terminal fragment 17–29 was not biologically active (Xu et al., 1990b). Thus, the receptor for galanin seems to recognize the N-, rather than the C-terminal. Since galanin appears to have an inhibitory function, its interaction with C-fiber CS of cutaneous and muscle afferents was examined. Intrathecal galanin inhibited the facilitation of the flexor reflex by CS of both cutaneous (Wiesenfeld-Hallin et al., 1989a) and muscle (Xu et al., 1991b) afferents.

Since reflex facilitation by CS of cutaneous and muscle afferents appears to involve the release of tachykinins and CGRP by primary afferents, we tested the interaction of galanin with SP and CGRP. Galanin preadministration antagonized the excitatory effect of SP and CGRP (Xu et al., 1989, 1990a). Thus, galanin appears to function as an antagonist of excitatory neuropeptides with which it coexists. No interaction between galanin and SOM or VIP was observed, which corresponds to a lack of coexistence between galanin and VIP or SOM in normal dorsal root ganglion cells. An inhibitory function of exogenous galanin was also indicated in behavioral and electrophysiological studies where it potentiated the analgesic effect of morphine (Wiesenfeld-Hallin et al., 1990d).

We have been able to demonstrate an inhibitory roll for endogenous galanin with some recently developed galanin receptor antagonists (Bartfai et al., 1991, 1993). The galanin antagonist M-35 significantly potentiated CS-induced reflex facilitation in rats with intact nerves (Wiesenfeld-Hallin et al., 1992), although the effect was much stronger after sciatic nerve section (see below). These results indicate that nociceptive transmission is under tonic galaninergic inhibitory influence, which is significantly increased after nerve injury.

The effects of cholecystokinin and oxytocin on the flexor reflex

Cholecystokinin (CCK) and oxytocin are two neuropeptides not present in normal dorsal root ganglion cells in the rat (Marley et al., 1982; Ju et al., 1986), but which are localized in dorsal horn interneurons or tracks descending from higher centers (Skirboll et al., 1983; Lundeberg et al., 1993). We have examined the effect of these two peptides in the flexor reflex since they have been described to have some interesting functional properties.

CCK may function as an endogenous opioid antagonist since systemically administered CCK reduces the analgesic effect of morphine and β-endorphin (Itoh et al., 1982; Faris et al., 1983). Antagonists of the CCK-B receptor, which predominates in the rat spinal cord, potentiate opioid analgesia and prevent the development of morphine tolerance (Dourish et al., 1990; Wiesenfeld-Hallin et al., 1990d). Intrathecal CCK dose-dependently facilitates the flexor reflex (Wiesenfeld-Hallin and Duranti, 1987b). CCK injected i.t. after morphine did not reverse morphine-induced reflex depression. However, if CCK was injected prior to i.t. morphine it enhanced the initial excitatory effect of morphine and reduced the subsequent inhibitory effect of the opioid. Thus, CCK antagonizes the analgesic effect of morphine on the flexor reflex by increasing mor-

phine-induced excitation, which may be due to the release of tachykinins from primary afferent terminals by the opioid (Wiesenfeld-Hallin et al., 1991b). Furthermore, CCK also reduced morphine-induced depression. We have tested the role of endogenous CCK with an antagonist of the CCK-B receptor, CI 988 (previously PD134308) (Wiesenfeld-Hallin et al., 1990d). CI 988 by itself caused a moderate naloxone-reversible depression of the flexor reflex. Since CI 988 has very low affinity to opioid receptors, it was presumably acting indirectly, indicating that the endogenous CCK system tonically antagonized the endogenous opioid system. CI 988 synergistically potentiated the analgesic effect of morphine, both on the flexor reflex and in behavioural tests in intact animals, further indicating that endogenous CCK is an opioid antagonist. In view of the fact that galanin synergistically potentiated the analgesic effect of morphine (Wiesenfeld-Hallin et al., 1990e), the effect of CI 988 combined with galanin was also evaluated. CI 988 intensely potentiated the inhibitory effect of galanin. Finally, a profound, long-lasting depression of the flexor reflex occurred when CI 988 was coadministered with galanin and morphine (Wiesenfeld-Hallin et al., 1990d)

Such results indicate that a convergence of the effect of μ opioids, galanin and CCK may occur in the dorsal horn. Convergence following activation of various receptors mediating analgesia is not universal, however. No such interaction was found between CCK and δ opioid actions (Magnuson et al., 1990). Furthermore, neither CCK nor galanin interacted with the α_2-adrenoceptor agonist clonidine, which is also an analgesic and depresses the flexor reflex (Xu and Wiesenfeld-Hallin, 1993). Like i.t. morphine, clonidine at low doses facilitates the flexor reflex, probably through the release of SP and NKA into the spinal cord (Luo and Wiesenfeld-Hallin, 1993).

Oxytocin, which has a documented effect in parturition and lactation, has been suggested to have an analgesic effect in rats following systemic (Uvnäs-Moberg et al., 1992) and i.t. (Lundeberg et al., 1993) administration. Intravenous oxytocin did not significantly influence the magnitude of the flexor reflex, but increased blood pressure and caused bradycardia (Xu and Wiesenfeld-Hallin, 1994a). Intrathecal oxytocin dose-dependently facilitated the flexor reflex (Xu and Wiesenfeld-Hallin, 1994b). It is therefore unlikely that oxytocin has an analgesic effect at spinal level.

The functional implications of messenger plasticity in primary sensory neurons following axotomy

Following peripheral axotomy, long-term changes occur in the expression of neuropeptides and their receptors in primary sensory neurons (for references, see Hökfelt et al., 1994). SP-LI, SOM-LI and CGRP-LI are down-regulated and galanin-LI and VIP-LI, which are normally found in few rat primary afferents, are up-regulated. Furthermore, CCK-LI and NPY-LI and receptor protein for CCK and NPY, two neuropeptides normally not found in rat primary afferents, are expressed following peripheral nerve section. Clear physiological correlates to these changes in neuropeptidergic phenotypes have been demonstrated with the flexor reflex model (Table 1).

After peripheral nerve section, myelinated (Wall and Devor, 1981) and unmyelinated (Wall, et al., 1981) afferents from the cut nerve are still able to excite central cells. However, the sensitization of the flexor reflex following CS of C-afferents is altered after axotomy (Wall and Woolf, 1986). The brief reflex hyperexcitability following CS of cutaneous afferents is maintained, but the prolonged effect of CS of muscle afferents is reduced. In view of the importance of SP and CGRP in the mediation of prolonged spinal cord hyperexcitability (Woolf and Wiesenfeld-Hallin, 1986), it is interesting to consider the role of neuropeptides following nerve injury. Within 2 weeks following sciatic nerve section, tachykinins totally lose their excitatory function in spinal reflex hyperexcitability (Wiesenfeld-Hallin et al., 1990c). The time course of this effect parallels the decline of SP-LI in dorsal root ganglion cells (Jessell et al., 1979). VIP, which normally has no role in spinal reflex sensitization (Xu

and Wiesenfeld-Hallin, 1991), is up-regulated after peripheral nerve injury (Shehab and Atkinson, 1986) and becomes a major excitatory mediator following section of the sciatic nerve (Wiesenfeld-Hallin, 1989; Wiesenfeld-Hallin et al., 1990c). Thus, there is a switch in the role of excitatory neuropeptides following peripheral nerve injury.

Galanin, which has a demonstrable inhibitory roll, is intensely up-regulated in dorsal root ganglion cells following peripheral nerve section (Hökfelt et al., 1987). This inhibitory role became enhanced after peripheral nerve section (Wiesenfeld-Hallin et al., 1989b). The reflex depressive effect of i.t. galanin was significantly increased, occurring at lower drug concentrations than in animals with intact peripheral nerves. Furthermore, the magnitude of reflex depression was significantly stronger with a more rapid onset after nerve section. The enhanced inhibitory role of galanin following nerve section was also demonstrated with the selective anagonist M-35 (Wiesenfeld-Hallin et al., 1992). In rats with intact nerves, M-35 moderately potentiated spinal cord sensitization following CS of a cutaneous nerve. This potentiation was significantly more pronounced after peripheral nerve section. These results indicate that the moderate tonic galaninergic control of nociceptive input to the spinal cord is enhanced after nerve injury. Thus, galanin agonists may be useful analgesics for the treatment of neuropathic pain following nerve injury.

Galanin was shown to function as an antagonist of the excitatory effect of SP and CGRP, but not VIP and SOM, when peripheral nerves were intact (Xu et al., 1989, 1990a). We examined the interaction of galanin with these neuropeptides after peripheral nerve section (Xu et al., 1990a). Galanin's antagonism of the excitatory effect of SP was totally abolished after axotomy, and its antagonism of the excitatory effect of CGRP was significantly reduced. Just as in rats with intact nerves, galanin did not interact with SOM. In contrast, after nerve section, galanin antagonized the excitatory effect of VIP. Interestingly, a strong coexistence between galanin-LI and VIP-LI was observed in dorsal root ganglion cells following axotomy. These results reinforce the conclusion that peptides that are colocalized have a functional interaction.

We have also examined the functional significance of the up-regulation of CCK-LI and CCK-B receptor mRNA in rat dorsal root ganglia (Xu et al., 1993; Zhang et al., 1993). In the clinic, pain arising after nervous tissue injury is difficult to treat and is usually insensitive to opioid analgesics (Arnér and Meyerson, 1988). In agreement with the clinical observation, chronic i.t. morphine administration was ineffective in blocking autotomy, a behavioural model of experimental neuropathic pain following peripheral nerve injury (Xu et al., 1993). Since CCK is an endogenous μ opioid antagonist, we examined whether morphine insensitivity could involve up-regulation of CCK. Chronic coadministration of the CCK-B receptor antagonist, CI 988, with morphine significantly reduced autotomy behavior (Xu et al., 1993). The effect of CI 988 and morphine on the flexor reflex in rats with sectioned sciatic nerves was evaluated (Xu et al., 1994). Morphine was significantly less effective in depressing the flexor reflex after axotomy than when peripheral neves were intact. However, the depressive effect of CI 988 was significantly enhanced in axotomized rats, which probably signifies increased tonic endogenous CCK activity. Combination of morphine and CI 988 resulted in significant potentiation of the analgesic effect of morphine, just as in rats with intact peripheral nerves (Wiesenfeld-Hallin et al., 1990d). Thus, coadministration of CCK antagonists in combination with opioids may offer a new approach for treating neuropathic pain.

Conclusions

From studies on the effect ot neuropeptides and their selective antagonists on the flexor reflex it has been possible to start to systematically examine the function of neuropeptides in spinal nociceptive processes. The flexor reflex is a robust model and represents a useful method among other methods to try to untangle the complexity of the pharmacology of spinal nociceptive mechanisms.

Acknowledgements

This work was supported by the Bank of Sweden Tercentenary Foundation, the Swedish Medical Research Council (project no. 07913), and Astra Pain Control AB.

References

Arnér, S. and Meyerson, B.A, (1988) Lack of analgesic effect of opioids on neuropathic and idiopathic forms of pain. *Pain*, 33: 11–23.

Bartfai, T., Bedecs, K., Land, T., Langel, U., Bertorelli, R., Girotti, P., Consolo, S., Xu, X.-J., Wiesenfeld-Hallin, Z., Nilsson, S., Pieribone, V.A. and Hökfelt, T. (1991) M-15: High affinity chimeric peptide that blocks the neuronal actions of galanin in the hippocampus, locus coeruleus, and spinal cord. *Proc. Natl. Acad. Sci. USA*, 88: 10961–10965.

Bartfai, T., Langel, U., Bedecs, K., Andell, S., Land, T., Gregersen, S., Ahrén, B., Girotti, P., Consolo, S., Corwin, R., Crawley, J., Xu, X.-J., Wiesenfeld-Hallin, Z. and Hökfelt, T. (1993) Galanin-receptor ligand M40 peptide distinguishes between putative galanin-receptor subtypes. *Proc. Natl. Acad. Sci. USA*, 90: 11287–11291.

Basbaum, A.I., Clanton, C.H. and Fields, H.L. (1978) Three bulbospinal pathways from the rostral medulla of the cat: an autoradiographic study of pain modulating pathways from the rostral medulla of the cat: an autoradiographic study of pain modulating systems. *J. Comp. Neurol.*, 178: 209–224.

Battaglia, G. and Rustioni, A. (1988) Coexistence of glutamate and substance P in dorsal root ganglion neurons of the rat and monkey. *J. Comp. Neurol.*, 277: 297–312.

Berge, O.-G., Garcia-Cabrera, I. and Hole, K. (1988) Response latencies in the tail flick test depend on tail skin temperature. *Neurosci. Lett.*, 86: 284–288.

Besson, J.-M. and Chaouch, A. (1987) Peripheral and spinal mechanisms of nociception. *Physiol. Rev.*, 67: 67–186.

Carstens, E., Hartung, M., Stelzer, B. and Zimmermann, M. (1990) Suppression of a hind limb flexion withdrawal reflex by microinjection of glutamate ormorphine into the periaqueductal gray in the rat. *Pain*, 1990: 105–112.

Chang, M.M. and Dallaier, M. (1989) Subjective pain sensation is linearly correlated with the flexion reflex in man. *Brain Res.*, 479: 145–150.

Ch'ng, J.L.C., Christofides, N.D, Anand, P., Gibson, S.J., Allen, Y.S., Su, H.C., Tatemoto, K., Morrison, J.F.B., Polak, J.M. and Bloom, S.R. (1985) Distribution of galanin immunoreactivity in the central nervous system and the response of galanin-containing neuronal pathways to injury. *Neuroscience*, 16: 343–354.

Cook, A.J., Woolf, C.J. and Wall, P.D. (1986) Prolonged C-fibre mediated facilitation of the flexion reflex in the rat is not due to changes in afferent terminal or motoneuron excitability. *Neurosci. Lett.*, 70: 91–96.

Dalsgaard, C.-J., Haegerstrand, A., Theodorsson-Norheim, E., Brodin, E. and Hökfelt, T. (1985) Neurokinin-A like immunoractivity in rat primary sensory neurons: coexistence with substance P. *Histochemistry*, 83: 37–40.

D'Amour, F.E. and Smith, D.L. (1941) A method for determining the loss of pain sensation. *J. Pharmacol. Exp. Ther.*, 72: 74–79.

Davies, S.N. and Lodge, D. (1987) Evidence for involvement of *N*-methylaspartate receptors in 'wind-up' of class 2 neurons in the dorsal horn of the rat. *Brain Res.*, 424: 402–406.

De Biasi, S. and Rustioni, A. (1988) Glutamate and substance P coexist in primary afferent terminals in the superficial laminae of spinal cord. *Proc. Natl. Acad. Sci. USA*, 85: 7820–7824.

De Biasi, S. and Rustioni, A. (1990) Ultrastructural immunohistochemical localization of excitatory amino acids in the somatosensory system. *J. Histochem. Cytochem.*, 38: 1745–1754.

Dourish, C.T., O'Neill, M.F., Coughlaan, J., Kitchenek, S.J., Hawley, D. and Iversen S.D. (1990) The selective CCK-B receptor antagonist L-365,260 enhances morphine analgesia and prevents morphine tolerance in the rat. *Eur. J. Pharmacol.*, 176: 35–44.

Faris, P.L., Komisaruk, B.R., Watkins, L.R. and Mayer, D.L. (1983) Evidence for the neuropeptide cholecystokinin as an antagonist of opiate analgesia. *Science*, 219: 211–222.

Fitzgerald, M., Millard, C. and MacIntosh, N. (1988) Cutaneous hypersensitivity following peripheral tissue damage in newbotn infants and its reversal with topical anaesthesia. *Pain*, 39: 31–36.

Fitzgerald, M., Shaw, A. and MacIntosh, N. (1989) The postnatal development of the cutaneous flexor reflex: comparative study of preterm infants and newborn rat pups. *Dev. Med. Child Neurol.*, 30: 520–526.

Fleetwood-Walker, S.M., Mitchell, R., Hope, P.J., El-Yassir, N., Molony, V. and Bladon, C.M. (1990) The involvement of neurokinin receptor subtypes in somatosensory processing in the superficial dorsal horn of the cat. *Brain Res.*, 519: 169–182.

Folkers, K., Hörig, J., Rosell, S. and Björkroth, U. (1981) Chemical design of antagonists of substance P. *Acta Physiol. Scand.*, 111: 505–506.

Folkers, K., Feng, D.-M., Asano, N., Håkanson, R., Wiesenfeld-Hallin, Z. and Leander, S. (1990) Spantide II, an effective tachykinin antagonist having high potency and negligible neurotoxicity. *Proc. Natl. Acad. Sci. USA*, 87: 4833–4835.

Henry, J.L. (1976) Effects of substance P on functionally identified units in cat spinal cord. *Brain Res.*, 114: 439–451.

Hökfelt, T., Elde, R., Johansson, O., Luft, R., Nilsson, G. and Arimura, A. (1976) Immunohistochemical evidence for separate populations of somatostatin-containing and substance P-containing primary afferent neurons in the rat. *Neuroscience*, 1: 131–136.

Hökfelt, T., Johansson, O., Ljungdahl, Å., Lundberg, J.M. and Schultzberg, M. (1980) Peptidergic neurons. *Nature*, 287: 515–521.

Hökfelt, T., Wiesenfeld-Hallin, Z., Villar, M.J. and Melander, T. (1987) Increase of galanin-like immunoractivity in rat dorsal root ganglion cells after peripheral axotomy. *Neurosci. Lett.*, 83: 217–220.

Hökfelt, T., Zhang, X. and Wiesenfeld-Hallin, Z. (1994) Messenger plasticity in primary sensory neurons following axotomy and its functional implications. *Trends Neurosci.*, 17: 22–30.

Itoh, S., Katsuura, G. and Maeda, Y. (1982) Caerulein and cholecystokinin suppress endorphin-induced analgesia in the rat. *Eur. J. Pharmacol.*, 80: 421–425.

Jessell, T., Tsunoo, A., Kanazawa, I. and Otsuka, M. (1979) Substance P: depletion in the dorsal horn of rat spinal cord after section of the peripheral processes of primary sensory neurons. *Brain Res.*, 168: 247–259.

Ju, G., Hökfelt, T., Fischer, J.A., Frey, P., Rehfeld, J.F. and Dockray, G.J. (1986) Does cholecystokinin-like immunoractivity in rat primary sensory neurons represent calcitonin-gene related peptide? *Neurosci. Lett.*, 68: 305–310.

Ju, G., Hökfelt, T., Brodin, E., Fahrenkrug, J., Fischer, J.A., Frey, P., Elde, R.P. and Brown, J.C. (1987) Primary sensory neurons of the rat showing calcitonin gene-related peptide immunoreactivity and their relation to substance P-, somatostatin-, galanin-vasoactive intestinal polypeptide- and cholecystokinin-immunoreactive ganglion cells. *Cell Tissue Res.*, 247: 417–431.

Le Grevés, P., Nyberg, F., Terenius, L. and Hökfelt, T. (1985) Calcitonin gene-related peptide is a potent inhibitor of substance P degradation. *Eur. J. Pharmacol.*, 115: 309–311.

Liebeskind, J.C., Guilbaud, G, Besson, J.-M. and Oliveras, J.-L. (1973) Analgesia from electrical stimulation of the periaqueductal gray matter in the cat: behavioral observations and inhibitory effects on spinal cord interneurons. *Brain Res.*, 50: 441–446.

Lundeberg, T., Meister, B., Björkstrand, E. and Uvnäs-Moberg, K. (1993) Oxytocin modulates the effects of galanin in carrageenan-induced hyperalgesia in rats. *Brain Res.*, 608: 181–185.

Luo, L. and Wiesenfeld-Hallin, Z. (1993) Low-dose intrathecal clonidine releases tachykinins in rat spinal cord. *Eur. J. Pharmacol.*, 235: 157–159.

Ma, O.P., Sivilotti, L.G., Nagy, I. and Woolf, C.J. (1993) Tachykinin receptor involvement in C-fiber evoked slow synaptic potentials in vitro and central sensitization in vivo. *Soc. Neurosci. Abstr.*, 19: 522.

Maggi, C.A., Patacchini,. R., Giuliani, S., Rovero, P., Dion, S., Regoli, D., Giachetti, A. and Meli, A. (1990) Competitive antagonists discriminate between NK$_2$ tachykinin receptor subtypes. *Br. J. Pharmacol.*, 100: 588–592.

Magnuson, D.S.K., Sullivan, A.F., Simonnet, G., Roques, B.P. and Dickenson, A.H. (1990) Differential interaction of cholecystokinin and FLFQPQRF-NH2 with μ and δ opioid antinociception in the rat spinal cord. *Neuropeptides*, 16: 213–218.

Marley, P.D., Nagy, J.E., Emson, P.C. and Rehfeld, J.F. (1982) Cholecystokinin in the rat spinal cord: distribution and lack of effect on neonatal capsaicin treatment and rhizotomy. *Brain Res.*, 238: 494–498.

Melzack, R. and Wall, P.D. (1988) Pain mechanisms: a new theory. *Science*, 150: 971–979.

Mendell, L.M. (1966) Physiological properties of unmyelinated fibre projections to the spinal cord. *Exp. Neurol.*, 16: 316–332.

Post, C. and Paulsson, I. (1985) Antinociceptive and neurotoxic actions of substance P analogues in the rat's spinal cord after intrathecal administration. *Neurosci. Lett.*, 57: 159–164.

Randić, M. and Miletić, V. (1978) Depressant actions of methionine-enkephalin and somatostatin in cat dorsal horn neurons activated by noxious stimuli. *Brain Res.*, 196–202.

Schouenborg, J. and Sjölund, B.H. (1983) Activity evoked by A- and C-afferent fibers in rat dorsal horn neurons and its relation to a flexion reflex. *J. Neurophysiol.*, 50: 1108–1121.

Shehab, S.A.S. and Atkinson, M.E. (1986) Vasoactive intestinal polypeptide (VIP) increases in the spinal cord after peripheral axotomy of the sciatic nerve originate from primary afferent neurons. *Brain Res.*, 372: 37–44.

Skirboll, L., Hökfelt, T., Dockray, G. and Rehfeld, J. (1983) Evidence for periaqueductal cholecystokinin-substance P neurons projecting to the spinal cord. *J. Neurosci.*, 3: 1151–1157.

Snider, M., Constantine, J.W., Lowe, J.A. III, Longo, K.P., Lebel, W.S., Woody, H.A., Drozda, S.E., Desai, M.C., Vinick, F.J., Spencer, R.W. and Hess, H.-J. (1991) A potent nonpeptide antagonist of the substance P (NK1) receptor. *Science*, 251: 435–437.

Uvnäs-Moberg, K., Bruzelius, G., Alster, P., Bilevicitue, I. and Lundeberg, T. (1992) Oxytocin increases and a specific oxytocin antagonist decreases pain threshold in male rats. *Acta Physiol. Scand.*, 145; 487–488.

Villar, M.J., Cortés, R., Theodorsson, E., Wiesenfeld-Hallin, Z., Schalling, M., Fahrenkrug, J., Emson, P.C. and Hökfelt, T. (1989) Neuropeptide expression in rat dorsal root ganglion cells and spinal cord after peripheral nerve injury with special reference to galanin. *Neuroscience*, 33: 587–604.

Wall, P.D. and Devor, M. (1981) The effect of peripheral nerve injury on dorsal root potentials and in transmision of afferent signals into the spinal cord. *Brain Res.*, 209: 95–111.

Wall, P.D. and Woolf, C.J. (1984) Muscle but not cutaneous C-afferent input produces prolonged increases in the excitability of the flexion reflex in the rat. *J. Physiol.*, 356: 443–458.

Wall, P.D. and Woolf, C.J. (1986) The brief and the prolonged facilitatory effects of unmyelinated afferent input on the rat spinal cord are independently influenced by peripheral nerve section. *Neuroscience*, 17: 1199–1205.

Wall, P.D., Fitzgerald, M. and Gibson, S.J. (1981) The response of rat spinal cord cells to unmyelinated afferents after peripheral nerve section and after changes in substance P levels. *Neuroscience*, 6: 2205–2215.

Wiesenfeld-Hallin, Z. (1985) Intrathecal somatostatin modulates spinal sensory and reflex mechanisms: behavioral and electrophysiological studies. *Neurosci. Lett.*, 62: 69–74.

Wiesenfeld-Hallin, Z. (1986a) Somatostatin and calcitonin gene-related peptide synergistically modulate spinal sensory and reflex mechanisms in the rat: behavioral and electrophysiological studies. *Neurosci. Lett.*, 67: 319–323.

Wiesenfeld-Hallin, Z. (1986b) Substance P and somatostatin modulate spinal cord excitability via physiologically different sensory pathways. *Brain Res.*, 372: 172–175.

Wiesenfeld-Hallin, Z. (1987) Intrathecal vasoactive intestinal polypeptide modulates spinal reflex excitability primarily to cutaneous thermal stimuli in rats. *Neurosci. Lett.*, 80: 293–297.

Wiesenfeld-Hallin, Z. (1989) Nerve section alters the interaction between C-fibre activity and intrathecal neuropeptides on the flexor reflex in rat. *Brain Res.*, 489: 129–136.

Wiesenfeld-Hallin, Z. and Duranti, R. (1987a) D-Arg[1],D-Trp[7,9], Leu[11]-substance P (Spantide) does not anagonize substance P-induced hyperexcitability of the nociceptive flexion withdrawal reflex in the rat. *Acta Physiol. Scand.* 129: 55–59.

Wiesenfeld-Hallin, Z. and Duranti, R. (1987b) Intrathecal cholecystokinin interacts with morphine but not substance P in modulating the nociceptive flexion reflex in the rat. *Peptides*, 8: 153–158.

Wiesenfeld-Hallin, Z. and Xu, X.-J. (1993) The differential roles of substance P and neurokinin A in spinal cord hyperexcitability and neurogenic inflammation. *Regul. Peptides*, 46: 165–173

Wiesenfeld-Hallin, Z., Hökfelt, T., Lundberg, J.M., Forsmann, W.G., Reinecke, M., Tschapp, F.A. and Fischer, J.A. (1984) Immunoractive calcitonin gene-related peptide and substance P co-exist in sensory neurons to the spinal cord and interact in spinal behavioural responses of the rat. *Neurosci. Lett.*, 52: 199–204.

Wiesenfeld-Hallin, Z., Villar, M.J. and Hökfelt, T. (1988) Intrathecal galanin at low doses increases spinal reflex excitability in rats more to thermal than mechanical stimuli. *Exp. Brain Res.*, 71: 663–666.

Wiesenfeld-Hallin, Z., Villar, M.J. and Hökfelt, T. (1989a) The effects of intrathecal galanin and C-fiber stimulation on the flexor reflex in the rat. *Brain Res.*, 486: 205–213.

Wiesenfeld-Hallin, Z., Xu, X.-J., Villar, M.J. and Hökfelt, T. (1989b) The effects of intrathecal galanin on the flexor reflex in rat: increased depression after sciatic nerve section. *Neurosci. Lett.*, 105: 149–154.

Wiesenfeld-Hallin, Z., Xu, X.-J., Håkanson, R., Feng, D.-M. and Folkers, K. (1990a) The specific antagonistic effect of intrathecal spantide II on substance P- and C-fiber conditioning stimulation-induced facilitation of the nociceptive flexor reflex in rat. *Brain Res.*, 526: 284–290.

Wiesenfeld-Hallin, Z., Xu, X.-J., Kristensson, K., Håkanson, R., Feng, D.-M. and Folkers, K. (1990b) Antinociceptive and substance P antagonistic effects of intrathecally injected spantide II in rat: no signs of motor impairment or neurotoxicity. *Regul. Peptides*, 29: 1–11.

Wiesenfeld-Hallin, Z., Xu, X.-J., Håkanson, R., Feng, D.-M. and Folkers, K. (1990c) Plasticity of the peptidergic mediation of spinal reflex facilitation after peripheral nerve section in the rat. *Journal Title*, 116: 293–298.

Wiesenfeld-Hallin, Z., Xu, X.-J., Hughes, J., Horwell, D.C. and Hökfelt, T. (1990d) PD134308, a selective antagonist of cholecystokinin type B receptor, enhances the analgesic effect of morphine and synergistically interacts with intrathecal galanin to depress spinal nociceptive reflexes. *Proc. Natl. Acad. Sci. USA*, 87: 7105–7109.

Wiesenfeld-Hallin, Z., Xu, X.-J., Villar, M.J. and Hökfelt, T. (1990e) Intrathecal galanin potentiates the spinal analgesic effect of morphine: electrophysiological and behavioural studies. *Neurosci. Lett.*, 109: 217–221.

Wiesenfeld-Hallin, Z., Xu, X.-J., Håkanson, R., Feng, D.-M. and Folkers, K. (1991a) Tachykinins mediate changes in spinal reflexes after activation of unmyelinated muscle afferents in the rat. *Acta Physiol. Scand.*, 141: 57–61.

Wiesenfeld-Hallin, Z., Xu, X.-J., Håkanson, R., Feng, D.-M. and Folkers, K. (1991b) Low-dose intrathecal morphine facilitates the spinal flexor reflex by releasing different neuropeptides in rats with intact and sectioned peripheral nerves. *Brain Res.*, 551: 157–162.

Wiesenfeld-Hallin, Z., Xu, X.-J., Langel, U., Bedecs, K., Hökfelt, T. and Bartfai, T. (1992) Galanin-mediated control of pain: enhanced role after nerve injury. *Proc. Natl. Acad. Sci. USA*, 89: 3334–3337.

Wiesenfeld-Hallin, Z., Luo, L., Xu, X.-J. and Maggi, C.A. (1994) Differential effects of selective tachykinin NK$_2$ receptor antagonists in rat spinal cord. *Eur. J. Pharmacol.*, 251: 99–102.

Willer, J.C. (1977) Comparative study of perceived pain and nociceptive flexion reflex in man. *Pain*, 3: 69–80.

Willis, W.D., Haber, L.H. and Martin, R.F. (1977) Inhibition of spinothalamic tract cells and interneurons by brain stem stimulation in the monkey. *J. Neurophysiol.*, 40; 968–981.

Woolf, C.J. (1983) Evidence for a central component of post-injury pain hypersensitivity. *Nature*, 306: 686–688.

Woolf, J.C. and Chong, M.-S. (1993) Preemptive analgesia: treating postoperative pain by preventing the establishment of central sensitization. *Anesth. Analg.*, 77: 362–379.

Woolf, C.J. and Thompson, S.W.N. (1991) The induction and maintenance of central sensitization is dependent on *N*-methyl-D-aspartic acid receptor activation: implications for the treatment of post-injury pain hypersensitivity states. *Pain*, 44: 293–300.

Woolf, C. and Wiesenfeld-Hallin, Z. (1986) Substance P and calcitonin gene-related peptide synergistically modulate the gain of the nociceptive flxor withdrawal reflex in the rat. *Neurosci. Lett.*, 66: 226–230.

Xu, X.-J. and Wiesenfeld-Hallin, Z. (1991) An analogue of growth hormone releasing factor (GRF), (Ac-Try[1], D-Phe[2]) GRF-(1–29), specifically antagonizes the facilitation of the flexor reflex induced by intrathecal vasoactive intestinal peptide in rat spinal cord. *Neuropeptides*, 18: 129–135.

Xu, X.-J. and Wiesenfeld-Hallin, Z. (1992) Intrathecal neurokinin A facilitates the spinal nociceptive flexor reflex evoked by thermal and mechanical stimuli and synergistically interacts with substance P. *Acta Physiol. Scand.*, 144: 163–168.

Xu, X.-J. and Wiesenfeld-Hallin, Z. (1993) Neither cholecystokinin nor galanin modulate intrathecal clonidine-induced depression of the nociceptive flexor reflex in the rat. *Brain Res.*, 621: 267–271.

Xu, X.-J. and Wiesenfeld-Hallin, Z. (1994a) Is systemically administered oxytocin hypoalgesic in rats? *Pain*, 57: 193–196.

Xu, X.-J. and Wiesenfeld-Hallin, Z. (1994b) Intrathecal oxytocin facilitates the spinal nociceptive flexor reflex in the rat. *NeuroReport*, 5: 750–752.

Xu, X.-J., Wiesenfeld-Hallin, Z., Villar, M.J. and Hökfelt, T. (1989) Intrathecal galanin antagonizes the facilitatory effect of substance P on the nociceptive flexor reflex in the rat. *Acta Physiol. Scand.*, 137: 463–464.

Xu, X.-J., Wiesenfeld-Hallin, Z., Villar, M.-J., Fahrenkrug, J. and Hökfelt, T. (1990a) On the role of galanin, substance P and other neuropeptides in primary sensory neurons of the rat: studies on spinal reflex excitability and peripheral axotomy. *Eur. J. Neurosci.*, 2: 733–743.

Xu, X.-J. and Wiesenfeld-Hallin, Z., Fisone, G., Bartfai, T. and Hökfelt, T. (1990b) The N-terminal 1–16, but not C-terminal 17–29, galanin fragment affects the flexor reflex in rats. *Eur. J. Pharmacol.*, 182: 137–141.

Xu, X.-J., Maggi, C.A. and Wiesenfeld-Hallin, Z. (1991a) On the role of the NK-2 tachykinin receptors in the mediation of spinal reflex excitability in the rat. *Neuroscience*, 44: 483–490.

Xu, X.-J., Wiesenfeld-Hallin, Z. and Hökfelt, T. (1991b) Intrathecal galanin blocks the prolonged increase in spinal cord flexor reflex excitability induced by conditioning stimulation of unmyelinated muscle afferents in the rat. *Brain Res.*, 541: 350–353.

Xu, X.-J., Dalsgaard, C.-J. and Wiesenfeld-Hallin, Z. (1992a) Intrathecal CP 96,345 blocks reflex facilitation induced in rats by substance P and C-fiber-conditioning stimulation. *Eur. J. Pharmacol.*, 216: 337–344.

Xu, X.-J., Dalsgaard, C.-J. and Wiesenfeld-Hallin, Z. (1992b) Spinal substance P and *N*-methyl-D-aspartate receptors are coactivated in the induction of central sensitization of the nociceptive flexor reflex. *Neuroscience*, 51: 641–648.

Xu, X.-J., Puke, M.J.C., Verge, V.M.K., Wiesenfeld-Hallin, Z., Hughes, J. and Hökfelt, T. (1993) Up-regulation of chole-cystokinin in primary sensory neurons is associated with morphine insensitivity in experimental neuropathic pain in the rat. *Neurosci. Lett.*, 152: 129–132.

Xu, X.-J., Hökfelt, T., Hughes, J. and Wiesenfeld-Hallin, Z. (1994) The CCK-B antagonist CI988 enhances the reflex depressive effect of morphine in axotomized rat. *NeuroReport*, 5: 718–720.

Zhang, X., Dagerlind, Å., Elde, R.P., Castel, M.-N., Broberger, C., Wiesenfeld-Hallin, Z. and Hökfelt, T. (1993) Marked increase in cholecystokinin B receptor messenger RNA levels in rat dorsal root ganglia after peripheral axotomy. *Neuroscience*, 57: 227–233.

F. Nyberg, H.S. Sharma and Z. Wiesenfeld-Hallin (Eds.)
Progress in Brain Research, Vol 104

CHAPTER 16

Proto-oncogenes: basic concepts and stimulation induced changes in the spinal cord

R. Munglani[1] and S.P. Hunt[2]

[1]*University Department of Anaesthesia, University of Cambridge Clinical School, Addenbrookes Hospital, Hills Road, Cambridge, England CB2 2QQ, UK and* [2]*Division of Neurobiology, Laboratory of Molecular Biology, MRC Centre, Hills Road, Cambridge, England, CB2 2QH, UK*

Introduction

Immediate early genes (IEGs) were originally described as a class of genes rapidly and transiently expressed in cells stimulated with growth factors without the requirement for de novo protein synthesis (Cochran et al., 1983). c-*fos* (Curran et al., 1987), c-*jun* (Angel et al., 1988; Ryseck et al., 1988; Sakai et al., 1989) and other IEGs have been shown to be transcription factors (Chiu et al., 1988; Halzonetis et al., 1988; Sassone-Corsi et al., 1988; Abate et al., 1990; Benbrook and Jones, 1990; Macgregor et al., 1990) and are differentially expressed in the central nervous system following specific types of stimulation (Hunt et al., 1987; Cole et al., 1989; Williams et al., 1989; Wisden et al., 1990; Morgan and Curran, 1991; Tolle et al., 1994). Indeed, evidence is accumulating to suggest that changes in immediate early gene expression within the nervous system signal long-term adaptation within particular neural pathways.

Rapid and transient expression are obviously ideal characteristics for putative cellular 'activity markers', in that the pattern of expression could, because of the rapidity of expression, be assumed to be generated directly by the stimulus and not mediated polysynaptically or by some other process or be the residual trace of previous stimulation.

However, while the value of IEGs as activity markers in vitro cannot be disputed, their appearance in vivo is under far greater control and appears to be tied to the physiological context of the stimulus. Here we argue that the localisation of IEG protein and mRNA in neurons and glial cells grown in vitro may accurately reflect that the cell has been recently stimulated in some way, while the appearance of IEG product in vivo does not simply reflect a pattern of evoked activity but a pattern which is crucially related to the type of stimulation and the physiological state of the animal. This is particularly so in the spinal cord response to noxious stimulation which is described in detail in the second half of the chapter. IEGs cannot be regarded simply as activity markers in vivo but perhaps as indicating the occurrence of a significant environmental stimulation that requires a long-term change in certain aspects of neuronal physiology.

In vitro studies

An enormous number of studies have now been published on the in vitro use of IEGs (particularly Fos) to map activity at the single cell level in cell cultures. In the examples given here, Fos expression has been used to confirm the presence of excitatory amino acid (EAA) receptors on glial cells and neurons and allow the dissection of intracellular pathways to the nucleus. It seems likely that this would not have been possible in vivo and, indeed, available evidence suggests that cells behave rather differently in vivo when stimulated in a comparable way.

For example, we have studied the effect of excitatory amino acids on the expression of mRNA for the immediate early genes c-*fos*, c-*jun*, *jun*-B and NGF-1A (zif 268) in isolated type 1 cortical astrocytes (McNaughton and Hunt, 1993). Excitatory amino acid receptors have been divided into a number of major subtypes; the metabotropic (quisqualic acid) receptor (QA, also known as GluR 1–6) , the AMPA receptor and low-affinity kainate receptor (GluR 1–4), and the high-affinity kainic acid (KA) receptor (GluR 5–7, KA-1 KA-2) and *N*-methyl-D-aspartate (NMDA) receptor (Young and Fagg, 1990; Nakanishi, 1992; Wisden and Seeberg, 1993).

Astrocytes have been shown to increase their levels of intracellular Ca^{2+} in response to the stimulation by quisqualate, kainate and glutamate, but not NMDA (Jensen and Chiu, 1990; McNaughton et al., 1990). Further, electrophysiological studies have shown the presence of quisqualate and kainate, but not NMDA receptors in cortical astrocytes, in vitro and suggests that the response may be mediated by the activation of receptor-linked ion channels (reviewed by Bowman and Kimelberg, 1984; Sontheimer et al., 1988; Barres 1991; Burnashev et al., 1992; Muller et al., 1992). In neuronal cell lines and neurons, elevation of Ca^{2+} levels is associated with the expression of genes such as c-*fos*. In PC12 cells, nicotinic or high K^+ stimulation results in the secondary activation of voltage-gated calcium channels which allow the entry of Ca^{2+} and a subsequent rise in intracellular Ca^{2+} levels (Greenberg et al., 1986; Bartel et al., 1989; Morgan and Curran, 1986, 1991).

In previous studies we (McNaughton et al., 1990) and others (Sontheimer et al., 1988; Jensen and Chiu, 1990; Wyllie et al., 1991) have been able to show that quisqualate and kainate, but not NMDA receptor, stimulation of glial cells results in an elevation of intracellular calcium

levels by two routes. Firstly, entry of calcium from the extracellular medium, presumably following opening of voltage-sensitive calcium channels as in PC12 cells (Morgan and Curren, 1986), and secondly by activation of the inositol phospholipid second messenger cascade, resulting in the generation of inositol triphosphate and the release of intracellular calcium from internal stores. The relationship between glutamate agonist stimulation and the expression of immediate early genes was therefore examined.

The expression of the different genes was induced by 100 mM kainate, quisqualate, AMPA and high concentrations of K^+ (140 mM). NMDA did not induce the expression of any of the genes studied. Elevated K^+ induced c-*fos* only when calcium was present in the external medium, implying calcium movement through voltage-dependent calcium channels. These findings also suggest that type-1 astrocytes lack NMDA receptors and that the induction of genes by quisqualate and kainate is mediated through second messenger pathways following metabotropic or ionotropic receptor activation.

Thus, while the expression of c-*fos* and, in fact, a large number of IEGs, can be predictably induced in glial cells in vitro and give significant insights into the intracellular mechanisms that accompany these receptor-mediated events, this is entirely different from the in vivo state. In vivo immediate early gene (IEG) activation in glial cells is never seen in either early postnatal or adult animals following comparable stimulation paradigms (unpublished observations). Thus, what is seen in culture may be entirely different from the pattern of gene expression found in the brain. Nevertheless, these in vitro phenomena are extremely useful as markers of single cell activity.

IEG activation has been used to chart the second messenger pathways leading to the nucleus following glutamate or other types of stimulation of hippocampal neurons (Bading et al., 1993; Lerea and McNamara, 1993). Primarily, these studies demonstrated that the two distinct pathways of calcium entry into the neuron (via the NMDA receptor channel or through the

285

opening of voltage-dependent calcium channels (VSCCs) following membrane depolarization) resulted in the activation of different intracellular pathways which converge upon the c-*fos* gene. Calcium entry through the NMDA receptor acts in part through a MAP kinase pathway (Bading et al., 1991) and induces changes in c-*fos* expression through the serum response element on the c-*fos* gene promoter, while calcium entry through VSCC appears to preferentially activate calcium-calmodulin-dependent kinase II which influences c-*fos* expression through the cyclic AMP response element on the c-*fos* gene. Thus, in vitro c-*fos* gene expression always follows EAA stimulation or high potassium treatment and appears to be borne out by these studies. However in the brain the situation appears to be rather more complicated. The induction of long-term potentiation in dentate gyrus granule cells following brief tetanic stimulation of the perforant pathway is dependent on NMDA activation and results in the induction of the IEG NGFl-A (also known as egr-1 and zif 268) but not, for the most part, c-*fos* or c-*jun* (Cole et al., 1989; Wisden et al., 1990; Worley et al., 1993)). While it could be argued that adjusting the stimulation intensity would result in the expression of other IEGs, the remarkable fact is that LTP is only associated in this stimulation paradigm with the expression of NGFI-A.

The spinal cord

In vivo studies

Some years ago we were able to demonstrate that *fos* is expressed postsynaptically in dorsal horn neurons of the spinal cord following noxious stimulation (Hunt et al., 1987). The protein product appears within 1–2 h post-stimulation and c-*fos*-positive neurons are restricted to layers 1 and 2 (the substantia gelatinosa) of the dorsal horn with some labelling in layer 5 (Fig. 1). We found that the type of stimulation was crucial for a change in gene expression within postsynaptic neurons of the dorsal horn. Thus, to achieve Fos expression

in superficial layers of the spinal cord it was essential to use noxious stimulation. Non-noxious stimulation was largely ineffective, although *fos* expression was seen in layer 3–4 neurons which are known to be non-nociceptive. No Fos expression was seen in dorsal column nuclei, ventral horn or, importantly, in the stimulated dorsal root ganglion cells themselves. In other words only a subset of stimulated neurons expressed c-*fos*.

Williams et al. extended these observations (Williams et al., 1989, 1990a, 1991). Using an easily reproducible technique of dipping the paw of the anaesthetised rat in water at 52°C for 20 sec, the Fos response was found to be remarkably consistent in that FOS protein appeared within 30 min following noxious thermal stimulation and peaked at 2 h in layers 1 and 2 ipsilateral to the injury. The pattern was similar to that seen by Hunt et al. (1987). However another peak of Fos expression was seen within the deep layers (5–7 and 10), commencing at 8 h, and peaking at 16 h, this second wave of labelling started ipsilaterally and spread to become bilateral (see Fig. 2).

The activation of deeper neurons is unlikely to be the result of a monosynaptic event. Thermal stimulation at 52°C stimulates unmyelinated C fibres which terminate in layers 1, 2 and 5. Fos-positive neurons were found in other layers and at much later time points indicating a polysynaptic mechanism. To examine whether this second wave of *fos* activity was dependent on continuous input from the site of thermal injury, three manoeuvres were performed. Firstly, a local anaesthetic block of the ipsilateral sciatic nerve was performed one hour post-thermal stimulation. These animals showed increased numbers of Fos-positive cells at 8 h (see Fig. 3). Secondly, the animals were kept constantly anaesthetised with equithesin (the composition of which includes sodium pentobarbitone, chloral hydrate, magnesium sulphate and ethanol) after thermal injury, and these animals showed fewer Fos-positive neurons than those allowed to recover from anaesthesia after thermal injury. Thirdly, those given both local and continuous general anaesthesia together, i.e., a combination of the first and second paradigm, showed a similar number and pattern of Fos-positive cells to those animals which had received only a single dose of equithesin, with no additional anaesthesia (see Fig. 3).

The use of the general anaesthetic equithesin reduced the Fos expression at 8 h. The increased Fos expression after afferent local anaesthetic blockade suggests that ongoing primary afferent

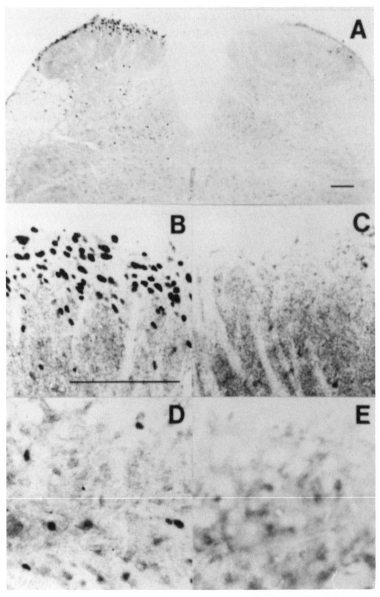

Fig. 1. (a) Section (40 μm) of rat spinal cord at L4 immunostained for FOS protein, 2 h after stimulation of the left hindpaw by immersion for 20 sec in gently stirred water at 52°C. *fos* expression in layers 1–2 (b) and layer 5 (d), respectively, in greater detail on the stimulated left hand side showing *fos* expression. No significant staining contralaterally in superficial (c) and deep layers (e) Scale = 100 μm. (From Williams, 1991.)

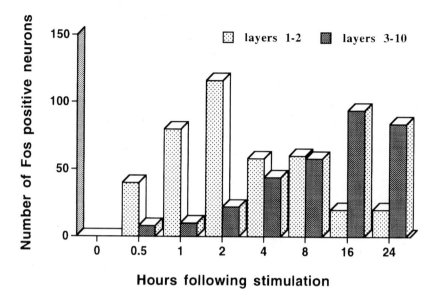

Fig. 2. *fos* cell counts after thermal stimulation in superficial (layers 1–2) and deep laminae (layers 3–10). This figure shows a superficial 'wave' of *fos* at 2 h and a second 'wave' of Fos peaking more deeply at 16 h. For clarity, only the response of the ipsilateral horn is shown and the SEMs have been omitted. After 4 h the Fos expression becomes bilateral with regard to depth, but there is little or no spread superficially. (Adapted from Williams et al., 1991.)

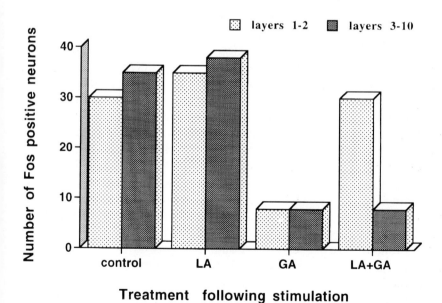

Fig. 3. *fos*-positive neurons per section of rat lumbar cord 8 h following heat stimulation of the left hind paw, with and without local anaesthetic blockade of the sciaitc nerve (LA), continuous general anaesthesia (GA), or both (LA + GA). For clarity the SEMs have been omitted. (Adapted from from Williams et al., 1991.)

activity is not required for the second wave, in fact the increase in Fos-positive cells suggests that a primary afferent tonic activity inhibits c-*fos* expression. This finding is matched by electro-physiological evidence for increased 'spontaneous activity' within layers 1 and 2 following surgical deafferentation (Basbaum and Wall, 1976). Animals which received both local and general anaesthesia suggests again that primary nerve activity was not required for the second wave effect and, in fact, the general anaesthetic which contains sodium pentobarbitone) may have reduced the deafferentation affect of the local anaesthetic.

Usefulness of fos expression as a long-term marker of nociception

The suggestion that c-*fos* expression in different layers of the spinal cord represents different processes is suggested by the studies of Abbadie and Besson (Abbadie and Besson, 1992, 1993a,b, 1994a,b). In this model, arthritis is induced by the injection of Freund's adjuvant into the base of the tail. After about 10 days, polyarthritis affects the hind limb joints and behavioural changes such as decreased locomotion and hyperalgesia to paw pressure appear. The symptoms peak at 3 weeks and continue for up to 11 weeks post-inoculation. The Fos-positive neurons were greatest in the lumbar segments L3/4 (corresponding to the innervation of the arthritic hind limbs) at 3 weeks (corresponding to the behavioural data). It must be emphasised that these Fos-positive cells were seen in arthritic animals in the basal state, i.e., with no further extra-peripheral stimulation applied. The pattern of Fos-positive neurons was very interesting, with most of the *fos*-positive cells in layers 5 and 6 and less than 5% of the total in layers 1–2 (see Fig. 4a); these latter layers are normally associated with large increases in *fos* in response to nociceptive intensity input. Interestingly the best correlation with behaviour was also with *fos* count in layers 5 and 6 rather than 1 and 2. Electrophysiological evidence indicates that afferent input from the inflamed joints and tissues continues in the adjuvant induced arthritis

model (AIA) (Menetrey and Besson, 1982), and so Fos protein might be expected to be seen in layers 1–2. To further examine this point, AIA rats were given a mechanical stimulus over the arthritic ankle joints under anaesthesia. These rats showed a normal pattern of *fos* response with large increases in layers 1 and 2 as well as layer 5 (see Fig. 4b). When these rats were treated with morphine before the stimulation, the greatest suppression of Fos was in the superficial layers (see Fig. 4c) (Abbadie and Besson, 1993b).

These results contrast with those studies looking at *fos* in acute pain situations where the suppression of the *fos* response with morphine is greatest in the deeper layers (Presley et al., 1990; Tolle et al., 1990; Gogas et al., 1991). High dose morphine was ineffective in reducing this 'basal' *fos* expression in the unstimulated AIA model. Furthermore if unstimulated AIA rats are given repeated doses of naloxone, there is a trend for increases in Fos count in the deeper layers, this suggests that there may be tonic activity of endogenous antinociceptive systems in situations of chronic pain (Abbadie and Besson, 1993b). The arthritis seen in AIA can prevented by inducing immunological tolerance using an injection of dilute FCA given 1–3 weeks before the main injection (Gery and Waksman, 1967). In these animals the Fos count in layer 5 is reduced but still shows a high degree of correlation with the disease state (Abbadie and Besson, 1994a,b). However, if the symptoms of the arthritis are ameliorated in the AIA model after 3 weeks with the administration of non-steroidal anti-inflammatory drugs (NSAIDs) (aspirin or acetaiminophen), there is no decrease in Fos count in the spinal cord (Abbadie and Besson, 1994a,b). It is unclear why *fos* expression and symptoms do not correlate after treatment, but the authors point out that, although the animals were less hyperalgesic, the arthritic joints showed very little decrease in size. However, NSAIDs do decrease Fos count (and symptoms) if started early in the disease (at 1 week), and the suppression is greatest in layers 5–6. Similarly NSAIDs suppress the Fos increase in layers 1–2 in response to mechanical stimula-

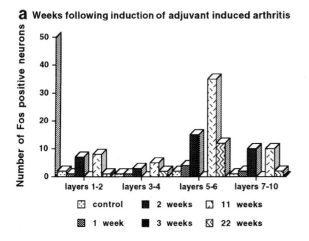

a Weeks following induction of adjuvant induced arthritis

Number of Fos positive neurons

layers 1-2   layers 3-4   layers 5-6   layers 7-10

control   2 weeks   11 weeks
1 week   3 weeks   22 weeks

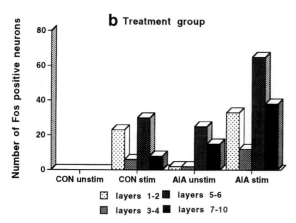

b Treatment group

Number of Fos positive neurons

CON unstim   CON stim   AIA unstim   AIA stim

layers 1-2   layers 5-6
layers 3-4   layers 7-10

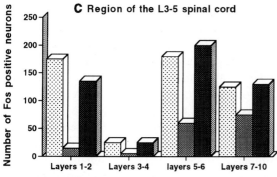

C Region of the L3-5 spinal cord

Number of Fos positive neurons

Layers 1-2   Layers 3-4   layers 5-6   Layers 7-10

AIA stimulated
AIA stimulated + morphine (3mg/Kg)
AIA stimulated +morphine (3mg/Kg) + naloxone (0.3mg/kg)

Fig. 4. (a) *fos*-positive neurons in L3 and L4 at different times post-Freund's adjuvant injection, in different layers of the spinal cord. *fos* expression was greatest in layers 5–6 at all time points. The peak counts were at 3 weeks, correlating with clinical signs of the arthritis in the animal. (b) *fos*-positive

tion in the AIA model. We can suggest, on the basis of these results, that the control of Fos in this chronic pain model in layers 5–6 is dependent on the afferent barrage at 1 week, but is less dependent on peripheral stimulation (and perhaps more self sustaining?) at 3 weeks. We postulate that the initial monosynaptic pathway into the deeper layers has now been replaced by a more dominant polysynaptic pathway. Furthermore, Fos expression in layers 1–2 in the AIA model at 3 weeks does not reflect the continued afferent barrage, but when an increase in the barrage occurs with mechanical stimulation, an increase in *fos* does occur, and this increase is responsive to morphine and NSAIDs. This may imply that layers 1 and 2 in the spinal cord had adapted to the basal level of afferent input from the polyarthritis, and so showed little or no Fos expression. With further afferent stimulation, there was an increase in the level of input to the spinal cord and consequently an increase in Fos expression.

Expression of fos after nerve injury

We also have been looking at Fos expression in a neuropathic model developed by Bennett and Xie (1988). In this chronic constriction injury (CCI) model, one sciatic nerve is loosely ligated with chromic cat gut and ipsilateral hyperalgesia and allodynia (perception of non-painful stimulation

neurons in L3 and L4 in control (CON) and arthritic (AIA) rats. There are four groups CON and AIA; each either unstimulated or stimulated with mechanical pressure. The stimulus for the AIA animals was performed under anaesthesia. There are large increases, greater in the AIA than the CON animals, both superficially and in the deeper layers. Thus, despite the paucity of *fos* expression superficially in the unstimulated AIA animal, there are appropriate increases with stimulation. See text for further discussion. (c) The suppressive effect of morphine on mechanical stimulus-evoked *fos* expression in AIA animals. The effect of morphine is greater in layers 1–2. This is unlike studies of acute pain, where the greatest decreases are in the deeper layers. The effect is reversed by naloxone. For clarity the SEMs have been omitted. (From Abbedie and Besson, 1992, 1993a,b.)

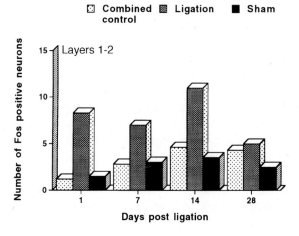

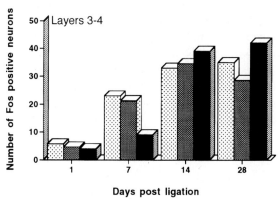

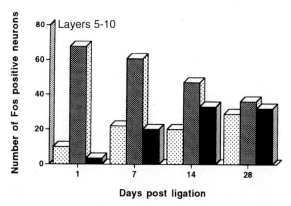

Fig. 5. Changes in *fos* expression with time in the Bennett and Xie (1988) mononeuropathic chronic constriction model. Layers 1-2 and 5-10 show intial increases, which then decrease to about control levels by 28 days. In contrast, layers 3-4 show an increase in *fos* numbers which persists at 28 days along with the hyperalgesic behaviour of the animals. Contrast this pattern of *fos* expression with that seen in Fig. 4a.

such as light touch as painful) develops over the following 7–10 days and persists for up to 7–8 weeks. This CCI model is known to be associated with partial loss of both myelinated and unmyelinated nerve fibres at the site of injury, but with a preferential loss of the myelinated fibres (Nuytten et al., 1992; Coggeshall et al., 1993). In some studies, the time course of the hyperalgesia corresponds to the loss of myelinated fibres (Gautron et al., 1990; Basbaum et al., 1991). Resolution of the hyperalgesia occurs as the myelinated fibres, including the A δ-fibres, appear histologically normal again (Guilbaud et al., 1993).

We have examined Fos expression in the spinal cord during development of the hyperalgesic state and attempted to relate it with behaviour. After the initial surge in Fos on the ipsilateral side at the time of ligation in layers 1–2 and 5–10, there was a decline in the numbers to control values by 28 days despite continuing hyperalgesia (see Fig. 5). Ectopic discharges from neuromas and dorsal root ganglia (DRG) are known to occur in this model (Kajander and Bennett, 1992; Kajander et al., 1992; Utzschneider et al., 1992). Yet, like the AIA model, there are no increases in Fos in the superficial layers. However, at 2 weeks, Fos-positive cells showed a bilateral increase in layers 3–4 in both sham and ligated animals. This increase was still present at 28 days (see Fig. 5). We also found that there was a striking inverse correlation between the ipsilateral *fos* count in layers 3 and 4 and the degree of mechanical hyperalgesia at 14 and 28 days in all animals (see Fig. 6).

This correlation is reminiscent of the correlation of Fos in layer 5 in the AIA model with 'disease state'. Layers 3 and 4 are the site of termination of the myelinated afferents, and the lower *fos* counts seen in the ligated CCI animals, compared to sham-operated animals, may reflect the greater damage to these myelinated fibres in the ligated animals. The trauma of a sham operation is known to be considerable with changes in levels of dorsal horn neuropeptides and transynaptic cell death (Nachemson and Bennett, 1993; Munglani et al., unpublished data). The increases in *fos* in the sham animals may relate to the greater numbers of myelinated fibres which are still intact. Normally, Fos expression in layers 3 and 4 is low (Hunt et al., 1987), but the up-regulation of second messenger pathways in the spinal cord in CCI may allow enhanced Fos expression (Mao et al., 1992). Molander et al. (1992) have shown how, after sciatic nerve injury, A-β strength stimulation will elicit more *fos* expression than in the uninjured nerve (Herdegen et al., 1991).

The data presented suggest that the fairly direct association of *fos* with nociceptive intensity seen with acute pain may not hold in chronic pain or after chronic nerve injury. Chronic pain state *fos* expression is, however, long-lasting rather than transient and may reflect the persistent molecular changes that underlie the physiological changes in these states.

Consequences of fos activation: relationship to preprodynorphin expression

Increases in Fos are seen in the dorsal horn in both arthritic and the nerve injury models. Similarly, increases in dynorphin have also been seen in both models (Millan et al., 1986; Iadarola et al., 1988; Kajander et al., 1990; Noguchi et al., 1991; Dubner and Ruda, 1992; Hunt et al., 1993). The increased expression of dynorphin is thought to occur in both local circuit and projection neurons which receive nociceptive afferent input (Takahashi et al., 1988; Nahin et al., 1989; Noguchi et al., 1991; Dubner and Ruda, 1992). Dynorphin is known to cause hyperalgesia when directly applied to the spinal cord (Knox and Dickenson, 1987; Dubner and Ruda, 1992), and it has been suggested that hyperalgesia seen in these pain states is due to the expression of dynorphin. Since the preprodynorphin gene has several AP1-like binding sites and may bind Fos (as a component of the AP1 transcription factor complex) it was tempting to speculate that Fos, as a component of the AP1, might directly lead to dynorphin expression. Certainly, Fos is expressed in the same dorsal horn cells as those expressing dynorphin

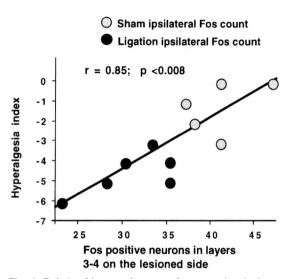

Fig. 6. Relationship seen between *fos* expression in layers 3–4 and mechanical hyperalgesia in the Bennett and Xie (1988) mononeuropathic chronic constriction model at 14 and 28 days post-ligation. Hyperalgesia is worse with more negative numbers. There is an inverse correlation between *fos* count and hyperlagesia. (Data adapted from Munglani et al., 1994.)

following noxious stimulation (Naranjo et al., 1991b; Noguchi et al., 1991), but it has not been possible to confirm that Fos expression leads to activation of an AP1 site on preprodynorphin.

The *jun* proto-oncogene and regeneration

Jun protein like Fos is induced *transynaptically* in the spinal cord after afferent nerve injury or noxious stimulation (Wisden et al., 1990). However *fos* is not seen in the DRG of the primary afferent fibre or motorneuron nuclei, even after intense afferent electrical stimulation. However *jun* expression is seen in motorneurons and DRG after peripheral axon section or block of axoplasmic transport. Since there is no Fos under these conditions, Jun may act via homodimerization, dimerizing with *fos*-related antigens (Sonnenberg et al., 1989), or via cyclic AMP response element-binding protein (Brenner et al., 1989; Naranjo et al., 1991a) The kinetics of this induction are also different from that seen after transynaptic activation. After sciatic nerve section and ligation, c-*jun* mRNA increases in the injured nerve at 24 h (but not 2 h) were maintained until the end of the experiment (up to 100 days later) (Jenkins and Hunt, 1991; Leah et al., 1991) (see Fig. 7). In the CCI model, *jun* was present in the ipsilateral DRG at one day and continued to be seen until 28 days, and even 100 days (Hunt et al., 1993; Munglani et al., 1994).

In contrast to peripheral nerve injury, sciatic nerve injury proximal to the L4/5 DRG, i.e., dorsal root rhizotomy has much less of an effect in causing Jun expression (Jenkins et al., 1993a). This poor Jun response to central denervation is also associated with a poor response of the neuron in growing back towards the spinal cord (see Fig. 8). It is known that, after either peripheral axotomy or dorsal root rhizotomy, peripheral or central nerve sprouting can take place from adjacent nerve roots. The L3 dorsal root ganglia does not supply the sciatic, but contributes to the adjacent saphenous nerve, and is known to sprout in response to sciatic nerve damage (McMahon, 1992). If this L3 ganglia is analysed after sciatic

nerve axotomy, it too shows good peripheral sprouting and a strong Jun response after 7 days (see Fig. 8).

Thus, it is nerve growth rather than, or as well as, nerve injury that is associated with *jun* activation. Other neuronal markers also increase after nerve injury, for example actin, tubulin (Wong and Oblinger, 1990), GAP-43 (Van der Zee et al., 1989), and the neuropeptides galanin (Hökfelt et al., 1987), NPY (Wakisaka et al., 1991) and VIP (Shehab and Atkinson, 1986). However, most of these other neuronal markers change only in subsets of neurons at specific time points after injury. GAP-43, for example, increases in small-diameter sensory neurons initially, and only later includes the large-diameter DRG (Sommervaille et al., 1991). In contrast, *jun* expression is rapid and appears in all sensory neurons within 24 h (Jenkins and Hunt, 1991).

jun may act as a 'switch' for new patterns of responsiveness for the nerve to its environment, perhaps facilitating regrowth (Diamond et al., 1990; Berko-Flint et al., 1994). Further evidence linking Jun activation to regrowth, comes from the CNS lesion studies (Jenkins et al., 1993b,c); if

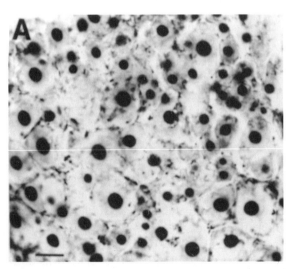 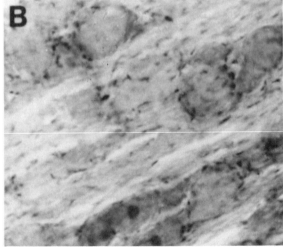

Fig. 7. *jun* activation in the L5 DRG in response to sciaitic nerve axotomy at one day. 'A' is the control side DRG and 'B' is the lesioned side. Bar = 100 μm.

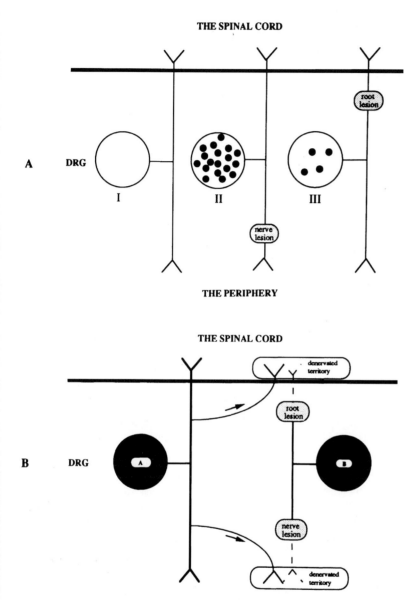

Fig. 8. Relationship between Jun activation in the DRG and nerve injury. (a) There is a greater Jun response in the DRG with distal nerve lesion than with dorsal root rhizotomy. (b) Jun activation in a DRG adjacent to an injured nerve. Again there is better Jun activation with distal nerve lesion than with dorsal root rhizotomy. The sprouting from the adjacent uninjured nerve correlates with the degree of Jun activation. See text for further details. (With permission, from Jenkins et al., 1993a.)

the nigro-striatal pathway is chemically axotomised with 6-hydroxydopamine, there is a substantial increase in Jun expression (but no Fos expression) in the substantia nigra pars compacta; unlike in the periphery, however, the increase peaks at 4–8 days and then declines by 14 days. Furthermore, regeneration in the CNS is known to be incomplete and collapse by day 14 (Björk-

294

land and Stenevi, 1979), and the transience of the
Jun response seen in the CNS may reflect this.
The Jun response in other parts of the CNS
varies. Neurones in the rubrospinal tract lesioned
at C3 show a Jun response at 8 days, while those
lesioned at T10 did not. There was also no GAP
43 or tα_1-tubulin response with the T10 lesion
(Jenkins et al., 1993). This finding may correlate
with the observation that peripheral nerve trans-
plants into the hemisected cord resulted in growth
of cut rubrospinal axons only when transplanted
at C3 but not at T10 (Richardson and Issa, 1984).
These findings indicate that failure of regeneration in the CNS is not due to a failure to initiate
gene expression characteristic of regeneration, but
a failure to maintain the regenerative processes
presumably because of inhibition from the glial
environment.

The nerve sprouting in the spinal cord that
accompanies Jun expression in the DRG after
peripheral nerve injury may contribute to the
setting up and maintenance of chronic pain states
(Woolf et al., 1992). This central sprouting leads
to central reorganisation of the spinal cord,
whereby the myelinated afferents from layers 3
and 4 (which are not considered to contain nociceptive input) grow into the area originally occu-
pied by the unmyelinated largely nociceptive fibres in the substantia gelatinosa. These sprouts
from the myelinated fibres may form synaptic
contacts within the more superficial layers and so
excite second order neurons in the spinothalamic
pain pathways. Thus non-noxious afferent stimulation carried by the myelinated input may be
perceived as noxious. This may be part of the
explanation of the phenomenon of allodynia in
chronic pain states.

Acknowledgements

We acknowledge other members of our laboratory, past and present; Bob Jenkins, Carmen De-
Felipe, James Palmer, Annette Bond, Judith Al-
lanson, Kerrie Thomas and Linda McNaughton,
from whose work we have drawn ideas for this
chapter. We would especially like to acknowledge
the work of Simon Williams who died in 1992.

References

Abate, C., Luk, D., Gentz, R., Rauscher, F.J., III, and Curran,
T. (1990) Expression and purification of the leucine zipper
and DNA-binding domains of Fos and Jun: both Fos and
Jun contact DNA directly. Proc. Natl. Acad. Sci. USA, 87:
1032–1036.
Abbadie, C. and Besson, J.M. (1992) C-fos expression in rat
lumbar spinal cord during the development of adjuvant-induced arthritis. Neuroscience, 48: 985–993.
Abbadie, C. and Besson, J.M. (1993a) C-fos expression in rat
lumbar spinal cord following peripheral stimulation in adjuvant-induced arthritic and normal rats. Brain Res., 607:
195–204.
Abbadie, C. and Besson, J.M. (1993b) Effects of morphine and
naloxone on basal and evoked Fos-like immunoreactivity in
lumbar spinal cord neurons of arthritic rats. Pain, 52:
29–39.
Abbadie, C. and Besson, J.M. (1994a) C-fos expression in the
spinal cord and pain related symptoms induced by chronic
arthritis in the rat are prevented by pretreatment with
Freunds adjuvant. J. Neurosci., in press.
Abbadie, C. and Besson, J.M. (1994b) Chronic treatments with
asprin or acetaminophen reduce both the development of
poly arthritis and Fos-like immunoreactivity in the rat
lumbar spinal cord. Pain, in press.
Abraham, W., Mason, S., Williams, J., Richardson, C., Tate,
W., Lawlors, P. and Dragunow, M. (1993) Corelations
between immediate early gene induction and the persis-
tance of long term potentiation. Neuroscience, 56: 717–727.
Angel, P., Hattori, K., Smeal, T. and Karin, M. (1988) The jun
proto-oncogene is positively autoregulated by its product,
Jun/AP-1. Cell, 55: 875–885.
Bading, H., Ginty, D.D. and Greenberg, M.E. (1993) Regulation of gene expression in hippocampal neurons by distinct
calcium signaling pathways. Science, 260: 181–186.
Barres, B.A. (1991) New roles for glia. J. Neurosci., 11(12):
3685–3694.
Bartel, D.P., Sheng, M., Lau, L.F. and Greenberg, M.E. (1989)
Growth factors and membrane depolarization activate distinct patterns of early response genes: dissociation of fos
and jun induction. Genes Dev., 3: 304–313.
Basbaum, A.I. and Fields, H.L. (1984) Endogenous pain control systems: brain stem spinal pathways and endorphin
circuitry. Annu. Rev. Neurosci., 7: 309–388.
Basbaum, A.I. and Wall, P.D. (1976) Chronic changes in the
response of cells in the adult cat dorsal horn following
partial deafferentation: the appearence of responding cells
in a previously non-responsive region. Brain Res., 116:
181–204.

Basbaum, A.I., Gautron, M., Jazat, F., Mayes, M. and Guilbaud, G. (1991) The spectrum of fibre loss in a model of neuropathic pain in the rat: An electron microscopic study. *Pain*, 47: 359–367.

Benbrook, D.M. and Jones, N.C. (1990) Heterodimer formation between CREB and JUN proteins. *Oncogene*, 5: 295–302.

Bennett, G.J. and Xie, Y.-K. (1988) A peripheral neuropathy in rat that produces disorders of pain sensation like those seen in man. *Pain*, 33: 87–108.

Berko-Flint, Y., Levkowitz, G. and Vardimon, L. (1994) Involvement of c-Jun in the control of glucocorticoid receptor transcriptional activity during the development of chicken retinal tissue. *EMBO J.*, 13: 646–654.

Berridge, M.J. (1993) Inositol trisphosphate and calcium signalling. *Nature*, 361: 315–325.

Bjorkland, A. and Stenevi, U. (1979) Regeneration of the monoaminergic and cholinergic neurons in the mammalian central nervous system. *Physiol. Rev.*, 59: 62–100.

Bowman, C.L. and Kimelberg, H.K. (1984) Excitatory amino acids directly depolarize rat brain astrocytes in primary culture. *Nature*, 311: 656–659.

Brenner, D.A., O'Hara, M., Angel, P., Chojkier, M. and Karin, M. (1989) Prolonged activation of *jun* and collagenase genes by tumour necrosis factor-α. *Nature*, 337: 661–663.

Burnashev, N., Khodorova, A., Jonas, P., Helm, P.J., Wisden, W., Monyer, H., Seeburg, P.H. and Sakmann, B. (1992) Calcium-permeable AMPA/kainate receptors in fusiform glial cells. *Science*, 256: 1566–1570.

Chiu, R., Angel, P. and Karin, M. (1989) Jun-B differs in its biological properties from, and is a negative regulator of, c-Jun. *Cell*, 59: 979–986.

Chiu, R., Boyle, W.J., Meek, J., Smeal, T., Hunter, T. and Karin, M. (1988) The c-*fos* protein interacts with c-*jun*/AP-1 to stimulate the transcription of AP-1 responsive genes. *Cell*, 54: 541–552.

Christy, B.A., Lau, L.F. and Nathans, D. (1988) A gene activated in mouse 3T3 cells by serum growth factors encodes a protein with 'zinc finger' sequences. *Proc. Natl. Acad. Sci. USA*, 85: 7857–7861.

Coggeshall, R.E., Dougherty, P.M., Pover, C.M. and Carlton, S.M. (1993) Is large myelinated fibre loss associated with hyperalgesia in a model of experimental peripheral neuropathy in the rat? *Pain*, 52: 233–242.

Cole, A.J., D.W. Saffen, J.M. Baraban and P.F. Worley (1989).Rapid increase of an immediate early gene messenger RNA in hippocampal neurons by synaptic NMDA receptor activation. *Nature*, 340: 474–476.

Curran, T., Gordon, M.B., Rubino, K.L. and Sambucetti, L.C. (1987) Isolation and characterization of the c-*fos* (rat) cDNA and analysis of post-translational modification in vitro. *Oncogene*, 2: 79–84.

De Felipe, C. and Hunt, S.P. (1994) The differential control of

c-Jun expression in regenerating sensory neurons and their associated glial cells. *J. Neurosci.*, 14:

Diamond, M.I., Miner, J.N., Yoshinaga, S.K. and Yamamoto, K.R. (1990) Transcription factor interactions: selectors of positive or negative regulation from a single DNA element. *Science*, 249: 1266–1271.

Dubner, R. and Ruda, M.A. (1992) Activity dependent neuronal plasticity following tissue injury and inflammation. *TINS* 15(3): 96–103.

Gautron, M., Jazat, F., Ratinahirana, H., Hauw, J.J. and Guilbaud, G. (1990) Alterations in myelinated fibres in the sciatic nerve of rats after constriction: Possible relationships between the presence of abnormal small myelinated fibres and pain-related behaviour. *Neurosci. Lett.*, 111: 28–33.

Gery, I. and Waksman, B.H. (1967) Studies of the mechanism where by adjuvant disease is supressed in rats pre treated with myobacteria. *Int. Arch. Allergy*, 31: 57–68.

Gogas, K.R., Presley, R.W., Levine, J.D. and Basbaum, A.I. (1991) The antinociceptive action of supraspinal opoids results from an increase in descending inhibitory control:correlation of behaviour and c-*fos* expression. *Neuroscience*, 42: 617–628.

Gold, B.G., Storm-Dickerson, T. and Austin, D.R. (1993) Regulation of the transcrition factor c-JUN by nerve growth factor in adult sensory neuron. *Neurosci. Lett.*, 154: 129–133.

Greenberg, M.E., Ziff, E.B. and Greene, L.E. (1986) Stimulation of neuronal acetylcholine receptor induces rapid gene expression. *Science*, 234: 80–83.

Guilbaud, G., Gautron, M., Jazat, F., Ratinahirana, H., Hassig, R. and Hauw, J.J. (1993) Time course of degeneration and regeneration of myelinated nerve fibres following chronic loose ligatures of the rat sciatic nerve: Can nerve lesions be linked to the abnormal pain-related behaviors? *Pain*, 53: 147–158.

Halzonetis, T.D., Georgeopoulos, K., Greenberg, M.E. and Leder, P. (1988) c-*jun* dimerizes with itself and with c-*fos* forming complexes of different DNA binding abilities. *Cell*, 55: 917–924.

Hebb, N.O. (1949) *The Organisation of Behaviour*. New York, Wiley.

Hengerer, B., Lindholm, D., Heumann, R., Ruther, U., Wagner, E. and Thoenen, H. (1990) Lesion inuced increase in nerve growth factor mRNA is mediated by c-*fos*. *Proc. Natl. Acad. Sci. USA*, 87: 3899–3903.

Herdegen, T., Kovary, K., Leah, J. and Bravo, R. (1991) Specific temporal and spatial distribution of JUN, FOS, and KROX-24 proteins in spinal neurons following noxious transsynaptic stimulation. *J. Comp. Neurol.*, 313: 178–191.

Hökfelt, T., Wiesenfeld-Hallin, Z., Villar, M. and Melander, T. (1987) Increase of galanin-like immunoreactivity in rat dorsal ganglion cells after peripheral axotomy. *Neurosci. Lett.*, 83: 217–220.

Hunt, S.P., Pini, A. and Evan, G. (1987) Induction of c-*fos* like protein in spinal cord neurons following sensory stimulation. *Nature*, 328: 632–634.

Hunt, S., Smith, G., Bond, A., Munglani, R., Thomas, T. and Elliot, P. (1993) Changes in immediate early genes, neuropeptides immunoreactivity and other neuronal markers in the spinal cord and dorsal root ganglion in a rat model of neuropathic pain. In: T. Hökfelt, H.-G. Schaible and R.F. Schmidt (Eds.) *Neuropeptides, Nociception and Pain*, Chapman Hall, London, 329–349.

Iadarola, M.J., Brady, L.S., Draisci, G. and Dubner, R. (1988) Enhancement of dynorphin gene expression in spinal cord following experimental inflammation: stimulus specificity, behavioural parameters and opioid receptor binding. *Pain*, 35: 313–326.

Jenkins, R. and Hunt, S. (1991) Long term increases in the levels of c-*jun* mRNA and Jun protein like immunoreactivity in motor and sensory neurons following axon damage. *Neurosci. Lett.*, 129: 107–111.

Jenkins, R., McMahon, S.B., Bond, A.B. and Hunt, S.P. (1993a) Expression of c-Jun as a response to dorsal root and peripheral nerve section in damaged and adjacent intact primary sensory neurons in the rat. *Eur. J. Neurosci.*, 5: 751–759.

Jenkins, R., O'Shea, R., Thomas, K.L. and Hunt, S.P. (1993b) c-Jun expression of immediate early genes in substantia nigra neurons following striatal 6-OHDA lesions in the rat. *Neuroscience*, 53: 447–457.

Jenkins, R., Tetzlaff, W. and Hunt, S.P. (1993c) Differential expression of immediate early genes in rubrospinal neurons following axotomy in the rat. *Eur. J. Neurosci.*, 5: 203–209.

Jensen, A.M. and Chiu, S.Y. (1990) Fluorescence measurement of changes in intracellular calcium induced by excitatory amino acids in cultured cortical astrocytes. *J. Neurosci.*, 10: 1165–1175.

Kajander, K.C. and Bennett, G.J. (1992) Onset of a painful peripheral neuropathy in rat: A partial and differential deafferentation and spontaneous discharge in Abeta and Adelta primary afferent neurons. *J. Neurophysiol.*, 68: 734–744.

Kajander, K.C., Sahara, Y., Iadarola, M.J. and Bennett, G.J. (1990) Dynorphin increases in the dorsal spinal cord in rats with a painful peripheral neuropathy. *Peptides*, 11: 719–728.

Kajander, K.C., Wakisaka, S. and Bennett, G.J. (1992) Spontaneous discharge originates in the dorsal root ganglion at the onset of a painful peripheral neuropathy in the rat. *Neurosci. Lett.*, 138: 225–228.

Knox, R. and Dickenson, A. (1987) Effects of selective and non-selective kappa-opioid receptor agonists on cutaneous C-fibre evoked responses of the rat dorsal horn neurones. *Brain Res.*, 415: 21–29.

Kouzarides, T. and Ziff, E. (1988) The role of the leucine zipper in the *fos-jun* interaction. *Nature*, 336: 646–651.

Lau, L.F. and Nathans, D. (1985) Identification of a set of genes expressed during G0/G1 transition of cultured mouse cells. *EMBO J.*, 4: 3145–3151.

Leah, J.D., Herdegen, T. and Bravo, R. (1991) Selective expression of Jun proteins following axotomy and axonal transport block in peripheral nerves in the rat; evidence for a role in the regeneration process. *Brain Res.*, 566: 198–207.

Lerea, L.S. and McNamara, J.O. (1993) Ionotropic glutamate receptor subtypes activate c-*fos* transcription by distinct calcium-requiring intracellular signaling pathways. *Neuron*, 10: 31–41.

Lucibello, F.C., Lowag, C., Neuberg, M. and Muller, R. (1988) Trans-repression of the c-*fos* promoter: a novel mechanism of *fos*-mediated trans-regulation. *Cell*, 59: 999–1007.

Macgregor, P.F., Abate, C. and Curran, T. (1990) Direct cloning of leucine zipper proteins: Jun binds cooperatively to the CRE with CRE-BP1. *Oncogene*, 5: 451–458.

Mao, J., Price, D.D., Mayer, D.J. and Hayes, R.L. (1992) Pain-related increases in spinal cord membrane-bound protein kinase C following peripheral nerve injury. *Brain Res.*, 588: 144–149.

McMahon, S.B. (1992) Plasticity of central terminations of primary sensory neurons in the adult animal. In: *Sensory Neurons. Diversity, Development and Plasticity*. New York, Oxford University Press. 333–362.

McNaughton, L.A., Lagnado, L., Socolovsky, M., Hunt, S.P. and McNaughton, P. (1990) Glutamate elevates free $[Ca_i]$ in type 1 astrocytes cultured from rat cerebral cortex. *J. Physiol.*, 424: 48P.

Menetrey, D. and Besson, J.D. (1982) Electrophysiological characterisitics of dorsal horn cells in rats with cutaneous inflammation resulting from chronic arthritis. *Pain*, 13: 343–364.

Milbrandt, J. (1987) A nerve growth factor-induced gene encodes a possible transcriptional regulatory factor. *Science*, 238: 797–799.

Millan, M.J., Millan, M.H., Czlonkowski, A., Hollt.V., Pilcher, C.W.T., Herz, A. and Colpaert, F.C. (1986) A model for chronic pain in the rat: response of multiple opioid systems to adjuvant-induced arthritis. *J. Neurosci.*, 6: 899–906.

Molander, C., Hongpaisan, J. and Grant, G. (1992) Changing pattern of c-*fos* expression in spinal cord neuron after electrical stimulation of the chronically injured sciatic nerve in the rat. *Neuroscience*, 50: 223–236.

Morgan, J.I., Cohen, D.R., Hempstead, J.L. and Curran, T. (1987) Mapping patterns of c-*fos* expression in the central nervous system after seizure. *Science*, 237: 192–197.

Morgan, J.I. and Curran, T. (1989) Stimulus-transcription coupling in neurons: role of cellular immediate-early genes. *TINS*, 12: 459–462.

Morgan, J.I. and T. Curran (1991) Stimulus transcription coupling in the nervous system: involvement of the inducible proto oncogenes c-*fos* and c-*jun*. *Annu. Rev. Neurobiol.*, 14: 421–451.

Muller, R., Bravo, D., Muller, D., Kurz, C. and Reiz, M. (1987) Different types of modification of c-*fos* and its associated protein p39: modulation of DNA binding by phosphorylation. *Oncogene Res.*, 2: 19–32.

Nachemson, A.K. and Benett, G.J. (1993) Does pain damage spinal cord neurons? Transsynaptic degeneration in rat following a surgical incision. *Neurosci. Lett.*, 162: 78–80.

Nahin, R.I., Hylden, J.L.K., Iadarola, M.J. and Dubner, R. (1989) Peripheral inflammation is associated with increased dynorphin immunoreactivity in both projection and local circuit neurons in the superficial dorsal horn of the rat lumbar spinal cord. *Neurosci. Lett.*, 96: 241–252.

Naranjo, J.R., Mellström, B., Achaval, M., Lucas, J.J., Del Rio, J. and Sassone-Corsi, P. (1991a) Co-induction of *jun* B and c-*fos* in a subset of neurons in the spinal cord. *Oncogene*, 6: 223–227.

Naranjo, J.R., Mellstrom, B., Achaval, M. and Sassone-Corsi, P. (1991b) Molecular pathways of pain: Fos/Jun-mediated activation of a noncanonical AP-1 site in the prodynorphin gene. *Neuron*, 6: 607–617.

Noguchi, K., Kowalski, K., Traub, R., Solodkin, A., Iadarola, M. and Ruda, M. (1991) Dynorphin depression and Fos-like immunoreactivity following inflammation induced hyperalgesia are colocalized in spinal cord neurons. *Mol. Brain Res.*, 10: 229–234.

Nakanishi, S. (1992) Molecular diversity of glutamate receptors and implications for brain function. *Science*, 258: 597–603.

Nuytten, D., Kupers, R., Lammens, M., Dom, R., Van, H.J. and Gybels, J. (1992) Further evidence for myelinated as well as unmyelinated fibre damage in a rat model of neuropathic pain. *Exp. Brain Res.*, 91: 73–78.

Peunova, N. and Enikolopov, G. (1993) Amplification of calcium induced gene transcription by nitric oxide in neuronal cells. *Nature*, 364: 450–457.

Presley, R.W., Menetrey, D., Levine, J.D. and Basbaum, A.I. (1990) Systemic morphine suppresses noxious stimulus-evoked Fos protein-like immunoreactivity in the rat spinal cord. *J. Neurosci.*, 10: 323–335.

Rauscher, F.J., III, Voulaslas, P.J., Franza, B.R., Jr. and Curran, T. (1988) Fos and Jun bind cooperatively to AP-1 site: reconstitution in vitro. *Genes Dev.*, 2: 1687–1699.

Richardson, P. and Issa, V.M.K. (1984) Peripheral injury enhances central regeneration of primary sensory neurons. *Nature*, 309: 791–793.

Ryseck, R.-P., Hirai, S.I., Yaniv, M. and Bravo, R. (1988) Transcriptional activation of c-*jun* during the G_0/G_1 transition in mouse fibroblasts. *Nature*, 334: 535–537.

Sakai, M., Okuda, A., Hatayama, I., Sato, K., Nishi, S. and Muramatsu, M. (1989) Structure and expression of the rat c-*jun* messenger RNA: tissue distribution and increase during chemical hepatocarcinogenesis. *Cancer Res.*, 49: 563–567.

Sassone-Corsi, P., Ransone. L.J., Lamph, W.W. and Verma, I.M. (1988) Direct interaction between *fos* and *jun* nuclear oncoproteins: role of the 'leucine zipper' domain. *Nature*, 336: 692–695.

Schutte, J., Viallet, J., Nau, M., Segal, S., Fedorko, J. and Minna, J. (1989) *jun*-B inhibits and c-*fos* stimulates the transforming and trans-activating activities of c-*jun*. *Cell*, 59: 987–997.

Shehab, S.A.S. and Atkinson, M.E. (1986) Vasoactive intestinal polypeptide increases in areas of the dorsal horn of the spinal cord from which other neuropeptides are depleted following peripheral axotomy. *Exp. Brain Res.*, 62: 422–430.

Smeyne, R.J., Montserrat, V., Hayward, M., Baker, S.J., Miao, G.G., Schilling, K., Robertson, L.M., Curran, T. and Morgan, J.I. (1993) Continuous c-*fos* expression precedes programmed cell death in vivo. *Nature*, 363: 166–169.

Sommervaille, T., Reynolds, M.L. and Woolf, C.J. (1991) Time-dependent differences in the increase in GAP-43 expression in dorsal root ganglion cells after peripheral axotomy. *Neuroscience*, 45: 213–230.

Sonnenberg, J.L., Macgregor-Leon, P.F., Curran, T. and Morgan, J.I. (1989) Dynamic alterations occur in the levels and composition of transcription factor AP-1 complexes after seizure. *Neuron*, 3: 359–365.

Sontheimer, H., Kettenmann, H., Backus, K.H. and Schachner, M. (1988) Glutamate opens Na^+/K^+ channels in cultured astrocytes. *Glia*, 1: 328–336.

Sukhatame, V.P., Cao, X., Chang, L.C., Rsai-Morris, C.-H., Stamenkovich, D., Ferreira, P.C.P., Cohen, D.R., Edwards, S.A., Shows, T.B., Curran, T., Le Beau, M.M. and Adamson, E.D. (1988). A zinc finger-encoding gene co-regulated with c-*fos* during growth and differentiation, and after cellular depolarisation. *Cell*, 53: 37–43.

Takahashi, O., Traub, R.J. and Ruda, M.A. (1988) Demonstration of calcitonin gene-related peptide immunoreactive axons contacting dynorphin A (1–8) immunoreactive spinal neurons in a rat model of peripheral inflammation and hyperalgesia. *Brain Res.*, 475: 168–172.

Tetzlaff, W. and Bisby, M.A. (1990) Cytoskeletal protein synthesis and regulation of nerve regeneration in PNS and CNS neurons of the rat. *Restorative Neurol. Neurosci.*, 1: 189–196.

Tetzlaff, W., Alexander, S., Miller, F. and Bisby, M. (1991) Response of facial and rubrospinal neurons to axotomy: changes in mRNA expression for cytoskeletal proteins and GAP-43. *J. Neurosci.*, 11: 2528–2544.

Tolle, T.R., Castro-Lopez, J.M., Evan, G. and Zieglgansberger, W. (1990). Opiates modify induction of c-*fos* proto-oncogene in the spinal cord following noxious stimulation. *Neurosci. Lett.*, 111: 46–51.

Tolle, T.R., Herdegen,T., Schadrack, J., Bravo,R., Zimmermann, M and Zieglgansberger, W. (1994) Application of morphine prior to noxious stimulation differentially modulates expression of Fos, Jun and Krox-24 proteins in rat spinal cord neurons. *Neuroscience*, 58: 305–321.

298

Utzschneider, D., Kocsis, J. and Devor, M. (1992) Mutual excitation among dorsal root ganglion neurons in the rat. *Neurosci. Lett.*, 146: 53–56.

Van der Zee, C.E.E.M., Nielander, H.B., Vos, J.P., Lopes da Silva, S., Verhaagen, J., Oestreicher, B., Schrama, L.H., Schotman, P. and Gispen, W.H. (1989) Expresssion of growth-associated protein B-50 (GAP43) in dorsal root ganglia and sciatic nerve during regenerative sprouting. *J. Neurosci.*, 9: 3505–3512.

Wakisaka, S., Kajander, K.C. and Bennett, G.J. (1991) Increased neuropeptide Y (NPY)-like immunoreactivity in rat sensory neurons following peripheral axotomy. *Neurosci. Lett.*, 124: 200–203.

Williams, S. (1991) *C-Fos Induction in Spinal Neurons by Sensory Stimulation*. Cambridge University Press, Cambridge.

Williams, S., Pini, A., Evan, G. and Hunt, S.P. (1989) Molecular events in the spinal cord following sensory stimulation. In: *Processing of Sensory Information in the Superficial Dorsal Horn of the Spinal Cord*. New York, Plenum Press, pp. 273–284.

Williams, S., Evan, G. and Hunt, S. (1990a) Spinal c-*fos* induction by sensory stimulation in neonatal rats. *Neurosci. Lett.*, 109: 309–314.

Williams, S., Evan, G.I. and Hunt, S.P. (1990b) Changing patterns of c-*fos* induction in spinal neurons following thermal cutaneous stimulation in the rat. *Neuroscience*, 36: 73–81.

Williams, S., Evan, G. and Hunt, S.P. (1991) C-*fos* induction in the spinal cord after peripheral nerve lesion. *Eur. J. Neurosci.*, 3: 887–894.

Wisden, W. and Seeburg, P.H. (1993) Mammalian inotropic glutamate receptors. *Curr. Opin. Neurobiol.*, 3: 291–298.

Wisden, W., Errington, M.L., Williams, S., Dunnett, S.B., Waters, C., Hitchcock, D., Evan, G., Bliss, T.V. and Hunt, S.P. (1990) Differential expression of immediate early genes in the hippocampus and spinal cord. *Neuron*, 4: 603–614.

Wong, J. and Oblinger, M.M. (1990) A comparison of peripheral and central axotomy effects on neurofilament and tubulin gene expression in rat dorsal root ganglion neurons. *J. Neurosci.*, 10: 2215–2222.

Woolf, C.J., Shortland, P. and Coggeshall, R.E. (1992) Peripheral nerve injury triggers central sprouting of myelinated afferents. *Nature*, 355: 75–78.

Worley, P.F., Bhat, R.V., Baraban, J.M., Erickson, C.A., McNaughton, B.L. and Barnes, C.A. (1993) Thresholds for synaptic activation of transcription factors in hippocampus: correlation with long-term enhancement. *J. Neurosci.*, 13: 4776–4786.

Wyllie, D.J., Mathie, A., Symonds, C.J. and Cull-Candy, S.G. (1991) Activation of glutamate receptors and glutamate uptake in identified macroglial cells in rat cerebellar cultures. *J. Physiol.*, 432: 235–258.

Young, A.B. and Fagg, G.E. (1990) Excitatory amino acid receptors in the brain: membrane binding and receptor autoradiographic approaches. *Trends Pharmacol. Sci.*, 11: 126–133.

F. Nyberg, H.S. Sharma and Z. Wiesenfeld-Hallin (Eds.)
Progress in Brain Research, Vol 104
© 1995 Elsevier Science BV. All rights reserved.

CHAPTER 17

Immediate early genes (IEGs) encoding for inducible transcription factors (ITFs) and neuropeptides in the nervous system: functional network for long-term plasticity and pain

T. Herdegen and M. Zimmermann

University of Heidelberg, II. Institute of Physiology, Im Neuenheimer Feld 326, 69120 Heidelberg, Germany

Introduction

Lasting biochemical and functional changes in the nervous system following physiological or pathophysiological stimulation often involve mechanisms at the level of gene expression. Among the earliest steps of these processes is the rapid induction of immediate early genes (IEGs). In vitro studies on neuronal and non-neuronal cells have established that IEGs are induced by growth factors, hormones or peptides. Among the best studied IEGs are those of *fos* (c-*fos*, *fos*B, fra-1, fra-2), *jun* (c-*jun*, *jun*B, *jun*D) and krox (krox-20, krox-24) families. These IEGs encode for inducible transcription factors (ITFs), a group of nuclear proteins that bind to regulatory DNA promotor and enhancer sites and control the transcription of numerous target or effector genes. This sequence of events turned out to be a fairly universal master switch of stimulation-transcription coupling. Apart from ITFs, IEGs also encode for secretory proteins, enzymes or membrane receptors.

Hunt and his colleagues (1987) were the first to discover that the c-Fos protein was expressed in spinal neurons of rats in vivo within one hour of sensory stimulation of the skin. More recent research has provided evidence that at least 20 ITFs can be induced by stimuli in the adult nervous system in vivo. Therefore, the question naturally arose whether activation of ITFs is a clue underlying those long-lasting changes in the nervous system that are associated with a diversity of systemic functions such as learning, physiological adapation to new environments and persistent neurological diseases including spasticity or chronic pain.

In this article we review findings on ITFs in the nervous system, and our particular emphasis is on their relationship with neuropeptides contributing to the processes of neuronal plasticity during pain and nerve fiber damage.

Functions of inducible transcription factors (ITFs)

ITFs are proteins encoded by IEGs that become induced within a few minutes when an eukaryotic cell is exposed to a stimulus such as growth hormones, transmitters, peptides or transmembraneous ion fluxes (Krujier et al., 1984; Lau and Nathans, 1985; Bravo et al., 1987; Almendral et al., 1988; Bartel et al., 1989; Bading et al., 1993). At present some 100 IEGs have been identified by screening in vitro systems, the majority encoding for transcription factors. Some of them are homologous to viral (v-) oncogenes and have therefore been termed cellular (c-) or proto-oncogenes such as c-*fos* and c-*jun* (Curran et al., 1984; Bohmann et al., 1987; Angel et al., 1988; Ryder et al., 1988; Ryseck et al., 1988). Viral oncogenes induce abnormal deregulated growth resulting in oncogenesis, whereas their cellular counterparts and the remaining ITFs have general functions in gene control affecting the regulation of growth, differentiation and alterations in the cellular programme (reviewed by Angel and Karin, 1991; see also Bravo, 1990; He and Rosenfeld, 1990; Ransone et al., 1990; Sheng and

Greenberg, 1990; Vogt and Bos, 1990; Herschman, 1991; Morgan and Curran, 1991).

Sequence of events in stimulation-transcription coupling

The special feature of ITFs is their de novo expression induced by external stimuli. The sequence of events between an external stimulus to a neuron and the expression of genes is comprised by the concept of 'stimulation-transcription-coupling' (Morgan and Curran, 1991). This sequence consists of several steps (Fig. 1). First, a synaptic or humoral stimulus results in increased intraneuronal levels of second messengers, e.g., of calcium, cAMP, cGMP or diacylglycerol. Subsequently, cytoplasmic protein kinases, such as PKA,

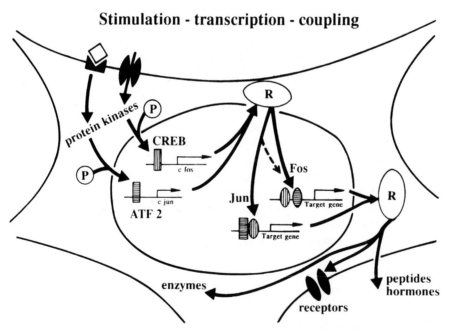

Fig. 1. Sequence of cytoplasmic and nuclear events between transmembrane stimulation and expression of effector/target genes: 'stimulation-transcription-coupling'. (1) Binding of ligands to membrane receptors or transynaptic ion fluxes activate cascades of protein kinases (2), which in turn phosphorylate (P) constitutively expressed transcription factors, i.e., CREB, SRF or ATF-2, in the nucleus. (3) Phosphorylated CREB, SRF or ATF-2 initiate transcription of c-*jun* and c-*fos* genes encoding for proteins that act as transcription factors. (4) Following translation in the ribosomes ®, Jun and Fos proteins form variable heterodimers and trans-activate the promotors of target genes which (5) finally encode for various effector proteins.

PKC, PKG, CaMK or casein kinases, are activated and/or translocated to the nucleus. These enzymes catalyse the phosphorylation of constitutive (i.e., already present) transcription factors, e.g. CREB (calcium response element-binding protein), SRF (serum response factor) and/or ATF-2 (activating transcription factor 2) which, in turn, bind to high-affinity DNA consensus sequences in the promotor region of ITFs and activate the mRNA polymerase II (Gonzalez et al., 1989; Sheng et al., 1990; Treisman, 1990; Ginty et al., 1992, 1993; Bading et al., 1993; van Dam et al., 1993).

Dimerization and post-translational modifications of Jun and Fos proteins

Jun and Fos proteins, also termed AP-1 proteins, tend to form heterodimers and thereby enhance their DNA binding affinity and the transactivation of their target genes (Angel et al., 1988; Halazonites et al., 1988; Nakabeppu et al., 1988; Rauscher et al., 1988; Gentz et al., 1989; Ryseck and Bravo, 1991). Furthermore, by interacting with other transcriptionally operating proteins such as ATF proteins or steroid hormone receptors, Jun and Fos proteins form a nuclear link between independent second messenger systems (Hai and Curran, 1991; Hagmeyer et al., 1993).

Jun and Fos proteins can also act as suppressors of gene transcription depending on the structure of their DNA binding sites (Schütte et al., 1989; Deng and Karin, 1993) or on alterations in the sequence of amino acids, as reported for the truncated form of *fos*B (Lazo et al., 1991; Nakabeppu and Nathans, 1991). Thus, the late and persistent FosB immunoreactivity following noxious stimulation, epileptic seizures and ischemia (Herdegen et al., 1991a,b, 1994b; Gass et al., 1993a,b) might also label the truncated FosB that can terminate the transcriptional operations initiated by its homologous family member c-Fos.

Finally, the formation of dimers, the binding to DNA regulatory sites and the transactivation of

ITFs are efficiently controlled by post-translational modifications. For example, phosphorylation of the C-terminus of c-Jun inhibits its binding to the DNA, and phosphorylation of the N-terminus of c-Jun increases its potency of transactivation (Pulverer et al., 1991; Boyle et al., 1992; Papavassiliou et al., 1992).

Inducible transcription factors in the nervous system

Because of their known general function in the control of the cell cycle, ITFs were originally associated with the development and differentiation of neurons (He and Rosenberg, 1991; Ingraham et al., 1989; Wilkinson et al., 1989). It was a matter of general excitement in the neurosciences some years ago to see expression of ITFs as a cellular and physiological response of neurons to exogenous stimuli (Hunt et al., 1987; Morgan et al., 1987; Sagar et al., 1988). Particularly, expression of c-Fos induced by sensory stimuli or pathophysiological conditions has been used, for metabolic mapping at the nuclear level, to explore the topographical distribution of nervous system activity (Sagar et al., 1988), e.g., following epileptic seizures (Morgan et al., 1987), noxious stimulation (Hunt et al., 1987; Bullitt, 1989; Menetrey et al., 1989) or stress (Ceccatelli et al., 1989).

Comparative studies show different temporo-spatial patterns of ITF expression. For instance, the zinc finger protein, Krox-24 (synonyms are NGFI-A, Egr-1, Zif/268), shows a strong expression in the brain of untreated rats that partially depends on NMDA-mediated synaptic input and can also be induced by axotomy. In contrast, the expression of the partially homologous protein, Krox-20 (synonym is Egr-2), is restricted to few neuronal populations and is up-regulated only following most intense stimuli such as epileptic seizures or displacement of neurons for cell culture experiments (Cole et al., 1989; Mack and Mack, 1992; Gass et al., 1993b; Herdegen et al., 1990, 1993a,c, 1995). Therefore, the comprehensive and comparative investigations of the expression of related ITFs provide a more complete insight into the genetic changes following experimental stimuli or manipulations.

In systematic studies we have addressed the induction of c-Jun, JunB, JunD, c-Fos, FosB, Krox-20 and Krox-24 proteins. Here we summarize our findings that are mainly related to ITF expression by noxious stimuli or axotomy and to subsequent alterations in peptide expression.

The study of ITF expression to map the central pain system

Hunt and his colleagues (1987) were the first to show, by immunocytochemistry, that expression of c-Fos protein occurs in vivo in the nuclei of dorsal horn neurons after noxious stimulation. This finding has been repeatedly confirmed (Bullitt et al., 1989; Menetrey et al., 1989; Presley et al., 1990). More recently, it was shown that nociceptive input to spinal and medullary neurons also results in the expression of other ITFs such as c-Jun, JunB, JunD, FosB, Nur77 or their mRNAs (Herdegen et al., 1990, 1991a,b, 1994b; Wisden et al., 1990; Walther et al., 1991; Naranjo et al., 1991a; Honkaniemi et al., 1992; Chan et al., 1993; Traub et al., 1993; Lanteri-Minet et al., 1993b, 1994; Tölle et al., 1994). The question arises whether these expressions are universal or whether they show specific patterns and relationships that depend on the context of pathophysiological events?

Pain related ITF expression in the spinal cord

In order to study the contribution of the different somatosensory afferent fibers to ITF expression in spinal dorsal horn neurons, we performed repetitive electrical stimulation of the sciatic nerve at various stimulation intensities. Stimulation of large A-fibers alone did not induce ITFs beyond base expression in the area of termination of sciatic nerve fibers (Herdegen et al., 1991a). However, when electrical stimulation also included Aδ- and C-fibers, many neurons of the ipsilateral dorsal horn showed nuclear labelling

for Jun, Fos and Krox proteins. c-Jun, JunB, c-Fos and Krox-24 were detected between 30 and 45 min after the start of repetitive sciatic nerve stimulation; their levels of expression were at maximum between 2 and 3 h and declined to base levels between nociceptors in anesthetized (noxious skin heating) or awake (formalin injection) rats (Herdegen et al., 1991b, 1994b; Tölle et al., 1994) that revealed patterns of spinal ITF expression which were rather congruent to those evoked by electrical stimulation of sciatic fibers described in the preceeding paragraph.

The numbers of neuronal nuclei labelled for c-Fos, JunD and Krox-24 were fairly equally distributed between superficial and deep dorsal horn, whereas c-Jun and FosB were predominantly expressed in the superficial layers (Table I). Thus, provided that ITFs are colocalized in neuronal nuclei (Naranjo et al., 1991a), varying compositions of Jun and Fos complexes can be formed depending on the specific temporo-spatial expression of the individual partners (Fig. 2): within the first 2 h, dimers containing c-Jun, JunB and c-Fos can be formed in the superficial layers and JunB:c-Fos dimers in the deep layers. Later, between 10 and 24 h, AP-1 complexes may predominantly consist of FosB:JunD dimers. It is noteworthy that c-Jun and FosB, which have the highest DNA binding affinity and transactivation potency in vitro (Ryseck and Bravo, 1991), are expressed in a fairly low number of neurons in vivo compared to c-Fos or JunB. These findings suggest a meaningful control of ITF expression dependent on their transcriptional potency.

Pain-related ITF expression in the brain

Fos, Jun and Krox proteins induced by noxious cutaneous stimulation were also found in the brain (Bullitt, 1989, 1990; Herdegen et al., 1990; Honkaniemi et al., 1992; Lanteri-Minet et al., 1993b, 1994; Pertovaara et al., 1993; Walther et al., 1993). Importantly, the distribution of their immunoreactivities was only partially homologous to what is generally considered the central pain system (Fig. 3). Several areas with definite electrophysiological neuronal excitation by non-noxi-

TABLE I

Selective expression of Jun, Fos and Krox-24 proteins in different brain areas 2–4 h following injection of formalin into one hindpaw

	c-Jun	JunB	JunD	c-Fos	FosB	Krox-24
LRt	+	−	+ +	+ +	+	+
LC	+	−	+ +	+ +	+	+
PAG	+ +	+ +	+ + +	+ + +	+ +	+ + +
PV/CM	+	+ +	+ + +	+ + +	+	+ +

LRt, lateral reticular nucleus of medulla; LC, locus coeruleus; PAG, periaqueductal gray; PV/CM, periventricular and centromedial nucleus of thalamus. −, no labelled nuclei, +, 5–20, + +, 20–50, + + +, > 50 labelled neuronal nuclei per 50-μm section.

ous and noxious somatosensory stimulation do not express ITFs, including the dorsal column nuclei, ventrobasal complex of thalamus, hippocampus and cerebellum (Bullitt, 1990; Molander et al., 1992; Pertovaara et al., 1993; Herdegen, unpublished observations). Moreover, the neuronal distribution of ITFs did not reveal a distinct unilaterality, as should be expected from the neuroanatomical architecture of the lemniscal or extralemniscal systems (comprehensively reviewed by Besson and Chaouch, 1987).

Similar to the expression in the spinal cord,

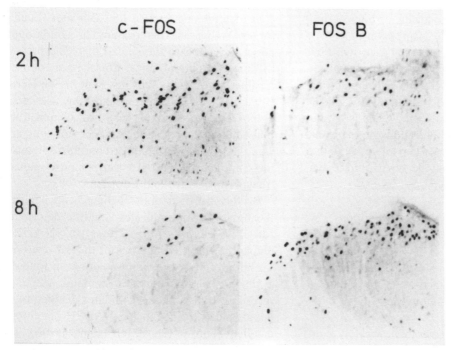

Fig. 2. Expression of c-Fos and FosB in the neurons of lumbar dorsal horn, 2 and 8 h following injection of 5% formalin into the ipsilateral hindpaw. In contrast to c-Fos, which reaches its maximum within 2 h and thereafter declines, levels of FosB expression are maximal not before 4 h and persist for up to 8 h. (From Herdegen et al., 1991b, 1994a.)

c-fos, JunD and Krox-24 showed the greatest numbers of labelled neurons in the brain areas studied, whereas c-Jun, JunB and FosB showed low prevalence or were even absent in some areas where c-Fos and JunD were strongly induced (Table I).

The pattern of supraspinal ITF expression described above is not specific for the application of cutaneous noxious stimulation and therefore does not map the 'pain system'. Expression of ITFs in the lateral reticular area of medulla, periaqueductal grey and medial thalamic or medial hypothalamic nuclei can be related to the stress and aversive components associated with the noxious condition. Handling of rats (Chan et al. 1993), activation of the baroreceptor reflex and changes in osmolarity (Sharp et al., 1991; McKitrick et al., 1992) evoke patterns of ITF expression in thalamic and hypothalamic nuclei similar to those observed following noxious events.

Interestingly, expression of ITFs can be seen in numerous brain areas in the untreated rat (Herdegen et al., 1994a) which show elevated levels of ITF expression following noxious peripheral stimulation. Thus, the expression of ITFs is not just a marker for neuronal activity; ITFs specifically indicate that processes have been activated at the nuclear level in selective neuronal populations. Therefore, the immunohistochemical detection of de novo synthetized ITFs is a valuable new tool to map alterations in neuronal functions that involve activation of transcription processes with subsequent de novo protein synthesis.

Expression of ITFs following persistent noxious stimulation and / or increase of stimulation intensity

Expression of ITFs in neurons depends on the intensity of transynaptic activation and other facilitatory or inhibitory conditions.

Facilitation of IEG expression

Conditioning treatments can affect the inducibility of ITFs. Thus, electrical stimulation of the proximal stump of the sciatic nerve 20 days after nerve transection was highly effective in inducing expression of c-Fos in neurons of spinal Lamina III and nucleus gracilis, whereas expression of c-Fos was not detectable in these areas following identical electrical stimulation paradigms of the intact sciatic nerve (Molander et al., 1992). Injection of formalin into the hindpaw 3 weeks following dorsal rhizotomy evoked an enhanced c-Fos expression in spinal neurons adjacent to the segment related to the transected root, compared with the injection of formalin only 2 days following the partial rhizotomy (Sugimoto et al., 1994). These observations suggest that, under pathophysiological conditions, neurons do not only alter their electrophysiological properties but also the activation of intraneuronal pathways, resulting in novel patterns of gene expression, and it is conceivable that these changes are interrelated.

In experiments using double noxious stimulations, we have shown that a first noxious stimulus enhances the induction of c-Fos that occurred in response to a second identical stimulus on the contralateral side applied 1.5–12 h later (Leah et al., 1992) (Fig. 3). This 'priming' or 'conditioning' effect is related to the spread of ITF expression to the contralateral spinal dorsal horn following noxious stimulation (Williams et al., 1990; Herdegen et al., 1991a). Interestingly, the use of the 2-deoxyglucose method has also demonstrated that unilateral noxious input does not only activate the ipsilateral spinal cord but also spreads to the contralateral cord at lower response intensity (reviewed by Porro and Cavazzuti, 1993).

By the use of double-labelling histochemistry, the functional prerequisites could be determined for ITF expression. Thus, in NADPH-diaphorase-labelled neurons of the rat deep dorsal horn, c-Fos expression was not seen following a single noxious cutaneous stimulus, whereas a second noxious stimulus 24 h later resulted in the appearance of c-Fos in the NADPH-diaphorase-labelled neurons (Herdegen et al., 1994b). This finding suggests that temporal summation or facilitation contributes to the induction of ITFs in these neurons. Following auditory stimulation

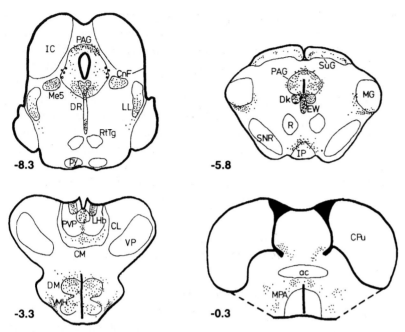

Fig. 3. Locations of c-*fos* immunoreactive cell nuclei in the brain 2 h following injection of 5% formalin into one hindpaw of awake rats. Each dot represents one immunopositive nucleus in a representative 50-μm section. The distribution of c-Fos-IR is symmetrical, i.e., does not show preference for the ipsi- or contralateral side of formalin injection. The numbers indicate the distances (mm) of frontal brain sections with reference to Bregma. (Herdegen, Leah and Zimmermann, unpublished observations) (Abbreviations are according to Paxinos and Watson, *The Rat Brain in Stereotaxic Coordinates*, Academic Press, 1989.)

numerous neurons expressed c-Fos in the auditory cortex, whereas cortical neurons that contain parvalbumin, a calcium binding protein, remained immunonegative (Zuschratter et al., 1994). This observation demonstrates that the effect of transmembrane stimulations on gene expression may depend on intervening biochemical variables that are also under the control of neuronal activity.

Inhibition or decrease of ITF expression

There is experimental evidence that the inducibility of ITFs can dramatically decrease in spite of ongoing sensory input or persistent stimulation of neurons. (i) Newborn cats exposed to visual stimuli show a strong expression of c-Fos in the visual cortex, whereas with increasing age and normal visual experience, c-Fos is no longer inducible by visual stimuli (Mower, 1993). (ii) Chronic monoarthritic inflammation of the hindpaw induces a strong ITF expression in the spinal cord within the first 48 h. Afterwards, expression of ITFs returns to basal levels at the time when reflex hyperalgesia and pain-related behavioral symptoms are at their maximum (Lanteri-Minet et al., 1993a). (iii) During daily seizures evoked by electrical shocks for 10 days, the inducibility of c-*fos* mRNA faded out in the brain, whereas the first electrical stimulation provoked a strong c-*fos* mRNA (Winston et al., 1990).

Thus, during ongoing neuronal stimulation the nuclear response typically decreases and eventually may be totally absent. This phenomenon is reminiscent of habituation observed at the behavioral and physiological levels during repeated administration of a stimulus.

The control of ITF expression by neurotransmitters and neuropeptides

Electrical activity of neurons per se is not a

sufficient condition for the expression of ITFs. KCl-induced membrane depolarisation is not followed by an increase of c-*jun* mRNA in fibroblasts (Bartel et al., 1989) and, similarly, cortical spreading depression elicited by topical KCl administration is almost ineffective in enhancing the levels of c-Jun and JunD (Herdegen et al., 1993d). However, under both conditions, c-Fos and JunB are expressed at high levels. Other examples of selective ITF expression depend on the activation of postsynaptic adenosine and adrenergic receptors in neurons (Gubits et al., 1989; Carter, 1992).

In vitro experiments

Superfusion of neuronal and non-neuronal cells with neuropeptides, neurotransmitters and trophic factors interacting with membrane-bound receptors have demonstrated that IEGs are induced by a variety of intracellular pathways.

Stimulation of quiescent fibroblasts by trophic factors such as EGF (epidermal growth factor), NGF (nerve growth factor) or PDGF (platelet-derived growth factor) results in the induction of numerous IEGs, including the genes encoding for ITFs. This rapidly emerging wave of induced genes is followed by alterations in metabolism, progress through the cell cycle and/or differentiation (Lau and Nathans, 1985; Bravo et al., 1987; Almendral et al., 1988; Bartel et al., 1989). Block of expression or inhibition of function of Fos and Jun proteins resulted in severe disturbances of cell cycle and cell growth, and also interfered with the cellular differentiation (Nishikura and Murray, 1987; Kovary and Bravo, 1991; Schlingensiepen et al., 1993; Pfarr et al., 1994).

Peptides, such as neurokinin A, have been described as efficient inducers of c-Fos and c-Jun in muscle cells. Thus, in this type of cell, the effects of neuropetides on differentiation and growth may involve ITF expression (Hultgardh-Nilsson et al., 1990). In cortical neurons, c-Fos is induced by VIP (vasoactive intestinal peptide) via NMDA-de-

pendent pathways suggesting that the trophic actions of VIP are associated with the activation of gene transcription (Hisanaga et al., 1992).

Dissociation and maintenance in culture of adult rat dorsal root ganglia provokes an eruptive expression of ITFs, including JunB, c-Fos, FosB, and Krox-20. These alterations have not been observed in vivo (Herdegen et al., 1993c; Herdegen and Zimmermann, 1994), which suggests that in vitro stimulation threshold and pathways for ITF induction are very different from the in situ conditions.

Mediators of ITF expression in spinal neurons following noxious afferent stimulation

Many studies over the past years have focussed on ITF expression in the spinal cord following noxious and non-noxious stimulation. Several synaptic input systems could be identified that contribute to the activation of rapidly inducible transcription factors (Zieglgänsberger and Tölle, 1993).

Apart from Krox-24 in Lamina III of the lumbar spinal cord, and a constitutive expression of JunD (Herdegen et al., 1991a; Tölle et al., 1994), ITFs are absent in the dorsal horn under normal physiological conditions, i.e., during activation by physiological extero- and proprioceptive input of daily life. A significant increase in the levels of ITFs depends on the activation of afferent Aδ- and C-fibers (Hunt et al., 1987; Herdegen et al., 1991a; Molander et al., 1992).

Neuropeptides and neurotransmitters as transynaptic inducers of ITFs

The importance of nociceptive afferent fibers in transynaptic induction of ITFs has suggested the involvement of peptidergic transmission to the spinal neurons. Peptides such as substance P, CGRP and galanin are predominantly expressed in small-diameter dorsal root ganglion (DRG) neurons and transported within the non-myelinated afferent fibers (Lawson et al., 1993).

Destruction of substance P-containing afferent fibers, by neonatal application of capsaicin, attenuates c-Fos expression following noxious cutaneous stimulation in adult animals (Hylden et al., 1992).

For ITF induction, neuropeptides cooperate with glutamate, since both compounds are co-released following C- but not A-fiber stimulation (Xu et al., 1990, 1992; Al-Ghoul et al., 1993). Behavioral symptoms, nociception and central sensitization following acute inflammation are mediated by NMDA-receptor operated calcium channels (Coderre and Melzack, 1992; Wu et al., 1992). However, block of NMDA-operated channels by the non-competitive antagonist, MK-801, does not reduce the subsequent expression of ITFs by noxious peripheral stimulation (Tölle et al., 1991, 1994). Because MK-801 reduces only the late tonic behavior, but not the acute phase behavior, following subcutaneous formalin application (Coderre and Melzack, 1992), and because ITFs are induced and expressed within 30–40 min (Herdegen et al., 1991a; Demmer et al., 1993), ITFs are concluded to be driven by the input from the acute phase that is not sensitive to blockade of NMDA receptors. Thus, other rapidly acting processes have to be involved in ITF induction.

Substance P and serotonin are released in the spinal cord by afferent noxious stimulation (Duggan et al., 1988), and electron microscopy has shown that varicosities containing substance P or serotonin directly contact those spinal dorsal horn neurons which express c-Fos following cutaneous application of mustard oil (Pretel and Pierkut, 1991).

Endogenous opioids can contribute to the suppression of ITFs following painful events: systemic application of morphine reduces the ITF expression in spinal cord neurons in a naloxone-reversible manner following peripheral noxious stimulation (Presley et al., 1990; Abaddie and Besson, 1993; Tölle et al., 1994). Thus, apart from acute analgesic effects, the release of opioids and the increase of opioid binding sites (Besse et al.,

1992) might also display a further delayed component of opioid functions, e.g., the inhibition of transcriptional operations.

Nitric oxide (NO) and nitric oxide synthase (NOS)

The gas molecule nitric oxide has become a focus of attention in neurobiology because it represents a novel class of neurotransmitter that, alone or in concert with glutamate, stimulates neurons (reviewed by Bredt and Snyder, 1992; see also Moncada, 1991) and evokes lasting alterations in the function of neurons. NO and its catalyzing enzyme NOS are most likely involved in a spinal neuronal network contributing to IEG expression, as suggested by the following findings: (1) the induction of c-Fos in spinal neurons following noxious cutaneous stimulation can be diminished by inhibition of NO synthesis prior to noxious stimulation (Lee et al., 1992); (2) immunohistochemical double labelling for reduced nicotinamide-adenine dinucleotide phosphate (NADPH) diaphorase (indicating the presence of NOS) and Jun, Fos and Krox proteins has revealed that many dorsal horn neurons labelled by ITFs, following subcutaneous application of formalin, are in close proximity to fibers labelled by NADPH diaphorase (Herdegen et al., 1994b); (3) on the other hand, ITFs might be involved in the transcriptional control of the NOS gene because subcutanous formalin increases NOS expression in neurons of the superficial dorsal horn that express the highest levels of ITFs and show co-expression of NOS and ITFs (Herdegen et al., 1994b).

Thus, induction of NOS and ITFs may be multiply interrelated in spinal cord neurons, and this interaction might be part of the hyperalgesic effects of NO (Haley et al., 1992). From the findings reported above we hypothesize the following cascade of events: afferent noxious stimulation evokes the release of neuropeptides and NO from primary afferents resulting in the expression of ITFs in dorsal horn neurons and, subsequently, in the up-regulation of NOS expression after 10 and 24 h in some of these neurons. The ensuing increased synthesis of NO then results in hyper-excitation of spinal neurons with concomitant hyperalgesia (Meller and Gebhart, 1993).

Intracellular messengers involved in mediation of stimulation-transcription coupling

The cascade of post-synaptic events between neuronal surface receptors and transcription of genes encoding for ITFs has been extensively reviewed as it emerges from in vitro experiments (Sheng and Greenberg, 1990; Treisman, 1990; Ginty et al., 1992; Delmas et al., 1994). In summary, three major pathways were identified that terminate onto the promotor sites of *jun*, *fos* and K*rox* genes: (i) stimulation of protein kinase A (PKA) or calcium/calmodulin kinases (CaMK) by calcium or cAMP with subsequent phosphorylation of CREB and activation of CRE promotor sites, (ii) stimulation of protein kinase C (PKC) by diacylglycerol and subsequent activation of the TRE promotor sites, (iii) stimulation of casein kinase II and subsequent phosphorylation of SRF and activation of SRE promotor sites.

The activation of either of these pathways results in preferential induction of genes encoding for ITFs: phosphorylation of CREB and/or SRF are potent activators of c-*fos* (Treisman, 1991; Ginty et al., 1993) but not of c-*jun*. Similarly, stimulation of cGMP and cAMP pathways by NO and/or calcium induce c-*fos* and *jun*B but not c-*jun* and *jun*D (Peunova and Enikopolov, 1993; Purkiss et al., 1993; Haby et al., 1994). Thus, phosphorylation of CREB presumably is a crucial step in the activation of ITFs following transynaptic stimulation of neurons with a dominant expression of c-Fos and JunB ('c-Fos type' of induction) (Herdegen et al., 1991a,b, 1993d, 1994b; Gass et al., 1992, 1993a,b). In contrast, the transcriptional operations during the cell body response of axotomized neurons (see below, p. 309) are dominated by expression of c-Jun and JunD, and their selective and stable transcription might be independent of those second messenger pathways that terminate at the SRE, CRE and TRE consensus sequences (Herdegen et al., 1994c).

Transcription control of neuropeptides by Jun and Fos proteins

The genes of several neuropeptides and neurotransmitters contain binding sites for Jun and Fos (AP-1) proteins in their promotors, and therefore might belong to the pool of target genes controlled by these transcription factors. Dependent on their partner in dimerization, Jun and Fos proteins can activate AP-1 and/or CRE binding sites (Hai and Curran, 1991; Ryseck and Bravo, 1991), and these DNA consensus sequences have been found in genes encoding for somatostatin (Montminy and Bilezikjian, 1987), cholecystokinin

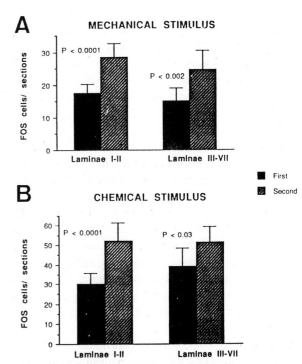

Fig. 4. 'Priming' of c-Fos expression by repeated noxious stimulation. Squeezing of the palmar hindpaw skin with a hemostat for 3 min (A) or injection of formalin into the hindpaw (B) induces c-Fos in the ipsilateral dorsal horn of lumbar spinal cord (first stimulus, black bars). Application of the same stimulus on the contralateral hindpaw 90 min after the first one (second stimulus, hatched bars) yields enhanced numbers of c-Fos labelled neurons by up to 80% compared to the numbers evoked by the first stimulus. (From Leah et al., 1992.)

(Monstein, 1993), preproenkephalin (Sonnenberg et al., 1989; Kobierski et al., 1991) and preprodynorphin (Naranjo et al., 1991b).

In addition, histochemical findings about sequential expression and colocalization of ITFs and neuropeptides have yielded evidence that Fos and/or Jun proteins are involved in the transcription control of neuropeptides in vivo. The rapid induction of c-*fos* mRNA and protein synthesis is followed, after a delay of one hour, by expression of preprodynorphin (Höllt et al., 1987; Draisci and Iadarola, 1989; Naranjo et al., 1991b). Preproenkephalin, which is only moderately induced following noxious stimulation (Draisci and Iadarola, 1991), exhibits a high co-localization with Fos proteins in spinal dorsal horn neurons following hindlimb inflammation (Noguchi et al., 1992). Because dynorphin and enkephalin have modulatory effects on the excitability of spinal neurons (reviewed by Dubner and Ruda, 1992; Coderre et al., 1993), the sequence of noxious input, ITF expression and increase in levels for these endogenous opioids can be considered as an example for the functional consequences of stimulation-transcription coupling (see Fig. 4).

Transection of nerve fibers induces long-lasting alterations in the expression of ITFs and neuropeptide peptides

Alterations in axotomized neurons

In nerve transection experiments we found a pattern of ITF expression that is in striking contrast to that observed following afferent noxious stimulation (see above, p. 302). Following transection of sciatic, vagus, facial or hypoglossal nerve fibers, increase in c-Jun and JunD expression starts in the axotomized neurons between 10 and 24 h following axotomy (Herdegen et al., 1992; Leah et al., 1991; Herdegen and Zimmermann, 1994), that is during the beginning of the chromatolysis, the major sign of the cell body response or axon response (Liebermann, 1971). Neither c-*fos* nor *fos*B mRNAs and proteins were detected in the injured neurons, whereas transient increases of

*jun*B mRNA without expression of JunB protein were reported in axotomized motoneurons of the facial nerve (Haas et al., 1993; Herdegen and Zimmermann, 1994). The Jun expression persisted for up to 20 days at maximal levels and, in the case of sciatic nerve transection, c-Jun was still suprabasal in small-diameter DRG neurons after 15 months. The selective expression of c-Jun and JunD in the absence of JunB, c-Fos and FosB proteins is a general finding in those peripheral and central neurons that show a cell body response following axotomy (Jenkins et al., 1991, 1993; Jones et al., 1991; Leah et al., 1991, Herdegen et al., 1992, 1993a; 1993; Koistinaho et al., 1993; reviewed by Herdegen and Zimmermann, 1994).

Most probably, the c-Jun response to nerve fiber lesion is mediated by the absence of target-derived signals normally transmitted retrogradely along axons, since blocking the axonal transport of the intact nerve with topical colchicine or vinblastine had similar results (Leah et al., 1991, 1993). Such signals would normally convey information on the intactness of the neuron-target axis, and thus suppress the regeneration-associated genes such as c-Jun, tubulin or GAP-43 (Tetzlaff et al., 1991; Strittmatter et al., 1992). Consequently, lack of these signals following nerve fiber transection results in disinhibition of c-*jun* transcription.

At the nuclear level, the selective induction of c-*jun* might be controlled by the ATF-2 transcription factor. ATF-2 is constitutively present in the rat nervous system (Herdegen and Gass, unpublished observations) and is activated following damage and/or disintegration of DNA organisation (van Dam et al., 1993). These pathological alterations are also part of the neuronal cell body response following axotomy. ATF-2 strongly activates the c-*jun* promotor (but is not effective for the c-*fos* promotor) and forms stable heterodimers with c-Jun. Thus, ATF-2 is a putative candidate for the induction of c-*jun* and the dimerization of the c-Jun protein (van Dam et al., 1993).

310

Functions of c-Jun *and its possible neuropeptide target genes during axonal regeneration*

The selective expression of c-Jun and JunD following axotomy suggests a crucial role for these ITFs in the regenerative response of neurons. In neurons that undergo neuronal cell death following axotomy, such as neurons of substantia nigra and retinal ganglion cells, decrease of c-Jun expression precedes the neuronal cell death. Rescue of the retinal ganglion cells, e.g., by grafting a peripheral nerve, evoked a prolonged up-regulation of c-Jun (Herdegen et al., 1993a; Herdegen and Zimmermann, 1994; Hüll and Bähr, 1994). The function of c-*jun* during the regenerative response might be related to its capacity to enhance the de novo protein synthesis. c-Jun is capable of accelerating the progression through the cell cycle and to generate neoplastic transformation not only in its viral (v-) but also in its cellular (c-) form (Angel and Karin, 1991; Pfarr et al., 1994). Increase of RNA turnover and protein synthesis is part of the cell body response (Lieberman, 1971; Grafstein, 1986) that could be triggered by the c-Jun transcription factor.

In order to explore the role of c-*jun* in the transcription control of effector genes, we investigated the association of this nuclear protein with the neuropeptides, galanin and CGRP, and the enzyme, nitric oxide synthase (NOS), in axotomized neurons. Many DRG neurons labelled for c-Jun after sciatic nerve transection also showed increased galanin immunoreactivity (IR) (Fig. 5), which is very low in untreated DRGs (Herdegen et al., 1993b). The time course of the increased galanin expression was nearly parallel to that of c-Jun, but it was clearly delayed (by 5–10 h). As to the possible function of galanin, this neuropeptide has been shown to exert inhibitory effects on spinal reflexes following deafferentation, and its increase in afferent fibers could contribute to a mechanism counteracting the hyperexcitability of spinal neurons following peripheral nerve lesion (Xu et al., 1990, 1992).

Sciatic nerve transection also increases the expression of CGRP in axotomized spinal motoneu-

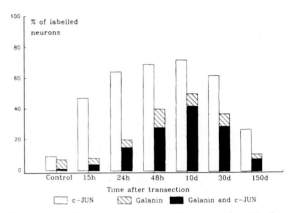

Fig. 5. Expression of c-Jun and galanin in neurons of ipsilateral L5 dorsal root ganglion following transection of the sciatic nerve in the rat. Open columns give the proportion of neurons labelled for c-Jun, hatched columns give the proportion of neurons labelled by galanin alone. Black columns give the percentage of neurons labelled for both galanin and c-Jun. Each column represents the mean of three sections each from three rats, selected at random (From Herdegen et al., 1993b.)

rons (Herdegen et al., 1993c). The increase in CGRP expression was preceded by a rise in c-*jun* levels by about 5 h, and c-Jun and CGRP had a high incidence of colocalization. CGRP regulates the synthesis of muscle acetylcholine receptors (New and Mudge, 1986), and thus contributes to the functional re-establishment of the neuromuscular junction after nerve regeneration.

These findings are in accordance with the hypothesis that the expressions of c-Jun and galanin as well as c-Jun and CGRP are functionally related and that the transcription of these neuropeptides are controlled by c-Jun as one of the transcription factors.

Axotomy also induces the expression of NOS which controls the synthesis of the novel messenger substance, NO, in many DRG neurons but not in motoneurons after sciatic nerve transection (Verge et al., 1992; Fiallos-Estrada et al., 1993). Histochemical double-labelling revealed that c-Jun and NOS were colocalized and were up-regulated by axotomy. The increase of c-Jun preceded the induction of NOS by 5 days, whereas the subsequent time courses of c-Jun-IR and NOS-IR were parallel for over 100 days. It is conceivable that c-Jun is involved in the control of NOS gene expression together with other, as yet unknown, transcription factors that are persistently up-regulated. The long time lag of 5 days suggests a more complex sequence of events being interposed between c-Jun and NOS transcription. The up-regulation of NOS in neurons of dorsal root ganglia, with the ensuing increased NO availability could be a mechanism to compensate for the decreased levels of substance P and CGRP in afferent neurons after nerve transection: both these peptides and NO have similar neurotransmitter effects in the periphery (neurogenic inflammation) and in the spinal dorsal horn (excitatory neurotransmission or neuromodulation) (Xu et al., 1990; Haley et al., 1992). Figure 6 summarizes these complex alterations in the associated expression and action of neuropeptides and ITFs.

Recent findings have extended the reaction patterns of neuropeptides following axotomy. The increase of NPY receptor mRNA and its shift from small- to large-diameter neurons in axotomized sciatic DRGs may reflect another adaptive response of damaged primary afferent neurons (Zhang et al., 1994), as well as the axotomy-triggered induction of VIP mRNA in sympathetic neurons (Mohney et al., 1993).

Altered expression of neuropeptides in deafferented spinal neurons

The experiments of Molander et al. (1992) have shown that spinal dorsal horn neurons alter their expressions of ITFs following axotomy (see above) afferent stimulation at an Aβ-fiber intensity that was ineffective for c-Fos induction in the normal rat, efficiently induced c-Fos following sciatic nerve transection. We have performed extensive investigations on changes of neuropeptide expression in spinal deafferented neurons (Leah

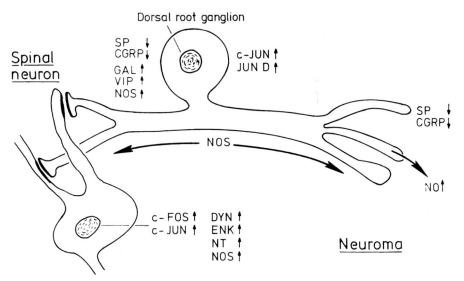

Fig. 6. Changes in protein expressions following sciatic nerve transection: schematic diagram of functional implications. In dorsal root ganglion neurons, the nuclear proteins c-Jun and JunD are expressed as the earliest genetic responses. They might control subsequent transcription of regeneration-associated genes. The transected axons start to regenerate by forming axonal sprouts. Contents in substance P (SP) and calcitonin gene-related peptide (CGRP) decrease over weeks, whereas galanin (GAL), vasoactive intestinal peptide (VIP) and nitric oxide synthase (NOS) are up-regulated over weeks. In dorsal horn neurons, c-Fos, c-Jun and Krox-24 are transynaptically induced following nerve transection, followed by up-regulations of dynorphin (DYN), enkephalin (ENK), neurotensin (NT) and NOS. Colocalizations, covariances and temporal order of expressions suggest that the IEG-encoded proteins act as transcription factors for the changes in biosynthesis of neuropeptides and NOS.

312

et al., 1988). Between 12 and 20 days after sciatic nerve cut, the lumbar spinal cord was exposed, colchicine was intrathecally applied and, after a further 24 h, the rats were killed. By means of immunocytochemistry, we observed significant increases in the number of neurons labelled for enkephalin, dynorphin and neurotensin in the ipsilateral lumbar dorsal horn (Herdegen et al.,

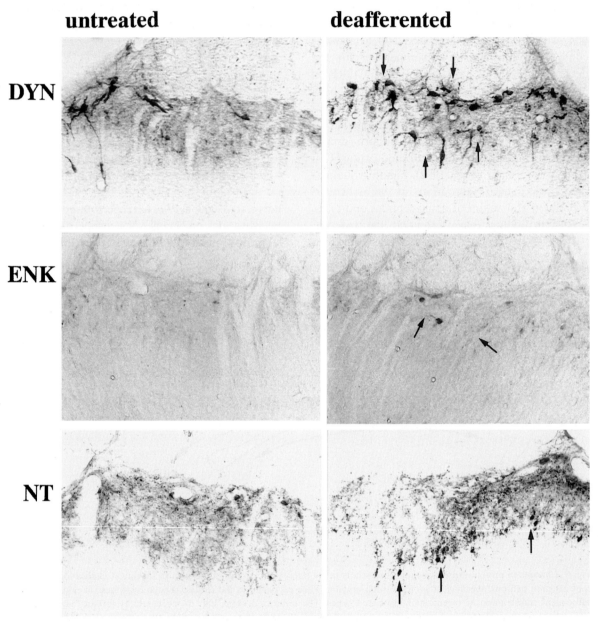

Fig. 7. Effect of sciatic nerve transection on the expression of neuropeptides in deafferented dorsal horn neurons. The numbers of dynorphin (DYN)- and enkephalin (ENK)- and neurotensin (NT)-labelled neurons in the medial superficial dorsal horn of L5 spinal cord is increased by 15 days following transection and ligation of the sciatic nerve (right hand side) compared to the contralateral untreated side (left hand side). Arrows mark neurons with increased immunoreactivities.

TABLE II

Increases in the numbers of neurons labelled for dynorphin (DYN), enkephalin (ENK) and neurotensin (NT) in Laminae I–III of rat L5 lumbar spinal cord 15 days following sciatic nerve transection

	n_1	n_2	Medial Laminae I–III		%	Lateral Laminae I–III		%
			untreated	transected		untreated	transected	
DYN	6	93	6.8 ± 2.0	9.9 ± 1.3	45.6**	7.0 ± 0.8	7.5 ± 1.2	7.7***
ENK	4	55	3.3 ± 1.1	5.1 ± 1.0	54.5**	5.3 ± 2.6	7.2 ± 2.3	35.8***
NT	5	69	2.5 ± 0.3	3.5 ± 1.0	40.0*	0.9 ± 0.4	1.2 ± 1.3	33.3***

For each neuropeptide, the mean $\pm$ S.D. was determined for both the medial and lateral parts of Laminae I–III on the side without (untreated) or with (transected) sciatic nerve transection.

n_1 = number of animals investigated; n_2 = total number of coronal 50-μm sections investigated; %, increase in the mean numbers of peptidergic neurons following sciatic nerve transection; *significant at $P < 0.05$; **significant at $P < 0.005$; ***not significant.

1988), (Fig. 7; Table II). We observed also an expression of ITFs in neurons of the superficial dorsal horn that is maximal within the first 24 h after nerve transection, and thereafter persists in a small number of neurons for up to 20 days (Leah et al., 1991). Taken together, these findings suggest a link of protein synthesis that begins with a rapid and rather transient expression of ITFs, and is followed by a delayed but persistent expression of neuropeptides.

Block of Jun and Fos expression by antisense-deoxynucleotides provokes alterations of stimulus-induced neuronal functions

The development of nuclease-resistant deoxynucleotides has opened a new stage in neurosciences. The design of deoxynucleotides complementary to RNA transcripts (antisense-deoxyoligonucleotides, ASO) offers the possibility to selectively block the translation of individual RNAs: extracellularly applied ASO pass through the cellular membrane by as yet unknown carriers, and associate selectively to its complementary native RNA strand. This association with ASO prevents the translation of the native mRNA, resulting in the loss of an individual protein with corresponding deficits in cell functions that can be studied by this assay.

Recent experiments have convincingly demonstrated the capability of ASO to selectively prevent expression of Jun and Fos proteins in vitro and in vivo. In cell culture of hippocampal neurons treated with ASO against c-jun or junB mRNA, the loss of c-Jun evokes an increase in neurite extension, whereas loss of JunB results in de-differentiation (Schlingensiepen et al., 1992, 1993). Overexpression of JunD and c-Jun in fibroblasts reveals that JunD normally has stabilizing effects on the cell cycle, whereas c-Jun accelerates the progress through the cell cycle that probably contributes to its potential for tumor transformation (Pfarr et al., 1994).

We have shown that superfusion of the lumbar spinal cord in anaesthetized rats with ASO against c-fos mRNA significantly reduces the expression of c-Fos, but not that of FosB or c-Jun proteins in the dorsal horn, when the ASO superfusion was performed several hours prior to noxious cutaneous stimulation (Gillardon et al., 1994) (Fig. 8). This experimental design offers the possibility to search for the functional role of ITFs in nociception and analgesia and in particular will help to identify target genes of ITFs under specific conditions.

In a recent experiment on rats, we have demonstrated that intraventricular injection of an ASO cocktail against c-fos and junB reduces the

c-fos ASO   **NSO**

c-Fos

c-Jun

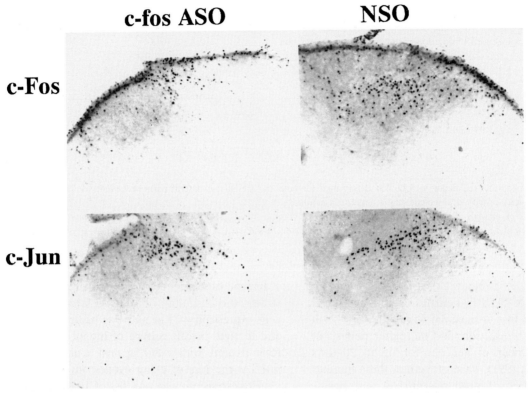

Fig. 8. Topical application of stabilized antisense-oligonucleotides against c-*fos* mRNA (anti-c-*fos* ASO) onto the lumbar spinal cord reduces the expression of c-Fos in dorsal horn neurons of rats following noxious skin heating of the hindpaws compared to topical application of nonsense-oligonucleotides (NSO) used as controls. In consecutive sections, application of anti-c-*fos*-ASO and NSO did not affect the expression of c-Jun.

expression of c-Fos and JunB in the suprachiasmatic nucleus. In animals that have been treated with these ASO, light cannot provoke a shift of the circadian rhythm as it does in control experiments (Wollnik et al., 1995). Figure 9 suggests a central position of ITF expression in the synchronisation of the circadian rhythms to the environmental light. This is the first demonstration of a physiological adaptation that can be prevented by interfering with transcription factors. Thus, local suppression of c-Fos and JunB that form the major AP-1 complexes following transynaptic stimulation can severely disturb fundamental biological processes in the nervous system.

Conclusions

The tenet of our contribution is that the induc-

tion of IEG-related ITFs indicates plasticity of function in the nervous system. This seems to be of great importance in relation to pain particularly to the transition from acute to chronic pain. Clinical observations suggest that an engram of pain may have formed in the CNS, e.g., in phantom pain or allodynia, which is thought to be due to persistent hyperexcitability of central neurons induced by a previous peripheral trauma. There is much support for this idea from animal experiments which have revealed that long-lasting modifications occur in the CNS in response to a noxious peripheral event or a lesion of a peripheral nerve. Experimental inflammation in the hindlimb is paralleled by slow biochemical and cellular processes in the spinal cord that may contribute to hyperalgesia. For example, tachykinin receptor mRNA and NOS are in-

315

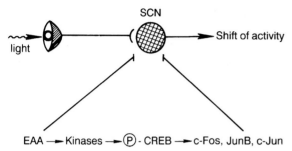

IEGs are part of the circadian synchronization

SCN

light → Shift of activity

EAA → Kinases → (P) - CREB → c-Fos, JunB, c-Jun

Fig. 9. Sequence between environmental stimuli, gene regulation and physiological neuronal responses in synchronization of diurnal rhythms: a one-hour light pulse applied to rats kept in constant darkness during the subjective night shifts the circadian locomotor. During this process, light pulses stimulate neurons in the suprachiasmatic nucleus (SCN) by presynaptic release of excitatory amino acid (EAA). In SCN neurons, activated protein kinases phosphorylate CREB (P-CREB) with subsequent induction of *jun* and *fos* genes resulting in expression of Jun and Fos transcription factors. Block of c-Fos and JunB expression by antisense-deoxy-oligonucleotides prevents the synchronization of the circadian rhythm with alterations of environmental stimuli. (From Wollnik et al., 1995.) These results demonstrate that c-Fos and JunB control the transcription of genes encoding for proteins which are responsible for the resetting of the 'zeitgeber' programme in SCN neurons.

creased in the spinal dorsal horn after a painful condition induced by subcutaneous injection of formalin (Noguchi and Ruda, 1992; Herdegen et al., 1993e). In the spinal cord of rats with an experimental arthritis, gene expression of prodynorphin mRNA and its product dynorphin is increased (Höllt et al., 1987; Ruda et al., 1988; Nahin et al., 1989) and opioid receptor binding is modified (Besse et al., 1992). Gene expression of prodynorphin and dynorphin in spinal dorsal horn neurons is dramatically increased after a peripheral nerve or spinal cord lesion (Przewlocki et al., 1988). Spinal neurons develop abnormal hyperactivity after transection of dorsal roots in rats (Lombard et al., 1979). The patterns of sympathetic reflexes to skin and muscle are persistently changed after transection of a peripheral nerve, an observation that has been associated with sym-

pathetic reflex dystrophy (Blumberg and Jänig, 1983).

It is likely that all of these experimental conditions which evoke long-term biochemical and physiological modifications also induce ITF expression. Thus, it is conceivable that the induction of IEGs and their proteins which function as ITFs represent early steps in these profound regulatory responses in the functional repertoire of nerve cells. A few of the relationships between an ITF and some of the target genes whose transcription it controls have been well established by direct molecular biological analysis (Hengerer et al., 1991).

Other relationships between ITFs and target genes can be concluded from the covariance of ITFs and neuropeptides in immunohistochemical or RNA analysis. Some of these have been reviewed in this article.

We do not know what determines the outcome of ITF induction by transient trauma or noxious stimulation. The same c-Fos/c-Jun transcription complex can be involved in the activation of hundreds of target genes, and the number of ITFs and other transcription controlling molecules currently known is too small to provide specificity of control in relation to the subsequent processes. Therefore, we do not know what happens beyond the few transcription factors we have been able to observe so far, and it might well be that what we can see today is a mere fraction of what will be discovered in our nervous system in the future.

References

Abbadie, C. and Besson, J.M. (1993) Effects of morphine and naloxone on basal and evoked *fos*-like immunoreactivity in lumbar spinal cord neurons of arthritic rats. *Pain*, 52: 29–39.

Almendral, J.M., Sommer, D., MacDonald-Bravo, H., Burckhardt, J., Perera, J. and Bravo R. (1988) Complexity of the early genetic response to growth factors in mouse fibroblasts. *Mol. Cell Biol.*, 8, 2140–2148.

Angel, P. and Karin, M. (1991) The role of Jun, Fos and the AP-1 complex in cell-proliferation and transformation. *Biochim. Biophys. Acta*, 1072: 129–157.

Angel P., Allegretto E.A., Okino, S.T., Hattori K., Boyle W.J., Hunter T. and Karin M. (1988) Oncogene jun encodes a

316

sequence-specific trans-activator similar to AP-1. *Nature*, 332: 166–171.

Anokhin, K.V. and Rose, S.P.R. (1991) Learning-induced increase of immediate early gene messenger RNA in the chick forebrain. *Eur. J. Neurosci.*, 3: 162–167.

Bading, H., Ginty, D.D. and Greenberg, M.E. (1993) Regulation of gene expression in hippocampal neurons by distinct calcium signaling pathways. *Science*, 260: 181–186.

Bartel, D.P., Sheng, M., Lau, L.F. and Greenberg, M.E. (1989) Growth factors and membrane depolarization activate distinct programs of early response gene expression: dissociation of *fos* and jun induction. *Gene Dev.*, 3: 304–313.

Bennett, G.H. and Xie, Y.K. (1988) A peripheral mononeuropathy in rat that produces disorders of pain sensation like those seen in man. *Pain*, 33: 87–107.

Besse, D., Weil-Fugazza, J., Lombard, M.C., Butler, S.H. and Besson, J.M. (1992) Monoarthritis induces complex changes in mu-, delta- and kappa-opioid binding sites in the superficial dorsal horn of the rat spinal cord. *Eur. J. Pharmacol.*, 223: 123–131.

Besson, J.M. and Chaouch, A. (1987) Peripheral and spinal mechanisms of nociception. *Physiol. Rev.*, 67: 67–154.

Blumberg, H. and Jänig, W. (1983) Changes of reflexes in vasoconstrictor neurons supplying the cat hindlimb following chronic nerve lesions: a model for studying mechanisms of reflex sympathetic dystrophy. *J. Autonom. Nerv. Syst.*, 7: 399–411.

Bohmann, D., Bos, T.J., Admon, A., Nishimura, T., Vogt, P.K. and Tjian, R. (1987) Human proto-oncogene *c-jun* encodes a DNA binding protein with structural and functional properties of transcription factor AP-1. *Science*, 238: 1386–1392.

Bravo, R. (1990) Growth factor inducible genes in fibroblasts. In: *Growth Factors, Differentiation Factors and Cytokines*. A. Herschman (Ed.), Springer-Verlag, Heidelberg, pp. 324–343.

Bravo, R., MacDonald-Bravo, H., Müller, R., Hübsch, D. and Almendral, J.M. (1987) Bombesin induces c-*fos* and *c-myc* expression in quiescent swiss 3T3 cells. *Exp. Cell Res.*, 170: 103–115.

Bredt, D.S. and Snyder, S.H. (1992) Nitric oxide, a novel neuronal messenger. *Neuron*, 8: 3–11.

Bullitt, E. (1989) Induction of c-*fos*-like protein in the lumbar spinal cord and thalamus of the rat following peripheral stimulation. *Brain Res.*, 493: 391–397.

Bullitt, E. (1990) Expression of c-*fos* like protein as a marker for neuronal activity following noxious stimulation in the rat. *J. Comp. Neurol.*, 296: 517–530.

Carter, D.A. (1992) Neurotransmitter-stimulated immediate-early gene responses are organized through differential post-synaptic receptor mechanisms. *Mol. Brain Res.*, 16: 111–118.

Casey, K.L. (Ed.) (1991) *Pain and Central Nervous System Disease: The Central Pain Syndrome.* Raven Press, New York.

Ceccatelli, S., Villar, M.J., Goldstein, M. and Hökfelt, T. (1989) Expression of c-Fos immunoreactivity in transmitter-characterized neurons after stress. *Proc. Natl. Acad. Sci. USA*, 86: 9569–9573.

Chan, R.K.W., Brown, E.R., Ericsson, A., Kovacs, K.J. and Sawchenko, P.E. (1993) A comparison of two immediate-early genes, c-*fos* and NGFI-B, as markers for functional activation in stress-related neuroendocrine circuitry. *J. Neurosci. Res.*, 13(12): 126–138.

Coderre, T.J. and Melzack, R. (1992) The contribution of excitatory amino acids to central sensitization and persistent nociception after formalin-induced tissue injury. *J. Neurosci.*, 12: 3665–3670.

Coderre, T.J., Katz, J., Vaccarino, A.L. and Melzack, R. (1993) Contribution of central neuroplasticity to pathological pain: review of clinical and experimental evidence. *Pain*, 52: 259–285.

Cole, A.J., Saffen, D.W., Baraban, J.M. and Worley, P.F. (1989) Rapid increase of an immediate early gene messenger RNA in hippocampal neurons by synaptic NMDA receptor activation. *Nature*, 340: 474–476.

Culp, W.J. and Ochoa, J. (Eds.) (1982) *Abnormal Nerves and Muscles as Impulse Generators.* Oxford University Press, New York, Oxford.

Curran, T., Miller, A.D., Zokas, L. and Verma, I.M. (1984) Viral and cellular *fos* proteins: a comparative analysis. *Cell*, 36: 259–268.

Delmas, V., Monlina, C.A., Lalli, E., de Groot, R., Foulkes, N.S., Masquillier, D. and Sassone-Corsi, P. (1994) Complexity and versatility of the transcriptional response to cAMP. *Rev. Physiol. Biochem. Pharmacol.*, 124: 1–28.

Demmer, J., Dragunow, M., Lawlor, P.A., Mason, S.E., Leah, J.D., Abraham, W.C. and Tate, W.P. (1993) Differential expression of immediate early genes after hippocampal long-term potentiation in awake rats. *Mol. Brain Res.*, 17: 279–286.

Deng, T. and Karin, M. (1993) Jun B differs from c-Jun in its DNA- binding and dimerization domains, and represses c-Jun by formation of inactive heterodimers. *Genes Dev.*, 7: 479–490.

Devor, M. (1988) Central changes mediating neuropathic pain. In: Dubner, R., Gebhart, G.F., Bond, M.R. (Eds.) *Proceedings of the Vth World Congress on Pain. Pain Research and Clinical Management, Vol. 3*, Elsevier, Amsterdam, pp. 114–128.

Dragunow, M. (1990) Presence and induction of FOS B-like immunoreactivity in neural, but not non-neural, cells in adult rat brain. *Brain Res.*, 533: 324–328.

Dragunow, M., Faull, R.L.M. (1990) MK-801 induces c-*fos* protein in thalamic and neocortical neurons of rat brain. *Neurosci. Lett.*, 113: 144–150.

Draisci, G. and Iadarola, M.J. (1989) Temporal analysis of increases in c-*fos*, preprodynorphin and preproenkephalin mRNAs in rat spinal cord. *Mol. Brain Res.*, 6: 31–37.

Dubner, R. (1991) Neuronal plasticity and pain following peripheral tissue inflammation or nerve injury. In: Bond, M.R., Charlton, J.E., Woolf, C.J. (Eds.) *Proceedings of the VIth World Congress on Pain. Pain Research and Clinical Management, Vol. 4*, Elsevier, Amsterdam, pp. 263–276.

Dubner, R. and Ruda, M.A. (1992) Activity-dependent neuronal plasticity following tissue injury and inflammation. *Trends Neurosci.*, 15: 96–103.

Duggan, A.W., Hendry, I.A., Morton, C.R., Hutchinson, W.D. and Zhao, Z.Q. (1988) Cutaneous stimuli releasing immunoreactive substance P in the dorsal horn of the cat. *Brain Res.*, 451: 261–273.

Fiallos-Estrada C.E., Kummer, W., Mayer, W., Bravo, R., Zimmermann, M. and Herdegen, T. (1993) Long-lasting increase of nitric oxide synthase immunoreactivcity and NADPH-diaphorase reaction, and co-expression with the nuclear c-Jun protein in rat dorsal root ganglion neurons following sciatic nerve transection. *Neurosci. Lett.*, 150: 169–173.

Gass, P., Spranger, M., Herdegen, T., Köck, P., Bravo, R., Hacke, W. and Kiessling, M. (1992) Induction of FOS and JUN proteins after focal ischemia in the rat: differential effect of the *N*-methyl-D-aspartate receptor antagonist MK-801. *Acta Neuropathol.*, 84: 545–553.

Gass, P., Herdegen, T., Bravo, R. and Kiessling, M. (1993a) Induction of six immediate-early gene encoded proteins in the rat brain after kainic acid induced limbic seizures: effects of NMDA receptor antagonist MK-801. *Eur. J. Neurosci.*, in press.

Gass, P., Herdegen, T., Bravo, R. and Kiessling, M. (1993b) Induction and suppression of immediate early genes (IEGs) in specific rat brain regions by the non-competitive NMDA receptor antagonist MK-801. *Neuroscience*, 53: 749–758.

Gentz, R., Rauscher, F.J., Abate, C. and Curran, T. (1989) Parallel association of Fos and Jun leucine zippers juxtaposes DNA binding domains. *Science*, 243: 1695–1699.

Gillardon, F., Beck, H., Herdegen, T., Sandkühler, J. and Zimmermann, M. (1994) Inhibition of c-Fos protein expression in rat spinal cord by antisense oligodeoxynucleotide superfusion. *Eur. J. Neurosci.*, 6: 880–884.

Ginty, D.D., Bading, H. and Greenberg, M.E. (1992) Transsynaptic regulation of gene expression. *Neurobiology*, 2: 312–316.

Ginty, D.D., Kornhauser, J.M., Thompson, M.A., Bading, H., Mayo, K.E., Takahashi, J.S. and Greenberg, M.E. (1993) Regulation of CREB phosphorylation in suprachiasmatic nucleus by light and a circadian clock. *Science*, 260: 238–241.

Gonzales, G.A., Yamamoto, K.Y., Fisher, W.H., Karr, D., Menzel, P., Biggs, W.I., Vale, W.W. and Montminy, M.R. (1989) A cluster of phosphorylation sites on the cyclic AMP-regulated nuclear factor CREB predicted by its sequence. *Nature*, 337: 749–752.

Grafstein, B. (1986) The retina as a regenerating organ. In: *The Retina: A Model for Cell Biology Studies*. R. Adler and D. Faber (Eds.), Academic Press, New York, pp. 275–335.

Gubits, R.M., Smith, T.M., Fairhurst, J.L. and Yu, H. (1989) Adrenergic receptors mediate changes in c-*fos* levels in brain. *Mol. Brain Res.*, 6: 39–45.

Haas, C.A., Donath, C. and Kreutzberg, G.W. (1993) Differential expression of immediate early genes after transection of the facial nerve. *Neuroscience*, 53, 91–99.

Haby, C., Lisovoski, F., Aunis, D. and Zwiller, J. (1994) Stimulation of the cyclic GMP pathway by NO induces expression of the immediate early genes c-*fos* and junB in PC12 cells. *J. Neurochem.*, 62: 496–501.

Hagmeyer, B.M., König, H., Herr, I., Offringa, R., Zantema, A., van der Eb, A.J., Herrlich, P. and Angel, P. (1993) Adenovirus E1A negatively and positively modulates transcription of AP-1 dependent genes by dimer-specific regulation of the DNA binding and transactivation activities of Jun. *EMBO J.*, 12: 3559–3572.

Hai, T. and Curran, T. (1991) Cross-family dimerization of transcription factors Fos/Jun and ATF/CREB alters DNA binding specificity. *Proc. Natl. Acad. Sci. USA*, 88: 3720–3724.

Halazonetis, T.D., Georgopoulos, K., Greenberg, M.E. and Leder, P. (1988) c-Jun dimerizes with itself and with c-Fos, forming complexes of different DNA binding affinities. *Cell*, 55: 917–924.

Haley, J.E., Dickenson, A.H. and Sacher, M. (1992) Electrophysiological evidence for a role of nitric oxide in prolonged chemical nociception in the rat. *Neuropharmacology*, 31: 251–258.

He, X. and Rosenfeld, M.G. (1991) Mechanisms of complex transcriptional regulation: implications for brain development. *Neuron*, 7: 183–196.

Herdegen, T. and Zimmermann, M. (1994) Induction of c-Jun and JunD transcription factors represents specific changes in neuronal gene expression following axotomy. *Progr. Brain Res.*, 103: 153–171.

Herdegen, T., Leah, J.D. and Zimmermann, M. (1988) Peripheral nerve injury induces changes in spinal peptidergic neurons. *Eur. J. Neurosci.*, Suppl. 1: 76.22.

Herdegen, T., Walker, T., Bravo, R., Leah, J.D. and Zimmermann, M. (1990) The KROX-24 protein, a new transcription regulating factor: expression in the rat nervous system following somatosensory stimulation. *Neurosci. Lett.*, 120: 21–24.

Herdegen, T., Kovary, K., Leah, J.D. and Bravo, R. (1991a) Specific temporal and spatial distribution of JUN, FOS and KROX-24 proteins in spinal neurons following noxious transynaptic stimulation. *J. Comp. Neurol.*, 313: 178–191.

Herdegen, T., Tölle, T., Bravo, R., Zieglgänsberger, W. and Zimmermann, M. (1991b) Sequential expression of JUN B,

318

JUN D and FOS B proteins in rat spinal neurons: cascade of transcriptional operations during nociception. *Neurosci. Lett.*, 129: 221–224.

Herdegen, T., Fiallos-Estrada, C.E., Schmid, W., Bravo, R. and Zimmermann, M. (1992) Transcription factors c-Jun, Jun D and Creb, but not Fos and Krox-24, are differentially regulated in neurons following axotomy of rat sciatic nerve. *Mol. Brain Res.*, 14: 155–165.

Herdegen, T., Brecht, S., Kummer, W., Mayer, B., Leah, J., Bravo, R. and Zimmermann, M. (1993a) Persisting expression of Jun and Krox transcription factors and nitric oxide synthase in rat central neurons following axotomy. *J. Neuroscience*, 13: 4130–4145.

Herdegen, T., Fiallos-Estrada, C.E., Bravo, R. and Zimmermann, M. (1993b) Colocalisation and covariation of the nuclear c-JUN protein with galanin in primary afferent neurons and with CGRP in spinal motoneurons following transection of rat sciatic nerve. *Mol. Brain Res.*, 17: 147–154.

Herdegen, T., Kiessling, M., Bravo, R., Zimmermann, M. and Gass, P. (1993c) The Krox-20 transcription factor in the adult brain: novel expression pattern of an immediate-early gene encoded protein. *Neuroscience*.

Herdegen, T., Sandkühler, J., Gass, P., Kiessling, M., Bravo, R. and Zimmermann, M. (1993d) Jun, Fos, Krox and Creb transcription factor proteins in the rat cortex: basal expression and expression by KCl-induced cortical spreading depression and bicuculline-induced seizures. *J. Comp. Neurol.*, 333: 271–288.

Herdegen, T., Kovary, K., Buhl, A., Bravo, R., Zimmermann, M. and Gass, P. (1995) Basal expression of c-Jun, JunB, JunD, c-Fos, FosB and Krox-24 transcription factors in the adult rat brain. *J. Comp. Neurol.*, 354: 39–56.

Herdegen, T., Rüdiger, S., Mayer, B., Bravo, R. and Zimmermann, M. (1994b) Increase in nitric oxide synthase and colocalization with Jun, Fos and Krox proteins in spinal neurons following noxious peripheral stimulation. *Mol. Brain Res.*, 22: 245–258.

Herdegen, T., Brecht, S., Neiss, W., Schmidt, W. and Gass, P. (1994c). The transcription factor CREB is not phosphorylated at serine 133 in axotomized neurons: implications for the expression of AP-1 proteins. *Mol. Brain Res.*, 26: 259–270.

Hisanaga, K., Sagar, S.M. and Sharp, F.R. (1992) *N*-Methyl-D-aspartate antagonists block *fos*-like protein expression induced via multiple signaling pathways in cultured cortical neurons. *J. Neurochem.*, 58: 1836–1844.

Honkaniemi, J., Kainu, T., Ceccatelli, S., Rechardt, L., Hoekfelt, T. and Pelto-Huiko, M. (1992) Fos and jun rat central amygdaloid nucleus after stress. *NeuroReport*, 3: 849–852.

Höllt, V., Haarmann, I., Millan, M.J. and Herz, A. (1987) Prodynorphin gene expression is enhanced in the spinal cord of chronic arthritic rats. *Neurosci. Lett.*, 73: 90–94.

Hüll, M. and Bähr, M. (1994) Regulation of immediate-early gene expression in rat retinal ganglion cells after axotomy

and during regeneration through a peripheral nerve graft. *J. Neurobiol.*, 25: 92–105.

Hunt, S.P., Pini, A. and Evan, G. (1987) Induction of c-*fos*-like protein in spinal cord neurons following sensory stimulation. *Nature*, 328: 632–634.

Hylden, J.L.K., Noguchi, K. and Ruda, M.A. (1992) Neonatal capsaicin treatment attenuates spinal *fos* activation and dynorphin gene expression following peripheral tissue inflammation and hyperalgesia. *J. Neurosci.*, 12: 1716–1725.

Ingraham, C.A., Cox, M.E., Ward, D.C., Fults, D.W. and Maness, P.F. (1989) C-src and other proto-oncogenes implicated in neuronal differentiation. *Mol. Chem. Neuropathol.*, 10: 1–14.

Jenkins, R. and Hunt, S.P. (1991) Long-term increase in the levels of c-jun mRNA and Jun protein-like immunoreactivity in motor and sensory neurons following axon damage. *Neurosci. Lett.*, 129: 107–110.

Jenkins, R., Tetzlaff, W. and Hunt, S.P. (1993) Differential expression of immediate early genes in rubrospinal neurons following axotomy in rat. *Eur. J. Neurosci.*, 5: 203–209.

Jones, K.J. and Evinger, C. (1991) Differential neuronal expression of c-*fos* proto-oncogene following peripheral nerve injury or chemically-induced seizure. *J. Neurosci. Res.*, 28: 291–298.

Kar, S., Rees, R.G. and Quirion, R. (1993) Altered calcitonin gene-related peptide, substance P and enkephalin immunoreactivities and receptor binding sites in the dorsal spinal cord of the polyarthritic rat. *Eur. J. Neurosci.*, 6: 345–354.

Kiessling, M. and Gass, P. (1993) Immediate early gene expression in experimental epilepsy. *Brain Pathol.*, 3: 381–393.

Kiessling, M. and Gass, P. (1994) Stimulus-transcription coupling in focal cerebral ischemia. *Brain Pathol.*, 4: 77–83.

Kobierski, LA., Chu, HM., Tan, Y. and Comb, M.J. (1991) cAMP-dependent regulation of proenkephalin by JunD and JunB: positve and negative effects of AP-1 proteins. *Proc. Natl. Acad. Sci. USA*, 88: 10222–10226.

Koistinaho, J., Hicks, K.J. and Sagar, S.M. (1993) Long-term induction of c-jun mRNA and Jun protein in rabbit retinal ganglion cells following axotomy or colchicine treatment. *J. Neurosci. Res.*, 34: 250–255.

Kovary, K. and Bravo, R. (1991) Expression of different JUN and FOS proteins during the G0 to G1 transition in mouse fibroblasts: in vitro and in vivo associations. *Mol. Cell Biol.*, 11 2451–2459.

Kruijer, W., Cooper, J.A., Hunter, T. and Verma, I.M. (1984) Platelet-derived growth factor induces rapid but transient expression of the c-*fos* gene and protein. *Nature*, 312: 711–716.

Lanteri-Minet, M., de Pommery, J., Herdegen, T., Weil-Fugazza, J., Bravo, R. and Menetrey, D. (1993a) Differential time-course and spatial expression of Fos, Jun and Krox-24 proteins in spinal cord of rats undergoing subacute or chronic somatic inflammation. *J. Comp Neurol.*, 333: 223–235.

Lanteri-Minet, M., Isnardon, P., de Pommery J. and Menetrey, D. (1993b) Spinal and hindbrain structures involved in visceroception and visceronociception as revealed by the expression of Fos, Jun and Krox-24 proteins. *Neuroscience*, 55: 737–753.

Lanteri-Minet, M., Weil-Fugazza, J., de Pommery, J. and Menetrey, D. (1994) Hind brain structures involved in pain processing as revealed by the expression of c-Fos and other immediate early gene proteins. *Neuroscience*, 58: 287–298.

Lau, L.F. and Nathans, D. (1985) Identification of a set of genes expressed during the G0/G1 transition of cultured mouse cells. *EMBO J.*, 4: 3145–3151.

Lawson, S.N., Perry, M.J., Prabhakar, E. and McCarthy, P.W. (1993) Primary sensory neurones: neurofilament, neuropeptides, and conduction velocity. *Brain Res. Bull.*, 30: 239–243.

Lazo, P.S., Dorfman, K., Noguchi, T., Mattei, M.G. and Bravo, R. (1991) Structure and mapping of the *fos*B gene. FosB downregulates the activity of the *fos*B promoter. *Nucleic Acids Res.*, 20: 343–350.

Leah, J., Herdegen, T. and Zimmermann, M. (1989) Physiological and pharmacological induction of c-*fos* protein immunoreactivity in superficial dorsal horn neurones. In: Cervero, F., Bennett, G.J., Headley, P.M. (Eds.) *Processing of Sensory Information in the Superficial Dorsal Horn of the Spinal Cord*. Plenum Press, New York, pp., 307–310.

Leah, J.D., Herdegen, T., Kovary, K. and Bravo, R. (1991) Selective expression of JUN proteins following peripheral axotomy and axonal transport block in the rat: evidence for a role in the regeneration process. *Brain Res.*, 566: 198–207.

Leah, J., Sandkühler, J., Herdegen, T., Murashov, A. and Zimmermann, M. (1992) Potentiated expression of FOS protein in the rat spinal cord following bilateral noxious cutaneous stimulation. *Neuroscience*, 48: 525–532.

Leah, J.D., Herdegen, T., Murashov, A., Dragunow, M. and Bravo, R. (1993) Expression of immediate-early gene proteins following axotomy and inhibition of axonal transport in the rat CNS. *Neuroscience*.

Liebermann, A.R. (1971) The axon reaction: a review of the principal features of perikaryal response to axon injury. *Int. Rev. Neurobiol.*, 14: 49–124.

Lee, J.H., Wilcox, G.L. and Beitz, A.J. (1992) Nitric oxide mediates Fos expression in the spinal cord induced by stimulation. *NeuroReport*, 3: 841–844.

Lombard, M.-C., Nashold, B.S.Jr., Albe-Fessard, D., Salman, N. and Sakr, C. (1979) Deafferentation hypersensitivity in the rat after dorsal rhizotomy: a possible animal model of chronic pain. *Pain*, 6, 163–174.

Mack, K.J. and Mack, P.A. (1992) Induction of transcription factors in somatosensory cortex after tactile stimulation. *Mol. Brain Res.*, 12: 141–147.

McKitrick, D.J., Krukoff, T.L. and Calaresu, F.R. (1992) Expression of c-*fos* protein in rat brain after electrical stimu-

lation of the aortic depressor nerve. *Brain Res.*, 599: 215–222.

McMahon, S.B., Lewin, G.R. and Wall, P.D. (1993) Central hyperexcitability triggered by noxious inputs. *Curr. Opin. Neurobiol.*, 3: 602–610.

Meller, S.T. and Gebhart, G.F. (1993) Nitric oxide (NO) and nociceptive processing in the spinal cord. *Pain*, 52: 127–136.

Menetrey, D., Gannon, A., Levine, J.D. and Basbaum, A.J. (1989) Expression of c-*fos* protein in interneurons and projection neurons of the rat spinal cord in response to noxious somatic, articular and visceral stimulation. *J. Comp. Neurol.*, 285: 177–195.

Minami, M., Kuraishi, Y., Kawamura, M., Yamagushi, T., Masu, Y., Nakanishi, S. and Satoh, M. (1989) Enhancement of preprotachykinin a gene expression by adjuvant-induced inflammation in the rat spinal cord: possible involvement of substance P-containing spinal neurons in nociception. *Neurosci. Lett.*, 98: 105–110.

Mohney, R.P., Siegel, R.E. and Zigmond, R.E. (1994) Galanin and vasoactive intestinal peptide messenger RNAs increase following axotomy of adult sympathetic neurons. *J. Neurobiol.*, 25: 108–118.

Molander, C., Hongpaisan, J. and Grant, G. (1992) Changing pattern of c-*fos* expression in spinal cord neurons after electrical stimulation of the chronically injured sciatic nerve in the rat. *Neuroscience*, 50: 223–236.

Moncada, S., Palmer, R.M.J. and Higgs, E.A. (1991) Nitric oxide: physiology, pathophysiology and pharmacology. *Pharmacol. Rev.*, 43: 109–142.

Monstein, H.J. (1993) Identification of an AP-1 transcription factor binding site within the human cholecystokinin (CCK) promoter. *NeuroReport*, 4: 195–197.

Montminy, M.R. and Bilezikjian, L.M. (1987) Binding of a nuclear protein to the cyclic-AMP response element of the somatostatin gene. *Nature*, 328: 175–178.

Morgan, J.I. and Curran, T. (1991) Stimulus-transcription coupling in the nervous system: involvement of the inducible proto-oncogenes *fos* and *jun*. *Annu. Rev. Neurosci.*, 14: 421–451.

Morgan, J.I., Cohen, D.R., Hempstead, J.L. and Curran, T. (1987) Mapping patterns of c-*fos* expression in the central nervous system after seizure. *Science*, 237: 192–196.

Mower, G.D. (1994) Differences in the induction of Fos protein in cat visual cortex during and after the critical period. *Mol. Brain Res.*, 21: 47–54.

Nahin, R.L., Hylden, J.L., Iadarola, M.J. and Dubner, R. (1989) Peripheral inflammation is associated with increased dynorphin immunoreactivity in both projection and local circuit neurons in the superficial dorsal horn of the rat lumbar spinal cord. *Neurosci. Lett.*, 96: 247–252.

Nakabeppu, Y. and Nathans, D. (1991) A naturally occurring truncated from of FosB that inhibits Fos/Jun transcriptional activity. *Cell*, 64: 751–759.

320

Nakabeppu, Y., Ryder, K. and Nathans, D. (1988) DNA binding activities of three different jun proteins: stimulation by Fos. *Cell*, 55: 907–915.

Naranjo, J.R., Mellström, B., Achaval, M., Lucas, J.J., Del Rio, J. and Sassone-Corsi, P. (1991a) Co-induction of Jun-B and c-Fos in a subset of neurons in the spinal cord. *Oncogene*, 6: 223–227.

Naranjo, J.R., Mellström, B., Achaval, M. and Sassone-Corsi, P. (1991b) Molecular pathways of pain: *fos*/jun-mediated activation of a noncanonical AP-1 site in the prodynorphin gene. *Neuron*, 6: 607–617.

New, H.V. and Mudge, A.W. (1986) Calcitonin gene-related peptide regulates muscle acetylcholine receptor synthesis. *Nature*, 323: 809–811.

Nishikura, K. and Murray, J.M. (1987) Antisense DNA of proto-oncogene c-*fos* blocks renewed growth of quiescent 3T3 cells. *Mol. Cell. Biol.*, 7: 639–649.

Noguchi, K. and Ruda, M.A. (1992) Inflammation induced increase in pre protachykinin mRNA in rat lamina I spinal projection neurons. *J. Neurosci.*, 12: 2563–2572.

Papavassiliou, A.G., Treier, M., Chavrier, C. and Bohmann, D. (1992) Targeted degradation of c-Fos, but not v-Fos, by a phosphorylation-dependent signal on c-Jun. *Science*, 258: 1941–1944.

Pertovaara, A., Herdegen, T. and Bravo, R. (1993) Induction and suppression of immediate-early genes by selective alpha-2-adrenoceptor agonist and antagonist in the rat brain following noxious peripheral stimulation. *Neuroscience*, 54: 117–126.

Peunova, N. and Enikolopov, G. (1993) Amplification of calcium-induced gene transcription by nitric oxide in neuronal cells. *Nature*, 364: 450–453.

Pfarr, C.M., Mechta, F., Spyrou, G., Lallemand, D., Carillo, S. and Yaniv, M. (1994) Mouse JunD negatively regulates fibroblast growth and antagonizes transformation by ras. *Cell*, 76: 747–760.

Porro, C. and Cavazzuti, M., Spatial and temporal aspects of spinal cord and brainstem activation in the formalin pain model. *Progr. Neurobiol.*, 41: 565–607.

Presley, R.W., Menetrey, D., Levine, J.D. and Basbaum, A.I. (1990) Systemic morphine suppresses noxious stimulus-evoked Fos protein-like immunoreactivity in the rat spinal cord. *J. Neurosci.*, 10: 323–335.

Pretel, S. and Piekut, D.T. (1991) Enkephalin, substance P, and serotonin axonal input to c-Fos-like immunoreactive neurons of the rat spinal cord. *Peptides*, 12: 1243–1250.

Przewlocki, R., Haarmann, I., Nikolarakis, K., Herz, A. and Höllt, V. (1988) Prodynorphin gene expression in spinal cord is enhanced after traumatic injury in the rat. *Brain Res.*, 464: 37–41.

Pulverer, B.J., Kyriakis, J.M., Avruch, J., Nikolakaki, E. and Woodgett, J.R. (1991) Phosphorylation of c-jun mediated by MAP kinases. *Nature*, 353: 670–674.

Purkiss, R.J., Legg, M.D., Hunt, S.P. and Davies, S.W. (1993)

Immediate early gene expression in the rat forebrain following striatal infusion of quinolinic acid. *Eur. J. Neurosci.*, 5: 1653–1662.

Ransone, L.J. and Verma, I.M. (1990) Nuclear proto-oncogenes FOS and JUN. *Annu. Rev. Cell Biol.*, 6: 539–557.

Rauscher, F.J., III, Voulaslas, P.J., Franza, B.R., Jr. and Curran T. (1988) Fos and jun bind cooperatively to the AP-1 site: reconstitution in vitro. *Genes Dev.*, 2: 1687–1699.

Ruda, M.A., Iadarola, M.J., Cohen, L.V. and Young, W.S. (1988) In-situ hybridisation histochemistry and immunohistochemistry reveal an increase in spinal cord dynorphin biosynthesis in a rat model of peripheral inflammation and hyperalgesia. *Proc. Natl. Acad. Sci. USA*, 85: 622–626.

Rusin, K.I., Jiang, M.C., Cerne, R. and Randic, M. (1993) Interactions between excitatory amino acids and tachykinins in the rat spinal dorsal horn. *Brain Res.*, 30: 329–338.

Ryder, K., Lau, LF. and Nathans, D. (1988) A gene activated by growth factors is related to the oncogene v-jun. *Proc. Natl. Acad. Sci. USA*, 85: 1487–1491.

Ryseck, P. and Bravo, R. (1991) c-Jun, Jun B, and Jun D differ in their binding affinities to AP-1 and CRE consensus sequences: effect of Fos proteins. *Oncogene*, 6: 533–542.

Ryseck, R., Hirai, S., Yaniv, M. and Bravo, R. (1988) Transcriptional activation of c-jun during the G0/G1 transition in mouse fibroblasts. *Nature*, 334: 535–537.

Sagar, S.M., Sharp, F.R. and Curran, T. (1988) Expression of c-*fos* proteins in brain: metabolic mapping at the cellular level. *Science*, 240: 1328–1331.

Schlingensiepen, K.H. and Brysch, W. (1992) Phosphorothioate oligomers: inhibitors of oncogene expression in tumor cells and tools of gene function analysis. In: *Gene Regulation: Biology of Antisense RNA and DNA*. R. Erickson and J. Izant, Eds. Raven Press, New York, pp. 317–328.

Schlingensiepen, K.H., Schlingensiepen, R., Kunst, M., Klinger, I., Gerdes, W., Seifert, W. and Brysch, W. (1993) Opposite functions of Jun-B and c-Jun in growth regulation and neuronal differentiations. *Dev. Genetics*, 14: 305–312.

Schütte, J., Viallet, J., Nau, M., Segal, S., Fedorko, J. and Minna, J. (1989) Jun-B inhibits and c-FOS stimulates the transforming and transactivating activities of c-jun. *Cell*, 59: 987–997.

Sharp, F.R., Sagar, S.M., Hicks, K., Lowenstein, D. and Hisanaga, K. (1993) c-*fos* mRNA, Fos and Fos-related antigen induction by hypertonic saline and stress. *J. Neurosci.*, 11: 2321–2331.

Sheng, M. and Greenberg, E. (1990) The regulation and function of c-*fos* and other immediate early genes in the nervous system. *Neuron*, 4: 477–485.

Sheng, M., McFadden, G. and Greenberg, M.E. (1990) Membrane depolarization and calcium induce c-*fos* transcription via phosphorylation of transcription factor CREB. *Neuron*, 4: 571–582.

Shin, C., McNamara, J.O., Morgan, J.I., Curran, T. and Cohen, D.R. (1990) Induction of c-*fos* mRNA expression by after-discharge in the hippocampus of naive and kindled rats. *J. Neurochem.*, 55: 1050–1055.

Simonato, M., Hosford D.A., Labiner, D.M., Shin, C., Mansbach, H.H. and McNamara, J.O. (1991) Differential expression of immediate early genes in the hippocampus in the kindling model of epilepsy. *Mol. Brain Res.*, 11: 115–124.

Sonnenberg, J.L., Rauscher III, F.J., Morgan, J.I. and Curran, T. (1989) Regulation of proenkephalin by Fos and Jun. *Science*, 246: 1622–1625.

Strittmatter, S.M., Vartanian, T. and Fishman, M.C. (1992) GAP-43 as a plasticity protein in neuronal form and repair. *J. Neurobiol.*, 23: 507–520.

Sugimoto, T., Yoshida, A., Nishijima, K. and Ichikawa, H. (1994) c-*fos* induction in the rat spinal dorsal horn partially deafferented by dorsal rhizotomy. *Neurosci. Lett.*, in press.

Tetzlaff, W., Alexander, S.W., Miller, F.D. and Bisby, M.A. (1991) Response of facial and rubrospinal neurons to axotomy: changes in mRNA expression for cytoskeletal proteins and GAP-43. *J. Neurosci.*, 11: 2528–2544.

Treisman, R. (1990) The SRE: a growth factor responsive transcriptional regulator. *Cancer Biol.*, 1: 47–58.

Tölle, T.R., Castro-Lopes, J.M., Evan, G. and Zieglgänsberger, W. (1991) C-*fos* induction in the spinal cord following noxious stimulation: prevention by opiates but not by NMDA antagonists. In: Bond, M.R., Charlton, J.E., Woolf, C.J. (Eds.) *Proceedings of the VIth World Congress on Pain. Pain Research and Clinical Management, Vol. 4*, Elsevier, Amsterdam, pp. 299–305.

Tölle, T., Herdegen, T., Bravo, R., Zimmermann, M. and Zieglgänsberger, W. (1994) Single application of morphine prior to noxious stimulation differentially modulates expression of Fos, Jun and Krox-24 in rat spinal cord neurons. *Neuroscience*, 58: 305–323.

Traub, R.J., Herdegen, T. and Gebhard, G.F. (1993) Differential expression of c-Fos and c-Jun in two regions of the rat spinal cord following noxious colorectal distension. *Neurosci. Lett.*, 160: 212–125.

van Dam, H., Duyndam, M., Rottier, R., Bosch, A., de Vries-Smits, L., Herrlich, P., Zantema, A., Angel, P. and van der Eb, A.J. (1993) Heterodimer formation of cJun and ATF-2 is reponsible for induction of c-jun by the 243 amino acid adenovirus E1A protein. *EMBO J.*, 12: 479–487.

Verge, V.K.M., Xu, Z., Xu, X.J. and Wiesenfeld-Hallin, S. (1992) Marked increase in nitric oxide synthase mRNA in rat dorsal root ganglia after peripheral axotomy: in situ hybridization and functional studies. *Proc. Natl. Acad. Sci. USA*, 89: 11617–11621.

Vogt, P.K. and Bos, T.J. (1990) JUN: oncogene and transcription factor. *Adv. Cancer Res.*, 55: 2–36.

Wall, P.D., Devor, M., Inbal, R., Scadding, J.W., Schonfeld, D., Seltzer, Z. and Tomkiewicz, M.M. (1979) Autotomy following peripheral nerve lesions: experimental anaesthesia dolorosa. *Pain*, 7: 103–113.

Walther, D., Takemura, M. and Uhl, G., Fos family member changes in nucleus caudalis neurons after primary afferent stimulation: enhancement of *fos* B and c-*fos*. *Mol. Brain Res.*, 17: 155–159.

Wilkinson, G., Bhatt, S., Ryseck, R. and Bravo, R. (1989) Tissue-specific expression of c-jun and jun B during mouse development. *Development*, 106: 464–473.

Williams, S., Evans, G.I. and Hunt, S.P. (1990) Changing patterns of c-FOS induction in spinal neurons following thermal cutaneous stimulation in the rat. *Neuroscience*, 36: 73–81.

Winston, S.M., Hayward, M.D., Nestler, E.J. and Duman, R.S. (1990) Chronic electroconvulsive seizures down-regulate expression of the immediate-early genes c-*fos* and c-*jun* in rat cerebral cortex. *J. Neurochem.*, 54: 1920–1925.

Wisden, W., Errington, M.L., Williams, S., Dunnett, S.B., Waters, C., Hitchcock, D., Evan, G., Bliss, T.V. and Hunt, S.P. (1990) Differential expression of immediate early genes in the hippocampus and spinal cord. *Neuron*, 4: 603–614.

Wollnik, F., Brysch, W., Uhlmann, E., Gillardon, F., Bravo, R., Zimmermann, M., Schlingensiepen, K.H. and Herdegen, T. (1995) Block of c-Fos and JunB expression by antisense-oligonucleotides inhibits light-induced phase shifts of the mammalian circadian clock. *Eur. J. Neurosci.*, 7: 388–393.

Woolf, C.J. (1984) Long term alterations in the excitability of the flexion reflex produced by peripheral tissue injury in the chronic decerebrate rat. *Pain*, 18: 325–343.

Xu, X.J., Wiesenfeld-Hallin, Z., Villar, M.J., Fahrenkrug, J. and Hökfelt, T. (1990) On the role of galanin, substance P and other neuropeptides in primary sensory neurons in the rat: studies on spinal reflex excitability and peripheral axotomy. *Eur. J. Neurosci.*, 2: 733–743.

Xu, X.-J., Dalsgaard, C.-J. and Wiesenfeld-Hallin, Z. (1992) Spinal substance P and *N*-methyl-D-aspartate receptors are coactivated in the induction of central sensitization of the nociceptive flexor reflex. *Neuroscience*, 51: 641–648.

Zhang, X., Wiesenfeld-Hallin, Z. and Hökfelt, T. (1994) Effect of peripheral axotomy on expression of neuropeptide Y receptor mRNA in rat lumbar dorsal root ganglia. *Eur. J. Neurosci.*, 6: 43–57.

Zieglgänsberger, W. and Tölle, T.R. (1993) The pharmacology of pain signalling. *Curr. Opin. Neurobiol.*, 3: 611–618.

Zimmermann, M. (1991) Central nervous mechanisms modulating pain-related information: do they become deficient after lesions of the peripheral or central nervous system? In: Casey, K.L. (Ed.) *Pain and Central Nervous System Disease: The Central Pain Syndrome*. Raven Press, New York, pp. 183–199.

Zuschratter, W., Gass, P., Herdegen, T. and Scheich, H. (1992) Parvalbumin containing neurons of the auditory cortex do not express c-Fos after acoustic stimulation classical conditioning or active avoidance training. *Eur. J. Neurosci.*, 5(Suppl.): 2118.

SECTION V

Pathophysiological Role of Neuropeptides in the Spinal Cord

F. Nyberg, H.S. Sharma and Z. Wiesenfeld-Hallin (Eds.)
Progress in Brain Research, Vol 104
© 1995 Elsevier Science BV. All rights reserved.

CHAPTER 18

Neuropeptides in neuroblastomas and ganglioneuromas

P. Kogner

Paediatric Oncology Unit, Department of Paediatrics, and Peptide Research Laboratory, Department of Clinical Chemistry, Karolinska Hospital, S-171 76 Stockholm, Sweden

Introduction

Neuroblastoma and ganglioneuroma are neural crest-derived childhood tumours which produce various neuropeptides. These peptides may cause symptoms and influence tumour growth and differentiation. Analysing neuropeptides in tissue and plasma may be useful for diagnosing, characterising and monitoring patients with these tumours and further indicate novel therapeutic modalities. The identification of specific neuropeptide receptors on tumour cells provides novel means for tumour imaging in vivo as well as innovative therapy. Furthermore, these tumours provide possibilities for studying the regulation of synthesis and specific actions of these peptides.

Neuropeptides are regulatory peptides produced by neuronal cells acting as neurotransmitters or neuromodulators in the peripheral and central nervous systems. Neuropeptides also act as hormones with paracrine and/or distant endocrine effects. Recently it has become evident that neuropeptides may play a role as trophic factors for both neuronal and non-neuronal cells (Hökfelt, 1991; Rozengurt, 1991; Gozes and Brenneman, 1993). Neuropeptides may act as paracrine or autocrine factors, stimulating growth or differentiation, and even having opposite actions in different cellular systems. Several neu-

ropeptides have been shown to be produced by tumour cells of neuroendocrine origin and the measurement of plasma concentrations of these peptides can be used for diagnosis and monitoring of disease (Theodorsson, 1989; Silen and Gardner, 1993). Proper sample handling (rapid cooling and freezing) is important for these purposes since most neuropeptides are labile in plasma (Theodorsson-Norheim et al., 1987). The purpose of this presentation is to review current knowledge concerning the biological and clinical significance of neuropeptide expression in childhood neuroblastoma and ganglioneuroma.

Neuroblastoma, an embryonal malignant tumour of neural crest origin, is the most common paediatric extracranial tumour, diagnosed mainly during infancy or early childhood. Neuroblastomas and their benign counterparts, ganglioneuromas, may arise wherever sympathetic tissue is present, including the adrenal medulla that is the most common site of primary neuroblastoma tumours. Clinical staging divides neuroblastomas into localised (stages 1 and 2), regional (3) and metastatic tumours (4), with a special subset of widespread but favourable tumours prone to spontaneous regression found in infants (4S) (Brodeur et al., 1993). The term 'ganglioneuroblastoma' refers to a sympathetic tumour with more differentiated morphological appearance than neuroblastoma. However, these tumours may still be highly malignant and are therefore commonly included under the general diagnosis neuroblastoma (Brodeur et al., 1993).

Neuroblastoma is the most frequent malignant spinal tumour in children, often described as a 'dumb-bell tumour' with growth extension from the sympathetic paravertebral ganglia through the intervertebral foramina into the spinal canal (Pasqual-Castroviejo, 1990). Neuroblastoma shows a remarkable clinical heterogeneity ranging from favourable outcome, due to spontaneous regression, complete remission after minimal therapy, to unfavourable outcome due to aggressive tumour growth in spite of intensive multimodal therapy (Berthold, 1992). Benign differentiated ganglioneuroma has an excellent clinical prognosis. Malignant but favourable neuroblastomas may undergo spontaneous or induced differentiation to ganglioneuromas or complete regression and disappearance similar to programmed cell death as described in the normal development of the sympathetic nervous system (Fig. 1). Recent findings indicate that the expression of functional high-affinity receptors for nerve growth factor (NGF) is critical for the commonly described spontaneous differentiation or regression of neuroblastoma (Kogner et al., 1993; Matsushima and Bogenmann, 1993), while loss of these receptors may constitute an early step in the evolution of neuroblastoma tumours with an aggressive clinical behaviour. Other common molecular features of unfavourable neuroblastomas include genetic amplification of the N-*myc* oncogene and deletion of the short arm of chromosome 1 (Brodeur et al., 1992).

Neuropeptide Y

Neuropeptide Y (NPY) is a 36-amino acid residue neurotransmitter or neuromodulator widely distributed in human central and peripheral nervous systems (Lundberg et al., 1982; Tatemoto et al., 1982; Adrian et al., 1983a). It has been shown that some tumours of neural crest origin contain high concentrations of NPY-like immunoreactiv-

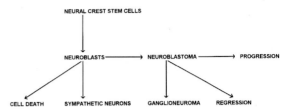

Fig. 1. Schematic outline of normal development of neural crest stem cells, either through differentiation to sympathetic neurons or programmed cell death of surplus cells. Similarly, the evolution of neuroblastoma tumours is indicated. Favourable neuroblastoma tumours may undergo induced or spontaneous regression or differentiation to ganglioneuromas. Aggressive neuroblastomas show progressive tumour growth and unfavourable clinical outcome, despite current intensive cytostatic therapy.

ity (NPY-LI) (Adrian et al., 1983b). We have previously reported that plasma concentrations of NPY-LI analysed by a competitive radioimmunoassay are elevated in children at diagnosis of neuroblastoma (Theodorsson-Norheim et al., 1985; Kogner et al., 1990). Increasing plasma NPY-LI during surgical tumour manipulation of neuroblastoma and high concentrations in tumour tissue give evidence for tumour origin of elevated systemic NPY (Kogner et al., 1993b). Furthermore, repeated determinations of plasma NPY-LI are useful and sensitive for follow up of these patients; in particular for early detection of tumour relapse (Kogner et al., 1990, 1991). However, renal failure may be a cause of elevated plasma NPY-LI of non-tumoural origin. Similar results regarding the usefulness of NPY as a tumour marker in neuroblastoma have subsequently been reported by groups in Japan as well as Germany (Hayashi et al., 1991; Mouri et al., 1992; Rascher et al., 1993).

In healthy children plasma NPY-LI decreases with age, while mild stress caused by the sampling procedure or general anaesthesia has no significant influence (Kogner et al., 1994a). An age-dependent reference level was established and a prospective study showed that children with ganglioneuroma have normal plasma NPY-LI at diagnosis; lower than that found in children with neuroblastoma ($P < 0.05$; Fig. 2). Furthermore, elevated NPY-LI in children with neuroblastoma indicates a poor prognosis, while those with normal concentrations at diagnosis have a favourable outcome ($P < 0.001$; Fig. 2) (Kogner et al., 1994a). These results show that a proper reference interval is necessary for the clinical interpretation of plasma neuropeptide concentrations as disease markers.

Primary neuroblastoma tumours contain high concentrations of NPY-LI, while ganglioneuromas and healthy adrenals show significantly lower levels (Kogner et al., 1993b, 1994b). Our results in primary tumours are summarised in Fig. 3. An association with tumour growth is implicated not only by the rapid increase in plasma NPY-LI at tumour relapse or metastatic spread but also by further increased concentrations of NPY-LI in metastases and relapsing tumour tissue compared to corresponding primary tumours (Kogner et al., 1994b). However, the most aggressive tumours

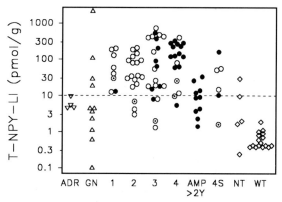

Fig. 3. Neuropeptide Y in tissue extracts (NPY-LI, pmol/g wet weight) of healthy adrenals (ADR, $n = 4$), ganglioneuromas (GN, $n = 11$), primary neuroblastomas of different clinical stages (1, 2, 3, 4 and 4S, $n = 83$), other neuroectodermal tumours (NT, $n = 5$) and Wilms' tumours (nephroblastomas, WT, $n = 16$). Neuroblastomas taken together had higher concentrations than adrenals ($P = 0.012$), ganglioneuromas ($P < 0.001$) and control tumours ($P < 0.001$). No differences were detected between different neuroblastomas with regard to age, stage or outcome. Neuroblastomas with amplification of the N-*myc* oncogene from children over 2 years of age (AMP, > 2Y) had significantly lower NPY-LI than other neuroblastomas ($P < 0.01–0.001$), and are reported separately. Filled circles, patients with neuroblastoma dead during follow-up: open circles, patients with neuroblastoma, alive without disease > 12 months from diagnosis; dotted circles, patients with neuroblastoma under treatment or followed < one year from diagnosis. Dashed line at 10 pmol/g indicates an arbitrary upper reference limit as obtained from the healthy adrenals analysed in this study. (From Kogner, 1993, with permission.)

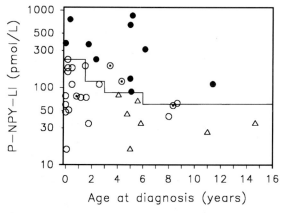

Fig. 2. Neuropeptide Y in plasma (NPY-LI) at diagnosis of neuroblastoma (circles, $n = 31$) and ganglioneuroma (triangles, $n = 7$). The line indicates the upper reference level for plasma NPY-LI in healthy children. Filled symbols, children dead from disease; dotted symbols, children still under treatment; open symbols, children alive, without evidence of disease. Children with neuroblastoma had significantly lower concentrations compared to those with ganglioneuroma ($P = 0.038$). Children with neuroblastoma and normal NPY-LI had better prognosis than those with elevated NPY-LI ($P < 0.001$). (From Kogner, 1994a, with permission from Scandinavian University Press.)

analysed by us, N-*myc*-amplified tumours from children above 2 years of age, show significantly lower concentrations, possibly indicating that these tumours are the most undifferentiated in the spectrum of paediatric neural crest tumours (Fig. 3).

High tumour concentrations of NPY-LI correlated with high expression of NPY mRNA and, in most cases, coexpression of *trk* protooncogene mRNA and low-affinity NGF receptor mRNA (Kogner et al., 1994b). This indicates that NPY expression may be regulated by NGF in tumour cells in vivo as has been previously shown in vitro (Allen et al., 1987; Sabol and Higuchi, 1990).

However, NPY mRNA and high concentrations of NPY-LI were detected in some tumours without detectable NGF receptor mRNA expression, suggesting an alternative method of NPY gene regulation in vivo. Recent results in vitro show that NPY gene expression increases during differentiation, induced also by other means than NGF, and a complex interaction of multiple transcription factors during differentiation of human SH-SY5Y neuroblastoma cells was suggested (Andersson et al., 1994).

Previous analysis of NPY immunoreactivity from neural crest tumours showed mainly intact NPY(1–36) and a minor fraction of the precursor proNPY containing 69 amino acids (O'Hare and Schwartz, 1989a). However, the same authors reported minor molecular forms from neuroblastoma cell lines, although these were not further characterized (O'Hare and Schwartz, 1989b). We have characterised different molecular forms with NPY immunoreactivity in plasma and tumour tissue, using different chromatographic means and antisera specific for the N- and C-terminal parts of the NPY(1–36) molecule, respectively (Kogner, 1993; Kogner et al., 1993b). Neuroblastomas from all different clinical stages showed both proNPY and intact human NPY(1–36) similar to healthy adrenal tissue (see Fig. 4, peaks I and II). In contrast, ganglioneuroma and phaechromocytoma, both benign tumours, contained almost only fully processed NPY(1–36). Furthermore, from a primary neuroblastoma tumour we were able to characterise a homologue with smaller Stokes radius with NPY immunoreactivity only reacting with the C-terminal, but not with the N-terminal antiserum (Fig. 4, peak III). These results indicate the presence of a hitherto undescribed smaller NPY homologue with a C-terminal allowing biological activity and receptor interaction. The described differences in molecular processing between different tumours of neural crest origin are consistent with the discrepancy in symptoms between adult patients with phaeochromocytomas, presenting with hypertension, and children with neuroblastoma, presenting with normal blood pressure. Both these categories show elevated

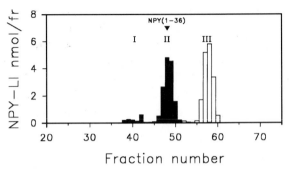

Fig. 4. Gel permeation chromatography of NPY-LI of a neuroblastoma tumour showing two components (I and II) detected with an N-terminal antiserum. Component II, with smaller Stokes radius, eluted at the position of intact NPY(1–36), and was also detected with a C-terminal antiserum. A third component (III) was only detected with the C-terminal antiserum (open bars). Elution position of synthetic NPY(1–36) is indicated. Component I was characterised as proNPY after enzymatic cleavage; component II amino acid sequence was identical to intact human NPY. Component III had a similar elution position to the C-terminal fragment NPY(26–36) on reversed-phase HPLC (From Kogner, 1993, with permission.)

plasma NPY-LI analysed with the same radioimmunoassay using an N-terminal antiserum (Theodorsson-Norheim et al., 1985; Lundberg et al., 1986; Kogner et al., 1990). However, phaeochromocytoma tumours contain only intact NPY with the ability to interact with the post-synaptic NPY-receptor Y1, which requires the complete NPY molecule for increased vascular tone (Wahlestedt et al., 1990). On the other hand, besides intact NPY(1–36), neuroblastoma tumours also contain proNPY and a smaller NPY homologue, neither of which are able to interact with the Y1 receptor and are consequently without any effect on blood pressure, except for the possibility that the smaller homologue may interact with the pre-synaptic Y2 receptor, thereby indirectly leading to a decrease in blood pressure.

Specific receptors for NPY, of both Y1 and Y2 types, have been detected on neuroblastoma cells in vitro (Sheikh et al., 1989). A simultaneous synthesis of NPY in some of these cell lines has made it possible to propose an autocrine role of NPY in neuroblastoma tumours (O'Hare and

Schwartz, 1989b; Sheikh et al., 1989). Specific effects of NPY, including calcium mobilisation and inhibition of adenylate cyclase, have been shown in human neuroblastoma cells in vitro (Aakerlund et al., 1990; Gordon et al., 1990). In SK-N-MC cells, NPY was shown to inhibit cyclic AMP accumulation stimulated by vasoactive intestinal peptide (VIP) (Gordon et al., 1990). However, a growth stimulatory function has hitherto not been described for NPY in tumour cells, such as the recently shown mitogenic effect on other non-neuronal cells (Zukowska-Grojec et al., 1993).

Vasoactive intestinal peptide

Vasoactive intestinal peptide (VIP) is a 28-amino acid residue neuropeptide with wide distribution in the central and peripheral nervous systems (Said and Mutt, 1970; Gozes and Brenneman, 1989). VIP is involved in a wide variety of biological actions and may act as a neurotransmitter, neuromodulator or a blood-borne hormone (Gozes and Brenneman, 1989; Said, 1991). It has been shown to promote neurite outgrowth and enhance survival of sympathetic neuroblasts (Pincus et al., 1990), and it is well known that neuroendocrine tumours may produce and secrete large amounts of VIP, causing severe watery diarrhoea (WDHA syndrome) (Said and Faloona, 1975). VIP-secreting neuroendocrine tumours have been shown to be associated with better differentiation and more favourable prognosis (Allen et al., 1985). Similarly, childhood neuroblastomas and ganglioneuromas associated with VIP secretion and severe diarrhoea were reported to have a favourable ultimate prognosis (Lacey et al., 1989). Furthermore, in vitro studies have shown that VIP may induce growth inhibition and differentiation of malignant neuroblastoma cell lines (Pence and Shorter, 1990). Growth inhibition and differentiation of human neuroblastoma cells require the intact VIP molecule (Pence and Shorter, 1991) and could not be induced by related peptides (e.g., glucagon, secretin or GRF(1–29)-amide). Hence, the expression of functional receptors specific for VIP are neces-

sary for VIP effects, and it has previously been detected on neuroblastoma cells (Muller et al., 1989). Binding studies have demonstrated VIP receptors on primary neuroblastoma tumours and cell lines, and it was indicated that expression of these receptors was regulated by VIP in an autocrine fashion (O'Dorisio et al., 1992). In neuroblastoma tumour samples, the presence of VIP receptors did not correlate with stage of disease. Recently, further data implicate that VIP-induced differentiation of neuroblastoma cells markedly increased VIP receptor expression (Pence and Shorter, 1993). Similarly, VIP synthesis is increased in neuroblastoma cells by differentiation induced by retinoic acid as well as by VIP (Agoston et al., 1992; Pence and Shorter, 1993). Furthermore, it was recently shown that, during neuroblastoma differentiation induced by retinoic acid, VIP increases tissue transglutaminase activity indicating that VIP potentiates programmed cell death, apoptosis, rather than enhancing differentiation under those circumstances (Goossens et al., 1993).

We have recently reported that ganglioneuroma tumours show high concentrations of VIP-LI when compared to neuroblastomas, healthy adrenals and control tumours (Kogner et al., 1992a), and also compared to mouse salivary glands, known to contain high levels of VIP (Kogner et al., 1992b). Aggressive neuroblastomas with N-*myc* amplification contained low concentrations of VIP-LI, whereas advanced neuroblastomas with high concentrations of VIP-LI had a significantly better clinical prognosis than those with low VIP-LI. Undifferentiated human neuroblastomas grown as xenografts in nude mice all showed low concentrations of VIP-LI. We have now extended this prospective study to 123 primary tumour samples, quick frozen at surgery and analysed for VIP-LI in tumour extracts using a competitive radioimmunoassay specific for VIP. All ganglioneuromas showed higher VIP-LI concentrations (7–471 pmol/g) than what was found in four healthy adrenals (0.8–5.5 pmol/g, $P < 0.001$). Ganglioneuromas contained more VIP than neuroblastomas and other control tumours

330

($P < 0.001$, Fig. 5). This strong correlation with differentiation indicates that VIP may be a useful marker for differentiation and may even have a functional significance for neuroblastoma differentiation in vivo, similar to what has been described in vitro. Furthermore, no patient in our material presented with diarrhoea, showing that it is worthwhile analysing VIP in tumours even though there are no signs of VIP secretion or associated symptoms. Similar results were obtained by Qualman and co-workers (1992), who found a correlation between VIP and morphological differentiation when investigating 16 neuroblastoma tumours. High VIP-LI was also associated with localised tumours, while most widespread tumours showed low or undetectable concentrations (Qualman et al., 1992).

The combined results in vivo and in vitro support a role of VIP in neuroblastoma differentiation, and it may be hypothesised that some aspect of this functional interaction might be deregulated in aggressive unfavourable tumours.

Somatostatin

Somatostatin (SOM), or somatotropin release-inhibiting factor (SRIF), is an extensively distributed peptide in the human body, including the central and peripheral nervous system, the gastrointestinal tract and various exocrine and endocrine glands (Reichlin, 1984). Somatostatin is a 14-amino acid peptide (SOM-14) which can be N-terminally extended to 28 amino acids (SOM-28). SOM has a wide range of physiological and pharmacological effects including inhibition of the release of GH and TSH from the pituitary gland and inhibition of the release of peptides from the gastrointestinal tract. Furthermore, SOM has growth inhibitory effects on malignant neuroendocrine cells in vitro, and a long-acting analogue is available and already used for treatment of neuroendocrine tumours in vivo (Schally, 1988; Öberg et al., 1991). The presence of high-affinity receptors for SOM (SS-R) seems to be necessary for the effect of somatostatin analogues in oncological treatment (Reubi et al., 1990). At least

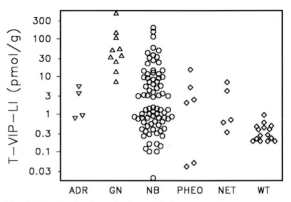

Fig. 5. Vasoactive intestinal peptide in tumour tissue extracts (VIP-LI, pmol/g wet weight) of ganglioneuromas (GN, $n = 10$) and neuroblastomas (NB, $n = 86$) compared to healthy adrenals (ADR, $n = 4$), and control tumours (six phaeochromocytomas (PHEO), five other neuroectodermal tumours (NET) and 16 Wilms' tumours (WT)). GN showed higher VIP-LI concentrations than all other tumours ($P < 0.001$), whereas NB had higher concentrations compared to WT ($P < 0.001$).

four distinct receptors for SOM have been cloned and characterised and are termed SSTR1–SSTR4, with differential distribution in rodent brain and peripheral tissues (SSTR1–SSTR3) and the pituitary gland (SSTR4) (for references, see Maggi et al., 1994). A preliminary study by Moertel and co-workers (1990) identified SS-R on neuroblastoma tumours, predominantly on tumours of localised stages with favourable prognosis. In two recent reports, the presence of SS-R has been characterised in human neuroblastoma tumours and cell lines (Maggi et al., 1994; O'Dorisio et al., 1994). SS-R on neuroblastoma tumours were found mainly in localised tumours (six of seven) compared to neuroblastomas of advanced stages (seven of 19, $P = 0.034$, one-sided Fisher exact test) (O'Dorisio et al., 1994). Down-regulation of SOM receptor binding was observed in five cases during disease progression and lack of SS-R was a poor prognostic sign correlated with advanced tumours and poor outcome. Furthermore, in that study O'Dorisio and co-workers (1994) showed that somatostatin and a long-acting synthetic analogue, octreotide, inhibited proliferation of

IMR32 neuroblastoma cells expressing SS-R, whereas no effect was noted on SK-N-SH neuroblastoma cells that did not express SS-R. Maggi et al. (1994) investigated a panel of eight neuroblastoma cell lines showing SOM high-affinity binding sites (SS_{R1}) in only three of these (CHP-134B, CHP-404 and CHP-382), while a low-affinity binding site (SS_{R2}) could be demonstrated in all cell lines. The low-affinity binding site SS_{R2} specifically bound SOM-14 and SOM-28 without any apparent biological activity. However, SS_{R1} mediated a slight antiproliferative effect of a somatostatin agonist, SMS-201995, in the nanomolar range, possibly linked to a decrease in Ca^{2+}.

The expression of somatostatin binding sites on tumour cells provides a novel opportunity for diagnostic imaging as well as therapeutic approaches in vivo. Clinical experience of SS-R scintigraphy for tumour imaging was reported using a radioactive isotope-labelled SOM analogue (Krenning et al., 1989). Detection in vivo of SS-R-expressing tumour cells is highly predictive for subsequent effect of somatostatin analogue therapy in patients with neuroendocrine tumours (Krenning et al., 1989; Lamberts et al., 1992). Recently SS-R scintigraphy has been used in children with neuroblastoma, and positive scintigrams were recorded at diagnosis or relapse in six of seven, and eight of 11 patients, respectively (Lamberts et al., 1992; Sautter-Bihl et al., 1994). There is a tendency that SS-R imaging detects more favourable tumours (Sautter-Bihl et al., 1994), while all children with SS-R-negative neuroblastoma succumbed to their disease. These results in vivo are highly consistent with those previously reported on SS-R detection by autoradiography in tumour samples (Moertel et al., 1990).

We have previously reported (Kogner et al., 1992b, 1993c) that high concentrations of SOM-LI may be detected in ganglioneuromas with a competitive radioimmunoassay using a specific antisera raised against SOM-14 (Efendic et al., 1978). SOM-LI was higher in ganglioneuromas compared to neuroblastomas, healthy adrenals and control tumours of neuroendocrine differentia-

tion; and tended to be associated with favourable outcome and inversely correlated with amplification of N-*myc*. This prospective series has now been extended, and a total of 121 samples has been analysed. SOM-LI in ganglioneuromas was higher ($P < 0.001$) compared to neuroblastomas, phaeochromocytomas, other neuroendocrine tumours as well as Wilms' tumours and healthy adrenals (Fig. 6a) (Kogner et al., unpublished observations). Neuroblastomas contained higher concentrations than the control tumours ($P < 0.001$). Although there was a significant correlation of high somatostatin expression with differentiated benign ganglioneuroma, there were no significant differences between neuroblastomas of localised and advanced stages (data not shown). However, in a subset of children with advanced neuroblastoma tumours (stages 3 or 4) and unfavourable age at diagnosis (> 12 months), all survivors showed high SOM-LI in tumour tissue comparable to what was found in ganglioneuromas (Fig. 6b). High tumour concentrations of SOM-LI in these children with unfavourable neuroblastomas indicated a better prognosis (44%, seven of 16, disease free > 12 months from diagnosis and off therapy) than in the whole subset (survival 22%) or those with lower SOM-LI (all died, $P < 0.001$). Chromatographic characterisation of SOM-LI in neuroblastoma tumour extract showed both SOM-14 and a component with larger Stokes radius, presumably SOM-28 (Kogner et al, unpublished observations). In another recent study comprising 16 neuroblastomas, higher tissue concentrations of SOM-LI were found in tumours with morphological differentiation and favourable clinical stage (Qualman et al., 1992). However, in that study, no correlation with clinical outcome could be found for SOM-LI.

The clinical significance of plasma SOM-LI as a marker in neuroblastoma remains to be investigated further. Our experience is that only a minority of children with neuroblastoma present with elevated plasma SOM-LI at diagnosis. Increasing plasma SOM-LI concentrations during surgical manipulation are detected in neuroblas-

332

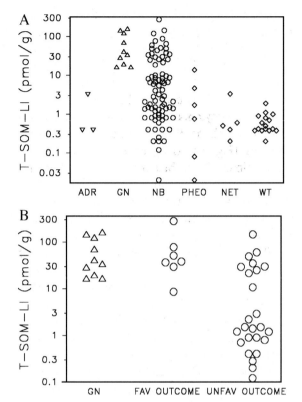

Fig. 6. (a) Somatostatin in tumour tissue extracts (SOM-LI, pmol/g wet weight) of ganglioneuromas (GN, $n = 10$) and neuroblastomas (NB, $n = 81$) compared to healthy adrenals (ADR, $n = 3$), and control tumours (six phaeochromocytomas (PHEO), five other neuroectodermal tumours (NET) and 16 Wilms' tumours (WT)). GN showed higher SOM-LI concentrations than all other tumours ($P < 0.001$), whereas NB had higher concentrations compared to control tumours ($P < 0.01-0.001$). (b) Somatostatin in tumour tissue extracts (SOM-LI, pmol/g wet weight) of ten ganglioneuromas (GN, triangles) and 32 neuroblastomas from children with poor clinical prognostic factors (advanced clinical stages 3 or 4, and age > 12 months at diagnosis, circles). Neuroblastomas are divided with respect to clinical outcome (FAV OUTCOME, alive and disease free > 12 months from diagnosis, $n = 7$; UNFAV OUTCOME, dead during follow-up, $n = 25$). GN and FAV OUTCOME had higher concentrations of SOM-LI than UNFAV OUTCOME ($P < 0.001$).

toma patients (Kogner et al., unpublished observations).

Considered together, high concentrations of somatostatin in favourable neuroblastomas and differentiated ganglioneuromas, suggest a possible autocrine function in tumour regression or differentiation in vivo as has been described in vitro, since both tumours and cell lines may express functional high-affinity receptors, SS-R. This may indicate a novel therapeutic modality in neuroblastoma using long-acting somatostatin agonists in children having neuroblastomas expressing SS-R. Furthermore, the recently demonstrated technique of in vivo detection of SS-R-containing tumour tissue enables not only a novel way of detecting neuroblastomas for diagnostic purposes, but also a way of selecting patients for a proposed treatment with somatostatin analogues. However, in vitro data imply that high concentrations of somatostatin agonists are necessary for the antiproliferative effect (in the nanomolar range) and, further, it has been shown in vitro that growth inhibition may only be to a limited degree, thereby probably limiting the therapeutic application of somatostatin analogues, as an adjunct to cytostatic drugs or other therapeutic means, to only a few selected patients.

Tachykinins

Tachykinins are neuropeptides with C-terminal amino acid homologies and characteristic biological properties, such as smooth muscle contraction, and sialogogic and hypotensive effects (Erspamer, 1981). The mammalian tachykinin family includes substance P (SP), neurokinin A (NKA), neuropeptide K (NPK) and neuropeptide γ (NPγ), derived from the preprotachykinin (PPT) I gene (Nawa et al., 1983; Krause et al., 1987; McDonald et al., 1989), and neurokinin B (NKB), derived from the PPT II gene (Kotani et al., 1986; Bonner et al., 1987). We analysed tachykinins in neuroblastomas, ganglioneuromas and control tissues using competitive radioimmunoassays and reverse-phase HPLC (Table I) (Svensson et al., 1992). Only five of 37 neuroblastomas and one of eight ganglioneuromas showed significant concentrations of tachykinin immunoreactivity (> 2 pmol/g). From our results it was evident that neuroblastomas show expression of the PPT I

TABLE I

Tachykinin immunoreactivity in tumour tissue

	n	All neg.	NKA+,SP−, SP−, NKB−, NPK−	NKA+, SP+, NKB−, NPK−	NKA+, SP+, NKB+, NPK−
ADR	3	2	0	0	1
GN	8	7	0	0	1
NB	37	32	4	1	0
NT	3	3	0	0	0
WT	1	0	0	0	1

Tachykinin immunoreactivities were analyzed in tissue extracts using antiseras raised against kassinin (K12, reacting with NKA, NKB and NPK) (Theodorsson-Norheim et al., 1984) and SP (SP2) and considered positive if > 2 pmol/g. Reversed phase HPLC characterized further extracts positive for K12. NKA, neurokinin A; SP, substance P; NKB, neurokinin B; NPK, neuropeptide K; ADR, healthy adrenal gland; GN, ganglioneuroma; NB, neuroblastoma; NT, control neuroendocrine tumours; WT, Wilms' tumour (nephroblastoma). (Results summarized from Svensson et al., 1992.)

gene containing NKA-LI, but not NKB-LI, while the ganglioneuroma, one healthy adrenal and one Wilms' tumour also expressed the PPT II gene and contained NKB-LI (Table I). However, these results were in contrast to those of McGregor et al. (1990), who reported elevated NKB in three neuroblastomas but absence of the tachykinins derived from the PPT I gene in all five tumours investigated.

Chromogranin A and pancreastatin

Chromogranin A (CGA) is a 439-amino acid acidic protein being the major soluble protein of catecholamine storage vesicles in adrenomedullary cells (Smith and Winkler, 1967; Helman et al., 1988). CGA has been proposed as a prohormone precursor for pancreastatin (PST) (Tatemoto et al., 1986) and several other biologically active peptides that have recently been shown to be produced by human neuroendocrine tumour cells (Iguchi et al., 1990, 1992; Conlon et al., 1992).

Plasma concentrations of CGA like immunoreactivity have been reported to be elevated in children with neuroblastoma with the highest levels recorded in those with widespread tumours (stages 3, 4 and 4-S) (Hsiao et al., 1990). High concentrations of CGA-LI (> 190 ng/ml) were associated with poor outcome in those with unfavourable tumours (stages 3 and 4). The majority of neuroblastoma cell lines analysed showed expression of CGA as reported by Cooper and co-workers (1990). Using immunohistochemistry, CGA can be detected in most paediatric tumours of neural crest origin, predominantly those with more differentiated morphology (Hachitanda et al., 1989; Molenaar et al., 1990).

Pancreastatin is a regulatory peptide consisting of 52 (human PST) or 49 amino acid residues (porcine PST) which inhibits glucose-induced insulin secretion and was recently shown to be produced by human small-cell lung carcinoma cells, and detected as elevated concentrations of PST-LI in plasma of most patients with this neuroendocrine tumour (Iguchi et al., 1990, 1992). In a recent study (Kogner et al., unpublished observations), we analysed PST-LI in plasma and tumour tissue from children with neuroblastoma and ganglioneuroma. All these children showed relatively low plasma concentrations of PST-LI (1.4–19 pmol/l). However, those with ganglioneuroma or neuroblastoma with favourable clinical stage had significantly higher concentrations compared to those with advanced unfavourable neuroblastoma ($P < 0.05$, data not shown). Significant correlations of PST with localized disease stage, differentiated tumours and favourable prognosis was shown when PST-LI concentrations were analysed in tumour tissue extracts (Fig. 7). These results imply the usefulness of PST-LI in plasma and tumours as a marker of differentiation and favourable clinical outcome.

Neurotensin

Neurotensin is a 13-amino acid peptide with a wide spectrum of biological activities (Carraway and Leeman, 1975; Granier et al., 1982). Using a

334

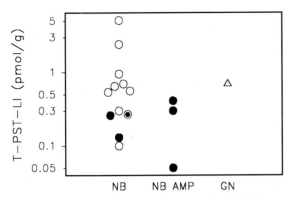

Fig. 7. Pancreastatin-like immunoreactivity (PST-LI) in extracts of 15 neuroblastomas (NB, circles) and one ganglioneuroma (GN, triangle). Three advanced neuroblastomas showed unfavourable amplification of the N-*myc* oncogene (NB AMP). Filled symbols, those who died during follow-up; dotted symbols, still under therapy or followed < 12 months. Tumours from children with favourable outcome had higher PST-LI concentrations than those from children who died ($P < 0.01$). N-*myc* amplified tumours had lower PST-LI concentrations than the other tumours ($P < 0.05$). Tumours of advanced clinical stage (3 and 4) had lower PST-LI concentrations than those of favourable stages ($P < 0.05$, data not shown). PST-LI was analysed using a competitive radioimmunoassay raised against porcine PST with 91% crossreactivity with human PST (Peninsula, Belmont, CA, USA).

competitive radioimmunoassay for neurotensin-like immunoreactivity (NT-LI), we analysed tumour extracts from 37 neuroblastomas and eight ganglioneuromas without detecting significant concentrations in any of these tumours (Kogner et al., unpublished observations). Similarly negative results were reported by Qualman and co-workers (1992) when analysing 16 neuroblastomas for NT-LI. In another study, plasma samples from 58 children with neuroblastoma were investigated for NT-LI, and only two showed higher concentrations than the controls (Becker and Berthold, 1992).

Conclusions

Several neuropeptides are produced and released by neuroblastoma and ganglioneuroma tumours, and may be significant with regard to symptoms, and growth or differentiation of tumour cells.

Furthermore, these peptides may provide clinically useful markers and also indicate novel therapeutic options in these patients. In addition, investigating these tumours and derived cell lines may provide further insight into biological characteristics of neuropeptides and their receptors.

In particular, accumulating data show that neuropeptide Y is associated with neuroblastoma growth and is a useful clinical marker with prognostic significance when analysed in plasma. Characterisation of NPY synthesis and processing has revealed significant differences between different tumours and tissues, and also indicated the presence of previously uncharacterised molecular forms. More detailed knowledge about the putative trophic significance of NPY for tumour cells may provide new possibilities of therapeutic interaction.

Vasoactive intestinal peptide, somatostatin and pancreastatin are associated with favourable differentiated sympathetic tumours. Furthermore, VIP and somatostatin have been shown to play a functional role in vitro and this gives hope for future design of novel treatment for children with neuroblastoma. Somatostatin agonists are already available for oncological treatment, although the clinical experience in neuroblastoma is very limited. New means of in vivo detection of tumours expressing specific receptors, like high-affinity somatostatin receptors, may provide better imaging and characterisation of neuroblastoma as well as better selection of patients for specific therapeutic measures.

Acknowledgements

The present work was supported by the Swedish Child Cancer Fund and the Swedish Cancer Society. Elvar Theodorsson and Carina Stenfors are acknowledged for critically revising the manuscript.

References

Aakerlund, L., Gether, U., Fuhlendorff, J., Schwartz, T.W. and Thastrup, O. (1990) Y1 receptors for neuropeptide Y are coupled to mobilization of intracellular calcium and inhibition of adenylate cyclase. *FEBS Lett.*, 260: 73–78.

Adrian, T.E., Allen, J.M., Bloom, S.R., Ghatei, M.A., Rossor, M.N., Roberts, G.W., Crow, T.J., Tatemoto, K. and Polak, J.M. (1983a) Neuropeptide Y distribution in human brain. *Nature*, 306: 584–586.

Adrian, T.E., Allen, J.M., Terenghi, G., Bacarese-Hamilton, A.J., Brown, M.J., Polak, J.M. and Bloom, S.R. (1983b) Neuropeptide Y in phaeochromocytomas and ganglioneuroblastomas. *Lancet*, ii: 540–542.

Agoston, D.V., Colburn, S., Krajniak, K.G. and Waschek, J.A. (1992) Distinct regulation of vasoactive intestinal peptide (VIP) expression at mRNA and peptide levels in human neuroblastoma cells. *Neurosci. Lett.*, 139: 213–216.

Allen, J.M., Hoyle, N.R., Yeats, J.C., Ghatei, M.A., Thomas, D.G. and Bloom, S.R. (1985) Neuropeptides in neurological tumors. *J. Neuro-Oncol.*, 3: 197–202.

Allen, J.M., Martin, J.B. and Heinrich, G. (1987) Neuropeptide Y gene expression in PC12 cells and its regulation by nerve growth factor: A model for developmental regulation. *Mol. Brain Res.*, 3: 39–43.

Andersson, G., Påhlman, S., Parrow, V., Johansson, I. and Hammerling, U. (1994) Activation of the human NPY gene during neuroblastoma cell differentiation-induced transcriptional activities of AP-1 and AP-2. *Cell Growth Diff.*, 5: 27–36.

Becker, K. and Berthold, F. (1992) Plasma neurotensin: lack of a differentiation and tumor marker in children with neuroblastoma. *Pediatr. Hematol. Oncol.*, 9: 269–272.

Berthold, F. (1990) Overview: biology of neuroblastoma. In C. Pochedly (Ed.), *Neuroblastoma: Tumor Biology and Therapy*, CRC Press, Boca-Raton, pp 1–27.

Bonner, T.I., Affolter, H.U., Young, A.C. and Young, W.S., III (1987) A cDNA encoding the precursor of the rat neuropeptide, neurokinin B. *Brain Res.*, 388: 243–249.

Brodeur, G.M., Azar, C., Brother, M., Hiemstra, J., Kaufman, B., Marshall, H., Moley, J., Nakagawara, A., Saylors, R., Scavarda, N., Schneider, S., Wasson, J., White, P., Seeger, R., Look, T. and Castleberry, R. (1992) Neuroblastoma; effect of genetic factors on prognosis and treatment. *Cancer*, 70: 1685–1694.

Brodeur, G.M., Pritchard, J., Berthold, F., Carlsen, N.L.T., Castel, V., Castleberry, R.P., De Bernardi, B., Evans, A.E., Favrot, M., Hedborg, F., Kaneko, M., Kemshead, J., Lampert, F., Lee, R.E.J., Look, A.T., Pearson, A.D.J., Philip, T., Roald, B., Sawada, T., Seeger, R.C., Tsuchida, Y. and Voûte, P.A. (1993) Revisions of the international criteria for neuroblastoma diagnosis, staging and response to treatment. *J. Clin. Oncol.*, 11: 1466–1477.

Carraway, R. and Leeman, S.E. (1975) The amino acid sequence of a hypothalamic peptide, neurotensin. *J. Biol. Chem.*, 250: 1907–1911.

Conlon, J.M., Hamberger, B. and Grimelius, L. (1992) Isolation of peptides arising from the specific posttranslational processing of chromogranin A and chromogranin B from human pheochromocytoma tissue. *Peptides*, 13: 639–644.

Cooper, M.J., Hutchins, G.M., Cohen, P.S., Helman, L.J., Mennie, R.J. and Israel, M.A. (1990) Human neuroblastoma tumor cell lines correspond to the arrested differentiation of chromaffin adrenal medullary neuroblasts. *Cell. Growth Diff.*, 1: 149–159.

Efendic, S., Nylén, A., Roovete, A. and Uvnäs-Wallenstein, K. (1978) Effects of glucose and arginine on the release of immunoreactive somatostatin from the isolated perfused rat pancreas. *FEBS Lett.*, 92: 33–35.

Erspamer, V. (1981) The tachykinin peptide family. *Trends. Neurosci.*, 4: 267–269.

Goossens, J.F., Manechez, D., Pommery, N., Formstecher, P. and Henichart, J.P. (1993) VIP potentiates retinoic-acid effect on tissue transglutaminase activity in human neuroblastoma, the SK-N-SH cells. *Neuropeptides*, 24: 99–103.

Gordon, E.A., Kohout, T.A. and Fishman, P.H. (1990) Characterization of functional neuropeptide Y receptors in a human neuroblastoma cell line. *J. Neurochem.*, 55: 506–513.

Gozes, I. and Brenneman, D.E. (1989) VIP: molecular biology and neurobiological function. *Mol. Neurobiol.*, 3: 201–236.

Gozes, I. and Brenneman, D.E. (1993) Neuropeptides as growth and differentiation factors in general and VIP in particular. *J. Mol. Neurosci.*, 4: 1–9.

Granier, C., van Rietschoten, J., Kitabgi, P., Poustis, C. and Freychet, P. (1982) Synthesis and characterization of neurotensin analogues for structure/activity relationship studies. Acetyl-neurotensin (8–13) is the shortest analogue with full binding and pharmacological activities. *Eur. J. Biochem.*, 124: 117–124.

Hachitanda, Y., Tsuneyoshi, M. and Enjoji, M. (1989) Expression of pan-neuroendocrine proteins in 53 neuroblastic tumors. An immunohistochemical study with neuron-specific enolase, chromogranin, and synaptophysin. *Arch. Pathol. Lab. Med.*, 113: 381–384.

Hayashi, Y., Ohi, R., Sone, M., Takahashi, K., Mouri, T., Watanabe, T., Yaoita, S. and Nakamura, M. (1991) Significance of plasma neuropeptide Y (NPY) in diagnosis and prognosis of neuroblastoma. In: A.E. Evans, G.J. D'Angio, A.G. Knudson, R.C. Seeger (Eds.), *Advances in Neuroblastoma Research, Vol. 3*, Wiley-Liss, New York, pp 359–365.

Helman, L.J., Ahn, T.G., Levine, M.A., Allison, A., Cohen, P.S., Cooper, M.J., Cohn, D.V. and Israel, M.A. (1988) Molecular cloning and primary structure of human chromogranin A (secretory protein I) cDNA. *J. Biol. Chem.*, 263: 11559–11563.

Hsiao, R.J., Seeger, R.C., Yu, A.L. and O'Connor, D.T. (1990) Chromogranin A in children with neuroblastoma. Serum concentration parallells disease stage and predicts survival. *J. Clin. Invest.*, 85; 1555–1559.

Hökfelt, T. (1991) Neuropeptides in perspective: the last ten years. *Neuron*, 7: 867–879.

Iguchi, H., Funakoshi, A., Tateishi, K., Ichinose, Y., Hara, N. and Ohta, M. (1990) Production of pancreastatin-like immunoreactivity, a presumed processing product of chromogranin A, in small cell lung carcinoma. *Cancer J.*, 3: 197–201.

Iguchi, H., Bannai, S., Takanashi, N. and Tsukada, Y. (1992) Production of chromogranin A and B derived peptides in human small cell lung carcinoma cell lines. *Eur. J. Cancer*, 28A: 1458–1462.

Kogner, P. (1993) *Neuropeptide Y and Nerve Growth Factor Receptors in Neuroblastoma and Leukemia in Children*. Karolinska Institute, Stockholm, 179 pp.

Kogner, P., Björk, O. and Theodorsson, E. (1990) Neuropeptide Y as a marker in pediatric neuroblastoma. *Pediatr. Pathol.*, 10: 207–216.

Kogner, P., Theodorsson, E. and Björk, O. (1991) Plasma neuropeptide (NPY); a novel marker of neuroblastoma. In: A.E. Evans, G.J. D'Angio, A.G. Knudson, R.C. Seeger (Eds.), *Advances in Neuroblastoma Research, Vol. 3*, Wiley-Liss, New York, pp 367–373.

Kogner, P., Björk, O., Dominici, C., Hedborg, F. and Theodorsson, E. (1992a) Vasoactive intestinal peptide (VIP) and somatostatin in childhood ganglioneuromas and neuroblastomas. *Proc. Am. Soc. Clin. Oncol.*, 11: 371.

Kogner, P., Rutgers, M. and Theodorsson, E. (1992b) Vasoactive intestinal peptide (VIP) in ganglioneuromas and neuroblastomas with favourable outcome indicating tumor differentiating activity of VIP in vivo. *Neuropeptides*, 22: 36–37.

Kogner, P., Barbany, G., Dominici, C., Castello, M.A., Raschella, G. and Persson, H. (1993a) Coexpression of messenger RNA for TRK protooncogene and low affinity nerve growth factor receptor mRNA in neuroblastoma with favorable prognosis. *Cancer Res.*, 53: 2044–2050.

Kogner, P., Björk, O. and Theodorsson, E. (1993b) Neuropeptide Y in neuroblastoma: Increased concentration in metastasis, release during surgery and characterization of plasma and tumor extracts. *Med. Pediatr. Oncol.*, 21: 317–322.

Kogner, P., Theodorsson, E. and Björk, O. (1993) Neuropeptides indicating growth, differentiation and outcome in childhood neuroblastoma and ganglioneuroma. *Clin. Chem. Enzym. Commun.*, 5: 289–294.

Kogner, P., Björk, O. and Theodorsson, E. (1994a) Plasma neuropeptide Y in healthy children; influence of age, anaesthesia, and the establishment of an age-adjusted reference interval. *Acta Paediatr.*, 83: 423–427.

Kogner, P., Nordenskjöld, A., Dominici, C., Hedborg, F., Barbany, G., Persson, H., Theodorsson, E. and Björk, O. (1994b) Neuropeptide Y immunoreactivity and mRNA expression in neuroblastoma; coexpression with nerve growth factor receptor mRNA and age dependent relationship with N-myc amplification. Submitted.

Kotani, H., Hoshimaru, M., Nawa, H. and Nakanishi, S. (1986) Structure and gene organization of bovine neuromedin K precursor. *Proc. Natl. Acad. Sci. USA*, 83: 7074–7078.

Krause, J.E., Chirgwin, J.M., Carter, M.S., Xu, Z.S. and Hershey, A.D. (1987) Three rat preprotachykinin mRNAs encode the neuropeptides substance P and neurokinin A. *Proc. Natl. Acad. Sci. USA*, 84: 881–885.

Krenning, E.P., Breeman, W.A.P., Kooij, P.P.M., Lameris, J.S., Bakker, W.H., Koper, J.W., Ausema, L., Reubi, J.C. and Lamberts, S.W. (1989) Localization of endocrine-related tumours with radioiodinated analogue of somatostatin. *Lancet*, i: 242–244.

Lacey, S.R., Gribble, T.J. and Kosloske, A.M. (1989) Favorable prognosis of vasoactive intestinal peptide-secreting ganglioneuroblastoma. *Pediatr. Surg. Int.*, 4: 217–219.

Lamberts, S.W., Reubi, J.C. and Krenning, E.P. (1992) Somatostatin receptor imaging in the diagnosis and treatment of neuroendocrine tumors. *J. Steroid Biochem. Mol. Biol.*, 43: 185–188.

Lundberg, J.M., Terenius, L., Hökfelt, T., Martling, C.R., Tatemoto, K., Mutt, V., Polak, J., Bloom, S.R. and Goldstein, M. (1982) Neuropeptide Y (NPY)-like immunoreactivity in peripheral noradrenergic neurons and effects of NPY on sympathetic function. *Acta Physiol. Scand.*, 116: 477–480.

Lundberg, J.M., Hökfelt, T., Hemsén, A., Theodorsson-Norheim, E., Pernow, J., Hamberger, B. and Goldstein, M. (1986) Neuropeptide Y-like immunoreactivity in adrenaline cells of adrenal medulla and in tumors and plasma of pheochromocytoma patients. *Regul. Peptides*, 13: 169–182.

Maggi, M., Baldi, E., Finetti, G., Franceschelli, F., Brocchi, A., Lanzillotti, R., Serio, M., Camboni, M.G. and Thiele, C.J. (1994) Identification, characterization, and biological activity of somatostatin receptors in human neuroblastoma cell lines. *Cancer Res.*, 54: 124–133.

Matsushima, H., Bogenmann, E. (1993) Expression of trkA cDNA in neuroblastoma mediates differentiation in vitro and in vivo. *Mol. Cell Biol.*, 13: 7447–7456.

McDonald, M.R., Takeda, J., Rice, C.M. and Krause, J.E. (1989) Multiple tachykinins are produced and secreted upon post-translational processing of three substance P precursor proteins, α-, β-, and γ-preprotachykinin. Expression of the preprotachykinins in AtT-20 cells infected with vaccinia virus recombinants. *J. Biol. Chem.*, 264: 15578–15592.

McGregor, G.P., Gaedicke, G. and Voigt, K. (1990) Neurokinin-immunoreactivity in human neuroblastomas. Evidence for selective expression of the preprotachykinin (PPT) II gene. *FEBS Lett.*, 277: 83–87.

Moertel, C.L., Reubi, J.C., Scheithauer, B., Schaid, D.J. and Kvols, L.K. (1990) Somatostatin receptors (SS-R) are expressed and correlate with prognosis in childhood neuroblastoma. *Proc. Am. Assoc. Cancer Res.*, Abstr. 306.

Molenaar, W.M., Baker, D.L., Pleasure, D., Lee, V.M.-Y. and Trojanowski, J.Q. (1990) The neuroendocrine and neural profiles of neuroblastomas, ganglioneuroblastomas and ganglioneuromas. *Am. J. Pathol.*, 136: 375–382.

Mouri, T., Sone, M., Takahashi, K., Itoi, K., Totsune, K., Hayashi, Y., Hasegawa, S., Ohneda, M., Murakami, O., Miura, Y., Katakura, R., Tachibana, S. and Maebashi, M. (1992) Neuropeptide Y as a plasma marker for phaeochromocytoma, ganglioneuroblastoma and neuroblastoma. *Clin. Sci.*, 83: 205–211.

Muller, J.M., Lolait, S.J., Yu, V.C., Sadée, W. and Waschek, J.A. (1989) Functional vasoactive intestinal polypeptide (VIP) receptors in human neuroblastoma subclones that contain VIP precursor mRNA and release VIP-like substances. *J. Biol. Chem.*, 264: 3647–3650.

Nawa, H., Hirose, T., Takashima, H., Inayama, S. and Nakanishi, S. (1983) Nucelotide sequences of cloned cDNAs for two types of bovine brain substamce P precursor. *Nature*, 306: 32–36.

Öberg, K., Norheim, I. and Theodorsson, E. (1991) Treatment of malignant midgut carcinoid tumors with a long acting somatostatin analogue (SMS 201–995). *Acta Oncol.*, 30: 503–507.

O'Dorisio, M.S., Fleshman, D.J., Qualman, S.J. and O'Dorisio, T.M. (1992) Vasoactive intestinal peptide: autocrine growth factor in neuroblastoma. *Regul. Peptides* 37: 213–226.

O'Dorisio, M.S., Chen, F., O'Dorisio, T.M., Wray, D. and Qualman, S.J. (1994) Characterization of somatostatin receptors on human neuroblastoma tumours. *Cell Growth Diff.*, 5: 1–8.

O'Hare, M.M.T. and Schwartz, T.W. (1989a) Expression and precursor processing of neuropeptide Y in human pheochromocytoma and neuroblastoma tumors. *Cancer Res.*, 49: 7010–7014.

O'Hare, M.M.T. and Schwartz, T.W. (1989b) Expression and precursor processing of neuropeptide Y in human and murine neuroblastoma and pheochromocytoma cell lines. *Cancer Res.*, 49: 7015–7019.

Pascual-Castroviejo, I. (1990) *Spinal Tumors in Children and Adolescents,* Raven Press, New York, 296 pp.

Pence, J.C. and Shorter, N.A. (1990) In vitro differentiation of human neuroblastoma cells caused by vasoactive intestinal peptide. *Cancer Res.*, 50: 5177–5183.

Pence, J.C. and Shorter, N.A. (1991) Further studies on the interaction between vasoactive intestinal peptide and neuroblastoma cell lines. In A.E. Evans, G.J. D'Angio, A.G. Knudson and R.C. Seeger (Eds.), *Advances in Neuroblastoma Research, Vol. 3,* Wiley-Liss, New York, pp 375–381.

Pence, J.C. and Shorter, N.A. (1993) The autocrine function of vasoactive intestinal peptide on human neuroblastoma cell growth and differentiation. *Arch. Surg.* 128: 591–595.

Pincus, D.W., DiCiccio-Bloom, E.M. and Black, I.B. (1990) Vasoactive intestinal peptide regulates mitosis, differentiation and survival of cultured sympathetic neuroblasts. *Nature*, 343: 564–567.

Qualman, S.J., O'Dorisio, M.S., Fleshman D.J., Shimada H. and O'Dorisio, T.M. (1992) Neuroblastoma. Correlation of neuropeptide expression in tumor tissue with other prognostic factors. *Cancer*, 70: 2005–12.

Rascher, W., Kremens, B., Wagner, S., Feth, F., Hunneman, H. and Lang, R.E. (1993) Serial measurements of neuropeptide Y in plasma for monitoring neuroblastoma in children. *J. Pediatr.*, 122: 914–916.

Reichlin, S. (1984) Somatostatin. *New Engl. J. Med.*, 309: 1495–1501 and 1556–1563 (two parts).

Reubi, J.C., Krenning, E., Lamberts, S.W.J. and Kvols, L. (1990) Somatostatin receptors in malignant tissues. *J. Steroid Biochem. Mol. Biol.*, 37: 1073–1077.

Rozengurt, E. (1991) Neuropeptides as cellular growth factors: role of multiple signalling pathways. *Eur. J. Clin. Invest.*, 21: 123–134.

Sabol, S.L. and Higuchi, H. (1990) Transcriptional regulation of the neuropeptide Y gene by nerve growth factor, antagonism by glucocorticoids and potentiation by adenosine 3′,5′-monophosphate and phorbol ester. *Mol. Endocrinol.*, 4: 384–392.

Said, S.I. (1991) Vasoactive intestinal polypeptide: Biological role in health and disease. *Trends. Endocrinol. Metab.*, 2: 107–112.

Said, S.I. and Faloona, G.R. (1975) Elevated plasma and tissue levels of vasoactive intestinal polypeptide in the watery-diarrhea syndrome due to pancreatic, bronchogenic and other tumors. *N. Engl. J. Med.*, 293: 155–160.

Said, S.I. and Mutt, V. (1970) Polypeptide with broad biological activity: isolation from small intestine. *Science*, 169: 1217–1218.

Sautter-Bihl, M.L., Dörr, U., Schilling, F.H., Koscielniak, E., Treuner, J. and Bihl, H. (1994) Somatostatin receptor imaging: a new horizon in the diagnostic management of neuroblastoma. *Semin. Oncol.*, in press.

Schally, A.V. (1988) Oncological applications of somatostatin analogues. *Cancer Res.*, 48: 6977–6985.

Sheikh, S.P., O'Hare, M.M.T., Tortora, O. and Schwartz, T.W. (1989) Binding of monoiodinated NPY to hippocampal membranes and human neuroblastoma cell lines. *J. Biol. Chem.*, 264: 6648–6654.

Silen, M.L. and Gardner, J.D. (1993) Gastrointestinal peptides and cancer. *Trends. Endocrinol. Metab.*, 4: 131–135.

Smith, A.D. and Winkler, H. (1967) Purification and properties of an acidic protein from chromaffin granules of bovine adrenal medulla. *Biochem J.*, 103: 483–492.

Svensson, T., Kogner, P. and Theodorsson, E. (1992) Tachykinin immunoreactivity in neuroblastoma and ganglioneuroma tissue represents neurokinin A (NKA) but not neurokinin B (NKB). *Neuropeptides*, 22: 64–65.

338

Tatemoto, K., Carlquist, M. and Mutt, V. (1982) Neuropeptide Y: a novel brain peptide with similarities to peptide YY and pancreatic polypeptide. *Nature*, 296: 659–660.

Tatemoto, K., Efendic, S., Mutt, V., Makk, G., Feistner, G.J. and Barchas, J.D. (1986) Isolation of pancreastatin, a novel pancreatic peptide that inhibits insulin secretion. *Nature*, 324: 476–478.

Theodorsson, E. (1989) Regulatory peptides as tumour markers. *Acta Oncol.*, 28: 319–324.

Theodorsson-Norheim, E., Brodin, E., Norheim, I. and Rosell, S. (1984) Antisera raised against eledoisin and kassinin detect immunoreactive material in rat tissue extracts: tissue distribution and chromatographic characterization. *Regul. Peptides*, 9: 229–244.

Theodorsson-Norheim, E., Hemsen, A. and Lundberg, J.M. (1985) Radioimmunoassay for neuropeptide Y (NPY): Chromatographic characterization of immunoreactivity in plasma and tissue extracts. *Scand. J. Clin. Lab. Invest.*, 45: 355–365.

Theodorsson-Norheim, E., Hemsen, A., Brodin, E. and Lundberg, J.M. (1987) Sample handling techniques when analyzing regulatory peptides. *Life Sci.*, 41: 845–848.

Wahlestedt, C., Grundemar, L., Håkanson, R., Heilig, M., Shen, G.H., Zukowska-Grojec, Z. and Reis, D.J. (1990) Neuropeptide receptor subtypes, Y1 and Y2. *Ann. NY Acad. Sci.*, 611: 7–26.

Zukowska-Grojec, Z., Pruszczyk, P., Colton, C., Yao, J., Shen, G.H., Myers, A.K. and Wahlestedt, C. (1993) Mitogenic effect of neuropeptide Y in rat vascular smooth muscle cells. *Peptides*, 14: 263–268.

F. Nyberg, H.S. Sharma and Z. Wiesenfeld-Hallin (Eds.)
Progress in Brain Research, Vol 104

CHAPTER 19

Effects of ankle joint inflammation on the proportion of calcitonin gene-related peptide (CGRP)-immunopositive perikarya in dorsal root ganglia

U. Hanesch and H.-G. Schaible

Physiologisches Institut, Universität Würzburg, Röntgenring 9, D-97070 Würzburg, Germany

The neuropeptide, calcitonin gene-related peptide (CGRP), was discovered, identified and characterized during the last decade using modern molecular biological techniques for the first time (Amara et al., 1982, 1985; Rosenfeld et al., 1983). This 37-amino acid peptide is widely distributed in the nervous system, including dorsal root ganglion (DRG) cells (Gibson et al., 1984; Gibbins et al., 1987; Ju et al., 1987) and, at the spinal level, the central branches of sensory primary afferents (Gibson et al., 1984; Carlton et al., 1987; McNeill et al., 1988), some local dorsal horn neurons (Conrath et al., 1989) and motoneurons (Arvidsson et al., 1989; Marlier et al., 1990). In the DRGs, CGRP is found in a higher proportion of cell bodies than substance P (SP), but both neuropeptides are also colocalized to a great extent, in that nearly all SP-positive neurons contain CGRP as well (Gibson et al., 1984; Wiesenfeld-Hallin et al., 1984; Gibbins et al., 1985; Lee et al., 1985a,b; Gulbenkian et al., 1986; Cameron et al., 1988). In a small proportion of DRG cells, CGRP is coexistent with somatostatin (SOM) and galanin (GAL) (Ju et al., 1987; Tuchscherer and Seybold, 1989). In articular nerves of cat's knee, we have shown (Hanesch et al., 1991) that the CGRP immunopositive cells form the largest proportion

among the neuropeptide-containing neurons so far tested. This population of CGRP-immunopositive neurons consists of afferents with unmyelinated group IV, and thinly myelinated group III fibers, whereas the proportion of thick myelinated fibers seems to be very low.

The functions of CGRP in afferent fibers are not well understood. This is, in part, due to the fact that the modality of CGRP-positive afferents is not known. The large proportion of CGRP-positive neurons with group III and IV fibers implies that the neuropeptide should also be contained in nociceptive afferents. In fact, immunoreactive CGRP (ir-CGRP) is released in the spinal cord by electrical stimulation of peripheral nerves, at stimulus intensities that are sufficient to activate unmyelinated fibers (Morton and Hutchison, 1989) and by application of noxious stimuli. With respect to mechanical noxious stimuli, it is not settled whether both heat and mechanical stimuli evoke release of ir-CGRP (Morton and Hutchison, 1989; Pohl et al., 1992). In the periphery, the neuropeptide can be released from peripheral terminals and, after release, it may contribute to neurogenic inflammation (Lam and Ferrell, 1991; Green et al., 1992). This action may have an influence on the severity of joint inflammation since the application of antibodies directed to CGRP prior to and during the development of polyarthritis results in a less dramatic inflammatory response in the limbs (Louis et al., 1989).

In the spinal cord, CGRP may excite dorsal horn neurons (Wiesenfeld-Hallin, 1986; Woolf and Wiesenfeld-Hallin, 1986; Cridland and Henry, 1988; Miletic and Tan, 1988; Ryu et al., 1988; Kawamura et al., 1989). Furthermore, CGRP acts synergistically with SP. At the behavioural level, CGRP enhances scratching and biting induced by intrathecal administration of SP (Wiesenfeld-Hallin et al., 1984), and CGRP and SP synergistically modulate the flexor reflex induced by noxious stimuli (Woolf and Wiesenfeld-Hallin, 1986). CGRP may enhance the action of SP by increasing release of SP (Oku et al., 1987) and/or by inhibiting endopeptidases, and therefore preventing the inactivation of this neurokinin (LeGrèves et al., 1985 1989; Mao et al., 1992; Schaible et al., 1992). Beyond that, CGRP may facilitate the release of the excitatory neurotransmitters, glutamate and aspartate, from dorsal horn nerve endings, probably through an increase of the Ca^{2+} level (Kangra and Randić, 1990; Oku et al., 1988).

There is evidence that the synthesis of neuropeptides may exhibit an up- or down-regulation under (experimental) pathological conditions. Peripheral axotomy results in a reduction of SP and CGRP in DRG cells (Jessel et al., 1979; Noguchi et al., 1989; Helke and Rabchevsky, 1991) and in an increased production of galanin and vasointestinal peptide in the same ganglia (Hökfelt et al., 1987; Villar et al., 1989). By contrast, chronic Freund's adjuvant-induced polyarthritis leads to enhanced levels of SP in peripheral nerves over weeks (Lembeck et al., 1981), and quantitative studies in polyarthritic rats showed a doubling of the CGRP level in the DRGs up to 26 days after inoculation (Kuraishi et al., 1989).

Whilst the polyarthritis model revealed an increase of CGRP synthesis, it is difficult in this model to define the population of afferent fibers involved in the up-regulation since polyarthritis is a multifocal disease affecting numerous organs.

Furthermore, it does not allow side-to-side comparisons within the same animal. More recently a chronic unilateral inflammation at the ankle joint, carpal joint or paw was developed that is restricted to a distinct region at the site of inoculation and does not cause secondary lesions, e.g., at the contralateral side (Stein et al., 1988; Grubb et al., 1991; Smith et al., 1992). This model now allows side-to-side comparison of neuropeptide levels. Smith and co-workers (1992) used the model of the inflammation at the carpal joint of the rat and measured CGRP levels by radioimmunoassay. They found an up-regulation of CGRP synthesis in the appropriate ganglia 15 days post-inoculation.

Whilst the former studies have focused on the synthesis of CGRP under chronic conditions, we have addressed the production of CGRP under acute (2 days) and chronic (20 days) conditions in order to define whether the up-regulation of the synthesis of CGRP displays an early and/or a late component of the inflammatory disease. As a model the unilateral inflammation of the rat ankle joint was used. The inflammation was induced by subcutaneous injections of Freund's complete adjuvant (FCA) around the left ankle joint under brief anesthesia. Swelling of the ankle region up to 134% of control, and an erythema of the overlying skin developed within hours and showed a maximum at about 2 days post-inoculation (early phase of inflammation) and persisted for at least 3 weeks (late phase of inflammation). Throughout the course of inflammation, the inflammatory signs were restricted to the proximal quarter of the foot and the distal quarter of the lower leg. Neither the contralateral ankle joint nor other parts of the body showed secondary lesions during the period observed. At the microscopic level, a cellular infiltration was seen in the skin, the subdermal connective tissue, muscles, tendons and joint capsule of the affected ankle. Within the 3 weeks of observation, the animals showed signs of hyperalgesia with a maximum in the first week. Pressing the inflamed ankle elicited vigorous withdrawal reflexes. Within the first week, half of the rats also showed disturbances of gait, i.e., limping, but these symptoms disappeared in the second and third week post-inoculation. The feeding behaviour appeared normal and the body weight of the animals increased with normal rate. In recordings from spinal cord neurons, differences were noted between neurons in control rats and neurons sampled in rats with inflammation. In neurons of rats with unilateral inflammation, the average mechanical threshold at the ankle was lowered, and fewer neurons appeared as nociceptive specific; more neurons exhibited very large receptive fields than those in control rats (Grubb at al., 1993).

In order to study changes in CGRP synthesis in primary afferent neurons, the dorsal root ganglia L4–L6 of both sides of perfused rats were dissected and processed for immunocytochemical localization of CGRP by the PAP method. For each ganglion, the ratio of CGRP-immunopositive cell bodies to the total number of cell bodies counted was determined by using a fractionator sampling method scheme, and was expressed as the percentage of neurons showing CGRP-like immunoreactivity (CGRP-LI). The percentages represent a relative frequency of CGRP-LI neurons, and these frequencies were then compared between control rats and rats with a 2-day- or 20-day-inflammation, and within the inoculated animals between the inflamed and non-inflamed side (for further details of staining and counting, see Hanesch et al., 1993a).

Stained CGRP-LI perikarya were found randomly distributed in the sections of all dorsal root ganglia. Identification of the CGRP-containing cell bodies was unequivocal, since the sections did not show background staining (Fig. 1). The particular staining pattern, however, varied between neurons. The perikarya showed either a dark and even staining across the cell body (this is also typical for SP-LI, SOM-LI and GAL-LI perikarya), or a granule-like staining forming a perinuclear ring (also seen in GAL-immunopositive neurons), or a punctate staining distributed over the cytoplasm. Morphometric studies on cell populations with different staining patterns performed on L5–L7 ganglia in the cat, showed no

correlation between staining pattern and cell size, although cells with punctate staining tended to be larger (unpublished observations). No difference in the staining pattern was seen between different lumbar levels and between the inflamed and non-inflamed side of rats.

In order to get a baseline, the relative frequencies of CGRP-immunopositive DRG neurons were determined in four control rats. In the 24 dorsal root ganglia, 20 419 perikarya were identified by our criteria and, within this sample, 24% of the neurons showed a CGRP-LI (Fig. 2). Significant differences in the proportion of CGRP-positive cell bodies were neither observed between the lumbar levels nor between the ganglia of the right and left side. Compared to the proportion (35%) of CGRP-immunopositive neurons in cats (Hanesch et al., 1991), the percentage in rats is apparently lower. The data in the rat are, however, comparable to data of other immunohistochemical studies showing percentages of 10–20% (Gibbins et al., 1987), 40% (Lee et al., 1985b) and 36–55% (McCarthy and Lawson, 1990) CGRP-immunopositive cells in corresponding segments in rats, and they are in line with in situ hybridization studies that reveal a percentage of 20–40% CGRP-mRNA expressing neurons in rats (Cortès et al., 1990).

To study quantitatively the effect of an acute and chronic unilateral inflammation, animals were inoculated with FCA and perfused for either 2 days (five rats) or 20 days (four rats) post-inoculation (see above). At each time point, more than 20 000 cell bodies were counted in ganglia L4–L6 from the inflamed and non-inflamed side, and the proportions of CGRP-immunopositive neurons were determined on both sides. In the ganglia of the non-inflamed (control) side of animals with inflammation lasting 2 days and 20 days, the percentages of CGRP-positive neurons were not different from those in control rats (Fig. 2). There was a small increase in the proportion of CGRP-LI cells at the noninflamed side at day 2 but this increase was not statistically significant.

By contrast, in the ganglia of the (left) inflamed side the proportion of CGRP-immunopositive

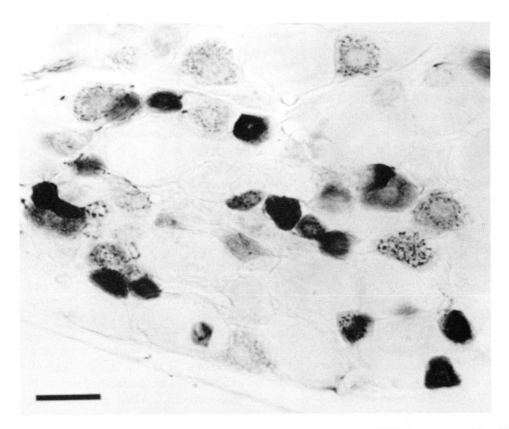

Fig. 1. Section of a dorsal root ganglion L5 of a control rat with neurons showing CGRP-like immunostaining. The reaction product is seen as even staining across the cell body, or as a granule-like staining forming a perinuclear ring, or as a punctate staining distributed across the cytoplasm. Scale bar: 50 μm.

cells showed a significant increase to 31.9% already 2 days post-inoculation and remained significantly enhanced to 28.6% at 20 days after induction of inflammation (Fig. 2). Thus the inflammation of the ankle region is associated with an increase in the percentage of CGRP-LI neurons in ipsilateral ganglia L4–L6. Setting the proportion of CGRP-positive cells in control rats to 100%, the acute and chronic phases of FCA-induced unilateral inflammation leads to a 20–30% increase in the number of DRG neurons synthetizing CGRP (Fig. 3).

The increase in the proportion of CGRP-positive neurons could either result from a de novo activation of the gene encoding for CGRP in neurons that do not express the peptide under normal conditions, or from an enhancement of the synthesis of CGRP in neurons that produce CGRP under normal conditions in amounts that are below the threshold for identification with immunohistochemical methods. The magnitude of the inflammation-induced increase in the number of CGRP-producing cells (30% at day 2 and 20% at day 20) is probably underestimated, since the dorsal root ganglia contain perikarya from afferents innervating different tissues, e.g., muscle, skin and viscera, which should not be affected by FCA. Cell bodies from articular afferents represent only a small portion of the neurons in ganglia L4–L6.

To study whether the inflammation-induced production of CGRP takes place in a distinct

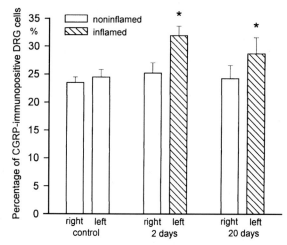

Fig. 2. Percentage of CGRP-immunopositive perikarya (mean values of ganglia L4–L6) from both sides in four control rats and from the inflamed (hatched bars) and the non-inflamed side (white bars) in four rats with acute inflammation (2 days), and in five rats with subchronic inflammation (20 days).

population of DRG cells, a morphometrical analysis was performed on L5 ganglia of both sides of three rats with an inflammation lasting 2 days. The immunopositive perikarya were drawn and

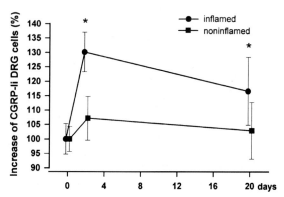

Fig. 3. Increase in the proportion of CGRP-like immunoreactive perikarya in ipsilateral DRGs L4–L6 of rats with unilateral inflamed ankle joints at days 2 and 20 post-inoculation. On the control side, the proportion of CGRP-positive neurons was set to 100% and the values obtained from each inflamed side at 2 days and 20 days were expressed as percentage of control. Differences between ganglia of the inflamed and non-inflamed side were tested using a paired t-test. *$P < 0.05$ was taken as significant.

the cross-sectional areas were measured using a computer-aided analysis system. The complete data of the inflamed and non-inflamed sides are represented in the histogram in Fig. 4. There is no difference in the distribution of the cross-sectional areas between the affected and non-affected side. Thus, the subset of neurons producing CGRP during inflammation is not different from neurons producing CGRP under normal conditions with regard to soma size.

In summary this study has shown that an inflammatory lesion activates the synthesis of CGRP in a portion of perikarya in the ipsilateral ganglia that do not (measurably) produce the peptide under normal conditions. This up-regulation occurs already at an early stage post-inoculation ($<$ 2 days) and remains stable for over at least 3 weeks. This suggests that the proportion of neurons actually synthetizing CGRP is not a constant but underlies 'plastic changes' within certain limits. The extent of this variability may depend on the type and duration of the stimulus applied as variations between individual animals are small.

It has been shown that, under experimental pathological conditions, the synthesis of other neuromodulators is changed as well. The production of SP in DRG cells is activated almost in parallel to the up-regulation of CGRP in chronic and acute phases of inflammation (Noguchi et al., 1988; Minami et al., 1989). In addition, we have recently demonstrated that this activation occurs not only in neurons in which SP is initially synthetized, but in a pool of cells in which the gene encoding for SP normally is not expressed (Hanesch et al., 1993b). This tempts the speculation that the induction of the CGRP- and SP-synthesis occurs in neurons in which both neuropeptides are colocalized.

The trigger of up-regulation of the neuropeptide synthesis in the perikarya is still unknown. Different mechanisms can be taken into consideration.

(1) Altered axonal transport rates or reduced degradation of neuropeptides. Both factors could

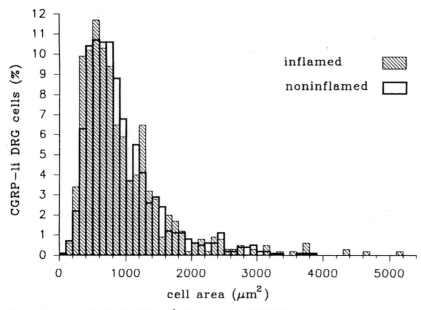

Fig. 4. Soma size distribution (50 μm^2-wide classes) of CGRP-like immunoreactive dorsal root ganglion cells from the L5 ganglia of three rats with an inflammation lasting 2 days. The cell area histograms of ganglia from the inflamed ($n = 649$ perikarya) and the non-inflamed ($n = 805$ perikarya) side are superposed.

be due to elevated peptide levels in the DRG cells.

(2) Induction of gene expression by messengers that are transported from the sensory endings in the inflamed region to the perikarya. The fast axonal transport of substances, however, may be too slow to account for the induction of rapid changes seen in acute phases of inflammation. This mechanism may contribute to the maintainance of up-regulation at chronic inflammatory stages.

(3) Compounds, e.g., nerve growth factor, that circulate in the blood might influence the changes in neuropeptide synthesis. The small but insignificant increase in the proportion of CGRP-LI cells at the non-inflamed side, seen in animals with an inflammation lasting 2 days, might be the result of gene-induction through circulating factors acting on perikarya. Considering the much larger increase in the proportion of CGRP-producing cells at the ipsilateral side, it is likely that circulating compounds cannot be exclusively re-

sponsible for the up-regulation of the neuropeptide synthesis.

(4) Enhanced release of the peptide in the spinal cord and the periphery might cause the induction of gene expression through feed-back mechanisms. In fact, the intraspinal release of CGRP is already enhanced within the first hours of inflammation (Schaible et al., 1994).

(5) Changes in the electrical activity of the neurons. Afferent fibers exposed to inflammatory stimuli are sensitized during the first few hours of an inflammation and they show enhanced responses to noxious stimuli and (in the case of high threshold and mechanoinsensitive units) lowering of mechanical threshold (Schaible and Schmidt, 1985, 1988). In consequence the enhanced number of action potentials might result in enhanced Ca^{2+} levels in the perikarya, and this could be a stimulus for activation of gene-expression.

The specific contribution of the different factors responsible for up-regulation in acute and chronic

inflammation remains to be clarified. We speculate that the early up-regulation of the synthesis
of CGRP favours a trigger role of the discharges
of afferents in (early) neurochemical changes. At
later stages several mechanisms may be at work.

References

Amara, S.G., Jonas, V., Rosenfeld, M.G., Ong, E.S. and Evans, R.M. (1982) Alternative RNA processing in calcitonin gene expression generates mRNA's encoding different polypeptide products. *Nature*, 298: 240–244.

Amara, S.G., Arriza, J.L., Leff, S.E., Swanson L.W., Evans R.M. and Rosenfeld, M.G. (1985) Expression in brain messenger RNA encoding a novel neuropeptide homologous to calcitonin gene-related peptide. *Science*, 229: 1094–1097.

Arvidsson, U., Cullheim, S., Ulfhake, B., Hökfelt, T. and Terenius, L. (1989) Altered levels of calcitonin gene-related peptide (CGRP)-like immunoreactivity of cat lumbar motoneurons after chronic spinal cord transection. *Brain Res.*, 489: 387–396.

Cameron, A.A., Leah, J.D. and Snow, P.J. (1988) The coexistence of neuropeptides in feline sensory neurons. *Neuroscience*, 27: 969–979.

Carlton, S.M., McNeill, D.L., Chung, K. and Coggeshall, R.E. (1987) A light and electron microscopic level analysis of calcitonin gene-related peptide (CGRP) in the spinal cord of the primate: an immunohistochemical study. *Neurosci. Lett.*, 82: 145–150.

Conrath, M., Taquet, H., Pohl, M. and Carayon, A. (1989) Immunocytochemical evidence for calcitonin gene-related peptide-like neurons in the dorsal horn and lateral spinal nucleus of the rat cervical spinal cord. *J. Chem. Neuroanat.*, 2: 335–347.

Cortès, R., Arvidsson, M., Schalling, M., Ceccatelli, S. and Hökfelt, T. (1990) In situ hybridization studies on mRNAs for cholecystokinin, calcitonin gene-related peptide and choline acetyltransferase in the lower brain stem, spinal cord and dorsal root ganglia of rat and guinea pig with special reference to motoneurons. *J. Chem. Neuroanat.*, 3: 467–485.

Cridland, R.A. and Henry, J.L. (1988) Effects of intrathecal administration of neuropeptides on a spinal nociceptive reflex in the rat: VIP, galanin, CGRP, TRH, somatostatin and angiotensin. *Neuropeptides*, 11: 23–32.

Gibbins, J.L., Furness, J.B., Costa, M., MacIntyre, J. Hillyard, C.J. and Grigis, S. (1985) Colocalization of calcitonin gene-related peptide-like immunoreactivity with substance P in cutaneous, vascular and visceral sensory neurons of guinea pigs. *Neurosci. Lett.*, 57: 125–130.

Gibbins, J.L., Furness, J.B. and Costa, M. (1987) Pathway-specific patterns of the co-existence of substance P, calcitonin gene-related peptide, cholecystokinin and dynorphin in neurons of the dorsal root ganglia of the guinea pig. *Cell Tissue Res.*, 248: 417–437.

Gibson, S.J., Polak, J.M., Bloom, S.R., Sabate, I.M., Mulderry, P.M., Ghatei, M.A., McGregor, G.P., Morrison, J.F. B., Kelly, J.S., Evans, R.M. and Rosenfeld, M.G. (1984) Calcitonin gene-related peptide immunoreactivity in the spinal cord of man and eight other species. *J. Neurosci.*, 4: 3101–3111.

Green, P.G., Basbaum, A.I. and Levine, J.D. (1992) Sensory neuropeptide interactions in the production of plasma extravasation in the rat. *Neuroscience*, 50: 745–749.

Grubb, B.D., Birrell, G.J., McQueen, D.S. and Iggo, A. (1991) The role of PGE2 in the sensitization of mechanoreceptors in normal and inflamed ankle joints of the rat. *Exp. Brain Res.*, 84: 383–392.

Grubb, B.D., Stiller, R.U. and Schaible, H.-G. (1993) Dynamic changes in the receptive field properties of spinal cord neurons with ankle input in rats with chronic unilateral inflammation in the ankle region. *Exp. Brain Res.*, 92: 441–452.

Gulbenkian, S., Merighi, A., Wharton, J., Varndell, I.M. and Polak, J.M. (1986) Ultrastructural evidence for the coexistence of calcitonin gene-related peptide and substance P in secretory vesicles of peripheral nerves in the guinea-pig. *J. Neurocytol.*, 15: 535–542.

Hanesch, U., Heppelmann, B. and Schmidt, R.F. (1991) Substance P and calcitonin gene-related peptide immunoreactivity in primary afferent neurons of the cat's knee joint. *Neuroscience*, 45: 185–193.

Hanesch, U., Pfrommer, U., Grubb, B.D. and Schaible, H.-G. (1993a) Acute and chronic phases of unilateral inflammation in rat's ankle are associated with an increase in the proportion of calcitonin gene-related peptide-immunoreactive dorsal root ganglion cells. *Eur. J. Neurosci.*, 5: 154–161.

Hanesch, U., Pfrommer, U., Grubb, B.D., Heppelmann, B. and Schaible, H.-G. (1993b) The proportion of CGRP-immunoreactive and SP-mRNA containing dorsal root ganglion cells is increased by a unilateral inflammation of the ankle joint of the rat. *Regul. Peptides*, 46: 202–203.

Helke, C.J. and Rabchevsky, A. (1991) Axotomy alters putative neurotransmitter in visceral sensory neurons of the nodose and petrosal ganglia. *Brain Res.*, 551: 44–51.

Hökfelt, T., Wiesenfeld-Hallin, Z., Villar, M. and Melander, T. (1987) Increase of galanin-like immunoreactivity in rat dorsal root ganglion cells after peripheral axotomy. *Neurosci. Lett.*, 83: 217–220.

Jessell, T., Tsunoo, A., Kanazawa, I. and Otsuka, M. (1979) Substance P: Depletion in the dorsal horn of rat spinal cord after section of the peripheral processes of primary sensory neurons. *Brain Res.*, 168: 247–259.

Ju, G., Hökfelt, T., Brodin, E., Fahrenkrug, J., Fischer, J.A., Frey, P., Elde, R.P. and Brown, J.C. (1987) Primary sensory neurons of the rat showing calcitonin gene-related peptide immunoreactivity and their relation to substance P-, somatostatin-, galanin-, vasoactive intestinal polypeptide-, and cholecystokinin-immunoreactive ganglion cells. *Cell Tissue Res.*, 247: 417–431.

Kangra, I. and Randić, M. (1990) Tachykinins and calcitonin gene-related peptide enhance release of endogenous glutamate and aspartate from the rat spinal dorsal horn slice. *J. Neurosci.*, 10: 2026–2038.

Kawamura, M., Kuraishi, Y., Minami, M. and Satoh, M. (1989) Antinociceptive effect of intrathecally administered antiserum against calcitonin gene-related peptide on thermal and mechanical noxious stimuli in experimental hyperalgesic rats. *Brain Res.*, 497: 199–203.

Kuraishi, Y., Nanayama, T., Ohno, H., Fuji, N., Ataka, A., Yajima, H. and Satoh, M. (1989) Calcitonin gene-related peptide increases in the dorsal root ganglia of adjuvant arthritic rat. *Peptides*, 10: 447–452.

Lam, F.Y. and Ferrell, W.R. (1991) Specific neurokinin receptors mediate plasma extravasation in the rat knee joint. *Br. J. Pharmacol.*, 103: 1263–1267.

Lee, Y., Kawai, Y., Shiosaka, S., Takami, K., Kiyanma, H., Hillyard, C.J., Girgis, S., MacIntyre, I., Emson, P.C. and Tohyama, M. (1985a) Coexistence of calcitonin gene-related peptide and substance P-like peptide in single cells of the trigeminal ganglion of the rat: immunohistochemical analysis. *Brain Res.*, 330: 194–196.

Lee, Y., Takami, K., Kawai, Y., Girgis, S., Hillyard, C.J., MacIntyre, I., Emson, P.C. and Tohyama, M. (1985b) Distribution of calcitonin gene-related peptide in the rat peripheral nervous system with reference to its coexistence with substance P. *Neuroscience*, 15: 1227–1237.

LeGrèves, P., Nyberg, F., Terenius, L. and Hökfelt, T. (1985) Calcitonin gene-related peptide is a potent inhibitor of substance P degradation. *Eur. J. Pharmacol.*, 115: 309–311.

LeGrèves, P., Nyberg, F., Hökfelt, T. and Terenius, L. (1989) Calcitonin gene-related peptide is metabolized by an endopeptidase hydrolyzing substance P. *Regul. Peptides*, 25: 277–286.

Lembeck, F., Donnerer, J. and Colpaert, F.C. (1981) Increase of substance P in primary afferent nerves during chronic pain. *Neuropeptides*, 1: 175–180.

Louis, S.M., Jamieson, A., Russell, N.J.W. and Dockray, G.J. (1989) The role of substance P and calcitonin gene-related peptide in neurogenic plasma extravasation in the rat. *Neuroscience*, 32: 581–586.

Marlier, L., Rajaofetra, N., Peretti-Renucci, R., Kachidian, P., Poulat, P., Feuerstein, C. and Privat, A. (1990) Calcitonin gene-related peptide staining intensity is reduced in rat lumbar motoneurons after spinal cord transection: a quantitative immunocytochemical study. *Exp. Brain Res.*, 82: 40–47.

Mao, J., Coghill, R.C., Kellstein, D.E., Frenk, H. and Mayer, D.J. (1992) Calcitonin gene-related peptide enhances substance P-induced behaviors via metabolic inhibition: in vivo evidence for a new mechanism of neuromodulation. *Brain Res.*, 574: 157–163.

McCarthy, P.W. and Lawson, S.W. (1990) Cell type and conduction velocity of rat primary sensory neurons with calcitonin gene-related peptide-like immunoreactivity. *Neuroscience*, 34: 623–632.

McNeill, D.L., Coggeshall, R.E. and Carlton, S.M. (1988) A light and electron microscope study of calcitonin gene-related peptide in the spinal cord of the rat. *Exp. Neurol.*, 99: 699–708.

Miletic, V. and Tan, H. (1988) Iontophoretic application of calcitonin gene-related peptide produces a slow and prolonged excitation of neurons in the cat lumbar dorsal horn. *Brain Res.*, 446: 169–172.

Minami, M., Kuraishi, Y., Kawamura, M., Yamaguchi, T., Masu, Y., Nakanishi, S. and Satoh, M. (1989) Enhancement of preprotachykinin A gene expression by adjuvant-induced inflammation in the rat spinal cord: possible involvement of substance P-containing spinal neurons in nociception. *Neurosci. Lett.*, 98: 105–110.

Morton, C.R. and Hutchison, W.D. (1989) Release of sensory neuropeptides in the spinal cord: studies with calcitonin gene-related peptides and galanin. *Neuroscience*, 31: 807–815.

Noguchi, K., Mortia, Y., Kiyama, H., Ono, K. and Tohyama, M. (1988) A noxious stimulus induces preprotachykinin-A gene expression in the rat dorsal root ganglion: a quantitative study using in situ hybridization histochemistry. *Mol. Brain Res.*, 4: 31–35.

Noguchi, K., Senba, E., Morita, Y., Sato, M. and Tohyama, M. (1989) Prepro-VIP and preprotachykinin mRNAs in the rat dorsal root ganglion cells following peripheral axotomy. *Mol. Brain Res.*, 6: 327–330.

Oku, R., Satoh, M., Fuji, N., Otaka, A., Yajima, H. and Takagi, H. (1987) Calcitonin gene-related peptide promotes mechanical nociception by potentiating release of substance P from the signal dorsal horn in rats. *Brain Res.*, 403: 350–354.

Oku, R., Nanayama, T. and Satoh, M. (1988) Calcitonin gene-related peptide modulates calcium mobilization in synaptosomes of rat spinal dorsal horn. *Brain Res.*, 475: 356–360.

Pohl, M., Collin, E., Bourgoin, S., Clot, A.M., Hamon, M., Cesselin, F. and Le-Bars, D. (1992) In vivo release of calcitonin gene-related peptide-like material from the cervicotrigeminal area in the rat. Effects of electrical and noxious stimulations of the muzzle. *Neuroscience*, 50: 697–706.

Rosenfeld, M.G., Mermod, J.-J., Amara, S.G., Swanson, L.W., Sawchenko, P.E., River, J., Vale, W.W. and Evans, R.M. (1983) Production of a novel neuropeptide encoded by the calcitonin gene via tissue-specific RNA processing. *Nature*, 304: 129–135.

Ryu, P.D., Gerber, G., Murase, K. and Randić, M. (1988) Actions of calcitonin gene-related peptide on rat spinal dorsal horn neurons. *Brain Res.*, 441: 357–361.

Schaible, H.-G. and Schmidt, R.F. (1985) Effects of an experimantal arthritis on the sensory properties of fine articular afferent units. *J. Neurophysiol.*, 54: 1109–1122.

Schaible, H.-G. and Schmidt, R.F. (1988) Time course of mechanosensitivity changes in articular afferents during a developing experimental arthritis. *J. Neurophysiol.*, 60: 2180–2195.

Schaible, H.-G., Hope, P.J., Lang, C.W. and Duggan, A.W. (1992) Calcitonin gene-related peptide causes intraspinal spreading of substance P released by peripheral stimulation. *Eur. J. Neurosci.*, 4: 750–757.

Schaible, H.-G., Freudenberger, U., Neugebauer, V. and Stiller, R.U. (1994) Intraspinal release of immunoreactive calcitonin gene-related peptide during development of inflammation in the joint in vivo — a study with antibody microprobes in cat and rat. *Neuroscience*, 62: 1293–1305.

Smith, G.D., Harmar, A.J., McQueen, D.S. and Seckl, J.R. (1992) Increase in substance P and CGRP, but not somatostatin content of innervating dorsal root ganglia in adjuvant monoarthritis in the rat. *Neurosci. Lett.*, 137: 257–260.

Stein, C., Millan, M.J. and Herz, A. (1988) Unilateral inflammation of the hindpaw in rats as a model of prolonged noxious stimulation: alterations in behavior and nociceptive thresholds. *Pharmacol. Biochem. Behav.*, 31: 445–451.

Tuchscherer, M.M. and Seybold, V.S. (1989) A quantitative study of the coexistence of peptides in varicosities within the superficial laminae of the dorsal horn of the rat spinal cord. *J. Neurosci.*, 9: 195–205.

Villar, M.J., Cortes, R., Theodorsson, E., Wiesenfeld-Hallin, Z., Schalling, M., Fahrenkrug, J., Emson, P.C. and Hökfelt, T. (1989) Neuropeptide expression in rat dorsal root ganglion cells and spinal cord after peripheral nerve injury with special reference to galanin. *Neuroscience*, 33: 587–604.

Wiesenfeld-Hallin, Z., Hökfelt, T., Lundberg, J.M., Forssmann, W.G., Reinecke, F.A., Tschopp, F.A. and Fischer, J.A. (1984) Immunoreactive calcitonin gene-related peptide and substance P coexist in sensory neurons to the spinal cord and interact in spinal behavioral responses of the rat. *Neurosci. Lett.*, 52: 199–204.

Wiesenfeld-Hallin, Z. (1986) Substance P and somatostatin modulate spinal cord excitability via physiologically different sensory pathways. *Brain Res.*, 372: 172–175.

Woolf, C.J. and Wiesenfeld-Hallin, Z. (1986) Substance P and calcitonin gene-related peptide synergistically modulate the gain of the nociceptive flexor withdrawal reflex in the rat. *Neurosci. Lett.*, 66: 226–230.

F. Nyberg, H.S. Sharma and Z. Wiesenfeld-Hallin (Eds.)
Progress in Brain Research, Vol 104

CHAPTER 20

Regulation of spinal neuropeptide genes in a rat model of peripheral inflammation and hyperalgesia

M.A. Ruda, K. Ren and D. Besse

Neurobiology and Anesthesiology Branch, National Institute of Dental Research, National Institutes of Health, Bldg 49, Rm 1A-11, 9000 Rockville Pike, Bethesda, MD 20892, USA

Introduction

A variety of neuropeptides have been identified at the spinal level. They act as neurotransmitters or neuromodulators and play important roles in the processing of nociceptive information. Recent studies indicate that, in the spinal cord, several neuropeptide genes and their resultant peptide products, including dynorphin, enkephalin and substance P, are up-regulated in response to peripheral tissue inflammation. Analysis of the neural circuits accessed by these peptides suggests that their regulation represents, in part, the mechanisms underlying neuronal hyperexcitability and behavioral hyperalgesia at the spinal level.

This chapter will focus on changes of three neuropeptides: dynorphin, enkephalin and substance P, especially with regard to their precursor mRNAs in the spinal cord. Analysis of mRNA regulation targets the response of intrinsic spinal cord neurons since mRNA transcription occurs in neuronal cell bodies, while analysis of peptide products can be confounded by the diverse origin of spinal axonal processes from primary afferents or descending axons from higher centers of the neuraxis. The molecular mechanisms of nociception will be addressed, and the neuronal regulation will be correlated to development of dorsal horn hyperexcitability and behavioral hyperalgesia.

Spinal opioid systems

Three genes which encode families of opioid peptides have been described. They are preprodynorphin (PPD), preproenkephalin (PPE) and preproopiomelanocortin (POMC). The main peptide products of each of these opioid genes, dynorphin (Kakidani et al., 1982), enkephalin (Noda et al., 1982) and β-endorphin (Nakanishi et al., 1981), respectively, have been identified in strikingly different amounts in the spinal cord. Although dynorphin and enkephalin are found in both cell bodies and numerous varicose axons, no neuronal cell bodies containing β-endorphin have been immunocytochemically labelled in the spinal cord of adult rats, although a few, scattered, varicose, immunoreactive axons have been observed (Tsou et al., 1986). Also, using a sensitive radioimmunoassay (RIA) method, Gutstein et al. (1992) have detected β-endorphin-immunoreactivity that persisted in the segments caudal to a thoracic spinal transection.

In situ hybridization histochemistry (ISHH) labelled PPD neurons in Laminae I, II, V and VI, and in the area around the central canal (Ruda et al., 1988; Noguchi et al., 1991). Dynorphin-like immunoreactive neurons and axons are concentrated in the same areas as the PPD mRNA cell bodies (Sasek et al., 1984; Cruz and Basbaum, 1985; Miller and Seybold, 1987), and originate predominantly from intrinsic neurons. Although there is immunocytochemical evidence for the presence of a small number of dynorphin-like immunoreactive primary afferent axons (Botticelli et al., 1981; Basbaum et al., 1986), it must be noted that, in lumbar dorsal root ganglia, no detectable amounts of PPD mRNA have been observed by ISHH and RNA blot analysis (Ruda, unpublished observations).

In situ hybridization histochemistry labelled PPE neurons in all laminae of the spinal cord, except for the motoneuronal cell groups (Noguchi et al., 1992). In contrast, immunocytochemistry (ICC) analysis has identified labelled neurons mainly in Laminae I, II, V and VI, and in the area around the central canal (for review, see Ruda et al., 1986). Most of the ENK-like immunoreactivity in the dorsal horn likely originates from intrinsic dorsal horn neurons, while a few ENK-like immunoreactive fibers may descend from the brainstem (Hökfelt et al., 1979) or originate from dorsal root ganglion neurons (Senba et al., 1982). This is confirmed by the presence of low levels of PPE mRNA expression in dorsal root ganglia which can be localized to a few smaller or medium-sized neurons (Ruda et al., 1989; also see Fig. 2). The pool of constitutive PPE mRNA expression in the spinal cord is substantially greater than PPD mRNA (see Figs. 1,2).

The endogenous opioid peptides act by binding to three main types of opioid receptors, μ, δ and κ, that are particularly abundant in Laminae I and II of the dorsal horn (e.g., Besse et al., 1991). The μ sites are the most numerous, while δ sites are intermediate and κ sites are very few (Morris and Herz, 1987; Besse et al., 1991, 1992). The endogenous ligands for the κ and δ opioid receptors appear to be dynorphin and enkephalin, respectively. Although β-endorphin binds to the μ site, it is not clear whether it represents the selective endogenous ligand. However, it must be noted that opioid peptides do not display strong selectivities for the three binding sites (Corbett et al., 1982; Paterson et al., 1983; Kosterlitz et al., 1986). It is likely that, under physiological conditions, ligand-receptor binding depends not only on the preferential affinity of the ligand for the receptor, but also on the amount of ligand and receptor available in a given tissue. Since, in the spinal cord, the proportions of the three types of opioid receptors do not match the respective concentrations of endogenous opioid peptides, caution is advised concerning the relationship between one particular opioid peptide and its 'preferential' binding site.

The response of spinal opioid systems to peripheral inflammation and hyperalgesia

Injection of inflammatory agents (complete Freund's adjuvant: CFA, carrageenan, yeast, or phorbol ester) into one hindpaw causes a rapid inflammation as demonstrated by the significant edema measured within 4 h after injection (Iadarola et al., 1988a). The edema displays a broad peak between days 1 and 6 after injection and returns to control values over the next 10 days. There is also a pronounced decrease in paw withdrawal latency to a radiant heat stimulus in the inflamed paw. This hyperalgesia develops within 4 h of injection, and persists for about 2 weeks. In this model of peripheral inflammation and hyperalgesia, alteration in mRNA and peptide contents can be assessed in individual neurons by using techniques such as ISHH and ICC, and quantified using RNA blot analysis and RIA.

PPD mRNA and dynorphin A(1–8) peptide

Four days after hindpaw CFA injection, a dramatic increase in both PPD mRNA and dynorphin peptide was observed on the ipsilateral side of the spinal cord in segments that receive innervation from the inflamed paw (Iadarola et al., 1988a,b; Millan et al., 1988; Ruda et al., 1988; Draisci and Iadarola, 1989; Noguchi et al., 1991). Neurons exhibiting the increase were concentrated in the medial portion of Laminae I and II, and in Laminae V and VI (Fig. 1). The superficial distribution corresponds to the projection site of nociceptive primary afferent fibers innervating the inflamed paw. An almost 3-fold increase in the number of labelled cell bodies in the side of the dorsal horn, ipsilateral to the inflammation, was observed with both ISHH and ICC labelling.

A time-course analysis using RNA blots showed a detectable increase in PPD mRNA as early as 4 h after hindpaw CFA injection, a time point that coincides with edema and hyperalgesia. The peak increase (approximatively 8-fold) is observed by 2 days after CFA injection (Iadarola et al., 1988a). PPD mRNA expression approaches control levels by 14 days, a point at which the inflammatory process has nearly completely resolved. The increase in dynorphin A(1–8), as measured by RIA, occurred later, peaking at a 3-fold increase by day 5. Both the time course and amount of increase differ for dynorphin peptide and PPD mRNA expression. One explanation for these differences is that dynorphin neurons may rapidly release their peptide products into the extracellular environment, and thereby offset any tendency towards peptide intracellular accumulation. Also, the PPD gene is a precursor for other neuropeptides, α- and β-neo-endorphin (Kakidani et al., 1982). These alternative peptides may be transcribed from the PPD gene, although their levels have not been determined in these animal models. Alternatively, the quantitated differences in mRNA versus peptide level may reflect dynamic molecular and cellular events that have not been determined.

PPE mRNA and enkephalin peptide

Whether peripheral inflammation and hyperalgesia induce increases in the synthesis of PPE-derived peptides in the dorsal horn has been controversial. An early RIA study indicating an increase of ENK-like immunoreactivity after injection of Freund's adjuvant into the paw (Faccini et al., 1984) has not been confirmed in more recent studies using the same inflammatory agent (Iadarola et al., 1988a; Millan et al., 1988). However, studies of PPE mRNA expression suggest a role for PPE in the response of spinal cord neurons to peripheral inflammation and hyperalgesia.

Using ISHH, 3 days after the beginning of the inflammation, an increase in PPE mRNA hybridization has been determined in a subpopulation of ipsilateral spinal cord neurons in Laminae I–II, V–VI and VII (Fig. 1) (Noguchi et al., 1992). This observation was facilitated by using a methodology which reduces the overall very high constitutive level of PPE hybridization signal. Quantification of RNA blots confirmed the presence of a slight but significant increase in PPE mRNA expression on the side ipsilateral to the inflammation. The induction represents 40–80% over constitutive values measured in naive animals (Fig. 2; see also Iadarola et al., 1988b). The increase in PPE mRNA also occurs rapidly, within the first hours of inflammation, and persists for about 5 days.

This apparently small change in PPE mRNA expression may be misleading as to the role of PPE neurons in the spinal response to peripheral inflammation and hyperalgesia. The in situ analysis showed that neurons involved in the increased expression likely represent only a subpopulation of spinal PPE neurons that may be distinct from those with a high constitutive expression of PPE mRNA. The hybridization signal is robustly increased in a subpopulation of PPE neurons (Noguchi et al., 1992; see also Fig. 1), suggesting a dynamic response to the noxious input. With the large number of spinal cord neurons observed to express PPE mRNA in so many different laminar locations that clearly are not part of nociceptive circuits, a diverse role for PPE in spinal cord function must be postulated.

Inflammation and opioid receptors

During the period of inflammation and hyperalgesia, there is no significant change in the number of κ, μ or δ opioid receptors in the dorsal horn (Iadarola et al., 1988a). The lack of detectable alteration in opioid binding sites in this acute model of hyperalgesia is in contrast to the decrease in κ opioid binding sites observed in rat after CFA-induced polyarthritis (Millan et al.,

352

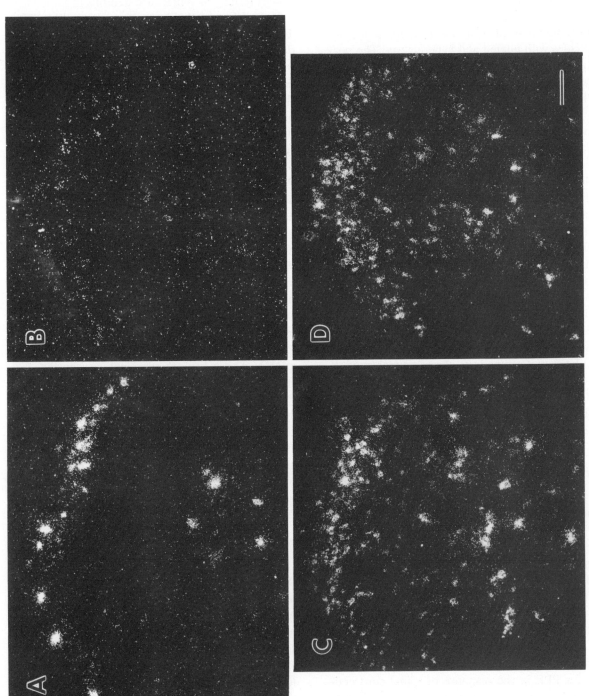

Fig. 1. Dark-field photomicrographs of the L5 segment of the spinal cord ipsilateral (A and C) and contralateral (B and D) to the inflamed paw using in situ hybridization with ^{35}S-labelled PPD (A and B) and PPE (C and D) probes. PPD mRNA expression is clearly increased from barely detectable constitutive levels while changes in PPE mRNA expression are difficult to detect over the high constitutive levels in a subpopulation of neurons in the superficial laminae and neck of the

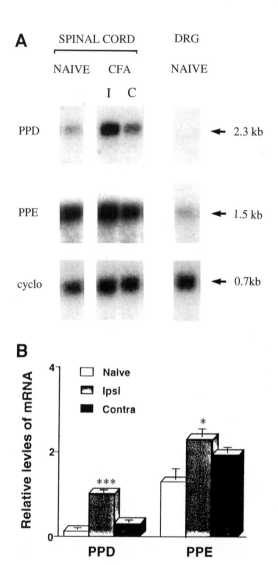

Fig. 2. Changes in PPD and PPE mRNA expression in the spinal cord of rats with hindpaw inflammation. A. Example of Northern blot obtained from 20 μg of total RNA of L4–L5 spinal segments in naive animals (NAIVE), and 2 days after CFA injection (CFA) on both ipsilateral (I) and contralateral (C) sides. L4 and L5 dorsal root ganglia (DRG) of naive rats were also analysed. The same blot has been hybridized successively with oligonucleotide probes specific to PPD and PPE mRNA, and with a cDNA probe specific to cyclophilin (cyclo) as a control for RNA lane loading. B. Quantification of three different blots obtained from distinct groups of rats. Data are expressed as mean (probe/cyclophilin) ratios ± SEM. *$P < 0.05$, ***$P < 0.001$, compared to naive value, t-test. Ipsi, ipsilateral; Contra, contralateral.

1986) or monoarthritis (Besse et al., 1992), as well as the changes in opioid binding sites in a model of chronic pain produced by unilateral footrot in sheep (Brandt and Livingston, 1990a,b). However, it must be emphasized that the differences may be due to events that occur over larger time periods, as the delays where alterations in opioid binding sites have been observed were in the range of 3–4 weeks. By this extended time point, inflammation, hyperalgesia and alterations in endogenous opioid biosynthesis have disappeared in the model of CFA inflammation of one hindpaw. These observations suggest that opioid receptor alterations may occur only in more long-term, persistent states of noxious stimulation.

Neuronal circuitry involved in inflammation-induced increase in PPD and PPE mRNA

The temporal and anatomical correlation of the increase in dynorphin and enkephalin biosynthesis, and the events related to peripheral inflammation and hyperalgesia, suggests a close association of the regulation of spinal opioid peptides with sensory processes. Dynorphin-containing neurons have been shown to be contacted by primary afferents (Cho and Basbaum, 1989), including putative nociceptive afferents that contain calcitonin gene-related peptide (Takahashi et al., 1988; Carlton and Hayes, 1989; Takahashi et al., 1990). These observations suggest a direct monosynaptic relationship between nociceptive primary afferents and dynorphin-containing neurons. Intact primary afferent axons innervating the inflamed hindpaw are necessary for up-regulation of spinal dynorphin neurons since previous studies, in which the sciatic and saphenous nerves or the spinal nerve was cut prior to induction of inflammation with CFA, resulted in no alteration in spinal dynorphin (Iadarola et al., 1988c).

A way to assess the role of different classes of primary afferent fibers in the events leading to opioid gene expression is by selectively destroying subpopulations of primary afferent fibers. Capsaicin is a neurotoxin that, when administered neonatally to rats, destroys almost all the unmyelinated nociceptive primary afferent fibers. In addition, the content of several neuropeptides, including substance P (SP) and calcitonin gene-related peptide (CGRP) are reduced in the dorsal root ganglia and subsequently in the spinal cord (Hammond and Ruda, 1991). In neonatal capsaicin-treated rats with CFA-induced hindpaw inflammation in adulthood, the number of neurons exhibiting PPD mRNA was reduced by over 80% in Laminae I–II, and by 50% in the neck of the dorsal horn, compared to neonatal vehicle-treated rats with hindpaw inflammation (Hylden et al., 1992). It appears that dynorphin gene expression is dependent on input from capsaicin-sensitive primary afferents. The concomitant loss of SP- and CGRP-containing primary afferents in these animals suggests that these neuropeptides participate in the initiation of synaptic events that lead to induction of dynorphin gene expression.

Morphine is known to produce analgesia in part by direct spinal mechanisms (see reviews by Duggan and North, 1984; Yaksh and Noueihed, 1985; Besson and Chaouch, 1987). This effect is mediated by the numerous μ opioid receptors in the superficial laminae of the dorsal horn (Besse et al., 1991), the majority of which occurs presynaptically (LaMotte et al., 1976; Ninkovic et al., 1981; Besse et al., 1990), presumably on nociceptive C- and Aδ-primary afferent fibers (Gamse et al., 1979; Fields et al., 1980; Nagy et al., 1980). Morphine is thought to inhibit the release of neuromediators such as SP (Jessel and Iversen, 1977; Yaksh et al., 1980) or CGRP (Pohl et al., 1989) from primary afferent fibers. We have recently observed that the robust ipsilateral increase in PPD mRNA expression occurring in the spinal cord 2 days after hindpaw inflammation is inhibited by analgesic doses of morphine administered via osmotic pumps implanted just before CFA injection (Besse et al., submitted). The inhibition of CFA-induced PPD mRNA expression reached 62% after subcutaneous (2 mg/kg/h, s.c.) and 45% after intrathecal (2 μg/kg/h) morphine infusion. Naltrexone co-administered at a dose 10-fold less than that of morphine abolished the morphine effect.

In contrast to PPD mRNA, we failed to detect a significant inhibition of morphine on the inflammation-induced increase in PPE mRNA occurring in the spinal cord. This result may be related to the sensitivity of the methodology employed since the percentage change in PPE mRNA expression was small and not easily quantifiable.

From both CFA-induced effects and morphine-induced effects, it is obvious that dynorphin and enkephalin systems are acting differentially in response to nociceptive stimuli. The dramatic changes in both dynorphin A(1–8) and PPD mRNA levels suggest that the dynamic response to inflammation and hyperalgesia in the spinal cord occurs in parallel with that of dynorphin. In contrast, the enkephalin system is differentially regulated and the response to inflammation and hyperalgesia likely involves only a subpopulation of enkephalin neurons.

Spinal preprotachykinin mRNA, substance P and neurokinin receptors

Substance P, a member of the tachykinin family, is an important neuropeptide involved in the nociceptive pathways within the spinal cord. Substance P is located in primary sensory neurons with axons terminating in superficial laminae and neck of the spinal dorsal horn, two regions important in the processing of nociceptive information. The release of SP from primary afferent terminals is the first synaptic event in the CNS related to transmission of nociceptive information. It is important to note that SP in the dorsal horn can originate from three sources: primary afferent axons, intrinsic spinal cord neurons and axons descending from brainstem cell groups. Since a significant number of SP fibers survive peripheral and supraspinal deafferentations (Nagy et al., 1980; Hammond and Ruda, 1991) the intrinsic spinal SP plays a significant role in SP-mediated events. Substance P-immunoreactive cell bodies are found in Laminae I–VI, Lamina X and the lateral spinal nucleus (for review, see Ruda et al., 1986). While there is a wealth of evidence indicating that SP-containing primary sensory neurons are involved in the transmission of nociceptive information, the nociceptive role of intrinsic spinal neurons that contain SP is less clear.

The mRNA encoding SP is derived from the preprotachykinin (PPT) A gene (Nawa et al., 1983; Krause et al., 1987). Alternative RNA splicing of the PPT A gene primary transcript results in the generation of three different mRNAs termed α-, β- and γ-PPT mRNA. Substance P precursor sequences are encoded by all three PPT mRNAs (for review, see Maggi et al., 1993). The other peptide products of the PPT A gene include neurokinin A, neuropeptide K and neuropeptide γ (for review, see Maggi et al., 1993). There are at least three distinct tachykinin receptors, called neurokinin (NK; NK_1, NK_2 and NK_3) (see Helke, this volume). The genes that encode the tachykinin receptors have been recently cloned and characterized (for review, see Nakanishi, 1991). Tachykinin receptors are differentially distributed. Using RNA blot analysis and radioligand binding, it has been found that NK_1 receptors are most abundant, in rat spinal cord, compared to the other two tachykinin receptors (Tsuchida et al., 1990; Yashpal et al., 1990). Substance P appears to act primarily at NK_1 receptors, although interactions with other tachykinin receptors are also possible (Maggi et al., 1993). Using molecular probes targeting PPT and tachykinin receptor genes, it is now clear that PPT mRNA (Minami et al., 1989; Noguchi and Ruda, 1992) and NK_1 receptor mRNA (Schäfer et al., 1993) are dramatically up-regulated in the spinal cord following peripheral tissue inflammation, suggesting a significant role of tachykinins in intrinsic spinal cord neurons in dorsal horn hyperexcitability and hyperalgesia.

Preprotachykinin mRNA expression in the spinal cord has been examined in a rat model of peripheral inflammation and hyperalgesia. Using either a cDNA (Minami et al., 1989) or oligonucleotide (Noguchi and Ruda, 1992) probe, it was found that PPT mRNA levels are significantly

increased, by 70–80%, in the hemisegment (L4–L6) ipsilateral to peripheral inflammation, when compared to the contralateral side or the same spinal segments from naive rats (Fig. 3).

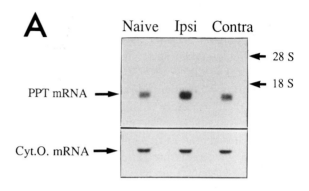

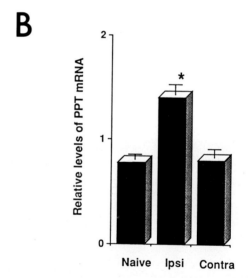

Fig. 3. Increased expression of PPT mRNA in rat lumbar spinal cord following peripheral inflammation and hyperalgesia. A. RNA blot analysis of L4,5 spinal cord total RNA 4 days after peripheral inflammation. The upper panel shows the blot hybridized with a PPT oligonucleotide probe labelled with ^{32}P-dATP, and the lower panel shows the same blot after stripping and rehybridization with a cDNA probe for cytochrome oxidase as a control for RNA lane loading. Locations of ribosomal RNA are marked. Ipsi, ipsilateral side; Contra, contralateral side. B. Quantification of RNA blot for PPT mRNA in rat lumbar spinal cord. Values are mean ± SEM. Five blots were used for quantification. ANOVA showed a significant increase on the side ipsilateral to the inflammation as compared to naive tissue or the contralateral side. *$P < 0.01$, ANOVA. (From Noguchi and Ruda, 1992.)

The induction of PPT mRNA at spinal levels appears to be selective to the noxious stimulus, as no significant changes in PPT mRNA levels are found in the striatum, midbrain or medulla oblongata in the hyperalgesia model (Minami et al., 1989).

In situ hybridization histochemistry can be used to further characterize the increase of PPT mRNA in subpopulations of spinal neurons. Spinal neurons expressing PPT mRNA are concentrated in the superficial dorsal horn (Laminae I and II), the neck of the dorsal horn (Laminae V/VI) and the lateral spinal nucleus. The most densely labelled neurons ipsilateral to the inflamed hindpaw are found in the middle two-thirds of the superficial laminae, especially Lamina I (Fig. 4). These densely labelled Lamina I neurons are typically larger than the PPT neurons in Lamina II. Compared to the contralateral non-inflamed side, both the number and intensity of labelled neurons ipsilateral to hindpaw inflammation are significantly increased in the superficial laminae and the neck

of the dorsal horn. In Lamina II, the ipsilateral increase in number of PPT neurons is relatively small (37%), an observation probably due to the high constitutive expression of many PPT neurons. The PPT neurons in Laminae V/VI represent less than 10% of the total number of PPT neurons in the spinal cord detected constitutively. A significant increase in the number of PPT neurons is also found in Laminae V/VI after hindpaw inflammation. In contrast, the population of PPT neurons in the lateral spinal nucleus does not appear to be regulated by peripheral inflammation.

Some PPT neurons in Lamina I and neck of the dorsal horn have recently been shown to be projection neurons. Using double-labelling methodology, combining ISHH with retrograde fluorogold tracer injected into the area surrounding the brachium conjunctivum at the pontomesencephalic junction, many double-labelled neurons are found in Laminae I and V, and the lateral spinal nucleus (Noguchi and Ruda, 1992).

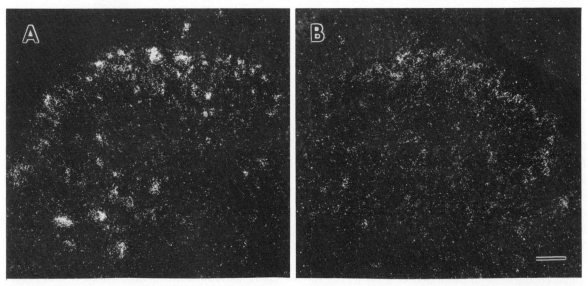

Fig. 4. Dark-field photomicrographs of tissue sections from the L5 segment of the lumbar spinal cord ipsilateral (A) and contralateral (B) to the inflamed paw. In situ hybridization histochemistry demonstrates PPT mRNA expressing neurons concentrated in Laminae I and II and the lateral part of Laminae V/VI. A subpopulation of the labelled neurons on the side ipsilateral to the inflammation exhibited increased silver grain density. Scale bar represents 100 μm. (Adapted from Noguchi and Ruda, 1992.)

This study demonstrates non-opioid neuropeptide-containing projection neurons in Lamina I, especially a subpopulation up-regulated in response to peripheral inflammation and hyperalgesia (Noguchi and Ruda, 1992). The double-labelled neurons in Lamina I are medium-sized and bipolar or polygonal cells with their dendrites extending medio-laterally along the superficial border of the dorsal horn. Most double-labelled neurons in Lamina I are concentrated in the area under the dorsal root entry zone. Lamina I projection neurons are almost exclusively nociceptive-specific, having small receptive fields and slow central conduction velocities (Hylden et al., 1986). On the side of the spinal cord ipsilateral to the inflammation, there is a significant increase in the number of retrogradely labelled Lamina I neurons that express PPT mRNA. Previous immunocytochemical studies using antisera to SP, one of the peptide products of the PPT A gene, had failed to detect SP-containing Lamina I projection neurons (Nahin, 1987). This may represent either differing sensitivities of the methodologies, especially related to the inflammation-induced increase in PPT expression, or alternative production of other peptide products of the PPT genes.

The cellular location of NK_1 receptor in the spinal cord has been determined recently by using a cRNA probe to the NK_1 receptor (Schäfer et al., 1993). The hybridization signal was expressed in subpopulations of neurons in the superficial dorsal horn, neck of the dorsal horn, the area surrounding the central canal, and in the ventral horn (Schäfer et al., 1993). Six days after CFA-induced unilateral hindpaw inflammation, NK_1 receptor mRNA levels in Laminae I/II of the dorsal horn ipsilateral to the inflamed paw increased significantly compared to the contralateral side (Schäfer et al., 1993). Further characterization of the cell types showing an increase of NK_1 receptor mRNA has not been done.

An increase in SP peptide in the spinal cord has been found in polyarthritic rats (Schoenen et al., 1985; Kar et al., 1991; Marlier et al., 1991), in rats with acute joint inflammation (Sluka and Westlund, 1993), and in rats receiving intraplantar injection of formalin (Kantner et al., 1985). Although some of this increase may originate from primary afferent axons terminating in the dorsal horn, based on the data reviewed here on increased levels of PPT mRNA and NK_1 receptor mRNA in the spinal cord, it is clear that the intrinsic spinal SP system is up-regulated in response to peripheral tissue injury. The identification of PPT mRNA and its regulation in Lamina I projection neurons provides strong evidence that substance P and/or other tachykinins are also involved in events that occur in secondary nociceptive pathways. It is not possible to exclude the fact that other tachykinins may play a role in nociceptive pathways, since the PPT A mRNA also encodes neurokinin A. Neurokinin A has been shown to be released upon peripheral noxious stimulation (Duggan et al., 1990; Duggan, this volume), and to have a facilitatory effect on the spinal flexor reflex (Wiesenfeld-Hallin and Xu, 1993; Wiesenfeld-Hallin, this volume).

Transcriptional regulation of gene expression during inflammation

Cellular immediate early genes code for proteins that bind to the promoter region of target genes to act as transcription factors. They are thought to regulate initial genetic events that lead to prolonged functional changes in the nervous system (Curran and Morgan, 1987; Morgan and Curran, 1989; Sheng and Greenberg, 1990). c-*fos* codes for one such nuclear phosphoprotein called Fos. Several immediate-early genes have now been identified in the spinal cord (Hunt et al., 1987; Menétrey et al., 1989; Wisden et al., 1990; Herdegen et al., 1991; Lanteri-Minet et al., 1993), and there appears to be a convergence of signal transduction pathways in the nucleus of spinal neurons leading to the regulation of target genes (Curran and Morgan, 1987; Morgan and Curran, 1989; Sheng and Greenberg, 1990; Wisden et al., 1990). Fos protein is thought to form a complex with the Jun transcription factor, and bind a DNA recognition site (called the AP-1 site) in the promoter region of target genes (Curran and Morgan, 1987;

Morgan and Curran, 1989; Sonnenberg et al., 1989; Sheng and Greenberg, 1990).

RNA blot analysis showed that the content of c-*fos* mRNA increases in the spinal cord within 30 min after injection of an inflammatory agent into the rat hindpaw (Draisci and Iadarola, 1989). There was a peak of induction at 2 h, and a near complete return to control values by 8 h after hindpaw injection. At the protein level, there is a rapid and robust elevation in the number of neurons expressing Fos-like immunoreactivity in the nuclei of dorsal horn neurons following inflammation, or noxious electrical and chemical stimulations (Hunt et al., 1987; Bullit, 1989; Draisci and Iadarola, 1989; Menétrey et al., 1989; Herdegen et al., 1991; Abbadie et al., 1992). These findings suggest that Fos may be used as a molecular marker of neuronal activity. Consistent with this idea, a single s.c. injection of morphine (20 mg/kg, dissolved in a slow release emulsion) almost totally blocked (84% inhibition) the ipsilat-

eral increase in c-*fos* mRNA observed in the spinal cord 2 h after CFA injection (Besse et al., submitted). The morphine-related reduction in c-*fos* mRNA expression results in fewer dorsal horn neurons with inflammation-induced Fos-like immunoreactivity (Presley et al., 1990).

In dorsal horn neurons, co-localization of Fos-immunoreactivity with PPD mRNA, or PPE mRNA, has been demonstrated by double-labelling techniques (Naranjo et al., 1991; Noguchi et al., 1991, 1992). Double-labelled neurons occur in both the superficial laminae and the neck of the dorsal horn, on the side of the spinal cord ipsilateral to the inflammation (e.g., Fig. 5). Over 80% of the neurons expressing PPD mRNA co-localized Fos-IR, although the number of neurons expressing PPD mRNA was substantially less than the number exhibiting induction of Fos protein (Noguchi et al., 1991). In addition, several AP-1-like binding sites have been found in the promoter region of the PPD gene (Naranjo et al.,

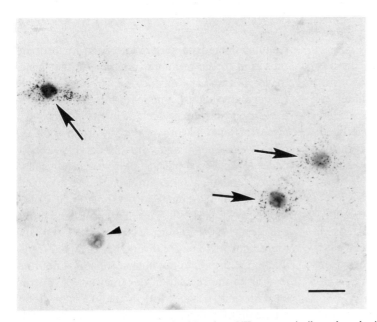

Fig. 5. Bright-field photomicrograph of Laminae VII neurons ipsilateral to the inflamed hindpaw using double-labelling methodology of in situ hybridization and immunohistochemistry. Neurons which co-localized Fos-immunoreactivity and PPE mRNA (arrows) exhibit a brown PAP-stained nucleus surrounded by a dense accumulation of silver grains for each marker. A cell nucleus with Fos-immunoreactivity labelling and no accumulation of silver grains is also visible (arrowhead). Scale bar represents 25 μm. (Adapted from Noguchi et al., 1992.)

1991; Iadarola and Messersmith, 1994). The promoter region of the PPD gene contains a specific enhancer element at -1545 upstream from the transcription start site, termed DYNCRE3, that differs from the consensus AP-1 site by one base, and also from the consensus cAMP response element by one base. This site has been shown to be a robust positive transcriptional element where Fos, Jun, CREB/ATF or other proteins may bind (Messersmith et al., in press). Also, a high percentage of neurons exhibiting PPE mRNA induction (69–90% depending on laminar location) co-localized Fos protein (Noguchi et al., 1992), and the Fos/Jun protein heterodimer has been found to activate the PPE gene (Sonnenberg et al., 1989). Although it is known that the promoter region of the PPT gene also contains an AP-1-like site (Carter and Krause, 1990), it has not yet been determined whether PPT mRNA and Fos induction occur in the same dorsal horn neurons following hindpaw inflammation.

Changes in neuropeptides and behavioral hyperalgesia

Changes in peptides and their precursor levels suggest an altered turnover rate. How would the alterations of dynorphin, enkephalin and tachykinins be involved in dorsal horn plasticity and hyperalgesia induced by peripheral inflammation? Based on anatomical, neurochemical and physiological evidence, both facilitation of nociceptive transmission and enhancement of endogenous pain control systems could be proposed to account for up-regulation of PPD, PPE and PPT gene expression in the spinal cord.

Dynorphin may have biphasic modulatory effects on neuronal activity (Kolaj et al., 1992) and interact with neuronal N-methyl-D-aspartate (NMDA) receptors (Caudle et al., 1993). At lower doses, dynorphin increases NMDA receptor-mediated current, while at higher doses it inhibits NMDA current in guinea pig hippocampal slices (Caudle et al., 1993). Dynorphin can be neurotoxic to spinal functions (Faden and Jacobs, 1984; Caudle and Isaac, 1987). This neurotoxicity is

likely to be related to the interaction of dynorphin peptide with NMDA receptors (Caudle and Isaac, 1988; Isaac et al., 1990). Recent studies suggest that activation of spinal NMDA receptors, and resulting excitotoxicity, is a key event in development of dorsal horn hyperexcitability and behavioral hyperalgesia (Dubner and Ruda, 1992). Some small local circuit inhibitory neurons may be very sensitive to NMDA receptor-mediated neurotoxicity. Loss or dysfunction of these neurons may lead to disinhibition of dorsal horn nociceptive neurons. On the other hand, induction of dynorphin is also found in Lamina I projection and Lamina II local circuit neurons (Nahin et al., 1989). It has been postulated that dynorphin-containing local circuit neurons are excitatory (Dubner and Ruda, 1992). Thus, the up-regulation of the PPD gene would enhance the activity of dynorphin-containing spinal neurons and facilitate nociceptive transmission in pain pathways. Consistent with dynorphin's excitatory effects, dynorphin can also increase glutamate-induced currents in isolated dorsal horn cells (Kolaj et al., 1992) and enhance NMDA receptor-mediated currents in rat spinal cord slice preparation (Caudle, unpublished observations). Direct application of dynorphin to the surface of the spinal cord produces expansion of the receptive fields in some dorsal horn nociceptive neurons (Hylden et al., 1991a) and antagonism of μ opioid receptor-mediated inhibition of nociceptive neurons (Dickenson and Knox, 1987). Intrathecal κ opioid agonists produce hyperalgesia in the guinea pig (Leighton et al., 1988) and low dose intrathecal dynorphin A(1–13) results in reduction of paw withdrawal latency to noxious heat in rats (Ren, unpublished observations).

Enkephalin, has a well-established role in the modulation of nociceptive transmission in the spinal cord (e.g., Dickenson et al., 1987). Most of the enkephalin-like immunoreactivity in the dorsal horn originates from intrinsic neurons (for review, see Ruda et al., 1986). Some enkephalin-containing neurons may be a population of inhibitory local circuit neurons (Dubner et al., 1984). Spinothalamic tract neurons receive synaptic con-

360

tacts from enkephalin-immunoreactive axon terminals (Ruda, 1982). Iontophoretically released enkephalin inhibits responses of spinothalamic tract cells to noxious and chemical stimulation (Willcockson et al., 1984). In the event of excessive depolarization, which can occur in inflammatory and nerve injured states, some local circuit inhibitory spinal neurons may be vulnerable to excitotoxicity. Abnormal function of such neurons could lead to a loss of inhibitory mechanisms and the disinhibition of pain transmission neurons, leading to dorsal horn hyperexcitability and hyperalgesia (Dubner and Ruda, 1992). The increased biosynthesis of enkephalin peptides may reflect an effort of surviving enkephalinergic inhibitory neurons to compensate for the loss of inhibitory machinery and potentiate the efficiency of endogenous pain control. Opioid agonists appear to be more effective in inhibiting nociceptive reflexes in an inflamed state. In studies of the analgesic effects of opioid receptor agonists on inflammatory hyperalgesia, it is found that the opioids are more potent at reversing hyperalgesia than in altering paw withdrawal latency above the normal baseline (Hylden et al., 1991b; Ren et al., 1992). This increased sensitivity of the endogenous opioid system may be induced by an initial reduction of opioid peptides resulting from dysfunction of opioidergic inhibitory local circuit neurons, an increase in receptor binding and/or an interaction with spinal noradrenergic systems (Hylden et al., 1991b).

A similar series of events are also possibly related to up-regulation of PPT mRNA and SP following peripheral inflammation. The demonstration of increased levels of PPT mRNA in intrinsic dorsal horn neurons suggests increased synaptic activity and nociceptive transmission. The increased activity in Lamina I projection neurons may activate descending pain modulatory systems, trigger affective responses to acute pain, and provoke somatovisceral reflexes (see discussion in Noguchi and Ruda, 1992). Increased biosynthesis of SP in Lamina II local circuit neurons may facilitate excitatory synaptic transmission in the dorsal horn (Dougherty et al., 1993). More impor-

tantly, spinal SP appears to be able to interact with excitatory amino acids. Glutamate and aspartate release from the dorsal horn by supramaximal electrical stimulation of the lumbar dorsal root is increased by the application of substance P (Kangrga and Randic, 1990). Responses of spinothalamic tract neurons to excitatory amino acids are facilitated by combined application with substance P (Dougherty et al., 1993).

It is of interest to note that, in neonatal capsaicin-treated rats, behavioral hyperalgesia still developed after CFA-induced inflammation, although from an elevated baseline nociceptive threshold (Fig. 6). Dorsal horn hyperexcitability is also present in neonatal capsaicin-treated rats with hindpaw inflammation (Ren et al., 1994). In this neonatal capsaicin model with inflammation, both the induction of Fos-like immunoreactivity

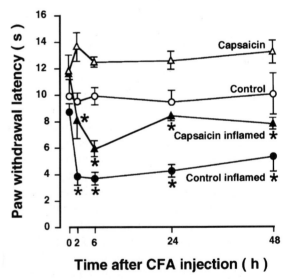

Fig. 6. Paw withdrawal latency before, and 2–48 h after, injection of CFA in one hindpaw of control ($n = 12$) and neonatal capsaicin-treated rats ($n = 24$). Inflamed paw withdrawal latencies were significantly lower ($P < 0.01$, ANOVA) than contralateral non-inflamed paw withdrawal latencies at 2–48 h for both control (solid circles) and capsaicin-treated rats (solid triangles). The time course and magnitude of the decrease in latency were not different in the two treatment groups. Contralateral non-inflamed paws in control (open circles) and capsaicin-treated rats (open triangles) showed no change in paw withdrawal latency. (From Hylden et al., 1992.)

and the enhanced expression of PPD mRNA normally seen following inflammation, are reduced (Hylden et al., 1992). The apparent dissociation of neurochemical changes and behavioral hyperalgesia probably reflects complex CNS plasticity which occurs in both capsaicin-treatment and inflammation states. Reorganization in the CNS, especially in the spinal dorsal horn, may have significant impact on nociceptive activity in capsaicin-treated animals. It has been shown that, after an early reduction due to neonatal capsaicin-treatment, CGRP-immunoreactivity and fluoride-resistant acid phosphatase activity increased after 8 weeks of age (Hammond and Ruda, 1991). Large myelinated primary afferent fibers terminating in naive rats in Laminae III/IV spread dorsally to the superficial laminae after capsaicin-treatment (Nagy and Hunt, 1983), and serotonergic fibers from the deep laminae sprout to innervate the inner part of Lamina II within a few days after capsaicin-treatment (Marlier et al., 1992). Ongoing reorganization in the spinal dorsal horn with possible compensation by large primary afferents may account for the behavioral hyperalgesia and dorsal horn hyperexcitability that occurs in capsaicin-treated rats with CFA-induced inflammation.

References

Abbadie, C., lombard, M.-C., Morain, F. and Besson, J.-M. (1992) Fos-like immunoreactivity in the superficial dorsal horn induced by formalin injection in the forepaw: effects of dorsal rhizotomies. *Brain Res.*, 578: 17–25.

Basbaum, A.I., Cruz, L. and Weber, E. (1986) Immunoreactive dynorphin B in sacral primary afferent fibers of the cat. *J. Neurosci.*, 6: 127–133.

Besse, D., lombard, M.-C., Zajac, J.-M., Roques, B.P. and Besson, J.-M. (1990) Pre- and postsynaptic distribution of μ, δ and κ opioid receptors in the superficial layers of the cervical dorsal horn of the rat spinal cord. *Brain Res.*, 521: 15–22.

Besse, D., lombard, M.-C. and Besson, J.-M. (1991) Autoradiographic distribution of mu, delta and kappa opioid binding sites in the superficial dorsal horn, over the rostrocaudal axis of the rat spinal cord. *Brain Res.*, 548: 287–291.

Besse, D., Weil-Fugazza, J., lombard, M.-C., Butler, S.H. and Besson, J.-M. (1992) Monoarthritis induces complex changes in m, d and k-opioid binding sites in the superficial dorsal horn of the rat spinal cord. *Eur. J. Pharmacol.*, 223: 123–131.

Besse, D., Ren, K. and Ruda, M.A. (1994) Action of morphine on preprodynorphin, preproenkephalin and c-*fos* gene expression in the spinal cord of rats with unilateral hindpaw inflammation. *Mol. Brain Res.,* (submitted).

Besson, J.-M. and Chaouch, A. (1987) Peripheral and spinal mechanisms of nociception. *Physiol. Rev.*, 67: 67–186.

Botticelli, L.H., Cox, B.M. and Goldstein, A. (1981) Immunoreactive dynorphin in mammalian spinal cord and dorsal root ganglia. *Proc. Nat. Acad. Sci. USA*, 78: 7783–7786.

Brandt, S.A. and Livingston, A. (1990a) Receptor changes in the spinal cord of sheep associated with exposure to chronic pain, *Pain*, 42: 323–329.

Brandt, S.A. and Livingston, A. (1990b) An autoradiographic investigation of the distribution of [^{3}H]DAGO and [^{3}H]DPDPE in the spinal cord of sheep and sheep experiencing chronic pain. In: J.M. Van Ree, A.H. Mulder, V.M. Wiegant and T.B. Van Wimersma Greidanus (Eds.), *New Leads in Opioid Research*, Elsevier Science, Amsterdam, pp. 51–52.

Bullit, E. (1989) Induction of c-*fos*-like protein within the lumbar spinal cord and thalamus of the rat following peripheral stimulation. *Brain Res.*, 493: 391–397.

Carlton, S.M. and Hayes, E.S. (1989) Dynorphin A(1–8) immunoreactive cell bodies, dendrites and terminals are postsynaptic to calcitonin gene-related peptide primary afferent terminals in the monkey dorsal horn. *Brain Res.*, 504: 124–128.

Carter, M.S. and Krause, J.E. (1990) Structure, expression, and some regulatory mechanisms of the rat preprotachykinin gene encoding substance P, neurokinin A, neuropeptide K, and neuropeptide γ. *J. Neurosci.*, 10: 2203–2214.

Caudle, R.M. and Isaac, L. (1987) Intrathecal dynorphin (1–13) results in an irreversible loss of the tail-flick reflex in rats. *Brain Res.*, 435: 1–6.

Caudle, R.M. and Isaac, L. (1988) A novel interaction between dynorphin (1–13) and an *N*-methyl-D-aspartate site. *Brain Res.*, 443: 329–332.

Caudle, R.M., Chavkin, C. and Dubner, R. (1993) Kappa$_2$ opioid receptors inhibit NMDA receptor-mediated synaptic currents in the CA3 of guinea pig hippocampus. *Soc. Neurosci. Abstr.*, 19: 1552.

Cho, H.J. and Basbaum, A.I. (1989) Ultrastructural analysis of dynorphin B-immunoreactive cells and terminals in the superficial dorsal horn of the deafferented spinal cord of the rat. *J. Comp. Neurol.*, 281: 193–205.

Corbett, A.D., Paterson, S.J., McKnight, A.T., Magnan, J. and Kosterlitz, H.W. (1982) Dynorphin$_{1-8}$ and dynorphin$_{1-9}$ are ligands for the kappa subtype of opiate receptor. *Nature*, 299: 79–81.

362

Cruz, L. and Basbaum, A.I. (1985) Multiple opioid peptides and the modulation of pain: immunohistochemical analysis of dynorphin and enkephalin in the trigeminal nucleus caudalis and spinal cord of the rat. *J. Comp. Neurol.*, 240: 331–348.

Curran, T. and Morgan, J.I. (1987) Memories of *fos. BioEssays*, 7: 255–258.

Dickenson, A.H. and Knox, R.J. (1987) Antagonism of μ-opioid receptor-mediated inibitions of nociceptive neurones by U50488H and Dynorphin A$_{1-13}$ in the rat dorsal horn. *Neurosci. Lett.*, 75: 229–234.

Dickenson, A.H., Sullivan, A.F., Fournie-Zaluski, M.C. and Roques, B.P. (1987) Prevention of degradation of endogenous enkephalins produces inhibition of nociceptive neurones in rat spinal cord. *Brain Res.*, 408: 185–191.

Dougherty, P.M., Palecek, J., Zorn, S. and Willis, W.D. (1993) Combined application of excitatory amino acids and substance P produces long-lasting changes in responses of primate spinothalamic tract neurons. *Brain Res. Rev.*, 18: 227–246.

Draisci, G. and Iadarola, M. (1989) Temporal analysis of increases in c-*fos*, preprodynorphin and preproenkephalin mRNAs in rat spinal cord. *Mol. Brain Res.*, 6: 31–37.

Dubner, R. and Ruda, M.A. (1992) Activity-dependent neuronal plasticity following tissue injury and inflammation. *Trends Neurosci.*, 15: 96–103.

Dubner, R., Ruda, M.A., Miletic, V., Hoffert, M.J., Bennett, G.J., Nishikawa, N. and Coffield, J. (1984) Neural circuitry mediating nociception in the medullary and spinal dorsal horns. In. L. Kruger and J.C. Liebeskind (Eds.), *Advances in Pain Research and Therapy, Vol. 6*, Raven Press, New York, pp. 151–166.

Duggan, A.W. and North, R.A. (1984) Electrophysiology of opioids. *Pharmacol. Rev.*, 35: 219–281.

Duggan, A.W., Hope, P.J., Jarrott, B., Schaible, H.-G. and Fleetwood-Walker, S.M. (1990) Release, spread and persistence of immunoreactive neurokinin A in the dorsal horn of the cat following noxious cutaneous stimulation. Studies with antibody microprobes. *Neuroscience*, 35: 195–202.

Faccini, E., Uzumaki, H., Govoni, S., Missale, C., Spano, P.F., Covelli, V. and Trabucchi, M. (1984) Afferent fibers mediate the increase of Met-enkephalin elicited in rat spinal cord by localized pain. *Pain*, 18: 25–31.

Faden, A.I. and Jacobs, T.P. (1984) Dynorphin-related peptides cause motor dysfunction in the rat through a non-opiate action. *Br. J. Pharmacol.*, 81: 271–276.

Fields, H.L., Emson, P.C., Leigh, B.K., Gilbert, R.F.T. and Iversen, L.L. (1980) Multiple opiate receptor sites on primary afferent fibers. *Nature*, 284: 351–353.

Gamse, R., Holzer, P. and Lembeck, F. (1979) Indirect evidence for presynaptic location of opiate receptors on chemosensitive primary sensory neurones, *Naunyn-Schmiedeberg's Arch. Pharmacol.*, 308: 281–285.

Gutstein, H.B., Bronstein, D.M. and Akil, H. (1992) β-En-

dorphin processing and cellular origins in rat spinal cord. *Pain*, 51: 241–247.

Hammond, D.L. and Ruda, M.A. (1991) Developmental alterations in the distribution of immunoreactive calcitonin gene-related peptide, substance P and fluoride-resistant acid phosphatase in the spinal cord of the rat after neonatal administration of capsaicin: relationship to nociceptive threshold. *J. Comp. Neurol.*, 312: 436–450.

Herdegen, T., Kovary, K., Leah, J. and Bravo, R. (1991) Specific temporal and spatial distribution of Jun, Fos, and Krox-24 proteins in spinal neurons following noxious transsynaptic stimulation. *J. Comp. Neurol.*, 313: 178–191.

Hökfelt, T., Terenius, L., Kuypers, H.G.J.M. and Dann, O. (1979) Evidence for enkephalin immunoreactive neurons in the medulla oblongata projecting to the spinal cord. *Neurosci. Lett.*, 14: 55–60.

Hunt, S.P., Pini, A. and Evan, G. (1987) Induction of c-*fos*-like proein in spinal cord neurons following sensory stimulation. *Nature*, 328: 632–634.

Hylden, J.L.K., Hayashi, H., Dubner, R. and Bennett, G.J. (1986) Physiology and morphology of the lamina I spinomesencephalic projection. *J. Comp. Neurol.*, 247: 505–515.

Hylden, J.L.K., Nahin, R.L., Traub, R.J. and Dubner, R. (1991a) Effects of spinal kappa-opioid receptor agonists on the responsiveness of nociceptive superficial dorsal horn neurons. *Pain*, 44: 187–193.

Hylden, J.L.K., Thomas, D.A., Iadarola, M.J., Nahin, R.L. and Dubner, R. (1991b) Spinal opioid analgesic effects are enhanced in a model of unilateral inflammation/hyperalgesia: possible involvement of noradrenergic mechanisms. *Eur. J. Pharmacol.*, 194: 135–143.

Hylden, J.L.K., Noguchi, K. and Ruda, M.A. (1992) Neonatal capsaicin treatment attenuates spinal Fos activation and dynorphin gene expression following peripheral inflammation and hyperalgesia. *J. Neurosci.*, 12: 1716–1725.

Iadarola, M.J. and Messersmith, D.J. (1994) Molecular biology of dynorphin gene expression in relationship to spinal cord processing of pain. In: L. Urban (Ed.), *The Cellular Mechanisms of Sensory Processing*, Springer-Verlag, Berlin, pp. 313–336.

Iadarola, M.J., Brady, L.S., Draisci, G. and Dubner, R. (1988a) Enhancement of dynorphin gene expression in spinal cord following experimental inflammation: stimulus specificity, behavioral parameters and opioid receptor binding. *Pain*, 35: 313–326.

Iadarola, M.J., Douglass, J., Civelli, O. and Naranjo, J.R. (1988b) Differential activation of spinal cord dynorphin and enkephalin neurons during hyperalgesia: evidence using cDNA hybridization. *Brain Res.*, 455: 205–212.

Iadarola, M.J., Ruda, M.A., Cohen, L.V., Flores, C.M. and Naranjo, J.R. (1988c) Enhanced dynorphin gene expression in spinal cord dorsal horn neurons during peripheral inflammation: behavioral, neuropeptide, immunocytochemical and mRNA studies. In: R. Dubner, G.F. Gebhart and M.R. Bond (Eds.), *Proceedings of the Vth World Congress on Pain*, Elsevier, Amsterdam, pp. 61–71.

Isaac, L., O'Malley, T.V.Z., Ristic, H. and Stewart, P. (1990) MK-801 blocks dynorphin A (1–13)-induced loss of the tail-flick reflex in the rat. *Brain Res.*, 531: 83–87.

Jessel, T.M. and Iversen, L.L. (1977) Opiate analgesics inhibit substance P release from rat trigeminal nucleus. *Nature*, 268: 549–551.

Kakidani, H., Furutani, Y., Takahashi, H., Noda, M., Morimoto, Y., Hirose, T., Asai, M., Inayama, S., Nakanishi, S. and Numa, S. (1982) Cloning and sequence analysis of cDNA for porcine beta-neo-endorphine/dynorphin precursor. *Nature*, 298: 245–249.

Kangrga, I. and Randic, M. (1990) Tachykinins and calcitonin gene-related peptide enhance release of endogenous glutamate and aspartate from the rat spinal dorsal horn slice. *J. Neurosci.*, 10: 2026–2038.

Kantner, R.M., Kirby, M.L. and Goldstein, B.D. (1985) Increase in substance P in the dorsal horn during a chemogenic nociceptive stimulus. *Brain Res.*, 338: 196–199.

Kar, S., Gibson, S.J., Rees, R.G., Jura, W.G.Z.O., Brewerton, D.A. and Polak, J.M. (1991) Increased calcitonin gene-related peptide (CGRP), substance P, and enkephalin immunoreactivities in dorsal spinal cord and loss of CGRP-immunoreactive motoneurons in arthritic rats depend on intact peripheral nerve supply. *J. Mol. Neurosci.*, 3: 7–18.

Kolaj, M., Cerne, R., Jiang, M.C., Lanthorn, t.H. and Randic, M. (1992) The effects of dynorphin A(1–13) on glutamate and synaptic responses of rat spinal dorsal horn neurons. *Soc. Neurosci. Abstr.*, 18: 281.

Kosterlitz, H.W., Corbett, A.D., Gillan, M.G.C., McKnight, A.T., Paterson, S.J. and Robson, L.E. (1986) Recent developments in bioassay using selective ligands and selective in vitro preparations. *Natl. Inst. Drug Abuse Res. Monogr. Ser.*, 70: 223–236.

Krause, J.E., Chirgwin, J.M., Carter, M.S., Xu, Z.S. and Hershey, A.D. (1987) Three rat preprotachykinin mRNAs encode the neuropeptides substance P and neurokinin A. *Proc. Natl. Acad. Sci. USA*, 84: 881–885.

LaMotte, C., Loh, H.H. and Li, C.H. (1976) Opiate receptor binding in primate spinal cord: distribution and changes after dorsal root section. *Brain Res.*, 112: 407–412.

Lantéri-Minet, M., de Pommery, J., Herdegen, T., Weil-Fugazza, J., Bravo, R. and Menétrey, D. (1993) Differential time-prolonged and spatial expression of Fos, Jun and Krox-24 proteins in spinal cord of rats undergoing subacute or chronic somatic inflammation. *J. Comp. Neurol.*, 333: 223–235.

Leighton, G.E., Hill, R.G. and Hughes, J. (1988) Intrathecal injection of a κ opioid agonist produces hyperalgesia in the guinea pig. *Eur. J. Pharmacol.*, 157: 241–242.

Maggi, C.A., Patacchini, R., Rovero, P. and Giachetti, A.

(1993) Tachykinin receptors and tachykinin receptor antagonists. *J. Auton. Pharmacol.*, 13: 23–93.

Marlier, L., Poulat, P., Rajaofetra, N. and Privat, A. (1991) Modifications of serotonin-, substance P- and calcitonin gene-related peptide-like immunoreactivities in the dorsal horn of the spinal cord of arthritic rats: a quantitative immunocytochemical study. *Exp. Brain Res.*, 85: 482–490.

Marlier, L., Poulat, P., Rajaofetra, N., Sandillon, F. and Privat, A. (1992) Plasticity of the serotonergic innervation of the dorsal horn of the rat spinal cord following neonatal capsaicin tretment. *J. Neurosci. Res.*, 31: 346–358.

Menétrey, D., Gannon, A., Levine, J.D. and Basbaum, A.I. (1989) Expression of c-fos protein in interneurons and projection neurons of the rat spinal cord in response to noxious somatic, articular and visceral stimulation. *J. Comp. Neurol.*, 285: 177–195.

Messersmith, D.J., Gu, J., Dubner, R., Douglass, J. and Iadarola, M.J. Basal and inducible transcriptional activity of an upstream AP-1/CRE element (DYNCRE3) in the prodynorphin promoter. *Cell. Mol. Neurosci.*, (in press).

Millan, M.J., Millan, M.H., Czlonkowski, V., Hsllt, V., Pilcher, W.T., Herz, A. and Colpaert, F.C. (1986) A model of chronic pain in the rat: response of multiple opioid systems to adjuvant-induced arthritis. *J. Neurosci.*, 6: 899–906.

Millan, M.J., Czlonkowski, A., Morris, B.J., Stein, C., Arendt, R., Huber, A., Hsllt, V. and Herz, A. (1988) Inflammation of the hindlimb as a model of unilateral localized pain: influence on multiple opioid systems in the spinal cord of the rat. *Pain*, 35: 299–312.

Miller, K.E. and Seybold, V.S. (1987) Comparison of met-enkephalin-, dynorphin A-, and neurotensin-immunoreactive neurons in the cat and rat spinal cords: I. lumbar cord. *J. Comp. Neurol.*, 255: 293–304.

Minami, M., Kuraishi, Y., Kawamura, M., Yamaguchi, T., Masu, Y., Nakanishi, S. and Satoh, M. (1989) Enhancement of preprotachykinin A gene expression by adjuvant-induced inflammation in the rat spinal cord: possible involvement of substance P-containing spinal neurons in nociception. *Neurosci. Lett.*, 98: 105–110.

Morgan, J.I. and Curran, T. (1989) Stimulus-transcription coupling in neurons: role of cellular immediate-early genes. *Trends Neurosci.*, 12: 459–462.

Morris, B.J. and Herz, A. (1987) Distinct distribution of opioid receptor types in rat lumbar spinal cord. *Naunyn-Schmiedeberg's Arch. Pharmacol.*, 336: 240–243.

Nagy, J.I. and Hunt, S.P. (1983) The termination of primary afferents within the rat dorsal horn: evidence for rearrangement following capsaicin treatment. *J. Comp. Neurol.*, 218: 145–158.

Nagy, J.I., Vincent, S.R., Staines, W.M.A., Fibiger, H.C., Reisine, T.D. and Yamamura, H.I. (1980) Neurotoxic action of capsaicin on spinal substance P neurons. *Brain Res.*, 186: 435–444.

364

Nahin, R.L. (1987) Immunocytochemical identification of long ascending peptidergic neurons contributing to the spinoreticular tract in the rat. *Neuroscience*, 23: 859–869.

Nahin, R.L., Hylden, J.L.K., Iadarola, M.J. and Dubner, R. (1989) Peripheral inflammation is associated with increased dynorphin immunoreactivity in both projection and local circuit neurons in the superficial dorsal horn of the rat lumbar spinal cord. *Neurosci. Lett.*, 96: 247–252.

Nakanishi, S. (1991) Mammalian tachykinin receptors. *Annu. Rev. Neurosci.*, 14: 123–136.

Nakanishi, S., Teranishi, Y., Watanabe, Y., Notake, M., Noda, M., Kakidani, H., Jingami, H. and Numa, S. (1981) Isolation and characterization of the bovine corticotropin/beta-lipotropin precursor gene. *Eur. J. Biochem.*, 115: 429–438.

Naranjo, J.R., Mellstrsm, B., Achaval, M., Lucas, J.J., Del Rio, J. and Sassone-Corsi, P. (1991) Pain stimulus co-induces jun B and c-*fos* in a subset of neurons in the spinal cord. *Oncogene*, 6: 223–227.

Nawa, H., Hirose, T., Takashima, H., Inayama, S. and Nakanishi, S. (1983) Nucleotide sequences of cloned cDNAs for two types of bovine brain substance P precursor. *Nature*, 306: 32–36.

Ninkovic, M., Hunt, S.P. and Kelly, J.S. (1981) Effect of dorsal rhizotomy on the autoradiographic distribution of opiate and neurotensin-like immunoreactivity within the rat spinal cord. *Brain Res.*, 230: 111–119.

Noda, M., Furutani, Y., Takahashi, H., Toyosato, M., Hirose, T., Inayama, S., Nakanishi, S. and Numa, S. (1982) Cloning and sequence analysis of bovine adrenal preproenkephalin. *Nature*, 295: 202–206.

Noguchi, K. and Ruda, M.A. (1992) Gene regulation in an ascending nociceptive pathway: inflammation-induced increase in preprotachykinin mRNA in rat lamina I spinal projection neurons. *J. Neurosci.*, 12: 2563–2572.

Noguchi, K., Kowalski, K., Traub, R., Solodkin, A., Iadarola, M.J. and Ruda, M.A. (1991) Dynorphin expression and Fos-like immunoreactivity following inflammation induced hyperalgesia are colocalized in spinal cord neurons. *Mol. Brain Res.*, 10: 227–233.

Noguchi, K., Dubner, R. and Ruda, M.A. (1992) Preproenkephalin mRNA in spinal dorsal horn neurons is induced by peripheral inflammation and is co-localized with Fos and Fos-related proteins. *Neuroscience*, 46: 561–570.

Paterson, S.J., Robson, L.E. and Kosterlitz, H.W. (1983) Classification of opioid receptors. *Br. Med. Bull.*, 39: 31–36.

Pohl, M., lombard, M.-C., Bourgoin, S., Carayon, A., Benoliel, J.J., Mauborgne, A., Besson, J.-M., Hamon, M. and Cesselin, F. (1989) Opioid control of the in vitro release of calcitonin gene-related peptide from primary afferent fibres projecting in the rat cervical cord. *Neuropeptides*, 14: 151–159.

Presley, R.W., Menétrey, D., Levine, J.D. and Basbaum, A.I. (1990) Systemic morphine suppresses noxious stimulus-evoked Fos protein-like immunoreactivity in the rat spinal cord. *J. Neurosci.*, 10: 323–335.

Ren, K., Williams, G.M., Hylden, J.L.K., Ruda, M.A. and Dubner, R. (1992) The intrathecal administration of excitatory amino acid receptor antagonists selectively attenuated carrageenan-induced behavioral hyperalgesia in rats. *Eur. J. Pharmacol.*, 219: 235–243.

Ren, K., Williams, G.M., Ruda, M.A. and Dubner, R. (1994) Inflammation and hyperalgesia in rats neonatally treated with capsaicin: effects on two classes of nociceptive neurons in the superficial dorsal horn. *Pain*, 59: 287–300.

Ruda, M.A. (1982) Opiates and pain pathways: Demonstration of enkephalin synapses on dorsal horn projection neurons. *Science*, 215: 1523–1525.

Ruda, M.A., Bennett, G.J. and Dubner, R. (1986) Neurochemistry and neural circuitry in the dorsal horn. In P.C. Emson, M.N. Rossor and M. Tohyama (Eds.), *Progress in Brain Research*, Elsevier, Amsterdam, Vol. 66, pp. 219–268.

Ruda, M.A., Iadarola, M.J., Cohen, L.V. and Young, W.S., III (1988) In situ hybridization histochemistry and immunocytochemistry reveal an increase in spinal dynorphin biosynthesis in a rat model of peripheral inflammation and hyperalgesia. *Proc. Natl. Acad. Sci. USA*, 85: 622–626.

Ruda, M.A., Cohen,L., Shiosaka, S., Takahashi, O., Allen, B., Humphrey, E. and Iadarola, M.J. (1989) In situ hybridization, histochemical and immunocytochemical analysis of opioid gene poducts in a rat model of peripheral inflammation. In: F. Cervero, G.J. Bennett and P.M. Headley (Eds.), *Processing of Sensory Information in the Superficial Dorsal Horn of the Spinal Cord*, Plenum, New York, pp. 383–394.

Sasek, C.A., Seybold, V.S. and Elde, R.P. (1984) The immunohistochemical localization of nine peptides in the sacral parasympathetic nucleus and the dorsal gray commissure in rat spinal cord. *Neuroscience*, 12: 855–874.

Schäfer, K.-H., Nohr, D., Krause, J.E. and Weihe, E. (1993) Inflammation-induced upregulation of NK1 receptor mRNA in dorsal horn neurones. *NeuroReport*, 4: 1007–1010.

Schoenen, J., Van Hees, J., Gybels, J., de Castro Costa, M., Vanderhaeghen, J.J. (1985) Histochemical changes of substance P, FRAP, serotonin and succinic dehydrogenase in the spinal cord of rats with adjuvant arthritis. *Life Sci.*, 36: 1247–1254.

Senba, E., Shiosaka, S., Hara, Y., Inagaki, S., Sakanaka, M., Takatsuki, K., Kawai, Y. and Tohyama, M. (1982) Ontogeny of the peptidergic system in the rat spinal cord: immunohistochemical analysis. *J. Comp. Neurol.*, 208: 54–66.

Sheng, M. and Greenberg, M.E. (1990) The regulation and function of c-*fos* and other immediate early genes in the nervous system. *Neuron*, 4: 477–485.

Sluka, K.A. and Westlund, K.N. (1993) Behavioral and immunohistochemical changes in an experimental arthritis model in rats. *Pain*, 55: 367–377.

Sonnenberg, J.L., Rauscher, F.J.III, Morgan, J.I. and Curran, T. (1989) Regulation of proenkephalin by Fos and Jun. *Science*, 246: 622–1625.

Takahashi, O., Traub, R.J. and Ruda, M.A. (1988) Demonstration of calcitonin gene-related peptide immunoreactive axons contacting dynorphin A(1–8) immunoreactive neurons in a rat model of peripheral inflammation and hyperalgesia. *Brain Res.*, 475: 168–172.

Takahashi, O., Shiosaka, S., Traub, R.J. and Ruda, M.A. (1990) Ultrastructural demonstration of synaptic connections between calcitonin gene-related peptide immunoreactive axons and dynorphin A(1–8) immunoreactive dorsal horn neurons in a rat model of peripheral inflammation and hyperalgesia. *Peptides*, 11: 1233–1237.

Tsou, K., Khachaturian, H., Akil, H. and Watson, S.J. (1986) Immunocytochemical localization of pro-opiomelanocortin-derived peptides in the adult rat spinal cord. *Brain Res.*, 378: 28–35.

Tsuchida, K., Shigemoto, R., Yokota, Y. and Nakanishi, S. (1990) Tissue distribution and quantitation of the mRNAs for three rat tachykinin receptors. *Eur. J. Biochem.*, 193: 751–757.

Wiesenfeld-Hallin, Z. and Xu, X-J. (1993) The differential roles of substance P and neurokinin A in spinal cord hyperexcitability and neurogenic inflammation. *Regul. Peptides*, 46: 165–173.

Willcockson, W.S., Chung, J.M., Hori, Y., Lee, K.H. and Willis, W.D. (1984) Effects of iontophoretically released peptides on primate spinothalamic tract cells. *J. Neurosci.*, 3: 741–750.

Wisden, W., Errington, M.L., Williams, S., Dunnett, S.B., Waters, C., Hitchcock, D., Evan, G., Bliss, T.V.P. and Hunt, S.P. (1990) Differential expression of immediate early genes in the hippocampus and spinal cord. *Neuron*, 4: 603–614.

Yaksh, T.L. and Noueihed, R. (1985) The physiology and pharmacology of spinal opiates. *Annu. Rev. Pharmacol. Toxicol.*, 25: 433–462.

Yaksh, T.L., Jessel, T.M., Gamse, R., Mudge, A.W. and Leeman, S.E. (1980) Intrathecal morphine inhibits substance P release from mammalian spinal cord in vivo. *Nature*, 286: 155–157.

Yashpal, K., Dam, T.-V. and Quirion, R. (1990) Quantitative autoradiographic distribution of multiple neurokinin binding sites in rat spinal cord. *Brain Res.*, 506: 259–266.

F. Nyberg, H.S. Sharma and Z. Wiesenfeld-Hallin (Eds.)
Progress in Brain Research, Vol 104

CHAPTER 21

Prostaglandin-induced neuropeptide release from spinal cord

M.R. Vasko

*Departments of Pharmacology and Toxicology, Anesthesia and Medicine, Indiana University School of Medicine,
Indianapolis, IN 46202-5120, USA*

Introduction

Activation of nociceptive sensory nerve endings throughout the body results in conduction of action potentials to their central terminals in the dorsal spinal cord and the subsequent release of neurotransmitters. This release is the first synaptic event in the conduction of the pain signal to the brain and represents a primary site for modulation of nociception. Inhibiting the release of transmitters from small-diameter sensory nerve terminals could be one mechanism for producing antinociception (Jessell and Iversen, 1977; Hamon et al., 1988). Conversely, acutely facilitating the release of putative nociceptive transmitters might be a way to enhance the perception of a noxious stimulus. The hyperalgesia associated with chronic inflammation also could result, in part, from a long-term facilitation of transmitter release from central terminals of sensory neurons.

Although a number of studies have assessed whether various analgesic agents inhibit transmitter release from sensory nerve endings in the spinal cord, little work has focused on the processes that could facilitate release at these sites. Recent studies, however, have demonstrated that inflammatory mediators, such as bradykinin and prostaglandins, augment transmitter release from peripheral endings of sensory neurons (for review, see Geppetti, 1993) and from isolated

preparations of these cells (MacLean et al., 1990; Vasko et al., 1993, 1994). In addition, inflammation caused by peripheral injection of chemical irritants results in an increase in the synthesis and release of the putative nociceptive transmitters, substance P (SP) and calcitonin gene-related peptide (CGRP), in the spinal cord (Oku et al., 1987; Nanayama et al., 1989; Donnerer et al., 1992; Garry and Hargreaves, 1992). Various chemical agents that are produced during inflammation, therefore, may augment transmitter release from central synapses of sensory neurons. The enhanced release, in turn, could contribute to the hyperexcitability of spinal nociceptive neurons that is observed during chronic inflammation (for review, see Dubner and Ruda, 1992).

Of the numerous inflammatory mediators that enhance the excitability of sensory neurons, prostaglandins are of primary importance. These metabolic products of arachidonic acid are synthesized and released at sites of tissue injury and inflammation (Trang et al., 1977; Higgs and Salmon, 1979; Bombardieri et al., 1981). Peripheral administration of these agents reduces the threshold for activation of sensory neurons by various noxious stimuli (Handwerker, 1976; Mense, 1981; Martin et al., 1987; Schaible and Schmidt, 1988) and produces hyperalgesia in laboratory animals and in man (Ferreira, 1972; Juan and Lembeck, 1974; Ferreira et al., 1978b;

Taiwo and Levine, 1989). Furthermore, inhibition of the synthesis of prostaglandins is believed to be the mechanism for the analgesic actions of non-steroidal anti-inflammatory drugs (NSAIDs; Vane, 1971; Smith and Willis, 1971).

Although it is well accepted that prostaglandins induce hyperalgesia by peripheral actions on sensory neurons, these eicosanoids also may modulate nociceptive input at the level of the spinal cord. The purpose of this chapter is to review the evidence supporting a role for prostaglandins in spinally-mediated pain modulation. Data will be summarized supporting the hypothesis that the mechanism for prostaglandin actions in the spinal cord is to increase the release of the putative nociceptive transmitters, SP and CGRP, from the central terminals of sensory neurons.

Evidence for actions of prostaglandins in the spinal cord

To substantiate that prostaglandins enhance nociception at the level of the spinal cord, several criteria need to be satisfied. First, prostaglandins should be localized in the spinal cord and prostaglandin production should increase with acute or chronic pain. Second, the exogenous administration of prostanoids onto the spinal cord should increase sensitivity to noxious stimulation, i.e., produce hyperalgesia. Finally, drugs that inhibit cyclooxygenase, the enzyme that catalyzes the conversion of arachidonic acid to prostaglandins, should act in the spinal cord to reduce pain associated with production of prostanoids.

Prostaglandin localization in the spinal cord

Because of the ubiquitous nature of arachidonic acid metabolism, it is not surprising that prostaglandins are found throughout the brain and spinal cord (Ogorochi et al., 1984; Leslie and Watkins, 1985). Binding sites for various prostaglandins, as well as the enzyme, cyclooxygenase, also are distributed in a number of regions of the central nervous system (Watanabe et al.,

1989; Breder et al., 1992; Matsumura et al., 1992). At the level of the spinal cord, however, a majority of the binding sites for PGE_2 are found in Laminae I and II of the dorsal horn (Matsumura et al., 1992). This distribution coincides with the terminals of the small diameter primary afferent neurons (for review, see Besson and Chaouch, 1987), suggesting that PGE_2 modulates sensory input in this region.

Prostaglandins are not stored in cells, but produced as needed. Therefore, if these autocoids influence nociceptive input, then levels of prostaglandins in the spinal cord might be expected to rise in response to peripheral noxious stimulation. Indeed, studies measuring prostaglandin release from spinal cord support this premise. Utilizing a perfused frog spinal cord preparation, Ramwell and co-workers demonstrated that electrical stimulation of the hindlimb evoked an increase in the outflow of PGE_1 and $PGF_{1\alpha}$ (Ramwell et al., 1966). Coderre et al. (1990) showed that immersion of the rat hindpaw into water at 50°C increased the outflow of PGE_2 from perfused lumbar spinal cord by approximately 2-fold compared to rats exposed to water at 35°C. Furthermore, nanomolar concentrations of the nociceptive sensory transmitter, SP, increase the production of PGE_2 and PGD_2 in astrocyte cultures derived from the rat spinal cord (Marriott et al., 1990). The release of SP in response to noxious stimulation (Kuraishi et al., 1985), therefore, may initiate prostaglandin synthesis in the spinal cord.

In general, the localization and production of prostaglandins in the spinal cord are compatible with the notion that these eicosanoids are involved in modulation of nociceptive input in this region. Whether there is a sustained elevation of prostaglandins in the central nervous system during chronic inflammation is yet to be determined.

Prostaglandin-induced hyperalgesia

Numerous studies have demonstrated that peripheral administration of prostaglandins produces hyperalgesia in laboratory animals

(Lembeck and Juan, 1974; Ferreira et al., 1978b; Taiwo and Levine, 1989) and in man (Ferreira, 1972). Administration of prostanoids into the central nervous system, especially onto the spinal cord, also reduces the threshold to noxious stimuli in various behavioral models of nociception. Ferreira and co-workers demonstrated that injection of nanogram amounts of PGE_2 into the cerebral ventricles of rats significantly enhanced the hyperalgesia induced by peripheral inflammation (Ferreira et al., 1978a). Conversely, intraventricular administration of a prostaglandin antagonist attenuated the hyperalgesia caused by peripheral injection of carrageenin. These results led to the conclusion that prostaglandins have both peripheral and central actions to augment nociception, although specific central nervous system sites of the prostaglandin effect were not determined.

Further studies, using intrathecal administration of various prostaglandins, support the premise that the spinal cord is an important site for the central hyperalgesic actions of these eicosanoids. Yaksh (1982) showed that injection of 100 ng of $PGF_{2\alpha}$ directly into the thecal space of rats significantly reduced the hot plate response latency, compared to intrathecal injection of a saline vehicle. In a similar manner, Ferreira (1983) and Taiwo and Levine (1986), demonstrated that the spinal injection of 100 ng of PGE_2 or $PGF_{2\alpha}$ produced hyperalgesia as indicated by a reduction in the paw pressure threshold. The $PGF_{2\alpha}$-induced hyperalgesia was attenuated by pretreatment with the cyclooxygenase inhibitor, indomethacin, suggesting that the actions of $PGF_{2\alpha}$ were caused by the production of other prostanoids (Taiwo and Levine, 1986). Using both the hot plate latency and acid writhing tests in mice, Uda and co-workers observed reductions in nociceptive thresholds after thecal injections of 1 pg to 10 ng of either PGE_2 or PGD_2, but not $PGF_{2\alpha}$ (Uda et al., 1990). The hyperalgesic actions of PGD_2 in the spinal cord were attenuated by co-injection of a SP antagonist with this eicosanoid, suggesting that the prostaglandin effect was secondary to increasing SP release.

These data make a strong case for the involvement of prostaglandins in augmenting pain sensitivity at the level of the spinal cord. In contrast, there is no mention in any of these studies that overt pain behaviors such as biting or scratching are elicited by intrathecal injection of prostaglandins. This suggests that prostaglandins do not produce pain when administered into the central nervous system, but only sensitize to noxious stimuli, an action analogous to the peripheral effects of these eicosanoids.

Central antinociceptive actions of NSAIDs

One of the major actions of the NSAIDs is the inhibition of cyclooxygenase, the enzyme that catalyzes the conversion of arachidonic acid to prostaglandins. By blocking the synthesis of prostaglandins at sites of tissue injury, these drugs presumably reduce prostaglandin-induced hyperalgesia and attenuate sensitization of nociceptive sensory neurons. Thus, their effectiveness as analgesics may depend on the production of prostaglandins. This could explain the observation that aspirin and aspirin-like drugs do not alter nociceptive thresholds in acute pain tests such as hot plate and tail-flick latency (Yaksh, 1982). During inflammation, however, prostaglandin levels increase and systemic administration of NSAIDs is antinociceptive (Lim et al., 1964; Moncada et al., 1975).

There is now substantial evidence to support the notion that a component of the analgesic actions of NSAIDs involves effects of these drugs in the central nervous system. Injection of microgram quantities of various NSAIDs into the cerebral ventricles of rats reduces the hyperalgesia induced by carrageenin injection into the hindpaw (Ferreira et al., 1978a). These central actions are additive with the antinociceptive effect of NSAIDs injected into peripheral sites of inflammation (Ferreira et al., 1978a), implying that the therapeutic effects of NSAIDs involve both peripheral and central sites of action. One potential site of action may be the thalamus. In this nucleus, neuronal firing evoked by inflammation or noxious peripheral stimulation is significantly reduced by systemic administration of NSAIDs (Guilbaud et al., 1982; Jurna and Brune, 1990).

At the level of the spinal cord, injection of NSAIDs also reduces nociceptive behaviors associated with inflammation. This was demonstrated by Yaksh (1982), who showed that intrathecal injection of microgram doses of aspirin or zomepirac diminished the writhing behavior induced by intraperitoneal injection of acetic acid (Yaksh, 1982). Recent studies by Malmberg and Yaksh (1992) have confirmed and expanded this initial work. They observed that the intrathecal injection of a variety of NSAIDs significantly diminished the late onset behavioral hyperalgesia caused by injection of formalin into rat paws, whereas the early phase of formalin-hyperalgesia was unaffected. This finding supports the idea that the antinociceptive actions of NSAIDs require an inflammatory state because the late phase of the formalin-induced hyperalgesia is a model for inflammation (Tjolsen et al., 1992).

The doses of intrathecal NSAIDs that Malmberg and Yaksh (1992) utilized were 100–1000-times less than those needed to produce antinociception after systemic injection. Thus, it is unlikely that the observed spinal actions of NSAIDs could result from redistribution of drug to peripheral sites of action. Furthermore, they demonstrated that the thecal injection of the R-enantiomer of ibuprofen was ineffective in reducing formalin-injected hyperalgesia, whereas the S-form was antinociceptive. Because only the S-enantiomer inhibits cyclooxygenase to a significant degree (Adams et al., 1976), these data suggest that the antinociception effects of spinal NSAIDs result from the inhibition of prostaglandin synthesis.

In humans, NSAIDs also appear to produce analgesia, in part, by actions in the central nervous system. Bromme and co-workers (1991) observed that the systemic administration of acetylsalicylic acid reduced the cerebral potentials and activation of the EEG induced by peripheral noxious stimulation. The drug did not affect auditory evoked potentials, spontaneous EEG, or reaction times. From this, they concluded that the drug had a direct action in the central nervous system. In two independent studies, investigators reported that intrathecal injection of low doses of lysine acetylsalicylate significantly diminished pain in cancer patients (Devoghel et al., 1984; Pellerin et al., 1987).

Using the antinociceptive effects of centrally administered NSAIDs as evidence that prostaglandins produce hyperalgesia by an action in the central nervous system is based on the assumption that inhibition of cyclooxygenase is the mechanism of action of these drugs. There is some debate as to whether this assumption is valid. Indeed, NSAIDs have other actions that might contribute to their analgesic effects (for review, see Biella and Groppetti, 1993). In addition, the potency of aspirin-like drugs as analgesics does not always parallel their ability to inhibit cyclooxygenase (McCormack and Brune, 1991). For example, Brune and co-workers recently showed that systemic administration of both the R- and S-enantiomers of fluribiprofen were nearly equipotent in blocking hyperalgesia induced by injecting interleukin-1 or yeast into the rat hindpaw. In contrast, the R-enantiomer was much less potent in inhibiting edema formation and in reducing prostaglandin formation (Brune et al., 1991). This suggests that the analgesic actions of NSAIDs are not secondary to inhibition of prostaglandin synthesis. Further work is warranted to elucidate the relationship between the effects of NSAIDs and prostaglandin production.

Possible sites of prostaglandin actions in the spinal cord

The specific mechanisms to account for the hyperalgesic actions of prostaglandins at the level of the spinal cord remain unknown. Based on the distribution of prostaglandin binding sites and the evidence that prostaglandins alter nociception, it is evident that one major site of action of these autocoids is at the level of sensory input in the dorsal horn.

Figure 1 illustrates four possible cellular targets for prostaglandin actions in the dorsal spinal cord. It is likely that prostanoids act on the terminals of sensory neurons to facilitate presynaptic release of transmitters (site 1, Fig. 1). Extensive evidence exists that prostaglandins enhance the excitability of sensory neurons, presumably by a receptor-mediated action on peripheral endings of these neurons (for review, see Treede at al., 1992). Because the peripheral and central terminals of sensory neurons are branches of the same cell, prostaglandin receptors should be found at both sites. In addition, recent studies in our laboratory and by others clearly demonstrate that prostaglandins can augment the release of the putative sensory transmitters, SP and CGRP, from various sensory nerve preparations (see below).

Prostaglandins could also act directly on nociceptive spinal cord neurons to enhance their excitability (sites 2 and 3, Fig. 1). Although few studies have directly addressed this possibility,

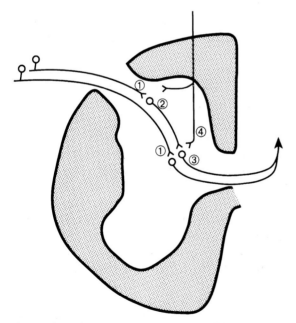

Fig. 1. Diagrammatic representation of possible cellular targets for prostaglandin actions in the dorsal spinal cord. See the text for a detailed discussion. (1) Sensory neurons; (2) interneurons; (3) projecting neurons; (4) descending neurons.

microiontophoresis of PGE_1 onto neurons in the isolated frog spinal cord significantly increases the firing rate of most neurons examined (Coceani and Viti, 1975). This indicates that prostaglandins are capable of exciting interneurons in the spinal cord. Furthermore, Chapman and Dickenson (1992) showed that the intrathecal administration of 250 μg of indomethacin significantly reduced the firing of nociceptive spinal cord neurons elicited by injection of formalin into peripheral receptive fields. When given systematically, however, this dose of indomethacin did not alter formalin-induced firing of neurons in the dorsal horn. These results suggest that the production of prostaglandins in the spinal cord augments synaptic activity between sensory terminals and receptive neurons in the dorsal spinal cord. Whether the eicosanoid action is presynaptic, postsynaptic, or both, has not been determined.

The spinally mediated actions of prostaglandins also might result from an action on terminals of descending bulbospinal fibers. These pathways, which are largely monoaminergic, are involved in descending inhibition of nociceptive inputs (for review, see Bausbaum and Fields, 1984). Prostaglandins could decrease the release of transmitter from these neurons, removing the inhibitory controls on the nociceptive signal. This mechanism was first proposed by Yaksh (1982) and is based, in part, on the fact that prostaglandins inhibit the release of norepinephrine (NE) from post-ganglionic sympathetic neurons (Bergstrom et al., 1973). By analogy, it is possible that prostaglandins in the spinal cord could reduce the release of NE from the terminals of descending noradrenergic fibers and diminish descending inhibitory control of nociceptive inputs. This is supported by a recent study of Taiwo and Levine (1988), who demonstrated that disruption of the bulbospinal noradrenergic pathway prevented the hyperalgesia induced by intrathecal administration of PGE_2.

Although prostaglandins could act at any or all of these sites to produce hyperalgesia, the available evidence best supports the hypothesis that these eicosanoids act at the central terminals of sensory neurons to augment the release of nociceptive transmitters. Experiments from my laboratory and work of others directly supporting this hypothesis are discussed in detail below.

Evidence that prostaglandins alter neuropeptide release from the spinal cord

The focus of this discussion is on the effects of prostaglandins on release of the neuropeptides, SP and CGRP, because abundant evidence supports that these peptides are important in nociception (for reviews, see Cuello, 1987; Poyner, 1992). In addition, release of these neuroactive peptides from peripheral endings of sensory neurons contributes to various components of inflammation (Payan, 1989; Poyner, 1992). Consequently, SP and/or CGRP are most often studied when evaluating the effects of prostaglandin on transmitter release from sensory neurons.

Prostaglandins increase the release of SP and CGRP

The initial evidence suggesting that prostaglandins increase SP release from sensory neurons was based on observations of prostaglandin actions in peripheral tissues. Butler and Hammond (1980) demonstrated that PGE_1, bradykinin or capsaicin caused ocular hypertension and miosis when infused into the posterior chamber of the rabbit eye. The effects of these agents were abolished by lesions of the fifth cranial nerves, whereas miosis induced by infusion of SP into the eye was not attenuated by nerve loss. They concluded that the actions of PGE_1, bradykinin and capsaicin on the eye were caused by activation of sensory nerves and the subsequent release of SP. In a similar manner, Ueda and co-workers showed that E series prostaglandins augmented the contractile responses of rabbit iris sphincter to transmural electrical stimulation (Ueda et al., 1985). The electrically stimulated contractions were attenuated by indomethacin, whereas neither prostaglandins nor indomethacin altered muscle contraction induced by exogenously administered SP. From these data the authors postulated that

the effects of prostaglandins on iris sphincter muscle were secondary to an increase in SP release from sensory neurons. A similar conclusion was reached by Mapp et al. (1991). In their study, infusion of PGI_2 caused a dose-dependent increase in contractions of isolated guinea pig bronchi. This action was significantly attenuated by pretreatment with either capsaicin, rutherium red or a tachykinin receptor antagonist, agents that disrupt the activity of sensory neurons.

Although limited studies have been performed to directly measure the prostaglandin-induced release of SP and/or CGRP from sensory neurons, results of this work support the premise that prostanoids enhance peptide release. Using the isolated guinea-pig heart preparation, Franco-Cereceda (1989) and Geppetti and co-workers (1991) demonstrated that prostaglandins increase the release of CGRP. Perfusing the isolated heart with either arachidonic acid (50 μM to 5 mM); PGE_2 (10 and 100 μM) or PGI_2 (10–100 μM) caused a significant increase in the outflow of CGRP compared to release in the absence of eicosanoid (Geppetti et al., 1991). The release induced by arachidonic acid was abolished by pretreating the tissues with indomethacin, suggesting that arachidonate is not directly altering release but serves as a substrate for prostaglandin synthesis. Capsaicin pretreatment also abolished the CGRP release induced by either arachidonic acid or prostaglandins indicating that the likely source of the peptide is sensory neurons.

In our laboratory, we examined whether selected prostaglandins could stimulate the release of SP and CGRP from dorsal root ganglia cells grown in culture. We demonstrated that exposing avian sensory neuronal cultures to micromolar concentrations of PGE_2 significantly increased the release of SP by 2–4-fold over basal release (Nicol et al., 1992). In a similar manner, treating isolated rat sensory neurons with 5 or 10 μM PGE_2 resulted in a small, but significant, increase in SP release (Vasko et al., 1993). Exposing these neuronal cultures to nanomolar concentrations of carba prostacyclin (a stable analog of PGI_2) also produced an approximate 2-fold increase in both SP and CGRP release (Hingtgen and Vasko,

1994). Treating either avian or mammalian sensory neurons with $PGF_{2\alpha}$ did not alter peptide release.

Taken together, these results indicate that prostaglandins can increase release of peptides from sensory neurons. The question remains, however, as to whether these autocoids act at central terminals of sensory neurons. To address this question, we examined the effects of various prostaglandins on the release of SP from rat spinal cord slices (Vasko et al., 1993). Exposing the spinal cord slices to 50 mM KCl resulted in a 2.5-fold increase in SP release above basal levels. Treating the tissues with 10 μM PGE_2 or 10 μM PGD_2 also significantly increased the release of SP, but to a lesser degree than 50 mM KCl, whereas 10 μM $PGF_{2\alpha}$ did not significantly alter the basal release. The prostaglandin-evoked peptide release was dependent on the presence of extracellular calcium in the perfusion buffer (Vasko et al., 1993), suggesting that prostanoids augment normal physiological release processes. The results of these slice experiments are important because they demonstrate that prostaglandins are involved in the regulation of sensory nerve function at synaptic terminals in the spinal cord, an action that may account for the hyperalgesic effects of these eicosanoids.

Prostaglandins augment neuropeptide release evoked by other stimuli

One major limitation of the studies described above is that the concentrations of prostaglandins needed to directly stimulate release are relatively large compared to the association constant for receptor binding in peripheral tissues (Halushka et al., 1989), and to the concentrations that sensitize sensory neurons. It is possible that more prostaglandins are required to affect release from isolated tissues (i.e., heart and spinal cord) because of diffusion, uptake, or metabolism. It is also possible that prostaglandins have two actions on sensory neurons; a direct stimulatory effect at high concentrations and a sensitizing action at lower concentrations.

A hallmark action of prostaglandins is their ability to sensitize sensory neurons to other stimuli. At a behavioral level this is manifest as hyperalgesia as opposed to overt pain (for review, see Treede et al., 1992). Thus, it seems likely that prostaglandins should facilitate the release of SP and CGRP evoked by other stimulating agents. This postulate is indirectly supported by a number of studies that measure bradykinin-evoked release of SP or CGRP in the absence or presence of indomethacin. Pretreatment with this NSAID either attenuated or abolished the bradykinin effect. This was observed with bradykinin-stimulated release of CGRP from the isolated tissues of guinea pig including the heart (Manzini et al., 1989; Geppetti et al., 1991), the bladder (Maggi et al., 1989), the trachea (Hua and Yaksh, 1993) and the dural sinuses (Geppetti et al., 1990). At the level of the spinal cord, indomethacin also prevented the bradykinin-induced facilitation of CGRP release (Andreeva and Rang, 1993). Because bradykinin increases the production of prostanoids in a number of tissues, (McGiff et al., 1972; Lembeck et al., 1976), the inhibitory actions of indomethacin likely result from the blockade of kinin-induced synthesis of prostaglandins. If this is the case, then prostaglandins are contributing to the increase in peptide release caused by bradykinin.

Recent studies performed in my laboratory have demonstrated a direct action of prostaglandins to enhance peptide release stimulated by other agents (Hingtgen and Vasko, 1994; Vasko et al., 1994). Using rat sensory neurons grown in culture, we demonstrated that pre-exposing the cultures to 100 nM or 1 μM PGE_2 augmented the peptide release induced by 100 nM bradykinin by approximately 2-fold compared to release evoked by bradykinin alone (Vasko et al., 1994). These concentrations of PGE_2 did not alter basal release of either SP or CGRP when given in the absence of bradykinin. Furthermore, pretreating the sensory neurons with indomethacin at a concentration that blocked prostaglandin synthesis attenuated bradykinin-evoked release of both SP and CGRP. In another study, we showed that exposing neuronal cultures to either 10 nM PGI_2 or 1 nM carba prostacyclin facilitated SP and

CGRP release evoked by capsaicin (Hingtgen and Vasko, 1994). When administered alone, these prostanoids did not alter peptide release at the concentrations used in the study. Furthermore, exposing sensory neurons in culture to 1 μM $PGF_{2\alpha}$ did not alter either the basal or stimulated release of either peptide.

To determine if prostaglandins also augment the release of SP and CGRP from the central terminals of sensory neurons, we performed experiments using an in vitro spinal cord slice preparation (for specific methods, see Pang and Vasko, 1986). Tissue slices from one half of each rat spinal cord were perfused with a Krebs-bicarbonate buffer containing 1 μM carba prostacyclin ($CPGI_2$), whereas slices from the other half were perfused with buffer that did not contain prostaglandin. In this way, each animal served as its own control. Basal release of SP and CGRP was measured from perfusate collected at 2 min

intervals for 12 min, after which time the slices were exposed to 250 nM capsaicin for 6 min to stimulate peptide release from the sensory nerve terminals (Gamse et al., 1981). Subsequently, the tissues were perfused for another 10 min with buffer to re-establish resting release. Peptide content in the perfusates and in the tissues was determined by radioimmunoassay and release expressed as a percent of the total peptide content in the spinal cord slices. Figures 2 and 3 illustrate the results of these experiments. Exposing the spinal cord tissue to 250 nM capsaicin causes a 2-fold increase in SP release from a basal value representing $0.5 \pm 0.1\%$ of the total tissue content released over 8 min (mean $\pm$ S.E.M.) to $1.0 \pm 0.1\%$ of total content (Fig. 2). Capsaicin also stimulates the release of CGRP by approximately 3-fold, from 0.8 ± 0.1 to $2.3 \pm 0.4\%$ of total CGRP content in the tissue per 8 min (Fig. 3). The evoked release of SP and CGRP (calculated

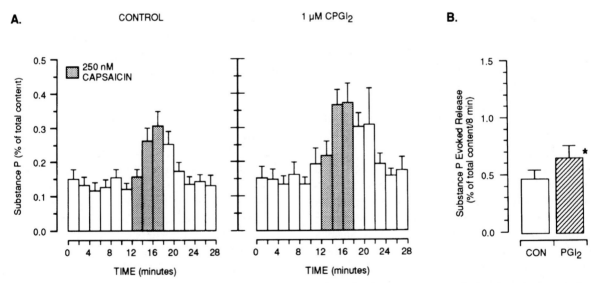

Fig. 2. Effect of carba prostacyclin on the release of substance P from rat spinal cord slices. A. Each column represents the mean $\pm$ S.E.M. ($n = 8$) of either resting release (open columns) or capsaicin-evoked release (shaded columns) of SP expressed as percent of the total SP content in the slices. The panel on the left (labelled control) represents the release of peptide in the absence of $CPGI_2$, whereas the panel on the right represents the release from tissues exposed to 1 μM $CPGI_2$ for 20 min prior to and throughout the first resting and capsaicin-stimulation periods. B. The evoked-release of SP is calculated by subtracting the resting release for the samples obtained during minutes 4–12 from the stimulated release for samples obtained during minutes 12–20. The columns represent the evoked release (mean $\pm$ S.E.M., $n = 8$) in the absence (open column), or presence (hatched column) of 1 μM $CPGI_2$. The asterisk indicates a significant difference between control and $CPGI_2$-treated tissue using a paired t-test ($P < 0.05$).

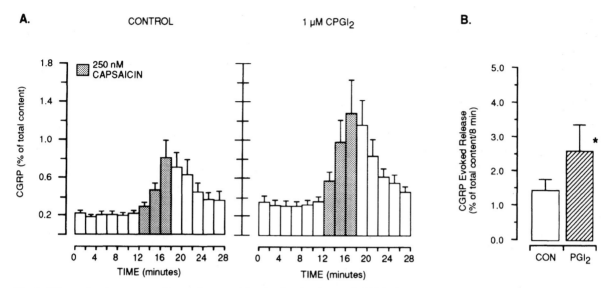

Fig. 3. Effect of carba prostacyclin on the capsaicin-stimulated release of CGRP from rat spinal cord slices. A. Each column represents the mean $\pm$ S.E.M. ($n = 8$) of either resting release (open columns) or capsaicin-evoked release (shaded columns) of CGRP expressed as percent of the total CGRP content in the slices. The panel on the left (labelled control) represents the release of peptide in the absence of $CPGI_2$, whereas the panel on the right represents the release from tissues exposed to 1 μM $CPGI_2$ for 20 min prior to and throughout the first resting and capsaicin-stimulation periods. B. The columns represent the evoked release of CGRP (mean $\pm$ S.E.M., $n = 8$) in the absence (open column), or presence (hatched column) of 1 μM $CPGI_2$. The asterisk indicates a significant difference between control and $CPGI_2$-treated tissue using a paired t-test ($P < 0.05$).

as the release for the 8-min stimulation period minus release for the 8 min preceding the stimulus) from eight experiments is 0.5 ± 0.1 and $1.4 \pm 0.3\%$, respectively (open columns, Figs. 2B and 3B).

Exposing the spinal cord slices to 1 μM $CPGI_2$ from the beginning of the perfusion through the capsaicin stimulation, results in a significant increase in the capsaicin-stimulated release of both SP and CGRP without altering basal release (Figs. 2A and 3A). The evoked release of SP in slices treated with $CPGI_2$ is enhanced 1.4-fold to a value representing $0.7 \pm 0.1\%$ of the total peptide content per 8 min when compared to matched controls (Fig. 2B). Capsaicin-evoked release of CGRP increased by 1.8-fold with $CPGI_2$ treatment to a value of $2.6 \pm 0.8\%$ of CGRP content per 8 min (Fig. 3B).

We assume that the capsaicin-stimulated release of SP and CGRP is originating largely from the central terminals of sensory neurons. This is based on the fact that capsaicin is relatively selec-

tive in activating small-diameter sensory neurons (Kenins, 1982; Szolcsanyi et al., 1988). Our data, therefore, suggest that $CPGI_2$ acts on sensory neurons at the level of the spinal cord to enhance peptide release. Furthermore, these data confirm the results of Andreeva and Rang (1993), who demonstrated that exposing spinal cord slices to various prostaglandins augmented the release of CGRP evoked by electrical stimulation of the dorsal roots. In their study, PGD_2 and PGE_2 were the most potent in facilitating release, whereas $PGF_{2\alpha}$ was only affective at 10 μM, and PGI_2 was ineffective. The apparent discrepancy between their lack of effect of PGI_2 and our results with the stable analog of PGI_2, might be explained by the fact that PGI_2 is highly unstable and rapidly oxidized in tissues.

Prostaglandins and enhanced peptide release in inflammation

Based on the studies discussed above, one can

conclude that prostaglandins facilitate the release of neuropeptides from sensory neurons. It is, therefore, interesting to speculate that the hyperalgesic actions of prostaglandins may be the result of an augmentation of transmitter release at nociceptive synapses in the dorsal spinal cord. It is also possible that the facilitatory action of these eicosanoids is one mechanism to account for the elevated content and release of SP and CGRP from spinal cord observed in experimental models of inflammation (Oku et al., 1987; Nanayama et al, 1989; Donnerer et al., 1992; Garry and Hargreaves, 1992).

To address the question of whether prostaglandins have long-term effects on sensory neurons during inflammation, we studied whether intrathecal administration of the NSAID, Ketorolac, could prevent the enhanced release of peptides that is observed during inflammation. For these studies, we induced unilateral inflammation in two groups of rats by injecting 150 μl of a 1:1 (v/v) solution of complete Freund's adjuvant (CFA) and saline into the plantar surface of one hindpaw. This resulted in a significant swelling and a reduced paw pressure threshold (i.e., enhanced sensitivity to a noxious stimulus) that lasted for at least 5 days. One group of animals was implanted with intrathecal cannulae connected to Alzet miniosmotic pumps containing Ketorolac so that they received 10 nmol of the drug per hour into the thecal space. The drug treatment started one day prior to inducing inflammation, and was maintained throughout the 5 days of experimental inflammation. This dosage of Ketorolac was selected because it significantly attenuates the late phase of hyperalgesia induced by formalin injection into the rat hindpaw (Malmberg and Yaksh, 1992).

On the fifth day after CFA injection, the rats were sacrificed and the lumbar region of the spinal cords were removed, divided midsagittally, chopped and perfused with a Krebs-bicarbonate buffer. In this way, in vitro release of SP from the spinal cord tissue on the side of the inflammation could be compared to release from the corresponding non-inflamed side. Tissues were perfused for 20 min to stabilize resting release, then

perfusate samples were collected every 3 min. After an additional 18 min of perfusion, the slices were exposed to 500 nM capsaicin for 9 min to stimulate peptide release from sensory nerve terminals. Tissues were then perfused with normal Krebs buffer for 15 min to re-establish the resting release. Substance P content in the perfusates was measured by radioimmunoassay. Upon completion of the release protocol, the peptide content in the tissues also was determined and release is expressed as percent of the total SP content in the spinal cord slices.

As can be seen in the top panels of Fig. 4, the capsaicin-stimulated release of SP is significantly elevated from the cord tissue on the side of the inflamed paw compared to the control side. Although there is no significant change in resting release, the capsaicin-stimulated release of SP is approximately 1.5-fold greater in cord tissue taken from the inflamed side. The total amount of SP released during exposure to capsaicin is 3.0 $\pm$ 0.9% of the tissue content per 9 min compared to 4.4 $\pm$ 1.0% for tissue from the control and inflamed side, respectively. These results confirm the work of others showing that inducing inflammation results in an enhanced release of SP and CGRP from sensory neurons (Oku et al., 1987; Nanayama et al., 1989; Donnerer et al., 1992; Garry and Hargreaves, 1992).

The intrathecal administration of Ketorolac prior to and throughout the period of inflammation completely abolishes the increase in SP release that occurs during inflammation (Fig. 4 right side, lower panel versus upper panel), without significantly altering the release profile of tissue from the non-inflamed side (lower panel, left). In rats treated with Ketorolac, capsaicin-evoked release from cord tissue on the non-inflamed side was 3.1 $\pm$ 0.8% of total content per 9 min; whereas stimulated release from the inflamed side was 2.4 $\pm$ 0.7% of total content per 9 min.

These results suggest a cause-effect relationship between the synthesis of prostaglandins at the level of the spinal cord and the enhanced release of neuropeptides from sensory neurons that occurs during inflammation. Indeed, the data show that a spinally administered NSAID can

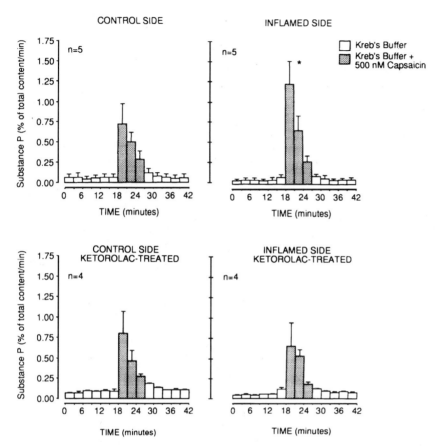

Fig. 4. Effects of Ketorolac on substance P release from spinal cord slices of rats with unilateral inflammation. Each column represents the mean ± S.E.M. (*n* = 5) of either resting release (open columns) or capsaicin-evoked release of SP (shaded columns) expressed as percent of the total SP content in the slices. The top panels represent release from cord tissues of untreated animals, whereas the bottom panels are release from animals treated with intrathecal Ketorolac for 6 days. The control side (left panels) represent release from the spinal cord tissue taken from the side with the non-inflamed paw. The right panels are release from tissue ipsilateral to the inflammation (see text for details). The asterisk indicates statistical significance compared to the control using ANOVA with Bonferroni's post hoc test.

block the elevation in peptide release observed during inflammation. Further studies, however, are needed to establish that prostanoid production in the spinal cord is a critical event in the long-term sensitization of sensory neurons.

Summary

The studies reviewed in this chapter present a convincing argument that prostaglandins have direct actions at the level of the spinal cord to enhance nociception. Furthermore, an increasing body of evidence supports the hypothesis that one

important site of action of these eicosanoids is the terminals of sensory neurons. Studies performed in our laboratory add to this evidence by demonstrating that relatively large concentrations of prostaglandins increase SP release, whereas lower amounts augment the capsaicin-stimulated release of both SP and CGRP from rat spinal cord slices. In neuronal cultures of rat dorsal root ganglia, prostaglandins also facilitate the evoked release of SP and CGRP, indicating a direct action of these autocoids on sensory neurons.

Based on these studies, it is interesting to speculate that the actions of prostaglandins on pep-

378

tide release are one mechanism to account for hyperalgesia produced by these eicosanoids. In addition, by a sustained action, prostaglandins may contribute to the enhanced excitability of sensory neurons during inflammation. Indeed, our observations that intrathecal Ketorolac abolished the elevation in SP release during inflammation support this possibility. Whether the effect of the NSAID are caused by the inhibition of prostaglandin synthesis in the spinal cord are yet to be determined.

Further work is necessary to establish a role for prostaglandins in the adaptive changes of nociceptive neurons that occur in chronic pain states and in inflammation. In addition, the cellular mechanisms underlying the effects of prostaglandins on sensory neurons are yet to be elucidated.

Acknowledgements

The author wishes to thank Dr. David Byers and Mr. Scott Grasso for their invaluable assistance in performing the experiments utilizing the spinal cord slices.

The data reported here were generated through the support of USPHS awards AR205882 and DA07176 and a grant from the Showalter Foundation.

References

Adams, S.S., Bresloff, P. and Mason, C.G. (1976) Pharmacological differences between the optical isomers of ibuprofen: evidence for metabolic inversion of the (−)-isomer. *J. Pharm. Pharmacol.*, 28: 256–257.

Andreeva, L. and Rang, H.P., Effect of bradykinin and prostaglandins on the release of calcitonin gene-related peptide-like immunoreactivity from the rat spinal cord in vitro. *Br. J. Pharmacol.*, 108 (1993) 185–190.

Basbaum, A.I. and Fields, H.L. (1984) Endogenous pain control systems: brainstem spinal pathways and endorphin circuitry. *Ann. Rev. Neurosci.*, 7: 309–338.

Bergstrom, S., Farnbeo, L.A. and Fuxe, K. (1973) Effect of prostaglandin E_2 on central and peripheral catecholamine neurons. *Eur. J. Pharmacol.*, 21: 362–368.

Besson, J.M. and Chaouch, A. (1987) Peripheral and spinal mechanisms of nociception. *Physiol. Rev.*, 67: 67–186.

Biella, G. and Groppetti A. (1993) Correlation between the antinociceptive effect of aspirin and central transmitters. *Progr. Pharmacol. Clin. Pharmacol.*, 10: 1–9.

Bombardieri, S., Cattani, P., Ciabattoni, G., Di Munno, O., Pasero, G., Patrono, C., Pinca, E. and Pugliese, F. (1981) The synovial prostaglandin system in chronic inflammatory arthritis: differential effects of steroidal and nonsteroidal anti-inflammatory drugs. *Br. J. Pharmacol.*, 73: 893–901.

Breder, C.D., Smith, W.L., Raz, A., Masferrer, J., Seibert, K., Needleman, P. and Saper, C.B. (1992) Distribution and characterization of cyclooxygenase immunoreactivity in the ovine brain. *J. Comp. Neurol.*, 322: 409–438.

Bromm, B., Rundshagen, I. and Scharein, E. (1991) Central analgesic effects of acetylsalicylic acid in healthy man. *Arzneim-Forsch / Drug Res.*, 41: 1123–1129.

Brune, K., Beck, W.S., Geisslinger, G., Menzel-Soglowek, S., Peskar, B.M. and Peskar, B.A. (1991) Aspirin-like drugs may block pain independently of prostaglandin synthesis inhibition. *Experientia*, 47: 257–261.

Butler, J.M. and Hammond, B.R. (1980) The effects of sensory denervation on the responses of the rabbit eye to prostaglandin E_1, bradykinin and substance P. *Br. J. Pharmacol.*, 69: 495–502.

Chapman, V. and Dickenson, A.H. (1992) The spinal and peripheral roles of bradykinin and prostaglandins in nociceptive processing in the rat. *Eur. J. Pharmacol.*, 219: 427–433.

Coceani, F. and Viti, A. (1975) Responses of spinal neurons to iontophoretically applied prostaglandin E_1 in the frog. *Can. J. Physiol. Pharmacol.*, 53: 273–284.

Coderre, T.J., Gonzales, R., Goldyne, M.E., West, J. and Levine, J.D. (1990) Noxious stimulus-induced increase in spinal prostaglandin E_2 is noradrenergic terminal-dependent. *Neurosci. Lett.*, 115: 253–258.

Cuello, A.C. (1987) Peptides as neuromodulators in primary sensory neurons. *Neuropharmacology*, 26: 971–979.

Devoghel, J.C. (1983) Small intrathecal doses of lysine-acetylsalicylate relieve intractable pain in man. *J. Int. Med. Res.*, 11: 90–91.

Donnerer, J., Schuligoi, R. and Stein, C. (1992) Increased content and transport of substance P and calcitonin gene-related peptide in sensory nerves innervating inflamed tissue: Evidence for a regulatory function of nerve growth factor in vivo. *Neuroscience*, 49: 693–698.

Dubner, R. and Ruda, M.A., (1992) Activity dependent neuronal plasticity following tissue injury and inflammation. *TINS*, 15: 96–103.

Ferreira, S.H. (1972) Prostaglandins, aspirin-like drugs and analgesia. *Nature*, 240: 200–203.

Ferreira, S.H. (1983) Prostaglandins: peripheral and central analgesia. In: *Advances in Pain Research and Therapy, Vol. 5* Bonica, J.J., Lindblom, U. and Oggo, A. (Eds.), Raven Press, New York, pp. 627–634.

Ferreira, S.H., Lorenzetti, B.B. and Correa, F.M.A. (1978a)

Central and peripheral antialgesic action of aspirin-like drugs. *Eur. J. Pharmacol.*, 53: 39–48.

Ferreira, S.H., Nakamura, M. and de Abreu Castro, M.S. (1978b) The hyperalgesic effects of prostacyclin and prostaglandin E$_2$. *Prostaglandins*, 16:31–37.

Franco-Cereceda, A. (1989) Prostaglandins and CGRP release from cardiac sensory nerves. *Naunyn-Schmiedeberg's Arch Pharmacol.*, 340: 140–184.

Gamse, R., Lackner, D., Gamse, G. and Leeman, S.E. (1981) Effect of capsaicin pretreatment on capsaicin-evoked release of immunoreactive somatostatin and substance P from primary sensory neurons. *Naunyn-Schmiedeberg's Arch. Pharmacol.*, 316:38–41.

Garry, M.G. and Hargreaves, K.M. (1992) Enhanced release of immunoreactive CGRP and substance P from spinal dorsal horn slices occurs during carrageenan inflammation. *Brain Res.*, 582: 139–142.

Geppetti, P. (1993) Sensory neuropeptide release by bradykinin: mechanisms and pathophysiological implications. *Regul. Peptides*, 47: 1–23.

Geppetti, P., Del Bianco, E., Santicioli, P., Lippe, I.Th., Maggi, C.A. and Sicuteri, F. (1990) Release of sensory neuropeptides from dural venous sinuses of guinea-pig. *Brain Res.*, 510: 58–62.

Geppetti, P., Del Bianco, E., Tramontana, M., Vigano, T., Folco, G.C., Maggi, C.A., Manzini, S. and Fanciullacci, M., (1991) Arachidonic acid and bradykinin share a common pathway to release neuropeptide from capsaicin-sensitive sensory nerve fibers of the guinea pig heart. *J. Pharmacol. Exp. Ther.*, 259: 759–765.

Guilbaud, G., Benoist, J.M., Gautron, M. and Kayser, V. (1982) Aspirin clearly depresses responses of ventrobasal thalamus neurons to joint stimuli in arthritic rats. *Pain*, 13: 153–163.

Halushka, P.V., Mais, D.E., Mayeux, P.R. and Morinelli, T.A. (1989) Thromboxane, prostaglandin and leukotriene receptors. *Annu. Rev. Pharmacol. Toxicol.*, 10:213–239.

Hamon, M., Bourgoin, S., LeBars, D and Cesselin, F. (1988) In vivo and in vitro release of central neurotransmitters in relation to pain and analgesia. *Progr. Brain Res.*, 77: 431–444.

Handwerker, H.O. (1976) Influences of algogenic substances and prostaglandins on the discharges of unmyelinated cutaneous nerve fibers identified as nociceptors. In: *Advances in Pain Research and Therapy, Vol. 1*, Eds. Bonica, J.J. and Albe-Fessard, D., Raven Press, New York. pp. 41–45.

Higgs, G.A. and Salmon, J.A. (1979) Cyclo-oxygenase products in carrageenin-induced inflammation. *Prostaglandins*, 17: 737–746.

Hingtgen, C.M. and Vasko, M.R. (1994) Prostacyclin enhances the evoked-release of substance P and calcitonin gene-related peptide from rat sensory neurons *Brain Res.*, 655: 51–60.

Hua, X.-Y. and Yaksh, T.L. (1993) Pharmacology of the

effects of bradykinin, serotonin, and histamine on the release of calcitonin gene-related peptide in the rat trachea. *J. Neurosci.*, 13: 1947–1953.

Jessell, T.M. and Iversen, L.L. (1977) Opiate analgesics inhibit substance P release from rat trigeminal nucleus. *Nature*, 268: 549–551.

Juan, H. and Lembeck, F. (1974) Action of peptides and other algesic agents on paravascular pain receptors of the isolated perfused rabbit ear. *Naunyn-Schmiedeberg's. Arch. Pharmacol.*, 283: 151–164.

Jurna, I. and Brune, K. (1990) Central effect of the non-steroid anti-inflammatory agents, indometacin, ibuprofen, and diclofenac, determined in C fibre-evoked activity in single neurones of the rat thalamus. *Pain*, 41: 71–80.

Kenins, P. (1982) Responses of single nerve fibers to capsaicin applied to the skin. *Neurosci. Lett.*, 29:83–88.

Kuraishi, Y., Hirota, N., Sato, Y., Hino, Y., Satoh, M. and Takagi, H., Evidence that substance P and somatostatin transmit separate information related to pain in the spinal dorsal horn. *Brain Res.*, 325 (1985) 294–298.

Lembeck, Popper, H. and Juan, H. (1976) Release of prostaglandins by bradykinin as an intrinsic mechanism of its algesic effect. *Naunyn-Schmiedeberg's Arch Pharmacol.*, 294: 69–73.

Leslie, J.B. and Watkins, W.D. (1985) Eicosanoids in the central nervous system. *J. Neurosurg.*, 63: 659–668.

Lim, R.K.S., Guzman, F., Rodgers, D.W., Groto, K., Braun, C., Dickerson, G.D. and Engle, R.J. (1964) Site of action of narcotic and non-narcotic analgesics determined by blocking bradykinin-evoked visceral pain. *Arch. Int. Pharmacodyn.*, 152: 25–58.

MacLean, D.B., Wheeler, F. and Hayes, L. (1990) Basal and stimulated release of substance P from dissocisted cultures of vagal sensory neurons. *Brain Res.*, 519: 308–314.

Maggi, C.A., Patacchini, R., Santicioli, P., Geppetti, P., Cecconi, R., Giuliani, S. and Meli, A. (1989) Multiple mechanism in the motor responses of the guinea-pig isolated urinary bladder to bradykinin. *Br. J. Pharmacol.*, 98: 619–629.

Malmberg, A.B. and Yaksh, T.L. (1992) Antinociceptive actions of spinal nonsteroidal anti-inflammatory agents on the formalin test in the rat. *J. Pharmacol. Exp. Ther.*, 263: 136–146.

Manzini, S., Perretti, F., De Benedetti, L., Pradelles, P., Maggi, C.A. and Geppetti, P. (1989) A comparison of bradykinin- and capsaicin-induced myocardial and coronary effects in isolated perfused heart of guinea-pig: involvement of substance P and calcitonin gene-related peptide release. *Br. J. Pharmacol.*, 97: 303–312.

Mapp, C.E., Fabbri, L.M., Boniotti, A. and Maggi, C.A. (1991) Prostacyclin activates tachykinin release from capsaicin-sensitive afferents in guinea-pig bronchi through a ruthenium red-sensitive pathway. *Br. J. Pharmacol.*, 104: 49–52.

Marriott, D., Wilkins, G.P., Coote, P.R. and Wood, J.N. (1990)

Eicosanoid synthesis by spinal cord astrocytens is evoked by substance P; possible implications for nociception and pain. *Adv. Prostaglandin Thromboxane Leukotriene Res.*, 21: 739–741.

Martin, H.A., Bausbaum, A.I., Kwiat, G.C., Goetzl E.J. and Levine, J.D. (1987) Leukotriene and prostaglandin sensitization of cutaneous high-threshold C- and A-delta mechanonociceptors in the hairy skin of rat hindlimbs. *Neuroscience*, 22: 651–659.

Matsumura, K., Watanabe, Y., Imai-Matsumura, K., Connolly, M., Koyama, Y., Onoe, H. and Watanabe, Y. (1992) Mapping of prostaglandin E_2 binding sites in rat brain using quantitative autoradiography. *Brain Res.*, 581: 292–298.

McCormack, K. and Brune, K. (1991) Dissociation between the antinociceptive and anti-inflammatory effects of the nonsteroidal anti-inflammatory drugs. *Drugs*, 41: 533–547.

McGiff, J.C., Terragno, N.A,, Malik, K.U. and Lonigro, A.J. (1972) Release of prostaglandin E-like substance from canine kidney by bradykinin. *Circ. Res.*, 31: 36–43.

Mense, S. (1981) Sensitization of group IV muscle receptors to bradykinin by 5-hydroxyttryptamine and prostaglandin E_2. *Brain Res.*, 225: 95–105

Moncada, S., Ferreira, S.H. and Vane, J.R. (1975) Inhibition of prostaglandin biosynthesis as the mechanism of analgesia of aspirin-like drugs in the dog knee joint. *Eur. J. Pharmacol.*, 31: 250–260.

Nanayama, T., Kuraishi, Y., Ohno, H. and Satoh, M. (1989) Capsaicin-induced release of calcitonin gene-related peptide from dorsal horn slices is enhanced in adjuvant arthritic rats. *Neurosci. Res.*, 6: 569–572.

Nicol, G.D., Klingberg, D.K. and Vasko, M.R. (1992) Prostaglandin E_2 increases calcium conductance and stimulates release of substance P in avian sensory neurons. *J. Neurosci.*, in press.

Ogorochi, T., Narumiya, S., Mizuno, N., Yamashita, K., Miyazaki, H. and Hayaishi, O. (1984) Regional distribution of prostaglandins D_2, E_2, $F_{2\alpha}$ and related enzymes in postmortem human brain. *J. Neurochem.*, 43: 71–82.

Oku, R., Satoh, M. and Takagi, H. (1987) Release of substance P from the spinal dorsal horn is enhanced in polyarthritic rats. *Neurosci. Lett.*, 74: 315–319.

Pang, I.H. and Vasko, M.R. (1986) Morphine and norepinephrine but not 5-hydroxytryptamine and γ-aminobutyric acid inhibit the potassium-stimulated release of substance P from rat spinal cord slices. *Brain Res.*, 376:268–279.

Payan, D.G. (1989) Neuropeptides and inflammation: the role of substance P. *Annu. Rev. Med.*, 40: 341–352.

Pellerin, M., Hardy, F., Abergel, A., Boule, D., Palacci, J.H., Babinet, P., Wingtin, L. NG., Glowinski, J., Amiot, J.-F., Mechali, D., Colbert, N. and Starkman, M. (1987) Douleur chronique rebelle des cancereux: interet de l'injection intrarachidienne d'acetylsalicylate de lysine soxante observations. *Presse Med.*, 16: 1465–1468.

Poyner, D.R. (1992) Calcitonin gene-related peptide: multiple actions, multiple receptors. *Pharmac. Ther.*, 56: 23–51.

Ramwell, P.W., Shaw, J.E. and Jessup,R. (1966) Spontaneous and evoked release of prostaglandins from frog spinal cord. *Am. J. Physiol.*, 211: 998–1004.

Schaible, H.-G. and Schmidt, R.F. (1988) Excitation and sensitization of fine articular afferents from cat's knee joint by prostaglandin E_2. *J. Physiol. (London)*, 403: 91–104.

Smith, J.B. and Willis, A.L. (1971) Aspirin selectively inhibits prostaglandin production in human platlets. *Nature*, 231: 235–237.

Szolcsanyi, J., Anton, F., Reeh, P.W. and Handwerker, H.O. (1988) Selective excitation by capsaicin of mechano-heat sensitive nociceptors in rat skin. *Brain Res.*, 466:262–268.

Taiwo, Y.O. and Levine, J.D. (1986) Indomethacin blocks central nociceptive effects of $PGF_{2\alpha}$. *Brain Res.*, 373: 81–84.

Taiwo, Y.O. and Levine, J.D. (1988) Prostaglandins inhibit endogenous pain control by blocking transmission at spinal noradrenergic synapses. *J. Neurosci.*, 8 :1346–1349.

Taiwo, Y.O. and Levine, J.D. (1989) Prostaglandin effects after elimination of indirect hyperalgesic mechanisms in the skin of the rat. *Brain Res.*, 492:397–399.

Tjolsen, A., Berge, O.-G., Hunskaar, S., Rosland, J.H. and Hole, K. (1992) The formalin test: an evaluation of the method. *Pain*, 51: 5–17.

Trang, L.E, Granstrom, E. and Lovgren, O. (1977) Levels of prostaglandins $F_{2\alpha}$ and E_2 and thromboxane B_2 in joint fluid in rheumatoid arthritis. *Scand. J. Rheum.*, 6: 151–154.

Treede, R.D., Meyer, R.A., Raja, S.N. and Campbell, J.N. (1992) Peripheral and central mechanisms of cutaneous hyperalgesia. *Progr. Neurobiol.*, 38: 397–421.

Uda, R., Horiguchi, S., Ito, S., Hyodo, M. and Hayaishi, O. (1990) Nociceptive effects induced by intrathecal administration of prostaglandin D_2, E_2, or $F_{2\alpha}$ to conscious mice. *Brain Res.*, 510: 26–32.

Ueda, N., Muramatsu, I. and Fujiwara, M. (1985) Prostaglandins enhance trigeminal substance P-ergic responses in the rabbit iris sphincter muscles. *Brain Res.*, 337:347–351.

Vane, J.R. (1971) Inhibition of prostaglandin synthesis as a mechanism of action for aspirin-like drugs. *Nature*, 231: 232–235.

Vasko, M.R., Zirkelbach, S.L. and Waite, K.J. (1993) Prostaglandins stimulate the release of substance P from rat spinal cord slices. *Progr. Pharmacol. Clin. Pharmacol.*, 10: 69–89.

Vasko, M.R., Campbell, W.B. and Waite, K.J. (1994) Prostaglandin E_2 enhances bradykinin-stimulated release of neuropeptides from rat sensory neurons in culture. *J. Neurosci.*, 14: 4987–4997.

Watanabe, Y., Watanabe, Y., Hamada, K., Bommelaer-Bayt, M.C., Dray, F., Kaneko, T., Yumoto, N. and Hayaishi, O. (1989) Distinct localization of prostaglandin D_2, E_2 and $F_{2\alpha}$ binding sites in monkey brain. *Brain Res.*, 478:143–148.

Yaksh, T.L. (1982) Central and peripheral mechanisms for the analgesic action of acetylsalicylic acid. In: Barett, H.J.M., Hirsh, J. and Mustard, J.F., Eds. *Acetylsalicylic Acid: New Uses for an Old Drug*, Raven Press, New York, pp. 137–151.

F. Nyberg, H.S. Sharma and Z. Wiesenfeld-Hallin (Eds.)
Progress in Brain Research, Vol 104

CHAPTER 22

The opioid receptor antagonist naloxone influences the pathophysiology of spinal cord injury

Y. Olsson[1], H.S. Sharma[1,2], F. Nyberg[2] and J. Westman[3]

[1]Laboratory of Neuropathology, University Hospital, Departments of [2]Pharmaceutical Biosciences and [3]Human Anatomy, Biomedical Centre, Uppsala University, Uppsala, Sweden

Introduction

A focal trauma to the spinal cord, for instance induced by a traffic accident, may lead to various degree of functional disturbances (Tator, 1990). The degree of permanent disability is influenced by several factors such as the extent and type of the initial physical injury, secondary or 'perifocal' changes around the site of the initial injury and the efficiency of medical treatment and rehabilitation (Balentine, 1978, 1988; Bracken et al., 1993).

The initial medical strategy may include surgery with decompression of the cord and stabilisation of the spine (Collins, 1984; Bracken and Holford, 1993; Young, 1993). Patients may also benefit from high doses of methylprednisolone in order to minimise the perifocal changes caused by microcirculatory alterations and edema. Methylprednisolone is the only compound which has gained widespread acceptance in the treatment of traumatic injuries of the human spinal cord (Young and Flamm, 1982; Editorial, 1990).

Due to the importance of spinal cord injuries, several groups of scientists are searching for additional agents which may influence the development of the perifocal lesions in spinal cord injury. To that end, a solid knowledge is needed about the pathogenesis of the perifocal changes. The significance of factors which may be formed or

released as a consequence of the initial physical injury has attracted a great deal of attention. Such injury factors include eicosanoids, platelet-activating factors, free radicals, neuropeptides, monoamines and cations (Tator and Fehlings, 1991; Faden and Salzman, 1992; Hayes et al., 1992; Lipton, 1993).

The spinal cord is very rich in opioid peptides, and opioid receptors of the spinal cord are involved in the regulation of sensory, autonomic and somato-motor functions (Hökfelt et al., 1978). The opioid peptides are often co-localised with various other neurotransmitters within the dorsal horn (Hökfelt et al., 1987). An injury to the spinal cord may thus induce a release of opioids and other neurotransmitters (Hogan and Banik, 1985).

The significance of opioids as injury factors in spinal cord trauma can be investigated in many different ways. Experimental studies can be performed by using opioid peptide antagonists. This chapter is focused on the influence of the important opioid peptide antagonist, naloxone in spinal cord injury. Naloxone is a competitive antagonist of μ, δ and κ opioid receptors (Martin, 1967). The effect of naloxone is rapid in onset and its half-life time in plasma is about 1 h (Misra, 1978).

Apart from a review of the literature on the action of naloxone in spinal cord injury we present some personal investigations in which naloxone has been used to explore the role of opioid peptides in the development of perifocal changes occurring after a focal trauma to the rat spinal cord.

Pathophysiology of spinal cord trauma

Studies on the pathophysiology of traumatic spinal cord injury is to a large extent based on animal experiments, and most models applied can be included in one of the following categories: weight drop technique, controlled contusion and maintained compression (de la Torre, 1981; Tator and Fehlings, 1991). As discussed in many excellent reviews, trauma to the spinal cord is associated with numerous reactions in the cells and the tracts of the cord, changes in their surrounding extracellular fluid and in the microcirculation (Faden and Salzman, 1992; Faden, 1993a).

After spinal cord injury, there is an immediate loss of electrical activity, increase in extracellular potassium, decrease in sodium-potassium ATP-ase, indicating membrane dysfunction, and failure of ionic pump mechanisms (Clendenon et al., 1978). Alterations in the fluid microenvironment of the spinal cord induced by trauma play important roles in the pathogenesis of the secondary cell changes, the so-called autodestructive process. The secondary injury processes include ischemia and impairment of autoregulation of blood flow (Lipton, 1993). These changes make the spinal cord vulnerable to reductions in arterial pressure and oxygen tension, both of which are frequent after cord injury (Sandler and Tator, 1976).

There are several 'injury factors' involved in the mechanisms of cell damage and edema following trauma to the spinal cord (de la Torre, 1981). Proposed factors include products of phospholipid hydrolysis such as polyunsaturated fatty acids, eicosanoids, free radicals, neuropeptides, monoamines and changes of cations and amino acids (Faden and Salzman, 1992). For many decades, various workers have tried to influence the secondary changes by agents which can interfere with the injury factors (de la Torre, 1981; Tator and Fehlings, 1991; Faden, 1993a). Nalox-one, nimodipine and thyrotropin-releasing hormone are examples of drugs which have the potential to minimise spinal cord injury of experimental animals (Faden et al., 1981a,b; Fehlings et al., 1989; Faden, 1993a,b).

Recent reports suggest that the κ opioid agonist, dynorphin, is involved in the pathophysiology of brain and spinal cord injury (Faden, 1993b) A possible mechanism of its action is via opioid and NMDA receptors (Bakshi et al., 1992). However, it may be that additional opioid receptors are involved in ameliorating the effects of experimental traumatic injury of the spinal cord.

Opioid peptides in the spinal cord

The spinal cord is very rich in opioid peptides which are co-localised with other transmitters (Hökfelt et al., 1978). Several classes of opioid receptors are present in the spinal cord. It has been suggested that opioid peptides are involved in the regulation of sensory, autonomic and somato-motor functions (Hökfelt et al., 1978; Herz et al., 1993).

Endogenous opioids have been implicated in the pathogenesis of secondary spinal cord injuries largely on the basis of findings demonstrating that the opioid receptor antagonist, naloxone, improves functional recovery after trauma (Bracken and Holford, 1993; Faden, 1993a,b). Furthermore, a lesion to the spinal cord results in a significant and progressive increase in dynorphin A immunoreactivity (Faden et al., 1981a,b; Faden, 1990; Sharma et al., 1992a, 1994b). The dynorphin alteration is localised in the vicinity of the injury and persists even 2 weeks after trauma (Faden et al., 1985). The levels of Leu- and Met-enkephalin immunoreactivity show a different spatial and temporal pattern following injury. There is a significant reduction in the levels of both peptides 24 h after moderate injury to the cord (Faden et al., 1981b). However, the level of Met-enkephalin-Arg-Phe (MEAP) increases in the cord rostral to injury site within a few hours after injury (Sharma et al., 1993a).

Endogenous opioids and opioid receptors in the spinal cord

The endogenous opioids are derived from three distinct prohormone precursors: (a) proenkephalin-derived peptides including methionine and leucine enkephalin; (b) pro-opiomelanocortin-derived peptides from which β-endorphin is formed; and (c) prodynorphin-derived peptides from which dynorphin A, dynorphin B and α-neoendorphin originate (Akil et al., 1984). These three classes of opioids are distributed differentially in the spinal cord, and their physiological and pharmacological functions probably differ from each other (Martin, 1983; Herz et al., 1993).

At least six classes of opioid receptors have been postulated (Herz et al., 1993). However, both in vivo and in vitro studies support the existence of three well-characterised types of receptors termed μ, δ and κ (Simons and Hiller, 1978). The pro-enkephalin-derived peptides have activities at μ and δ, and possibly at κ receptors, and prodynorphin-derived peptides act at κ sites (Mansour and Watson, 1993).

The concentration of all the three major classes of opioid binding sites is higher in the dorsal horn than in the ventral horn (Yaksh, 1993). In terms of relative levels of total spinal binding sites, μ and κ sites are less than δ sites (Yaksh, 1993). The location of the bindings is heterogeneous within the dorsal horn. Thus, μ binding is highest in the substantia gelatinosa and elevated in the neck of the nucleus proprius (Laminae III, IV, V and VIII). Delta binding sites are highest in the marginal layer (Lamina I) (Mansour and Warson, 1993); whereas κ binding has been shown to be highest in the substantia gelatinosa (Yaksh, 1993). Similar binding of opioids occur in the spinal cord of various mammalian species. In general, the highest binding sites are observed in the lateral aspects of the intermediolateral cell columns for the preganglionic sympathetics and in the sacral cord in the vicinity of the parasympathetic outflow (Akil et al., 1984; Mansour and Watson, 1993; Yaksh, 1993).

Electrophysiological effects of opioids

Opioid molecules such as meperidine, methadone, sufentanil and fentanyl produce a concentration-dependent reduction in the amplitude of the compound action potential of peripheral nerves and a slowing of their conduction velocity (Kosterlitz and Wallis, 1964). This action of opioids is not antagonised by naloxone. There is considerable evidence that μ, δ and κ opioids can reduce the terminal excitability and opening of voltage-sensitive Ca^{2+} channels which mediate terminal release (McDonald and Nelson, 1978; Attali et al., 1989). Whether opioids diminish depolarisation of terminals or act directly to inhibit the opening of voltage-gated Ca^{2+} channels is unknown (Yaksh, 1993). However, these events will alter the amount of neurotransmitter release that will follow after opioid-induced depolarisation (Duggan and Fleetwood-Walker, 1993).

Recently it has been shown that opioids can reduce the magnitude of the excitatory postsynaptic potentials in the spinal cord with no change in the resting membrane potential (McDonald and Nelson, 1978; Duggan and Fleetwood-Walker, 1993; Yaksh, 1993). The presence of opioids on the terminals, and the coupling of opioid receptors with voltage-sensitive Ca^{2+} channels, suggests that opioids may have the capacity to block directly the release of neurotransmitters contained in the respective terminals (North, 1993).

Iontophoretic experiments in which opioids are applied directly to circumscribed regions of the dorsal horn have shown that there is a dose-dependent reduction in the firing of neurons evoked by high-threshold stimuli (Duggan and Fleetwood-Walker, 1993; North, 1993; Yaksh, 1993). This activation of dorsal horn neurons by high-threshold mechanical, thermal and chemical stimuli is naloxone-reversible (Duggan and Fleetwood-Walker, 1993).

Opioid receptor antagonists in spinal cord trauma

A survey of experiments carried out in the past on the effects of naloxone in various trauma models to the central nervous system is presented in Tables I and II.

Previously, high doses of naloxone and other antagonists have been found to improve blood flow in some, but not in all, animal studies on spinal cord trauma (Faden, 1993a,b). Recent experiments indicate that both methylprednisolone and naloxone are potentially beneficial agents in the treatment of such injuries (Bracken, 1993; Bracken and Holford, 1993; Bracken et al., 1993; Faden, 1993b). However, clinical trials using naloxone in human spinal cord injury failed to reveal any improvement in neurological outcome.

In the trial, the drug was given at different post-injury intervals (Flamm et al., 1985; Bracken et al., 1993; Faden, 1993b). In patients receiving the drug within 8 h neurological function below the lesion was improved (Bracken, 1993; Bracken et al., 1993).

Treatment with naloxone initiated one hour after experimental injury, at doses of 2 mg/kg bolus followed by the same dose per hour during 4 h, significantly increased spinal cord blood flow and improved neurological outcome during a 6-week follow-up period (Faden et al., 1981a,b). Such beneficial effects of naloxone on feline spinal

TABLE I

Investigations indicating beneficial effects of naloxone treatment in spinal cord injury

Type of insult	Animal species	Naloxone dose (mg/kg)	Time of injection	Parameters evaluated	Survival	Results	References
Impact	cat	2 bolus + 2/h for 4 h	1 h after	SCBF	6 weeks	improved	Faden et al., 1981a,b
			4 h after	functional recovery	1−7 days		
Impact	cat		1 h after	SCBF, SSEP		improved	Young et al., 1981 Flamm et al., 1982
Compression	rat			SCEP		improved	Inoue et al., 1986
Impact	rat	3 + 3	45 min + 2 h after	motor recovery		improved	Arias, 1985
Compression	rat	0.8	45 min + 2 h	histopathology	72 h	protection	Akdemir et al., 1992
Impact	rat	10 bolus + 5/h	continuous 7 days	histopathology SSEP neurological function	6-weeks	protection improved improved	Baskin et al., 1993
Compression	rat	2−10	−10 to +45 min	neurological function	1−10 days	improved	Benzel et al., 1990
	rat	2	45 min after	histology neurological function	1−7 day	protection? improved	Benzel et al., 1992
Contusion	monkey	2−10	30 min after	motor function	1 week	improved	Cherian et al., 1992
Incision	rat	10	30 min before	edema, cell changes	5 h	protection	Olsson et al., 1992
Incision	rat	10	30 min before	SCEP, edema	5 h	improved	Winkler et al., 1994
Heat	rat	10	30 min before	edema, cell changes	4 h	protection	Sharma et al., 1994
Ischemia	rabbit	2 bolus + 2 /h	1 h after + every h, 4 h	motor recovery	1−7 days	improved	Faden et al., 1984

SCBF, spinal cord blood flow; SSEP, somatosensory-evoked potentials; SCEP, spinal cord-evoked poetentials.

TABLE II

Investigations indicating negative results with naloxone treatment in spinal cord injury

Type of insult	Animal species	Naloxone dose (mg/kg)	Time of injection	Parameters evaluated	Survival	Results	References
Compression	rat	40/day	24 h after 7 days	neurological function	1–7	no improvement	Hashimoto and Fukada, 1991
Weight-drop	rat	1–10	4–24 h after	neurological function histopathology	1–4 weeks	no improvement no protection	Black et al., 1991
							Hoerlein et al., 1985
							Wallace and Tator, 1986
							Haghighi and Chehrazi, 1987
				neurological function blood flow	1–7 days		Holtz et al., 1989
				neurological function			Robertson et al., 1986

cord injury were later confirmed by Young et al. (1981). It was further observed that naloxone treatment was effective in a cat spinal cord injury model when the drug given up to 4 h after the initial impact (Faden et al., 1982).

Protective effects of naloxone on spinal cord injury have been found in rats (Faden, 1993b). Thus, naloxone improved changes of spinal cord evoked potentials after compression-induced trauma (Inoue, 1986). Enhanced motor recovery in animals treated with naloxone (3 mg/kg at 45 min and 2 h after trauma) was observed in rats after impact trauma (Arias, 1985).

Another opioid peptide antagonist, WIN44441-3, with an increased potency, but similar selectivity as naloxone at opioid receptor sites, also enhanced long-term motor recovery in cats after impact trauma (Faden and Jacobs, 1985). Another compound, nalmefene, with increased potency and high selectivity at κ opioid receptors, as compared to naloxone, significantly improved recovery of somato-sensory evoked-responses, neurological function and histopathological changes in rats subjected to impact trauma to the thoracic cord (Faden et al., 1988). These observations indicate an involvement of κ opioid receptors in

spinal cord trauma. This is further supported by the experiments of Faden and co-workers, who injected intrathecally or systemically a selective κ opioid receptor antagonist, nor-binaltorphimine (norBNI), and observed enhanced neurological recovery after spinal cord trauma in rats (Faden et al., 1987).

Winkler et al. (1994) examined the influence of naloxone pretreatment on spinal cord-evoked potentials (SCEP) following an incision of the dorsal horn in the rat. The work of Winkler and his colleagues showed that naloxne (10 mg/kg) has the capacity to reduce the amplitude depression following trauma. The drug was ineffective in reducing late SCEP latency increase (Winkler et al., 1994). However, lower doses of naloxone (1 and 5 mg) were either ineffective or worsened the SCEP amplitude and latency changes (Winkler, 1994).

However, some laboratories (see Table II) failed to find beneficial effects of opioid receptor antagonists, particularly naloxone, given after traumatic spinal cord injury (Hoerlein et al., 1985; Robertson et al., 1986; Wallace and Tator, 1986; Haghighi and Chehrazi, 1987; Holtz et al., 1989; Black et al., 1991; Hashimoto and Fukada, 1991).

Opioid receptor antagonists also have been tried in experiments on brain trauma. Naloxone, at high doses (10 mg/kg), and WIN44441-3 significantly improved fluid-percussion injury-induced alterations in cardiovascular and respiratory functions, and in EEG and cerebral blood flow changes of cats (Hayes et al., 1983; McIntosh et al., 1987). Involvement of κ opioid receptor antagonist in improving early metabolic recovery in a rat model of fluid-percussion injury has been reported by Vink et al. (1990, 1991). These observations support the concept of a receptor-mediated action of opioids in brain injury.

Mechanisms of action of naloxone

In trauma, the opioid receptor antagonist naloxone improves local blood flow after injury (Faden et al., 1981a, 1982; Young et al., 1981; Sandòr et al., 1986; McIntosh et al., 1987; Tator and Fehlings, 1991). However, it remains to be seen to what extent this effect is related to reduced cell damage.

Another mechanism of action of naloxone is by the influence on calcium fluxes into cells. After trauma to dog spinal cord, naloxone treatment can restore extracellular calcium levels to normal levels (Stokes et al., 1984). High doses of naloxone in tissue cultures attenuate N-methyl-D-aspartate (NMDA) receptor-mediated neurotoxicity (Kim et al., 1987). The mechanism of such toxicity is thought to involve calcium influx through this channel (Choi, 1988). Intracellular accumulation of calcium may lead to cell death after ischemia (Siesjö and Bengtsson, 1989) and trauma (Fehlings et al., 1989). Alterations in magnesium level and magnesium-dependent enzymes, such as Na^+, K^+-ATPase, following trauma may also play important roles in naloxone-induced beneficial effects (Lemke et al., 1987). The data by Furui et al., showing a recovery of Na^+, K^+-ATPase in the ischemic hemisphere after occlusion of the middle cerebral artery in the rat by naloxone are in line with this concept (Furui et al., 1990).

Our investigations of naloxone pretreatment in spinal cord trauma

As is evident from Table II, most studies on the effects of naloxone in spinal cord trauma concern neurological outcome and blood flow alterations (Faden et al., 1981a,b 1982; Collins, 1984; Benzel et al., 1990, 1992; Furui et al., 1990; Cherian et al., 1992; Baskin et al., 1993; Bracken and Holford, 1993; Bracken et al., 1993; Faden, 1993a,b). Few previous investigations are focused on the effect of naloxone on trauma-induced edema and cell changes (Benzel et al., 1990, 1992; Akdemir et al., 1992; Olsson et al., 1992; Baskin et al., 1993; Sharma et al., 1994a).

We have been using a rat model of spinal cord injury which is quite reproducible in nature (Olsson et al., 1990). The injury is produced by making an incision into the right dorsal horn at the T10–11 segments. The deepest part of the lesion extends into Rexed's Lamina VIII. This model enables us to investigate the pathogenesis of edema and cell reactions around the primary injury by using the contralateral side and the other segments of the cord for our investigations on secondary changes. In this model the most pronounced injury occurs within the dorsal horn and the long tracts of the cord are to a great extent spared.

The phenomenology of cell and fluid changes following trauma can be investigated in our model of spinal cord trauma. However, we have used the model chiefly to study the pathogenesis of edema and cell alterations by pretreating the animals with various compounds, including naloxone, and compare the outcome between treated and untreated animals. We have given naloxone systemically in high doses (10 mg/kg, i.p.) 30 min before injury. With this dose, all three types of opioid receptors (μ, δ and κ) are blocked for about 4 h. We examined the effect of trauma 5 h after injury and recorded several parameters (Table III).

Naloxone and the stress protein response

Injury to the spinal cord is a severe stress at

TABLE III

Experimental protocol of naloxone treatment in rat spinal cord injury

Parameters investigated	Control	Spinal cord injury	Naloxone treatment	
			Normal	Spinal cord injury
Water content	6	7	5	5
Microvascular permeability (Evans blue [^{131}I]sodium)	5	5	4	6
Electron microscopy (lanthanum morphology)	5	5	3	5
Light microscopy (GFAP, MBP, H&E)	3	4	3	4
HSP (70 kDa)	3	5	3	3

Naloxone (10 mg/kg) was given intraperitoneally in rats 30 min before trauma. The animals were allowed to survive 5 h after injury. MBP, myelin basic protein; HSP, heat shock protein; GFAP, glial fibrillary acidic protein.

cellular and molecular levels (Faden, 1993a). Trauma to the central nervous system results in an up-regulation of intracellular stress proteins known as heat shock proteins (HSP) (Lindquist, 1986; Kaufmann, 1992). The mechanisms of up-regulation of the HSP response following trauma is not well understood. Available evidence suggests that this response is protective in nature (Kumar, 1992; Sloviter and Lowenstein, 1992).

We have started to investigate, by immunohistochemistry, the role of opioids in induction of the stress protein response following trauma to the cord. For this purpose, we pretreated rats with naloxone and divided them into two groups (Table III). In one group, the spinal cord was injured and, in another group of pretreated rats, the same injury was caused. The HSP response was examined in vibratome sections using one commercially available primary antibody (Sharma et al., 1992b, 1995).

Trauma to the spinal cord in untreated animals was associated with a marked up-regulation of HSP (70 kDa) response in the perifocal segments of the cord (Fig. 1a). Many neurons exhibited an increased reaction product in the cytoplasm and in the nucleus of the cells. Ultrastructural studies showed that the reaction product was present in the cytoplasm and attached to the endoplasmic reticulum of dendrites and neurons (Sharma et al., 1995).

Pretreatment with naloxone markedly reduced the HSP response seen after spinal cord injury of untreated rats (Fig. 1b). The naloxone-treated injured animals did not show any signs of reaction product in the cells of the cord. This suggests that blockade of opioid peptide receptors are capable of reducing the stress protein response following injury, indicating a beneficial effect of the drug in spinal cord injury. Since there was no difference in the HSP response between normal and drug-treated animals not subjected to trauma, a direct effect on HSP by naloxone is unlikely.

Naloxone and the astrocytic response

Astrocytes are constitutive elements of the central nervous system and are very important in the regulation of the fluid microenvironment (Arenander and Vellis, 1984). Astrocytes respond to various noxious insults, for instance trauma by increased production of glial fibrillary acidic protein (GFAP) (Bignami et al., 1980). This protein is a marker of astrocytic activation (Bignami et al., 1980; Duffy, 1984; Fedoroff and Vernadakis, 1986). In our experiments, using immunocytochemistry of GFAP, spinal cord injury induced

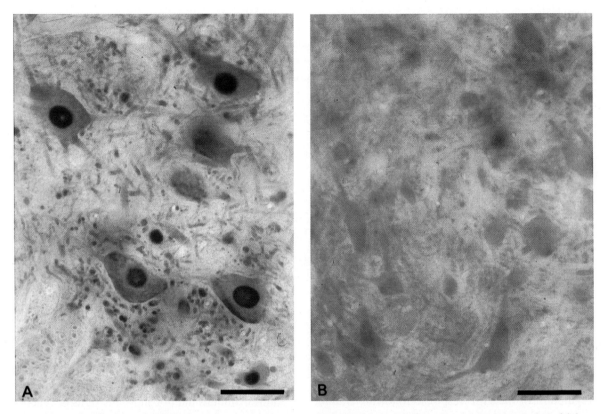

Fig. 1. Heat shock protein (HSP, 70 kDa) immunoreactivity in the ventral horn of the T9 segment 5 h after spinal cord injury (T10–11 segments) in one untreated (a) and in one naloxone-treated (b) rat. HSP immunostaining is present in the neuronal cytoplasm and nucleus of the untreated traumatised rat. The immunostaining is mainly absent in the naloxone-treated injured rat (bar = 25 and 50 μm, in (a) and (b), respectively).

an up-regulation of GFAP in the perifocal segments (Sharma et al., 1993c). This effect was reduced by pretreatment of the rats with p-CPA, an inhibitor of serotonin synthesis (Sharma et al., 1993c).

Opioid receptors are present on astrocytes (Arenander and Vellis, 1984). Astrocytes release many neuropeptides in pathological conditions (Murphy and Pearce, 1987). This release of pep-

tides is regulated by various hormones and neurochemicals (Orkand, 1983). However, the functional significance of such phenomena is largely obscure.

Our results with naloxone suggest that trauma-induced activation of the astrocytic response is inhibited, indicating a role of opioids in up-regulation of GFAP (Fig. 2). However, we did not observe any major change in GFAP immunoreac-

Fig. 2. Glial fibrillary acidic protein (GFAP) immunoreactivity in the ventral horn of the T9 segment 5 h after spinal cord injury (T10–11 segments) in one untreated (a) and in one naloxone-treated (b) injured rat. In the untreated rat, astrocytes exhibit a marked up-regulation of GFAP following injury. This activation of astrocytes is less pronounced in the naloxone-treated rat (bar = 50 μm).

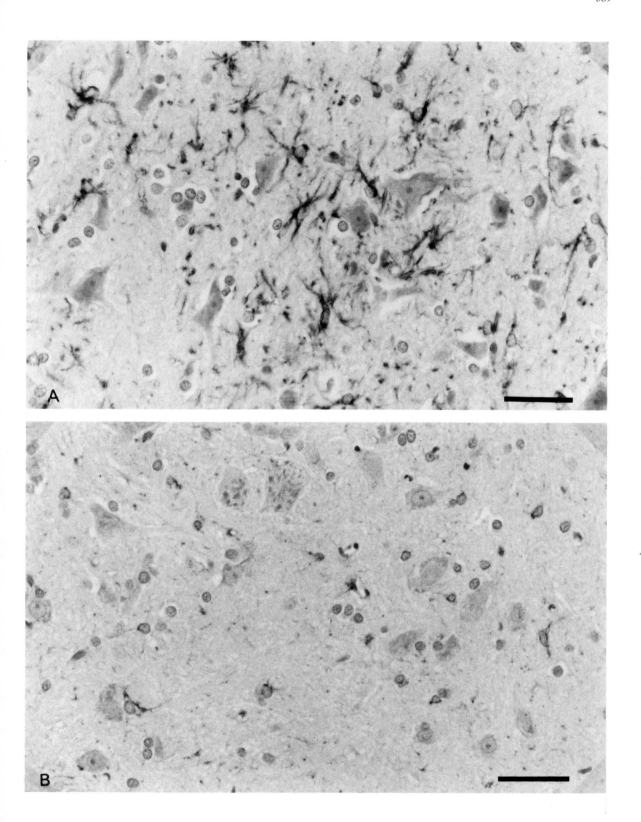

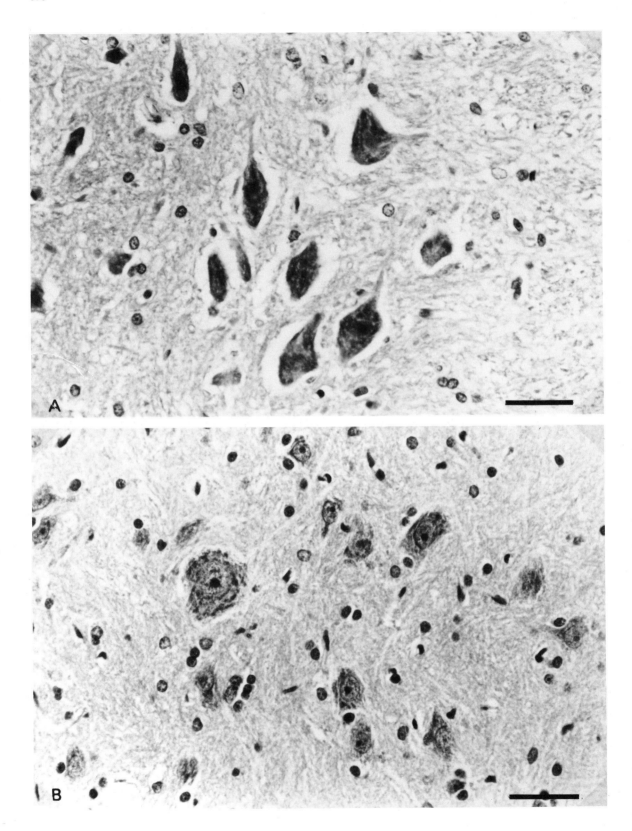

tivity in normal rats or in animals treated with naloxone alone. Thus, a direct inhibitory effect of opioids on GFAP response is unlikely.

Naloxone and neuronal injury

Our results indicate that opioid peptides are involved in the early pathological reaction of neurons after trauma. Thus, at 5 h, neurons in untreated animals showed profound pathological changes in the perifocal segments. Many neurons were dark and distorted, some were swollen and some were shrunken. A general sponginess and edema could be seen in the grey matter (Fig. 3a). Pretreatment with naloxone markedly reduced these changes (Fig. 3b).

It thus appears that blockade of opioid receptors before spinal cord injury reduces the nerve cell changes. The mechanisms of this protection by naloxone is unclear. However, it seems likely that reduced microcirculatory disturbances (Tator and Fehlings, 1991) in the drug-treated rats after trauma are important factors (Tator and Fehlings, 1991; Faden and Salzman, 1992; Sharma et al., 1993b). Additionally, blockade of κ opioid receptors at the high dose we used may attenuate a direct effect of the κ agonist, dynorphin, on the spinal cord cellular environment (Martin, 1967; Faden, 1990; Sharma et al., 1992a). Dynorphin levels are increased following trauma to the spinal cord, and this peptide has the capacity to induce blood flow abnormalities and cell changes (Faden, 1990; Sharma et al., 1992a, 1994a,b). Failure by some workers to get neuroprotection with naloxone in spinal cord injury may be related to the dose and the time interval after trauma. All these parameters obviously will affect the bioavailability of naloxone to produce beneficial effects in the spinal cord (Akil et al., 1984; Herz et al., 1993).

Naloxone and myelin damage

Spinal cord injury produces morphological alterations of myelinated axons (Balentine, 1978; Hogan and Banik, 1985; Fehlings et al., 1989). The degradation of myelin basic protein (MBP) following injury depends on the severity of the primary injury (Hogan and Banik, 1985). If injury is severe, loss of myelin basic protein is rapid (within 15 min of impact). This degradation is progressive and reaches its peak at about 6–8 h after injury (Balentine, 1988).

Our results with naloxone indicate that opioid peptides directly or indirectly are involved in degradation of MBP. Thus, 5 h after injury, loss of MBP immunoreactivity in untreated animal is evident (Balentine, 1988; Olsson et al., 1992; Sharma et al., 1993b). This loss of MBP staining is less apparent in naloxone-treated rats after injury (Fig. 4a,b).

Naloxone and microvascular permeability

Since opioid peptides influence microvascular reactions and permeability changes in the periphery (Akil et al., 1984), it appears that they may be equally important in the response to CNS trauma. Thus, we examined the influence of naloxone on microvascular permeability and edema following spinal cord injury.

Our investigations with naloxone suggest that opioid peptides contribute to the breakdown of the blood-spinal cord barrier (BSCB). Since opioid peptides are known modulators of neurochemical transmission, it appears that opioids, in synergy with other neurochemicals, may influence the microvascular permeability of the cord after trauma.

We observed a marked increase in the perme-

Fig. 3. Nerve cell changes in the ventral horn of the T9 segment 5 h after spinal cord injury (T10–11 segments) in one untreated (a) and in one naloxone-treated (b) injured rat. In the untreated rat many distorted nerve cells are present. A general sponginess and expansion of the gray matter are evident (a). Pretreatment with naloxone markedly reduced the nerve cell changes (b) (bar = 30 μm).

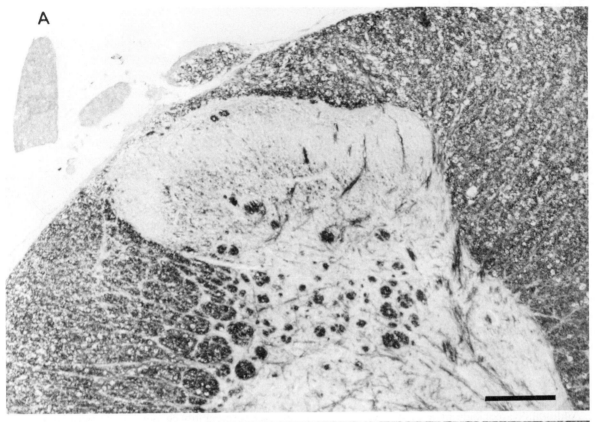

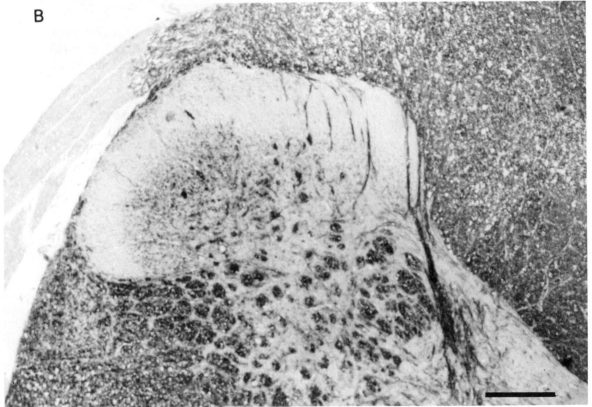

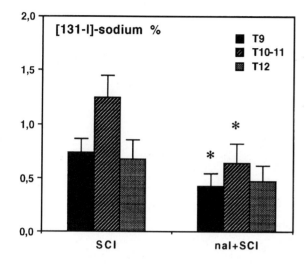

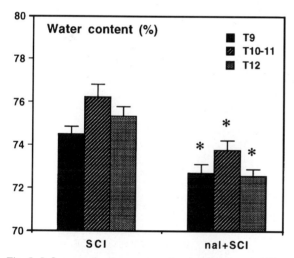

Fig. 5. Influence of naloxone on microvascular permeability (above) and edema (below) following spinal cord injury in rats. $*P < 0.05$, Dunnet test for multiple group comparison.

cantly reduced by naloxone treatment (Fig. 5). This suggests that opioids are involved. It seems likely that opioids either directly contribute to the permeability disturbances seen after trauma or they may modify the influence of other neurochemicals (cf. North, 1993; Yaksh, 1993).

The passage of tracer transport across microvessels was examined using lanthanum as an electron-dense tracer. We observed diffused penetration of lanthanum into the endothelial cell cytoplasm after trauma, but no opening of the tight junctions between the endothelial cells (Olsson et al., 1990, 1992). Pretreatment with naloxone markedly attenuated this response. Thus, in naloxone-treated rats, lanthanum remained in the lumen of the vessels. However, a few of vesicles contained lanthanum (Fig. 6). This suggests that endothelial cell membrane permeability is influenced by opioid peptides which could be blocked by naloxone.

Naloxone and vasogenic edema

Our results with naloxone suggest that opioids participate in the secondary injury factors and contribute to edema formation of the traumatised cord. There is a rapid increase in the water content 1 h after trauma in our model. This increase is progressive up to 5 h. Pretreatment with naloxone reduced the accumulation of cord water content in the perifocal segments at 5 h (Fig. 5). This indicates that opioids have the capacity to influence edema formation.

This effect of naloxone could be seen also by electron microscopy. In untreated rats with spinal cord injury, perivascular edema, synaptic damage, membrane disruption, swollen neuronal and glial cells and myelin disruption are very common (Frankel, 1969; Tator and Fehlings, 1991; Sharma

ability of Evans blue and radioactive sodium following trauma to the cord in perifocal segments (Fig. 5). The permeability increase was signifi-

Fig. 4. Myelin basic protein (MBP) immunostaining in the dorsal horn of the T9 segment 5 h after spinal cord injury (T10–11 segments) in one untreated (a) and in one naloxone-treated (b) rat. Loss of staining in many bundles of myelinated axons in the dorsal horn, as well as in the region of the dorsal gray matter, in the untreated injured rat is apparent, compared with the rat (b) given naloxone prior to injury (bar = 150 μm).

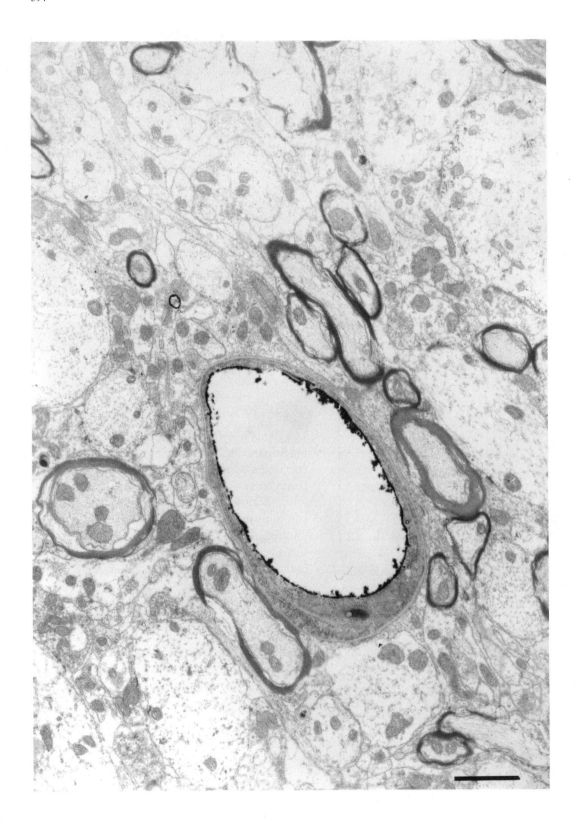

et al., 1993c,d, 1994a,b). Pretreatment with naloxone reduced these ultrastructural changes (Fig. 6).

General comments

Our investigations with naloxone show that this drug is beneficial in reducing the early consequences of spinal cord injury. This is in line with previous observation that opioids are involved in the pathophysiology of spinal cord injury (Faden, 1993a,b). In some clinical situations, neuroprotection of the spinal cord would be of advantage. In order to reach such an effect, many different compounds may be used. Naloxone is one compound which may be used for such protection.

However, various workers did not see beneficial effects of naloxone on trauma-induced changes on motor function, electrical activity and histology of the cord. The negative results obtained by various workers should be interpreted with great caution. In most of the investigations, naloxone was given several hours after the initial impact. Since the onset of naloxone effect is rapid, and the half-life of the drug in plasma is only about 1 h, the bioavailability of the drug at the desired level is of very short duration. The route and time of administration of naloxone are obviously very important. Clinical trial data have shown that, if naloxone is administered within 8 h of the primary insults, the outcome is definitely better than placebo (Bracken et al., 1993; Faden, 1993a,b).

Additionally, the degree of primary insult is also important. In some laboratories, who failed to observe beneficial effects of any drug including naloxone (see Table II), it seems that the degree of their primary insult is very severe. In such cases, no improvement in the outcome could be seen (Ducker, 1976).

Another most important parameter is dose response. The most beneficial effects of naloxone in various CNS injuries have been reported by Faden and his colleagues (Table I). They used a very high dose regimen of the compound and repeated the injections. They maintained a very high plasma concentration of the drug over long periods after injury. In our opinion this appears to be most important for the beneficial action of the compound. This idea is further supported by the more recent meticulous work of Baskin et al. (1993). In this investigation, Baskin et al. implanted a 'mini osmotic pump' to deliver naloxone continuously and was preceded by a bolus injection of the drug. The animals were allowed to survive for 6 weeks with slow infusion of the drug. In this experiment, the investigators found beneficial effects with regard to motor function and neuropathological score (Baskin et al., 1993).

The time of administration and the bioavailability of the drug are crucial in determining the final outcome in experiments on spinal cord trauma. Our pretreatment studies with naloxone in spinal cord injury adds new information that the drug is capable of reducing the early consequences of spinal cord injury. These results indicate that opioids participate in the pathophysiology of spinal cord trauma.

Future directions

Experimental investigations based on pretreatment with naloxone can add valuable information about the role of opioid peptides in spinal cord trauma. Our results do not give details of particular opioid receptors involved. It appears that, with high doses of naloxone, all three opioid receptor subtypes will be blocked. This does not exclude the possibility that μ or δ receptors are not involved. It may be that blockade of all opioid receptors are needed for beneficial effect. Blockade of only μ, δ or κ alone may not be sufficient

Fig. 6. Influence of naloxone on ultratsructural cell changes of the spinal cord 5 h after injury in the ventral horn of a T9 segment. Lanthanum is mainly confined to the lumen of the microvessel. Only a few vesicles contain lanthanum at the luminal cell border. Perivascular edema, distortion of myelin and of other cell structures are minimal (bar = 2 μm).

for neuroprotection. A careful study of blockade of different opioid receptors using specific antagonists are needed.

Studies in order to explore the potential role of naloxone in the treatment of spinal cord trauma should be performed in such a way that an early administration at a high and constant tissue concentration of the compound can be obtained. In this connection, the use of 'slow release capsules' seems to be a promising approach. Furthermore, the choice of experimental model of spinal cord trauma is crucial. We have until now restricted our investigations to the very early events occurring after spinal cord trauma, since we have used urethane anaestheisa for neurophysiological experiments. Our observations on the short-term effects are thus limited. It is difficult to delineate reversible from irreversible cell changes at an early period after trauma. Therefore, we are currently developing a model of controlled minor trauma to the cord with long-term survival. With such a model, clinically more relevant information may be obtained.

Acknowledgements

This investigation was supported by grants from the Swedish Medical Research Council projects no. 0320, 2710, 9459, Trygg-Hansa, Göran Gustafsson's Foundation, Hedlund's Foundation, Åhlén's Foundation, Thyring's Foundation, and O.E. and Edla Johnson's Foundation. We very much appreciate Törd Loving, Librarian, Physiological Library, Biomedical Centre, for his outstanding help. The skilful technical assistance of Mrs. Kärstin Flink, Kerstin Rystedt, Ingmarie Olsson in immunocytochemistry; Madeleine Thörnwall in radioachemical experiments; Madeleine Jarild and Gunilla Tibbling in electron microscopy; and Frank Bittkowski in photography is highly appreciated.

References

Akdemir, H., Pasaoglu, A., Öztürk, F. and Selcuklu, A. (1992) Histopathology of experimental spinal cord trauma. *Res. Exp. Med.*, 192: 177–183.

Akil, H., Watson, S.J., Young, E., Lewis, M.E., Khachaturian, H. and Walker, J.M. (1984) Endogenous opioids: biology and function. *Annu. Rev. Neurosci.*, 7: 223–255.

Arenander, A.T. and Vellis, J.D. (1984) Frontiers of glial physiology. In: R.N. Rosenberg, W.D. Willis, Jr. (Eds). *The Clinical Neurosciences, Vol V: Neurobiology*, Raven Press, New York: pp. 53–91.

Arias, M.J. (1985) Effect of naloxone on functional recovery after experimental spinal cord injury in the rat. *Surg. Neurol.*, 23: 440–442.

Attali, B., Saya, D., Nah, S.-Y. and Vogel, Z. (1989) κ-opiate agonists inhibit Ca^{2+} influx in rat spinal cord-dorsal root ganglion cocultures. Involvement of a GTP-binding protein. *J Biol Chem.*, 264: 347–353.

Bakshi, R., Ni, R. and Faden, A.I. (1992) N-Methyl-D-asparate and opioid receptors mediate dynorphin-induced spinal cord injury. *Brain Res.*, 580: 255–264.

Balentine, J.D. (1978) Pathology of experimental spinal cord trauma. I. the necrotic lesion as a function of vascular injury. *Lab Invest.*, 39: 236–253.

Balentine, J.D. (1988) Spinal cord trauma: in search of the meaning of granular axoplasm and vesiculation of myelin. *J Neuropathol Exp. Neurol.*, 47: 77–92.

Baskin, D.S., Jr., R.K.S., Browning, J.L., Dudley, A.W., Rothenberg, F. and Bouge, L. (1993) The effect of lomgterm high-dose naloxone infusion in experimental blunt spinal cord injury. *J. Spinal Disord.*, 6: 38–43.

Benzel, E.S., Lancon, J.A., Bairnsfather, S. and Kesterson, L. (1990) Effect of dosage and timimg of naloxone on outcome in the rat ventral compression model of spinal cord injury. *Neurosurgery.*, 27: 597–601.

Benzel, E.C., Khare, V. and Fowler, M.R. (1992) Effect of naloxone and nelmefene in rat spinal cord injury induced by the ventral compression technique. *J. Spinal Disord.*, 5: 75–77.

Bignami, A., Dahl, D. and Rueger, D.C. (1980) Glial fibrillay acidic protein (GFAP) in normal neural cells and in pathological conditions. *Adv. Cell Neurobiol.*, 1: 285–319.

Black, P., Markowitz, R.S., Gillespie, J.A. and Finkelstein, S.D. (1991) Naloxone and experimental spinal cord injury: effect of varying dose and intensity of injury. *J. Neurotrauma*, 8: 157–171.

Bracken, M.B. (1993) Pharmacological treatment of acute spinal cord injury: current status and future projects. *J. Emerg. Med.*, 11: 43–48.

Bracken, M.B. and Holford, T.R. (1993) Effects of timimg of methylprednisolone or naloxone administration on recovery of segmental and long-tract neurological function in NASCIS 2. *J. Neurosurg.*, 79: 500–507.

Bracken, M.B., Shepard, M.J., Collins, W.F., Holford, T.R., Baskin, D.S., Eisenberg, H.M., Flamm, E., Leo-Summers, L., Maroon, J.C., Marshall, L.F., Perot, P.L., Piepmeier, J., Sontag, V.K.H., Wagner, F.C., Wilberger, J.L., Winn, H.R. and Young, W. (1993) Methylprednisolone or naloxone treatment after acute spinal cord injury: 1-year follow-up data. Results of the second national acute spinal cord injury study. *J. Neurosurg.*, 76: 23–31.

Cherian, L., Kuruvilla, A., Abraham, J. and Chandy, M. (1992) Evaluation of drug effects on spinal cord injury: an experimental study in monkeys. *Indian J. Exp. Biol.*, 30: 509–511.

Choi, D.W. (1988) Calcium-mediated neurotoxicity: relationship to specific channel types and role in ischemic damage. *Trends Neurosci.*, 11: 465–469.

Clendenon, N.R., Allen, N. and Gordon, W.A., Bingham, W.G. Jr. (1978) Inhibition of Na^+, K^+-activated ATPase activity following experimental spinal cord trauma. *J. Neurosurg.*, 49: 563–568.

Collins, W.F. (1984) A review of treatment of spinal cord injury. *Br. J. Surg.*, 71: 974–975.

de la Torre, J.C. (1981) Spinal cord injury. Review of basic and applied research. *Spine*, 6: 315–335.

Ducker, T.B. (1976) Experimental injury of the spinal cord. *Handbook Neurol.*, 9: 26–68.

Duffy, P.E. (1984) *Astrocytes: Normal, Reactive and Neoplastic*. Raven Press, New York.

Duggan, A.W. and Fleetwood-Walker, S.M. (1993) Opioids and sensory processing in the central nervous system. *Handbook Exp. Pharmacol.*, 104 (II): 731–771.

Editorial (1990) Steroids after spinal cord injury. *Lancet*, 336: 279–280.

Faden, A.I. (1990) Opioid and nonopioid mechanisms may contribute to dynorphin's pathophysiological actions in spinal cord injury. *Ann. Neurol.*, 27: 67–74.

Faden, A.I. (1993a) Experimental neurobiology of central nervous system trauma. *Crit. Rev. Neurobiol.*, 7: 175–186.

Faden, A.I. (1993b) Role of endogenous opioids and opioid receptors in central nervous system injury. *Handbook Exp. Pharmacol.*, 104 (I): 325–341.

Faden, A.I. and Salzman, S. (1992) Pharmacological strategies in CNS trauma. *Trends Pharmacol. Sci.*, 13: 29–35.

Faden, A.I., Jacobs, T.P. and Holaday, J.W. (1981a) Opiate antagonists improve neurologic recovery after spinal injury. *Science.*, 211: 493–494.

Faden, A.L., Jacobs, T.P. and Holaday, J.W. (1981b) Endorphins in experimental spinal injury: therapeutic effect of naloxone. *Ann. Neurol.*, 10: 326–332.

Faden, A.I., Jacobs, T.P. and Holaday, J.W. (1982) Comparison of early and late naloxone treatment in experimental spinal injury. *Neurology*, 32: 677–681.

Faden, A.I., Jacobs, T.P., Smith, M.T. and Zivin, J.A. (1984) Naloxne in experimental spinal cord ischemia dose-response studies. *Eur. J. Pharmacol.*, 103: 115–120.

Faden, A.L. and Jacobs, T.P. (1985) Opiate antagonist WIN44,441-3 stereospecifically improves neurological recovery after ischemic spinal injury. *Neurology*, 35: 1311–1315.

Faden, A.I., Molineaux, C.J., Rosenberger, J.G., Jacobs, T.P. and Cox, B.M. (1985) Endogenous opioid immunoreactivity in rat spinal cord following traumatic injury. *Ann. Neurol.*, 17: 386–390.

Faden, A.I., Takemori, A.E. and Portoghese, T.S. (1987) κ-Selective opiate antagonist nor-binaltorphimine improves outcome after traumatic spinal cord injury in rats. *CNS Trauma*, 4: 227–237.

Faden, A.I., Sacksen, I. and Noble, L.J. (1988) Opiate-receptor nalmefene improves neurological recovery after traumatic spinal cord injury in rats through a central mechanism. *J Pharmacol. Exp. Ther.*, 245: 742–748.

Fedoroff, S. and Vernadakis, A. (1986) *Astrocytes, Vols. 1–3*. Academic Press, Orlando.

Fehlings, M.G., Tator, C.H. and Linden, R.D. (1989) The effect of nimodipine and dextran on axonal function and blood flow following experimental spinal cord injury. *J. Neurosurg.*, 71: 403–411.

Flamm, E.S., Young, W., Collins, W.F., Piepmeier, J., Clifton, G.L. and Fischer, B. (1985) A phase I trial of naloxone treatment in acute spinal cord injury. *J. Neurosurg.*, 63: 390–397.

Frankel, H.L. (1969) Ascending cord lesion in the early stages following spinal injury. *Paraplegia*, 7: 111–116.

Furui, T., Tanaka, I. and Iwata, K. (1990) Alterations in Na^+, K^+-ATPase activity and b-endorphin content in acute ischemic brain with and without naloxone treatment. *J. Neurosurg.*, 72: 458–462.

Haghighi, S.S. and Chehrazi, B. (1987) Effect of naloxone in experimental acute spinal cord injury. *Neurosurgery*, 20: 385–388.

Hashimoto, T. and Fukada, N. (1991) Effect of thyrotropin-releasing hormone on the neurologic impairments in rats with spinal cord injury: treatment starting 24 h and 7 days after injury. *Eur. J. Pharmacol.*, 203: 25–32.

Hayes, R.L., Galinet, B.J., Kulkarne, P. and Becker, D.P. (1983) Effects of naloxone on systemic and cerebral responses to experimental concussive brain injury in cats. *J. Neurosurg.*, 58: 720–728.

Hayes, R.L., Jenkins, L.W. and Lyeth, B.G. (1992) Neurotransmitter-mediated mechanisms of traumatic brain injury: acetylcholine and excitatory amino acids. *J. Neurotrauma*, 9 (Suppl. 1): S 173-S 187.

Herz, A., Akil, H. and Simon, E.J. (1993) Opioids. *Handbook Exp. Pharmacol.*, 104 (I/II).

Hoerlein, B.F., Redding, R.W., Hoff, E.J. and McGuire, J.A. (1985) Evaluation of naloxone, crocetin, thyrotrophin releasing hormone, methylprednisolone, partial myelotomy and hemilaminectomy in the treatment of acute spinal cord trauma. *J. Am. Anim. Hosp. Assoc.*, 2: 67–77.

Hogan, E.L. and Banik, N.L. (1985) Biochemistry of the spinal cord. *Handbook Neurochem.*, 10: 285–337.

Holtz, A., Nystrom, B. and Gerdin, B. (1989) Blocking weight-induced spinal cord injury in rats: effects of TRH or naloxone on motor function recovery and spinal cord blood flow. *Acta Neurol. Scand.*, 80: 215–220.

Hökfelt, T., Elde, R., Johansson, O., Ljungdahl, Å., Schultzberg, M., Fuxe, K., Goldstein, M., Nilsson, G., Pernow, B., Terenius, L., Ganten, D., Jeffocate, S.L., Rehfeld, J. and Said, S. (1978) Distribution of peptide containing neurons. In: M.A. Lipton, A. DiMascio, K.F. Killam (Eds). *Psychopharmacology: A Generation of Progress.*, Raven Press, New York, pp. 39–66.

Hökfelt, T., Johansson, O., Holets, V., Meister, B. and Melander, T. (1987) Distribution of neuropeptides with special reference to their coexistence with classical neurotransmitters. In M.H.Y. Meltzer (Ed) *Psychopharmacology: The Third Generation of Progress*, Raven Press, New York, pp. 401–416.

Inoue, Y. (1986) Evoked spinal potentials in the Wistar rat: effect of cord compression and drugs. *J. Jpn. Orthop. Assoc.*, 60: 777–785.

Kaufmann, S.H.E. (1992) Heat shock proteins in health and disease. *Int. J. Clin. Lab. Res.*, 21: 221–226.

Kim, J.P., Goldberg, M.P. and Choi, D.W. (1987) High concentrations of naloxone attenuate N-methyl-D-aspartate receptor mediated neurotoxicity. *Eur. J. Pharmacol.*, 138: 133–136.

Kosterlitz, H.W. and Wallis, D.I. (1964) The action of morphine like drugs on impulse transmission in mammalian nerve fibres. *Br. J. Pharmacol.*, 22: 499–510.

Kumar, K. (1992) Heat shock proteins in brain ischemia: role undefined as yet. *Metab. Brain Dis.*, 7: 115–123.

Lemke, M., Demediuk, P., McIntosh, T.K., Vink, R. and Faden, A.I. (1987) Alterations in tissue Mg^{2+}, Na^+ and spinal cord edema following impact trauma in rats. *Biochem. Biophys. Res. Commun.*, 147: 1170–1175.

Lindquist, S. (1986) The heat shock response. *Ann. Rev. Biochem.*, 55: 1151–1191.

Lipton, S.A. (1993) Molecular mechanisms of trauma-induced neuronal degenration. *Curr. Opin. Neurol. Neurosurg.*, 6: 588–596.

Mansour, A. and Watson, S.J. (1993) Anatomical distribution of opioid receptors in mammalians: an overview. *Handbook Exp. Pharmacol.*, 104 (II): 79–105.

Martin, W.R. (1967) Opioid antagonists. *Pharmacol. Rev.*, 19: 463–521.

Martin, W.R. (1983) Pharmacology of opioids. *Pharmacol. Rec.*, 35: 283–323.

McDonald, R.L. and Nelson, P.G. (1978) Specific-opiate-induced depression of transmitter release from dorsal root ganglion cells in culture. *Science*, 199: 1449–1451.

McIntosh, T.K., Hayes, R.L., Dewitt, D.S., Agura, V. and Faden, A.I. (1987) Endogenous opioids may mediate secondary damage after experimental brain injury. *Am. J. Physiol.*, 253: E565–E574.

Misra, A.L. (1978) Metabolism of opiates. In M.L. Adler, L. Manara, R. Samanin (Eds) *Factors Affecting the Action of Narcotics.* Raven Press, New York, pp. 297–343.

Murphy, S. and Pearce, B. (1987) Functional receptors for neurotransmitters on astroglial cells. *Neuroscience*, 22: 381–394.

North, A.R. (1993) Opioid actions in membrane channels. *Handbook Exp. Pharmacol.*, 104 (II): 773–797.

Olsson, Y., Sharma, H.S. and Pettersson, C.Å.V. (1990) Effects of p-chlorophenylalanine on microvascular permeability changes in spinal cord trauma. An experimental study in the rat using ^{131}I-sodium and lanthanum tracers. *Acta Neuropathol.*, 79: 595–603.

Olsson, Y., Sharma, H.S., Pettersson, C.Å.V. and Cervós-Navarro, J. (1992) Release of endogenous neurochemicals may increase vascular permeability, induce edema and influence cell changes in trauma to the spinal cord. *Progr. Brain Res.*, 91: 197–203.

Orkand, R.K. (1983) Glial cells. *Handbook Physiol.*, The Nervous System I Part 2, Chapter 23. American Physiological Society Bethesda, Maryland, 855–875.

Robertson, C.S., Foltz, R., Grossman, R.G. and Goodman, J.C. (1986) Protection against experimental ischemic spinal cord injury. *Neurosurgery*, 9: 40–47.

Sandler, A.N. and Tator, C.H. (1976) Review of the effect of spinal cord trauma on the vessels and blood flow in the spinal cord. *J. Neurosurg.*, 45: 638–646.

Sandòr, P., Gotoh, F., Tomita, M., Tanahashi, N. and Gogolak, I. (1986) Effects of a stable enkephalin analogue, (D-Met^2,Pro^5)-enkephalinamide, and naloxone on cortical blood flow and cerebral blood volume in experimental brain ischemia in anaesthetised cats. *J. Cereb. Blood Flow Metab.*, 6: 553–558.

Sharma, H.S., Nyberg, F. and Olsson, Y. (1992a) Dynorphin A content in the rat brain and spinal cord after a localized trauma to the spinal cord and its modification with p-chlorophenylalanine. An experimental study using radioimmunoassay technique. *Neurosci. Res.*, 14: 195–203.

Sharma, H.S., Westman, J. and Olsson, Y. (1992b) Increased heat shock protein (HSP-70 kD) immunoreactivity following acute spinal cord trauma in the rat. *Clin. Neuropathol.*, 11: 174–175.

Sharma, H.S., Nyberg, F., Thörnwall, M. and Olsson, Y. (1993a) Met-enkephalin-Arg6-Phe7 in spinal cord and brain following traumatic injury to the spinal cord. Influence of p-chlorophenylalanine. An experimental study in the rat using radioimmunoassay technique. *Neuropharmacology.*, 32: 711–717.

Sharma, H.S., Olsson, Y. and Cervós-Navarro, J. (1993b) Early perifocal cell changes and edema in traumatic injury of the spinal cord are reduced by indomethacin, an inhibitor of prostaglandins synthesis. *Acta Neuropathol.*, 85: 145–153:

Sharma, H.S., Olsson, Y. and Cervós-Navarro, J. (1993c) p-chlorophenylalanine, a serotonin synthesis inhibitor, reduces the response of glial fibrillary acidic protein induced by trauma to the spinal cord. *Acta Neuropathol.*, 86: 422–427.

Sharma, H.S., Olsson, Y. and Dey, P.K. (1993d) Early accumulation of serotonin in rat spinal cord subjected to traumatic injury. Relation to edema and blood flow changes. *Neuroscience*, 36: 725–730.

Sharma, H.S., Westman, J., Nyberg, F., Cervós-Navarro, J. and Dey, P.K. (1994a) Opioid peptides participate in the pathophysiology of heat stress in the rat. *Neuropeptides.*, 26: 44–45.

Sharma, H.S., Olsson, Y. and Nyberg, F. (1994b) Influenec of dynorphin A antibodies on the formation of edema and cell changes in spinal cord trauma. *Progr. Brain Res.*, 104: 401–416.

Sharma, H.S., Olsson, Y. and Westman, J. (1995) A serotonin synthesis inhibitor, p-chlorophenylalanine reduces the heat shock protein response following trauma to the spinal cord: an immunohistochemical and ultrastructural study in the rat. *Neurosci. Res.* 21: 241–249.

Siesjö, B.K. and Bengtsson, F. (1989) Calcium fluxes, calcium antagonists, and calcium-related pathology in brain ischemia, hypoglycemia, and spreading depression: a unifying hypothesis. *J. Cereb. Blood Flow Metab.*, 9: 127–140.

Simons, E.J. and Hiller, J.M. (1978) The opiate receptors. *Annu. Rev. Pharmacol. Toxicol.*, 18: 371–394.

Sloviter, R.S. and Lowenstein, D.H. (1992) Heat shock protein expression in vulnerable cells of the rat hippocampus as an indicator of excitation-induced neuronal stress. *J. Neurosci.*, 12: 3004–3009.

Stokes, B.T., Hollinden, G. and Fox, P. (1984) Improvement in injury-induced hypocalcia by high-dose naloxone intervention. *Brain Res.*, 290: 187–190.

Tator, C.H. (1990) Acute management of spinal cord injury. *Br. J. Surg.*, 77: 485–486.

Tator, C.H. and Fehlings, M.G. (1991) Review of the secondary injury theory of acute spinal cord trauma with emphasis on vascular mechanisms. *J. Neurosurg.*, 75: 15–26.

Vink, R., McIntosh, T.K., Romhanyi, R. and Faden, A.I. (1990) Opiate antagonist nalmefene improves intracellular free Mg^{2+}, bioenergetic state and neurologic outcome following traumatic brain injury in rats. *J. Neurosci.*, 10: 3524–3530.

Vink, R., Portoghese, P.S. and Faden, A.I. (1991) Kappa-opioid antagonist improves cellular bioenergetics and recovery after traumatic brain injury. *Am J Physiol.*, 261: R1527–R1532.

Wallace, M.C. and Tator, C.H. (1986) Failure of naloxone to improve spinal cord blood flow and cardiac output after spinal cord injury. *Neurosurgery*, 18: 428–432.

Winkler, T. (1994) Evaluation of spinal cord injuries using spinal cord evoked potentials. An experimental study in the rat. *Acta Univ. Ups.*, 467: 1–45.

Winkler, T., Sharma, H.S., Stålberg, E. and Olsson, Y. (1994) Naloxone reduces alterations in evoked potentials and edema in trauma to the rat spinal cord. *Acta Neurochir.*, 60(Suppl.): 511–515.

Yaksh, T.L. (1993) The spinal actions of opioids. *Handbook Exp. Pharmacol.*, 104 (I): 53–90.

Young, W. (1993) Secondary injury mechanisms in acute spinal cord injury. *J. Emerg. Med.*, 11: 13–32.

Young, W. and Flamm, E.S. (1982) Effect of high-dose corticosteroid therapy on blood flow, evoked potentials and extracellular calcium in experimental spinal injury. *J. Neurosurg.*, 57: 667–673.

Young, W., Flamm, E.S., Demopoulos, H.B., Tomasula, J.J. and DeCrescito, V. (1981) Naloxone ameliorates posttraumatic ischemia in experimental spinal contusion. *J. Neurosurg.*, 55: 209–219.

F. Nyberg, H.S. Sharma and Z. Wiesenfeld-Hallin (Eds.)
Progress in Brain Research, Vol 104

CHAPTER 23

Influence of dynorphin A antibodies on the formation of edema and cell changes in spinal cord trauma

H.S. Sharma[1,2], Y. Olsson[1] and F. Nyberg[2]

[1]*Laboratory of Neuropathology, University Hospital and* [2]*Department of Pharmaceutical Biosciences, Biomedical Center, Uppsala University, Uppsala, Sweden*

Introduction

Dynorphin is characterised as one of the important neurotransmitters of the mammalian brain and spinal cord (Vincent et al., 1982; Fallon and Ciofi, 1990; Herz et al., 1993; Weisskopf et al., 1993). This opioid peptide is present in a high concentration in the central nervous system (Hökfelt et al., 1978; Fallon and Ciofi, 1990). It is co-localised with other neurotransmitters and neuropeptides in various classes of neurons in the dorsal horn of the spinal cord (Bowker et al., 1983; Code and Fallon, 1986; Hökfelt et al., 1987). Dynorphin has many important physiological actions (Smith and Lee, 1988; Fallon and Ciofi, 1990; Herz et al., 1993) including modulation of neurochemical transmission and receptor function of the central nervous system (Kondo et al., 1993; Weisskopf et al., 1993).

Trauma to the spinal cord of experimental animals results in an increased content of dynorphin (Faden et al., 1985a,b; Sharma et al., 1992a). Intrathecal infusion of dynorphin into normal animals will induce ischemia, motor paralysis and cell changes (Long et al., 1988a,b, 1989; Thornhill et al., 1989). There are thus indications in the literature that the amount of dynorphin is changed as a result of physical injury to the spinal cord, and that this peptide may influence the outcome after injury.

This chapter is an overview of existing knowledge of the involvement of dynorphin in the pathophysiology of spinal cord trauma. In addition, information is provided about some new experiments in which we, by topical application of dynorphin antibodies, have influenced the development of edema and cell changes in the rat spinal cord subjected to a focal trauma. Our results indicate that dynorphin mediates some of the adverse consequences which develop during the first hours after an injury to the cord.

Pathophysiology of spinal cord injury

Research on the pathophysiology and therapy of spinal cord injury relies to a large extent on animal experiments. Anderson and Stokes (1992) have discussed the advantages and limitations of existing experimental models and commented that "there is no single ideal experimental injury model just as there is no stereotypic clinical spinal cord injury". Therefore, each scientific question should be approached with this limitation in mind.

Most models of spinal cord trauma can be grouped into one of the following categories: weight drop technique, controlled contusion and maintained compression (Anderson and Stokes, 1992). The weight drop technique produces a rapid kinetic impact to the cord, whereas the other two methods rely on compression over several minutes, mimicking the clinical situation with compression caused, for instance, by bony fragments, herniated discs or hematomas. Finally, models based on small surgical incisions into the thoracic cord of the rat have been widely used to investigate the very early pathophysiological events occurring immediately after an injury. Our investigations on the significance of various endogenous neurochemicals on the early pathophysiological consequences in spinal cord trauma are based on an incision model in which a small lesion is produced in the dorsal horn of rat thoracic cord (Olsson et al., 1990, 1992; Sharma and Olsson, 1990; Sharma et al., 1991, 1990a,b).

Trauma to the spinal cord is associated with numerous reactions in the cells and the tracts of the cord, changes in their surrounding extracellular fluid and in the microcirculation (Faden and Simon, 1988; Tator and Fehlings, 1991; Faden, 1993a). The outcome after injury is influenced by several mechanisms: (1) the severity of cell and fluid changes (edema, haemorrhages) at the site of the primary physical injury; (2) the degree of disruption and block of descending and ascending neuronal pathways, including axonal and myelin alterations; (3) additional lesions in the segments cranial and caudal to the primary injury caused by edema, circulatory disturbances and other factors, so-called perifocal or secondary injuries; and (4) repair mechanisms. In order to understand the pathogenesis and the effects of therapy of experimental spinal cord injury all these changes must be taken into account.

The degree of the initial impact is the major factor influencing the magnitude and severity of the various circulatory disturbances which occur around the primary injury in spinal cord trauma. Rheological disturbances occur very early (Young and Flamm, 1982; Faden, 1993a). Alteration of microvascular permeability in the perifocal segments of the spinal cord is evident within minutes after injury (Griffiths and Miller, 1974; Hsu et al.,

1985; Olsson et al., 1990). Edema of the cord is present as soon as 30 min after injury and progresses with time (Griffiths and Miller, 1974; Lewin et al., 1974; Wagner and Stewart, 1981; Sharma et al., 1990a,b; Olsson et al., 1992). The extracellular type of edema spreads in both longitudinal and transverse direction with advancement of time after injury (Griffiths and Miller, 1974).

It is widely believed that alterations in the fluid microenvironment of the spinal cord induced by trauma play important roles in the pathology of secondary cell and tissue changes, the so-called autodestructive process. However, there are several 'secondary injury factors' involved in the mechanisms of cell damage and edema following trauma to the spinal cord. Proposed injury factors include products of phospholipid hydrolysis, such as polyunsaturated fatty acids, eicosanoids, free radicals, neuropeptides, monoamines and changes of cations and amino acids (Tator and Fehlings, 1991; Faden and Salzman, 1992).

The concept that peptides may be involved in the production of cell and fluid alterations after trauma to the spinal cord has been examined in several studies, in which opioid antagonists have been used to reduce such secondary consequences (Faden et al., 1992; Faden, 1993a,b). There is evidence that naloxone (an opioid receptor antagonist) attenuates spinal cord dysfunction after trauma (Winkler et al., 1994). There are additional reports that the metabolism of neuropeptides, e.g., substance P, dynorphin A and Met-Enk-Arg[6]-Phe[7] is altered following a trauma to the rat spinal cord (Sharma et al., 1990a, 1992a, 1993).

Dynorphin-containing neurons in the spinal cord

The family of dynorphin peptides (α-neo-endorphin, dynorphin A, dynorphin B) represents one of the major groups of opioids which are present in the nervous system (Goldstein and Ghazarhosian, 1980; Vincent et al., 1982). Originally, dynorphins were discovered in the pituitary gland and were then found in many other regions of the nervous system (Cox et al., 1975). The distribution of dynorphin in the CNS is similar in many mammalian species (Hökfelt et al., 1978; Watson et al., 1983). High concentrations are found in the spinal cord (Hökfelt et al., 1978; Sasek and Elde., 1986; Fallon and Ciofi, 1990). Histochemical studies on the distribution of dynorphin-containing pathways are in good agreement with the findings of opioid receptor localisation in many parts of the brain and spinal cord (Cho and Basbaum, 1989). There is thus a close association between the anatomical distribution and the physiological functions.

In the entire spinal cord, dynorphin fibres are densely distributed in Lamina I (marginal zone) and outer Lamina II (substantia gelatinosa). Dynorphin fibres are more sparsely scattered in Laminae IV–VII, the dorsal grey commissure, Lamina X intermediolateral cell column and intermediolateral cell cluster (Fallon and Ciofi, 1990). Dynorphin B-containing cell bodies are located in Lamina I, the border between Laminae I and II and Laminae IV–VII, X, dorsal grey commissure and the intermediomedial cell cluster (Vincent et al., 1982; Miller and Seybold, 1989; Fallon and Ciofi, 1990).

Co-localisation of dynorphin with other peptides and neurotransmitters

There is evidence that dynorphins are co-localised with many other neuropeptides and neurotransmitters in neurons of the spinal cord (Hökfelt et al., 1978, 1987; Pohl et al., 1990). Many reports show that substance P, Met-enkephalin, calcitonin gene-related peptide (CGRP) and cholecystokinin (CCK) can be found in dynorphin A (1–8)-containing neurons in all levels of the spinal cord (Anderson and Reiner, 1990). The concentrations of these peptides are higher in the dorsal than in the ventral horns (Pohl et al., 1990).

It may well be that there are still other combinations of transmitters and dynorphins in spinal cord neurons. Convergence of serotonin-, enkephalin- and SP-fibres on single neurons has

been described in Laminae I and V (Tashiro et al., 1989). Therefore it appears that a functional interaction may exist between dynorphin and other neuropeptides and neurotransmitters (Hökfelt et al., 1978). Such relationships may be important for the normal function of the cord.

Dynorphin receptors

Dynorphin has numerous physiological and pharmacological actions which are mediated by various opioid receptor subtypes. In the spinal cord and brain, dynorphin interacts particularly with κ receptors (Mansour and Watson, 1993). Therefore, binding of the peptide with this receptor subtype appears to be most important for its physiological actions. Dynorphins also have the capacity to bind with μ and δ receptors (James and Goldstein, 1984). The shorter dynorphins such as (1–8) have particularly pronounced affinity with δ receptors (Garzon et al., 1984). In vivo, the actions of dynorphin is dependent on binding to several receptor subtypes.

There are indications that dynorphin receptors are coupled to ion channels. For instance, dynorphin has the capacity to inhibit transmitter release by depressing calcium conductance (Cherubini and North, 1985). This effect is mediated by κ opioid receptors because activation of μ and δ opioid receptors increases potassium conductance (Mihara and North, 1986). Very little is known about the possible second messengers by which dynorphin receptors may interact. It appears that the effects of dynorphin on calcium level may be mediated through GTP binding proteins which inhibit the adenyl cyclase activity and increase polyphosphoinositide (PI) turnover (Cockcroft and Gomperts, 1985; Nakamura and Ui, 1985). However, there is no direct evidence of opioid effects on PI turnover.

Basic functions of dynorphin

Dynorphin is implicated in many basic functions of the organism. It is involved in temperature regulation, in stress, pain and inflammation (Smith and Lee, 1988; Fallon and Ciofi, 1990). Administration of dynorphin into the hypothalamic nuclei induces many cardiovascular effects such as lowering of blood pressure and heart rate (Laurent and Schmitt, 1983). Furthermore, it has numerous electrophysiological effects in the nervous system.

Dynorphin has modulatory effects on opioid-induced alteration of body temperature. When given alone, the peptide has a slight hyperthermic effect and it potentiates morphine-induced hypothermia (Adler and Geller, 1993). There are indications that temperature changes can alter the levels of dynorphin in the brain. Morley et al. (1982) found that when rats were kept at 4°C for 2 h, hypothalamic levels of dynorphin were decreased. Subjection of animals to 4 h heat stress at 38°C results in a widespread alterations of dynorphin level in the brain and spinal cord (Sharma et al., 1992b). It may well be that temperature-induced changes in dynorphin levels may act as a feedback system in thermo-regulation (Adler and Geller, 1993).

The ability of dynorphin to potentiate morphine analgesia in morphine-tolerant animals suggests that the peptide is not analgesic by itself. However, it can modulate the effect of morphine-induced analgesia. Present data do not support the concept of a direct role of dynorphin in analgesia in the brain and the situation in the spinal cord appears to be different. When injected intrathecally, dynorphin (1–13) produces analgesia with a similar potency to that of morphine (Herman and Goldstein, 1985). This effect is not antagonised by naloxone, suggesting the involvement of some non-opioid mechanism.

Dynorphins appear to participate in some of the events of the inflammatory response. Sydbom and Terenius (1986) reported an increased release of histamine from mast cells caused by dynorphin in a dose-dependent manner. Chahl and Chahl (1986) found that dynorphin induced plasma extravasation in skin.

Several studies have shown that dynorphin has anticonvulsant activity. Przewlocka et al. reported that dynorphin antagonised the convulsant effects of pentylene tetrazole. An initial decrease in pituitary dynorphin levels occurred during amygdaloid kindling and was followed by an increase in hippocampal dynorphin (Przewlocka et al., 1983).

Electrophysiological effects of dynorphin

Dynorphin modulates synaptic transmission in the CNS and may act as a neurotransmitter (Weisskopf et al., 1993). This has been shown in the monosynaptic pathways of the mossy fibres in the hippocampus (Chavkin et al., 1985). These fibres are rich in glutamate and in opioid peptides, particularly dynorphin. Activation of mossy fibres generates a fast excitatory postsynaptic potential. This is supposed to be due to a release of glutamate, whereas a long-lasting inhibition of neighbouring mossy fibre synapses appears to be induced by a presynaptic release of dynorphin (Weisskopf et al., 1993).

In vitro, application of dynorphin in nanomolar concentrations (100–500 nM) inhibits mossy fibre synaptic response (Weisskopf et al., 1993). This effect is slow in onset and long lasting, requiring 30–60 min for recovery. Intracellular recording of mossy fibre excitatory postsynaptic potentials has revealed that dynorphin decreases the peak amplitude and the rate of rise of the potentials. In addition, dynorphin decreases the inhibitory postsynaptic potentials which follow the excitatory postsynaptic potential after mossy fibre activation (Werz and McDonald, 1982). These effects of dynorphin are reversed by the opioid antagonist, naloxone. This indicates that the action of dynorphin is mediated by opioid receptors. However, dynorphin has no consistent effect on membrane potential, input resistance and the threshold for action potential generation tested in CA3 pyramidal cells (Weisskopf et al., 1993).

Dynorphin affects the activity of individual neurons in many regions of the CNS. Both excitatory and inhibitory effects of dynorphin (1–17) on spontaneous and evoked activity have been described (North, 1993). The excitatory effects of dynorphin are usually antagonised by naloxone, whereas the inhibitory effects are not affected

(Duggan and Fleetwood-Walker, 1993). Werz and MacDonald (1982) reported that dynorphin decreased the duration of calcium-dependent action potential in dorsal root neurons in culture. This effect was blocked by naloxone (Werz and McDonald, 1982). The excitatory effects may be mediated by μ or δ receptors, whereas the inhibitory effects may be mediated by κ receptors (Duggan and Fleetwood-Walker, 1993).

The electrophysiological effects of dynorphin are blocked by naloxone, suggesting the involvement of multiple opioid receptors. The selective κ antagonist, nor-binaltrophimine (norBNI), completely blocks the inhibitory effect of dynorphin in a concentration of the drug which has no effect on μ or δ opioid receptors. This indicates that dynorphin selectively activates κ opioid receptors.

Further evidence of dynorphin-induced activation of κ opioid receptors comes from the peptide-induced EEG changes seen after application of morphine (Hong et al., 1988). Intraventricular administration of dynorphin (20 μg) into the rat brain 10 min before injection of morphine antagonises the changes of morphine-induced EEG power spectra and the latency of slow wave sleep (Young and Khazan, 1984). These results are quite similar to those which have been described after administration of a selective κ opioid antagonist. However, the mechanisms of the dynorphin-induced modulatory effect on EEG are not known in all their details.

In the spinal cord, application of dynorphin A (1–13) and U50488H (a specific κ agonist) near Laminae IV/V spinocervical tract neurons of the cat exerts potent naloxone-sensitive inhibition of both thermal and mechanical noxious stimuli from cutaneous origin, a feature not observed when the compounds are applied on substantia gelatinosa (Fleetwood-Walker et al., 1988).

There are several reports that dynorphin will be released from the spinal cord into an artificial cerebrospinal fluid superfusing the subarachnoid space following high-intensity electrical stimulation of peripheral nerves or during high-frequency electro-acupuncture analgesia (Fleetwood-Walker et al., 1988; Smith and Lee, 1988; Hutchinson et al., 1990; Duggan and Fleetwood-Walker, 1993). This release of dynorphin is most marked in the superficial dorsal horn in Lamina I. A less consistent release occurs in deep dorsal horn Laminae V and VI.

Though the precise functions of the dynorphin release in the spinal cord are not known, several lines of recent evidence suggest that the peptide is involved in spinal nociceptive mechanisms. Thus, micro-iontophoretic administration of dynorphin A (1–13) near spinocervical tract neurons selectively inhibits their nociceptive responses (Fleetwood-Walker et al., 1988). Similarly, chronic peripheral inflammation enhances spinal dynorphin gene expression (Weihe et al., 1989).

Dynorphin in spinal cord injury

Dynorphin levels of the central nervous system are altered in trauma, pain and in chronic stress situations (Smith and Lee, 1988). There are a few reports that this peptide is involved in the pathophysiology of brain injury and stroke (Faden, 1993b). Thus, dynorphin treatment of cats with experimental stroke prolongs the survival period (Baskin et al., 1984). The injury itself is associated with an up-regulation of opioid receptor activity (Faden et al., 1985a,b). The beneficial effect of dynorphin appears to be due to a reversal of opioid binding sites after injury (Krumins and Faden, 1986).

Dynorphins seem to be involved in the changes taking place after an injury to the spinal cord. Increased immunoreactivity of dynorphin was found following a focal injury and this reaction was limited to the site of injury and correlated in magnitude with the severity of trauma (Faden and Salzman, 1992; Sharma et al., 1992a).

Pharmacological studies with various opioid-receptor antagonists support the concept that dynorphin may contribute to the pathophysiology of tissue damage after CNS trauma (Faden, 1993a,b). This action of dynorphin seems to be mediated by influences at the κ opioid receptors (Faden, 1990). Thus, κ opioid receptors, but not

μ or δ receptors, are up-regulated after spinal cord injury (Faden et al., 1987). Opioid antagonists that are more potent or selective antagonists of κ receptors are more effective in reducing the consequences of injury than naloxone (Faden, 1990).

Dynorphin A (1–17), but not enkephalins and β-endorphins, accumulates at the injury site of traumatic spinal cord injury (Faden et al., 1985a,b). However, dynorphin fragments (2–17) and (3–13), which have no activity at opioid receptors, produce hind limb weakness, whereas κ opioid agonist do not (Faden et al., 1983). It seems likely that dynorphin-induced paralysis is mediated by both opioid and non-opioid mechanisms.

Intrathecal administration of dynorphin influences spinal cord function

In order to evaluate the role of dynorphin in spinal cord functions, several workers used intrathecal infusion of the peptide and recorded nociceptive, behavioural and pathological consequences to the cord. Intrathecal administration of dynorphin produces paralysis of the hind limbs and tail, loss of nociceptive response, atonic paralysis of bladder and bowel, and loss of motor and autonomic reflexes (Long et al., 1988a,b, 1989; Gaumann et al., 1990; Issac et al., 1990). The neurological deficits correlate well with neuropathological changes of the spinal cord (Long et al., 1989; Gaumann et al., 1990).

The deleterious effects of intrathecal infusion of dynorphin A in the rat appear to be mediated by ischemic injury (Thornhill et al., 1989). Specifically, dynorphin A (1–17) and dynorphin A (1–13) cause dramatic reductions in spinal cord blood flow that are associated with about a 3-fold increase in CSF lactic acid (Long et al., 1989). Widespread ischemic cell changes, neuronal loss, necrosis, cavitation, gliosis and vascular proliferation occur 72 h after intrathecal injection of dynorphin into the spinal cord (Long et al., 1989; Gaumann et al., 1990).

Several investigators believe that dynorphin A interaction with opioid receptor is not essential for the production of these neurological deficits (Stevens and Yaksh, 1986). Blockade of opioid receptors are not effective in reducing such deficits (Faden, 1993a,b). However, other investigators suggest an involvement of opioid receptors. Their conclusion is based on the observation that opioid antagonist, naloxone blocks the paralytic actions of dynorphin (Faden, 1990). Faden concluded that hind limb paralysis results from both opioid and non-opioid actions of dynorphin (Faden, 1993a,b).

Intrathecal injections of dynorphin will result in a non-selective exposure of the spinal cord and its vasculature to large concentrations of the peptide. After this mode of administration there will be a rapid degradation and a limited penetration of the peptide into the spinal cord parenchyma. This will prevent the injected dynorphin from reaching the sites where endogenous dynorphin may act following trauma. Therefore, intrathecal injection of dynorphin may not mimic the actions of endogenous dynorphin in the injured spinal cord. Divergent pharmacological results obtained with opioid or non-opioid antagonist in modulating dynorphin action on the spinal cord may be related to the various concentrations of dynorphin in the spinal cord after injury compared with that after intrathecal infusion of the peptide.

Influence of dynorphin antibodies on brain and spinal cord functions

The participation of dynorphin in various brain and spinal cord functions has been examined by several workers using dynorphin antiserum (Table I). It is believed that dynorphin antiserum in vivo will neutralise the action of endogenous dynorphin (Sander et al., 1989). Intrathecal administration of a dynorphin antibody, which binds dynorphin A (1–17), enhances inhibition of the tail flick response in mice produced by intraventricular administration of a number of analgesic agonists (Fujimoto et al., 1990).

TABLE I

Studies dealing with the effect of dynorphin (Dyn) given intrathecally to rats

Dynorphin analogue	Dosage used	Site of injection	Animal state	Parameters examined	Results	References
Dyn A (1–13)	20 nmol in 10 μl	intrathecal (T10–12)	anaesthetised	spinal cord blood flow (2 min after infusion) Blood pressure	reduced increased	Thornhill et al., 1989
Dyn A (3–13) Dyn A (1–13)	20 nmol in 10 μl	intrathecal (T10–12)	anaesthetised	spinal cord blood flow motor function (15 min after infusion)	reduced paralysis weakness of limbs	Long et al., 1988a,b Faden and Jacobs, 1983
Dyn A (1–13)	20 nmol in 10 μl	intrathecal (T10–12)	conscious unrestrained	blood pressure reflex bradycardia (10 min after infusion)	increased present	Thornhill et. al, 1989
Dyn A (1–17)	20 nmol in 10 μl	intrathecal (T8)	anaesthetised	motor function (15 min after infusion)	complete paralysis	Faden, 1990
Dyn A (2–17)	20 nmol in 10 μl	intrathecal (T8)	anaesthetised	motor function	weakness of limbs	Faden, 1990
Dyn A (1–17)	30 nmol in 10 μl	intrathecal (T8)	spinal cord injured	motor function (4 weeks after SCI)	severe paralysis	Faden, 1990
Dyn A (2–17)	30 nmol in 10 μl	intrathecal (T8)	spinal cord injured	motor function	weakness of limbs	Faden, 1990
Dyn A (1–17)	20 nmol in 10 μl	intrathecal (T10–12)	anaesthetised rat	motor function (15 min after infusion) CSF-lactate (10 min after infusion) spinal cord pathology (72 h after infusion)	motor paralysis increased cell loss, necrosis degeneration	Long et al., 1989 Long et al., 1989 Long et al., 1989
Dyn A (1–13)	25 nmol in 10 μl	intrathecal level unknown	conscious unrestrained	tail flick response (15, 30 min after infusion)	loss of tail flick response	Issac et al., 1990

SCI = spinal cord injury.

Han and Xie (1984) reported that intrathecal administration of dynorphin antibody reduced electro-acupuncture analgesia in rabbits. Sander et al. (1989) injected dynorphin antibodies intrathecally in pregnant rats to examine whether dynorphin is the endogenous opioid ligand responsible for mediating the analgesia during pregnancy following foot electroshock. The data of Sander et al. show that dynorphin antibodies reduce the jump thresholds following elec-troshock during pregnancy to an extent that is comparable to that which has been observed following the intrathecal administration of naltrexone. The lack of an effect following intrathecal application of pre-adsorbed antisera demonstrates that the effects are due to dynorphin-specific antibodies and not to other constituents or impurities (Sander et al., 1989). These authors concluded that the significant reduction in jump thresholds, observed following the intrathecal application of the dynorphin antisera, most probably results from the neutralisation of the physiological effects of dynorphin and indicates that dynorphin is a major substrate for the spinal analgesia that occurs during pregnancy.

Injection of antibodies to dynorphin A (1–17) into the lateral cerebral ventricle elevates the feeding threshold which is naloxone sensitive (Carr and Bak, 1990). The authors feel that the injected antibodies may affect behaviour by inactivating peptides that are released into the CSF or into the neural tissue.

Studies on dynorphin antibodies in spinal cord injury

Previously, Faden was the only one having reported experiments on the effects of dynorphin antibodies in spinal cord trauma on neurological outcome (Table II). Faden injected 10 μl dynorphin A (1–17) antiserum 15 min before spinal cord injury, followed by a second dose of the antiserum 4 h after injury (Faden, 1990). Motor function was analysed 4 weeks after the initial trauma. Treatment with dynorphin A (1–17) antiserum significantly improved chronic neurological recovery in walking ability, although the angle difference on the inclined plane test did not improve. Faden attributed this effect of Dyn A (1–17) antiserum as specific because similar treatment with leucine-enkephalin antiserum or normal rabbit serum did not produce these beneficial effects (Faden, 1990).

We are interested in the effects of dynorphin antiserum on the formation of edema and cell changes occurring around a focal spinal cord trauma (Sharma et al., 1994). Therefore we applied dynorphin antibodies topical 2 min after spinal cord injury in the rat and evaluated edema and cell changes 5 h after trauma. As shown in Table II, application of dynorphin antibodies reduced the consequences of edema and cell changes compared with animals treated with normal rabbit serum (Sharma et al., 1994). In the following sections our new results are described in detail and the possible mechanisms underlying

TABLE II

Effect of dynorphin antibodies on some spinal cord and brain functions

Antibodies to dynorphin analogue	Dosage used	Site of injection	Animal species	Parameters examined	Results	References
Dyn A (1–17) antiserum	10 μl (15 min before and 4 h after SCI)	intrathecal (T8)	anaesthetised rat	motor paralysis (4 weeks after trauma)	good recovery	Faden, 1990
Dyn A (1–13) antiserum	5 μl	intrathecal (L1–4)	conscious rat unrestrained	footshock induced jumping (10–60 min after infusion)	reduction in threshold	Sander et al., 1989
Dyn A (1–13) antiserum	4–5 μl	intrathecal	conscious mice unrestrained	drug-induced analgesia (10 min before infusion)	increased	Fujimoto et al., 1990
Dyn A (1–13) antiserum	10 μl (1:10)	lateral cerebral ventricle	conscious rats unrestrained	hypothalamic self stimulation	increased	Carr and Bak, 1990
Dyn A (1–17) antiserum	10 μl (2 min after SCI)	topical (T10–11)	anesthetised rat	edema, cell changes (5 h after SCI)	reduced	Sharma et al., 1994

SCI = spinal cord injury.

the protective effect of dynorphin antibodies on cell changes after spinal cord injury are discussed.

Spinal cord injury model

We have a model of spinal cord injury in the rat in which a minimal lesion is induced in the dorsal horn occupying about 2% volume (Fig. 1). Under urethane anaesthesia (1.5 g/kg, i.p.), one segment laminectomy is done over the T10–11 segments (Olsson et al., 1990). The lesion is limited mainly to the Rexed Laminae VII.

Dynorphin antiserum

Dynorphin A (1–17) antiserum was produced by the method of Hollt et al. (1978). This antibody, produced by immunisation of rabbits with the conjugated dynorphin A (1–17) antigen, crossreacts with dynorphin A (1–17) by 100%, with dynorphin (1–13) by 83%, with dynorphin (2–17) by 37%, with dynorphin (1–8) by < 0.002%, with β-endorphin by < 0.006%, with Met-Enk by < 0.001% and with Leu-Enk by < 0.001%. The binding capacity of the antiserum for dynorphin

A (1–17) was determined by displacement of ^{125}I-dynorphin A (1–17) in the radioimmunoassay procedure. Antiserum, prebound with dynorphin A (1–17) (attenuated antiserum) was evaluated for non-specific actions of the antiserum. The attenuated antiserum did not bind ^{125}I-dynorphin A (1–17). However, the procedure, performed on antiserum without the addition of dynorphin A (1–17), showed that the ability of the antiserum to bind dynorphin A (1–17) was unaffected (Christensson-Nylander et al., 1985; Nyberg et al., 1990).

Application of dynorphin antiserum

Using a microliter syringe, 10 μl of dynorphin antiserum (undiluted $n = 17$; 1:100 $n = 6$; 1:500 $n = 4$) was applied topically on the injured spinal cord 2 min after the injury for 10 sec. The injury to the cord probably facilitates the penetration of the dynorphin antibodies into the tissue. The animals were allowed to survive for 5 h after injury. A control group ($n = 17$) received normal rabbit serum (Table III).

At 5 h, water content, microvascular permeability to ^{125}I-BSA (bovine serum albumin), and morphology of the spinal cord treated with either dynorphin antiserum or normal rabbit antiserum, were examined (Table III).

Spinal cord edema

Application of dynorphin antiserum resulted in a marked reduction in the visual swelling of the spinal cord as compared to the control animals (Fig. 2). The gross expansion of the spinal cord was significantly reduced in the dynorphin antiserum-treated group (Fig. 2).

Measurement of water content showed a significant reduction in the T9 and the injured spinal cord segments; however, no significant reduction in the water content was seen in the T12 segment (Fig. 3). This effect of dynorphin antiserum was dose dependent. Our results show that dynorphin antiserum has the capacity to reduce water con-

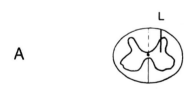

A

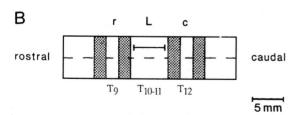

B

Fig. 1. Schematic diagram of spinal cord lesion (L) in cross section (a) and in longitudinal section (b). Stippled bars denote sampling of spinal cord tissue for the study of microvascular permeability, edema and ultrastructural investigations (bar = 5 mm).

TABLE III

Experimental protocol of dynorphin A (1–17) antiserum treatment (10 µl in 10 sec) given 2 min after spinal cord injury (SCI) and the parameters measured

Type of experiment	No. of animals	Parameters measured
Treatment with dynorphin A (1–17) antiserum (n = 26)		
Undiluted antiserum	17	Gross expansion (6)
		Electron microscopy (3)[a]
		Water content (5)
		Permeability (6)
Antiserum 1: 100	5	Gross expansion (5)
		Water content (5)[a]
Antiserum 1:500	4	Gross expansion (4)
		Water content (4)[a]
Control treatment with normal rabbit serum (n = 17)		
Rabbit serum	17	Gross expansion (6)
		Electron microscopy (3)[a]
		Water content (5)
		Permeability (6)

SCI was made in the T10–11 segments and the parameters were examined in the T9, T10–11, and T12 segments 5 h after injury. Figures in parentheses indicate number of animals in each group.

SCI = spinal cord injury.

a Same group of animals.

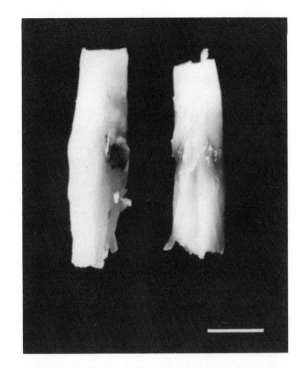

Fig. 2. Gross pathology of the injured spinal cord in one rat treated with normal rabbit serum (left) and another rat given dynorphin A (1–17) antiserum (right), 2 min after spinal cord injury of the right dorsal horn of the T10–11 segments (bar = 5 mm).

tent of the injured segment if applied in concentrated form after injury. This suggests that dynorphin may induce edema of the spinal cord by some unknown mechanisms. It may be that dynorphin-induced spinal cord ischemia plays an important role in edema formation. An increased dynorphin content seen after spinal cord injury in the T9 segment is in line with this assumption (Sharma et al., 1992a).

Microvascular permeability

Application of dynorphin antiserum significantly reduced the extravasation of ^{125}I-BSA in spinal cord injured rats compared with animals which received normal rabbit serum alone. This effect of dynorphin antiserum was most marked in the perifocal T9 segment. The reduction of microvascular permeability changes to albumin in the spinal cord segments after injury showed a close parallelism with reduction in the water content (see Fig. 3).

A breakdown of the microvascular permeability is an important factor in inducing cell reactions in the injured cord. Obviously, various serum constituents, which are normally prevented by the blood-spinal cord barrier, may enter the neuronal microenvironment after a breakdown of the microvascular permeability (Beggs and Waggner, 1976). An alteration in the neurochemical, immunological and ionic environment will lead to abnormal cell reactions and may lead to permanent damage if the situation prevails for a long period of time. It remains to be seen whether application of dynorphin antiserum several hours

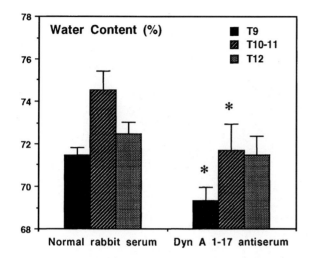

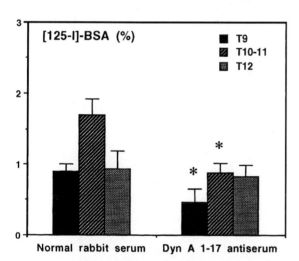

Fig. 3. Influence of dynorphin antiserum on water content and microvascular permeability to ^{125}I-labelled bovine serum albumin after spinal cord injury compared with normal rabbit serum. Each bar over the column represents standard deviations of the mean. *$P < 0.01$ (Student's unpaired t-test).

after the primary insult to the spinal cord is still effective in minimising the injury.

Structural changes of the spinal cord

That application of dynorphin antiserum reduces the cell changes is seen after trauma to the spinal cord. Electron microscopy of the injured spinal cord of rats not given dynorphin antiserum shows membrane disruption, perivascular edema, neuronal damage, and vesiculation of myelin. These cell reactions are most marked in the perifocal T9 and T12 segments. However, treatment with dynorphin antiserum markedly reduced membrane disruption, stuctural signs of edema and cell damage (Fig. 4b).

The observed reduction in the cell reactions by dynorphin antiserum shows that the actions of dynorphin can be antagonised with an antiserum to dynorphin. Several factors, such as local haemorrhages, CSF flow and tissue swelling, will interfere with the transport and binding of antiserum into the deeper tissues. Further studies using application of antiserum labelled with radiotracers are needed to evaluate the transport of the compounds within the spinal cord tissue in different spinal cord segments over a 5-h survival period.

Prospect for future research

Dynorphin has the capacity to produce motor paralysis, ischemia and cell changes in the spinal cord if given locally (Long et al., 1988a,b, 1989). Our studies using dynorphin antiserum indicate that: (i) dynorphin has the capacity to induce edema of the spinal cord; and (ii) this edema-inducing capacity is related to the ability of dynorphin to influence microvascular permeability. To further test this hypothesis, studies on edema formation and alteration in the microvascular permeability of the normal spinal cord following intrathecal infusion of dynorphin in normal animals are needed.

Our studies do not clarify the involvement of specific opioid receptors in the action of dynorphin-induced pathology of the spinal cord. To investigate the role of opioid versus non-opioid mechanisms involved in the action of dynophin on the spinal cord selective κ antagonists should be used. It seems that the effect of spinal dynorphin on motor paralysis is mediated by non-opioid mechanisms. However, the other action of dynor-

412

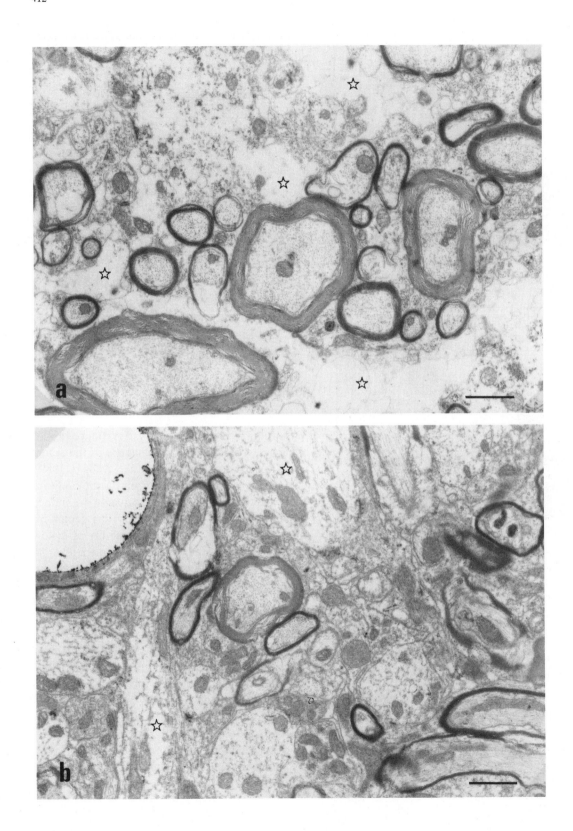

phin on the spinal cord, e.g., cell changes, edema and microvascular permeability are mediated by some opioid mechanisms.

Acknowledgements

This investigation was supported by grants from the Swedish Medical Research Council projects no. 0320, 9457, Trygg-Hansa, Göran Gustafsson's Foundation, Hedlund's Foundation, Åhlén's Foundation, Thyring's Foundation, and O.E. and Edla Johnson's Foundation. We very much appreciate the outstanding help of Törd Loving for library facilities and Aruna Misra for secretarial assistance. The skilful technical assistance of Mrs Margaretta Einarson, Madeleine Thörnwall in radioachemical experiments; Madeleine Jarild, Gunilla Tibbling in electron microscopy; and Frank Bittkowski in photography, is highly appreciated.

References

Adler, M.W. and Geller, E.B. (1993) Physiological functions of opioids: Temperature regulation. *Handbook Exp. Pharmacol.*, 104 (I): 205–238.

Anderson, K.D. and Reiner, A. (1990) Extensive co-occurrence of substance P and dynorphin in striatal projection neurons: An evolutionary conserved feature of basal ganglia organization. *J. Comp. Neurol.*, 295: 339–369.

Anderson, T.E. and Stokes, B.T. (1992) Experimental models for spinal cord injury research: Physical and physiological considerations. *J. Neurotrauma*, 9 (Suppl. 1): S135–S142.

Baskin, D.S., Hosobuchi, Y., Loh, H.H. and Lee, N.M. (1984) Dynorphin (1–13) improves survival in cats with focal cerebral ischemia. *Nature*, 312: 551–552.

Beggs, J. and Waggener, J. (1976) Transendothelial vesicular transport of protein following compression injury to the spinal cord. *Lab. Invest.*, 34: 428–439.

Bowker, R.M., Westlund, K.N., Sullivan, M.C., Wilber, J.F. and Coutler, J.D. (1983) Descending serotonergic, peptidergic and cholinergic pathways from the raphe nuclei: a multiple transmitter complex. *Brain Res.*, 288: 33–41.

Carr, K.D. and Bak, T.H. (1990) Rostral and caudal ventricular infusion of antibodies to dynorphin A (1–17) and dynorphin A (1–8): effects on electrically-elicited feeding in the rat. *Brain Res.*, 507: 289–294.

Chahl, L.A. and Chahl, J.S. (1986) Plasma extravasation induced by dynorphin (1–13) in rat skin. *Eur. J. Pharmacol.*, 124: 343–347.

Chavkin, C., Shoemaker, W.J., McGinty, J.F., Bayon, A. and Bloom, F.E. (1985) Characterization of the prodynorphin and proenkephalin neuropeptide systems in rat hippocampus. *J. Neurosci.*, 5: 808–813.

Cherubini, E. and North, R.A. (1985) μ and κ opioids inhibit transmitter release by different mechanisms. *Proc. Natl. Acad. Sci. USA*, 82: 1860–1863.

Cho, H.J. and Basbaum, A.I. (1989) Ultrastructural analysis of dynorphin B-immunoreactive cells and terminals in the superficial dorsal horn of the deafferented spinal cord of the rat. *J. Comp. Neurol.*, 281: 193–201.

Christensson-Nylander, I., Nyberg, F., Ragnarsson, U. and Terenius, L. (1985) A general procedure for analysis of proenkephalin B derived opioid peptides. *Regul. Peptides*, 11: 65–76.

Cockcroft, S. and Gomperts, B.D. (1985) Role of guanine nucleotide binding proteins in the activation of polyphosphoinositide phosphodiesterase. *Nature*, 314: 315–318.

Code, R.A. and Fallon, J.H. (1986) Some projections of dynorphin-immunoreactive neurons in the rat central nervous system. *Neuropeptides*, 8: 165–175.

Cox, B.M., Opheim, K.E., Teschemacher, H. and Goldstein, A. (1975) A peptide-like substance from pituitary that acts like morphine. *Life Sci.*, 16: 1777–1780.

Duggan, A.W. and Fleetwood-Walker, S.M. (1993) Opioids and sensory processing in the central nervous system. *Handbook Exp. Pharmacol.*, 104 (II): 731–771.

Faden, A.I. (1990) Opioid and non opioid mechanisms may contribute to dynorphin's pathophysiological actions in spinal cord injury. *Ann. Neurol.*, 27: 64–74.

Faden, A.I. (1993a) Experimental neurobiology of central nervous system trauma. *Crit. Rev. Neurobiol.*, 7: 175–186.

Faden, A.I. (1993b) Role of endogenous opioids and opioid receptors in central nervous system injury. *Handbook Exp. Pharmacol.*, 104 (I): 325–341.

Faden, A.I. and Jacobs, T.P. (1983) Dynorphin induces partially reversible paraplegia in the rat. *Eur. J. Pharmacol.*, 91: 321–324.

Faden, A.I. and Simon, R. (1988) A potential role of excitotox-

Fig. 4. Low power electron micrograph of the ventral horn of the T9 segment of one rat treated with normal rabbit serum (a) or dynorphin antiserum (b), given 2 min after spinal cord injury to the T10–11 segments. The animals were allowed to survive 5 h after injury. In the rat given normal rabbit serum, vacuolation and edema (*) are frequent. The structural changes and edema are less apparent in the rat treated with dynorphin antiserum (bar = 2.5 μm).

ins in the pathophysiology of spinal cord injury. *Ann. Neurol.*, 23:

Faden, A.I. and Salzman, S. (1992) Pharmacological strategies in CNS trauma. *TIPS*, 13: 29–35.

Faden, A.I., Molineaux, C.J., Rosenberger, J.G., Jacobs, T.P. and Cox, B.M. (1985a) Endogenous opioid immunoreactivity in rat spinal cord following traumatic injury. *Ann Neurol.*, 17: 386–390.

Faden, A.I., Molineaux, C.J., Rosenberger, J.G., Jacobs, T.P. and Cox, B.M. (1985b) Increased dynorphin immunoreactivity in spinal cord after traumatic injury. *Regul. Peptides*, 11: 35–41.

Faden, A.I., Takemori, A.E. and Portoghese, T.S. (1987) κ-Selective opiate antagonist norbinaltorphimine improves outcome after traumatic spinal cord injury in rats. *CNS Trauma*, 4: 227–237.

Fallon, J.H. and Ciofi, P. (1990) Dynorphin-containing neurons. *Handbook Chem. Neuroanat.*, 9 (Part II): 1–130.

Fleetwood-Walker, S.M., Hope, P.J., Mitchell, R., El-Yassir, N. and Molony, V. (1988) The influence of opioid receptor subtypes on the processing of nociceptive inputs in the spinal dorsal horn of the cat. *Brain Res.*, 451: 213–226.

Fujimoto, J.M., Arts, K.S., Rady, J.J. and Tseng, L.F. (1990) Spinal dynorphin A (1–17): possible mediator of antianalgesic action. *Neuropharmacology*, 29: 609–617.

Garzon, J.G., Sanchez-Blazquez, P., Gerhart, J., Loh, H.H. and Lee, N.M. (1984) Dynorphin 1–13: interaction with other opiate ligand bindings in vitro. *Brain Res.*, 302: 392–396.

Gaumann, D.M., Grabow, T.S., Yaksh, T.L., Casy, S.J. and Rodriguez, M. (1990) Intrathecal somatostatin, somatostatin analogs, substance P analog and dynorphin A cause comparable neurotoxicity in rats. *Neuropharmacology*, 39: 761–774.

Goldstein, A. and Ghazarhosian, V. (1980) Immunoreactive dynorphin in pituitary and brain. *Proc. Natl. Acad. Sci. USA*, 77: 6207–6210.

Griffiths, I.R. and Miller, R. (1974) Vascular permeability to protein and vasogenic oedema in experimental concussive injuries to the canine spinal cord. *J. Neurol. Sci.*, 22: 291–304.

Han, J. and Xie, G. (1984) Dynorphin: important mediator for electroacupuncture analgesia in the spinal cord of the rabbit. *Pain*, 18: 367–376.

Herman, B.H. and Goldstein, A. (1985) Antinociception and paralysis induced by intrathecal dynorphin-A. *J. Pharmacol. Exp. Ther.*, 232: 27–32.

Herz, A., Akil, H. and Simon, E.J. (1993) Opioids I, II. In: *Handbook of Experimental Pharmacology*, 104 (I/II): Springer-Verlag, Berlin.

Hökfelt, T., Elde R., Johansson, O., Ljungdahl, Å., Schultzberg, M., Fuxe, K., Goldstein, M., Nilsson, G., Pernow, B., Terenius, L., Ganten, D., Jeffocate, S.L., Rehfeld, J. and Said, S. (1978) Distribution of peptide containing neurons. In M.A.

Lipton, A. DiMascio and K.F. Killam (Eds.) *Psychopharmacology: A Generation of Progress*, Raven Press, New York, pp. 39–66.

Hökfelt, T., Johansson, O., Holets, V., Meister, B. and Melander, T. (1987) Distribution of neuropeptides with special reference to their coexistence with classical neurotransmitters. In: H.Y. Meltzer (Ed.) *Psychopharmacology: The Third Generation of Progress*, Raven Press, New York, pp. 401–416.

Hollt, V., Przewlocki, R. and Herz, A. (1978) Radioimmunoassay of β-endorphin basal and stimulated levels in extracted rat plasma. *Arch. Pharmacol.*, 303: 171–174.

Hong, O., Young, G.A. and Khazan, N. (1988) Modulation of morphine-imduced EEG and behavioural effects by dynorphin A (1–13) in non-tolerant and morphine tolerant rats. *Neuropharmacology*, 27: 807–812.

Hsu, C.Y., Hogan, E.L., Gadsden, R.H., Spicer, K.M., Shi, M.P. and Cox, R.D. (1985) Vascular permeability in experimental spinal cord injury. *J. Neurol. Sci.*, 70: 275–282.

Hutchinson, W.D., Morton, C.R. and Terenius, L. (1990) Dynorphin A: in vivo release in the spinal cord of the cat. *Brain Res.*, 532: 299–306.

Issac, L.I., O'Malley, T.V.Z., Ristic, H. and Stewart, P. (1990) MK-801 blocks dynorphin A (1–13) induces loss of tail flick reflex in the rat. *Brain Res.*, 531: 83–87.

James, I.F. and Goldstein, A. (1984) Site directed alkylation of multiple opioid receptors. I. Binding selectivity. *Mol. Pharmacol.*, 25: 337–342.

Kondo, Y., Ogawa, N., Asanuma, M., Hirata, H., Tanaka, K., Kawada, Y. and Mori, A. (1993) Regional changes in neuropeptide levels after 5,7-dihydroxytryptamine-induced serotonin depletion in the rat brain. *J. Neural Transm. Gen. Sect.*, 92: 151–157.

Krumins, S.A., Faden, A.I. (1986) Traumatic injury alters opiate receptor binding in spinal cord. *Ann Neurol.*, 19: 498–501.

Laurent, S. and Schmitt, H. (1983) Central cardiovascular effects of κ-agonists dynorphin (1–13) and ethylketocyclazocine in the anaesthetised rat. *Eur. J. Pharmacol.*, 96: 165–169.

Lewin, M.G., Hansebout, R.R. and Pappius, H.M. (1974) Chemical characteristics of traumatic spinal cord edema in cats. *J. Neurosurgery*, 40: 65–75.

Long, J.B., Martinez-Arizala, A., Echevarria, E.E., Tidwell, R.E. and Holaday, J.W. (1988a) Hindlimb paralytic effects of prodynorphin-derived peptides following spinal subarachnoid injection in rats. *Eur. J. Pharmacol.*, 153: 45–54.

Long, J.B., Petras, J.M., Mobley, W.C. and Holaday, J.W. (1988b) Neurological dysfunction after intrathecal injection of dynorphin A (1–13) in the rat. II. Nonopioid mechanisms mediate loss of motor, sensory and autonomic function. *J. Pharmacol. Exp. Ther.*, 246: 1167–1174.

Long, J.B., Rigamonti, D.R., deCosta, B., Rice, K.C. and Martinez-Arizala, A. (1989) Dynorphin A-induced rat hindlimb paralysis and spinal cord injury are not altered by the κ-opioid antagonist nor-binaltorphimine. *Brain Res.*, 497: 155–162.

Mansour, A. and Watson, S.J. (1993) Anatomical distribution of opioid receptors in mammalians: an overview. *Handbook Exp. Pharmacol.*, 104 (II): 79–105.

Mihara, S. and North, R.A. (1986) Opioids increase potassium conductance in submucous neurons of guinea-pig caecum by activating delta-receptors. *Br. J. Pharmacol.*, 88: 315–322.

Miller, K.E. and Seybold, V.S. (1989) Comparison of Met-En-kephalin, dynorphin A, and neurotensin immunoreactive neurons in the cat and rat spinal cords. II. Segmental differences in the marginal zone. *J. Comp. Neurol.*, 279: 619–628.

Morley, J.E., Elson, M.K., Levin, A.S. and Shafer, R.B. (1982) The effects of stress on central nervous system concentrations of the opioid peptide, dynorphin. *Peptides*, 3: 901–906.

Nakamura, T. and Ui, M. (1985) Simultaneous inhibition of inositol phospholipid breakdown, arachidonic acid release and histamine secretion in mast cells by islets activating protein, pertussis toxin. *J. Biol. Chem.*, 260: 3584–3588.

North, R.A. (1993) Opioid actions on membrane ion channels. *Handbook Exp. Pharmacol.*, 104 (II): 773–797.

Nyberg, F. and Silberring, J. (1990) Conversion of the dynorphins to leu-enkephalins in human spinal cord. *Progr. Clin. Biol. Res.*, 328: 261–265.

Olsson, Y., Sharma, H.S. and Pettersson, C.Å.V. (1990) Effects of p-chlorophenylalanine on microvascular permeability changes in spinal cord trauma. An experimental study in the rat using ^{131}I-sodium and lanthanum tracers. *Acta Neuropathol. (Berlin)*, 79: 595–603.

Olsson, Y., Sharma, H.S., Pettersson, C.Å.V. and Cervós-Navarro, J. (1992) Release of endogenous neurochemicals may increase vascular permeability, induce edema and influence cell changes in rauma to the spinal cord. *Progr. Brain Res.*, 91: 197–203.

Pohl, M., Benoliel, J.J., Bourgoin, S., Lombard, M.C., Mauborgne, A., Taquet, H., Carayon, A., Besson, J.M., Cesselin, F. and Hamon, M. (1990) Regional distribution of calcitonin gene related peptide-. substance P-, cholecystokinin-, Met^5-Enkephalin-, and dorsal root ganglia in the spinal cord and dorsal root ganglia of adult rats: effects of dorsal rhizotomy and neonatal capsaicin. *J. Neurochem.*, 55: 1122–1130.

Przewlocka, B., Stala, L., Lason, W. and Przewlocka, R. (1983) The effect of various opiate receptor agonist on the seizure threshold in the rat. Is dynorphin an endogenous anticonvulsant? *Life Sci.*, 33 (Suppl 1): 595–598.

Sander, H.W., Kream, R.M. and Gintzler, A.R. (1989) Spinal dynorphin involvement in the analgesia of pregnancy: effects of intrathecal dynorphin antisera. *Eur. J. Pharmacol.*, 159: 205–209.

Sasek, C.A. and Elde, R.P. (1986) Coexistence of enkephalin and dynorphin immunoreactivities in neurons in the dorsal grey commissure of the sixth lumbar and first sacral spinal cord segments. *Brain Res.*, 381: 8–15.

Sharma, H.S. and Olsson, Y. (1990) Edema formation and celular alteration in spinal cord injury in the rat and their modification with p-chlorophenylalanine. *Acta Neuropathol. (Berlin)*, 79: 604–610.

Sharma, H.S., Nyberg, F., Olsson, Y. and Dey, P.K. (1990a) Alteration of substance P after trauma to the spinal cord. An experimental study in the rat. *Neuroscience*, 38: 205–212.

Sharma, H.S., Olsson, Y. and Dey, P.K. (1990b) Early accumulation of serotonin in rat spinal cord subjected to traumatic injury. Relation to edema and blood flow changes. *Neuroscience*, 36: 725–730.

Sharma, H.S., Winkler, T., Stålberg, E., Olsson, Y. and Dey, P.K. (1991) Evaluation of traumatic spinal cord edema using evoked potentials recorded from the spinal epidural space. An experimental study in the rat. *J. Neurol. Sci.*, 102: 150–162.

Sharma, H.S., Nyberg, F. and Olsson, Y. (1992a) Dynorphin A content in the rat brain and spinal cord after a localized trauma to the spinal cord and its modification with p-chlorophenylalanine. An experimental study using radioimmunoassay technique. *Neurosci. Res.*, 14: 195–203.

Sharma, H.S., Nyberg, F. and Cervós-Navarro, J. (1992b) Acute systemic heat stress alters dynorphin A contents in the rat brain and spinal cord. *Neuropeptides*, 22: 62–63.

Sharma, H.S., Nyberg, F., Thörnwall, M. and Olsson, Y. (1993) Met-Enkephalin-Arg^6-Phe^7 in spinal cord and brain following traumatic injury to the spinal cord: influence of p-chlorophenylalanine. An experimental study in the rats using radioimmunoassay technique. *Neuropharmacology*, 32: 711–717.

Sharma, H.S., Nyberg, F. and Olsson, Y. (1994) Topical application of dynorphin-A antibodies reduces edema and cell changes in traumatised rat spinal cord. *Regul. Peptides*, Suppl. 1: S91–S92.

Smith, A.P. and Lee, N.M. (1988) Pharmacology of dynorphin. *Ann. Rev. Pharmacol. Toxicol.*, 28: 123–140.

Stevens, C.W. and Yaksh, T.L. (1986) Dynorphin A and related peptides administered intrathecally in the rat: a search for putative kappa opiate receptor activity. *J. Pharmacol. Exp. Ther.*, 238: 833–838.

Sydbom, A. and Terenius, L. (1985) The histamine releasing effect of dynorphin and other opioid peptides possessing arg-pro sequences. *Agents Actions*, 16: 269–272.

Tashiro, T., Ruda, M.A., Satoda, T., Matsushima, R. and Mizuno, N. (1989) Convergence of serotonin-, enkephalin- and substance P-like immunoreactive afferent fibers onto cat medullary dorsal horn projection neurons: a triple immunocytochemical staining technique combined with the retrograde HRP-tracing method. *Brain Res.*, 491: 360–365.

Tator, C. and Fehlings, M. (1991) Review of the secondary injury theory of acute spinal cord trauma with emphasis on vascular mechanism. *J Neurosurg.*, 75: 15–26.

416

Thornhill, J.A., Gregor, L., Mathison, R. and Pittman, Q. (1989) Intrathecal dynorphin A administration causes pressor responses in rats associated with an increased resistance to spinal cord blood flow. *Brain Res.*, 490: 174–177.

Vincent, S.R., Hökfelt, T., Christensson, I. and Terenius, L. (1982) Dynorphin-immunoreactive neurons in the central nervous system of the rat. *Neurosci. Lett.*, 33: 185–190.

Wagner, F. and Stewart, W.B. (1981) Effect of trauma dose on spinal cord edema. *J. Neurosurg.*, 54: 802–806.

Watson, S.J., Khachaturian, H., Akil, H., Coy, D.H. and Goldstein, A. (1983) Prodynorphin peptides are found in the same neurons throughout rat brain. Immunocytochemical study. *Proc. Natl. Acad. Sci. USA*, 80: 891–896.

Weihe, E., Millan, M.J., Holt, V., Nohr, D. and Herz, A. (1989) Induction of the gene encoding pro-dynorphin by experimentally induced arthritis enhances staining for dynorphin in the spinal cord of rats. *Neuroscience*, 31: 77–95.

Weisskopf, M.G., Zalutsky, R.A. and Nicoll, R.A. (1993) The opioid peptide dynorphin mediates heterosynaptic depression of hippocampal mossy fibre synapses and modulates long-term potentiation. *Nature*, 362: 423–427.

Werz, M.A. and McDonald, R.L. (1982) Dynorphin and neoendorphin peptides decrease dorsal root ganglion neuron calcium-dependent action potential duration. *J. Pharmacol. Exp. Ther.*, 234: 49–56.

Winkler, T., Sharma, H.S., Stålberg, E., Olsson, Y. and Nyberg, F. (1994) Naloxone reduces alterations in evoked potentials and edema in trauma to the rat spinal cord. *Acta Neurochir. (Wien)*, Suppl. 60: 511–514.

Young, G.A. and Khazan, N. (1984) Differential neuropharmacological effects of mu, kappa and sigma opioid agonists on cortical EEG power spectra. Stereospecificity and naloxone antagonism. *Neuropharmacology*, 23: 1161–1165.

Young, W. and Flamm, R.S. (1982) Effect of high dose corticosteroid therapy on blood flow, evoked potentials, and extracelluler calcium in experimental spinal cord injury. *J. Neurosurg.*, 57: 667–673.

Subject Index